AF478351

Cognitive Plasticity in Neurologic Disorders

Cognitive Plasticity in Neurologic Disorders

EDITED BY

Joseph I. Tracy, PhD, ABPP/CN

*Jefferson Hospital for Neuroscience, Department of Neurology,
Thomas Jefferson University/Jefferson Medical College,
Philadelphia, PA*

Benjamin M. Hampstead, PhD, ABPP/CN

*Atlanta VAMC RR&D Center of Excellence for Visual
and Neurocognitive Rehabilitation,
Decatur, GA
Department of Rehabilitation Medicine,
Emory University,
Atlanta, GA*

K. Sathian, MD, PhD, FANA

*Departments of Neurology,
Rehabilitation Medicine and Psychology, Emory University,
Atlanta, GA
Atlanta VAMC RR&D Center of Excellence for Visual and
Neurocognitive Rehabilitation
Decatur, GA*

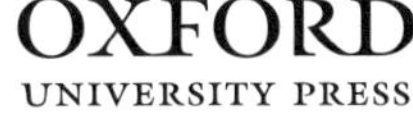

OXFORD
UNIVERSITY PRESS

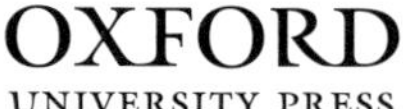

OXFORD
UNIVERSITY PRESS

Oxford University Press is a department of the University of Oxford.
It furthers the University's objective of excellence in research,
scholarship, and education by publishing worldwide.

Oxford   New York
Auckland   Cape Town   Dar es Salaam   Hong Kong   Karachi
Kuala Lumpur   Madrid   Melbourne   Mexico City   Nairobi
New Delhi   Shanghai   Taipei   Toronto

With offices in
Argentina   Austria   Brazil   Chile   Czech Republic   France   Greece
Guatemala   Hungary   Italy   Japan   Poland   Portugal   Singapore
South Korea   Switzerland   Thailand   Turkey   Ukraine   Vietnam

Oxford is a registered trademark of Oxford University Press
in the UK and certain other countries.

Published in the United States of America by
Oxford University Press
198 Madison Avenue, New York, NY 10016

Library of Congress Cataloging-in-Publication Data
Cognitive Plasticity in Neurologic Disorders / edited by Joseph I. Tracy, Benjamin M. Hampstead,
K. Sathian.
    p. ; cm.
Includes bibliographical references.
ISBN 978–0–19–996524–3 (alk. paper)
I. Tracy, Joseph, editor.   II. Hampstead, Benjamin, editor.   III. Sathian, K., editor.
[DNLM: 1.   Nervous System Diseases—physiopathology.   2.   Cognitive Reserve—physiology.
3.   Neuronal Plasticity—physiology.   4.   Recovery of Function. WL 140]
RC394.N47
616.8′4—dc23
2014016378

The science of medicine is a rapidly changing field. As new research and clinical experience
broaden our knowledge, changes in treatment and drug therapy occur. The author and publisher
of this work have checked with sources believed to be reliable in their efforts to
provide information that is accurate and complete, and in accordance with the standards accepted at the
time of publication. However, in light of the possibility of human error or changes in the
practice of medicine, neither the author, nor the publisher, nor any other party who has been
involved in the preparation or publication of this work warrants that the information contained
herein is in every respect accurate or complete. Readers are encouraged to confirm the
information contained herein with other reliable sources, and are strongly advised to check the
product information sheet provided by the pharmaceutical company for each drug they plan to
administer.

9 8 7 6 5 4 3 2 1
Printed in the United States of America
on acid-free paper

To my wife, Carol, for her unwavering love and friendship. To my children Ryan,
Lauren, Nicole (and also Chris), who inspire all that I do.
Joseph Tracy

With my love and deep appreciation to Sara, A, K, and X as well as our parents, who
are our role models, and families. Many thanks to the outstanding mentors, including
KS and JT, who have patiently guided and advised.
Ben Hampstead

Dedicated to my amazing parents with everlasting gratitude; my wife Usha for her
indefatigable love and support; to our wonderful children, Tejas Aditya and Sanjena
Anshu, who have brought us immeasurable joy; and to my sterling brothers Suresh,
Sudhir, and Subash, growing up with whom was an incomparable experience.
K. Sathian

Contents

PART TWO   Plasticity of Cognition in Neurologic Syndromes

**PART THREE   Plasticity of Cognition and the New
                Emerging Technologies**

Foreword

Plasticity refers to the property of a material to undergo alterations. Of all human organs, the brain is the most plastic, and it is continually undergoing alterations. The brain senses and perceives; it learns, stores, and manipulates knowledge; and, based on goals and drives, it plans and executes mental and physical actions. The brain is most plastic during youth, but it is the mature and aging brain that is more likely to be injured by disorders such as vascular, autoimmune, infectious, metabolic, endocrine, deficiency, neoplastic, and degenerative diseases, while head trauma can affect the brain at any age. These diseases often induce neurobehavioral disorders with serious disability.

Some people with these injuries and diseases spontaneously recover. This recovery may be related to several factors. For example, the injured neuronal networks, which initially were not functioning, may recover, or other areas that can perform the functions of the injured portion of the brain may substitute for the injured areas. With acute injury to a portion of the brain, uninjured but connected areas may become inhibited and dysfunctional. Von Monakow called this phenomenon "diaschisis." With time, this inhibition may remit, and functionally impaired networks may perform normally. Since the human brain is plastic, after an injury there may be remyelination, dendritic and axonal sprouting, and an increase of dendritic spines with the formation of new synaptic connections in uninjured areas of the brain, as well as alterations in neurotransmitter and neuromodulator systems. These changes may allow recovery of function. This "spontaneous" improvement of function shortly after an acute brain injury usually abates after several months, and many patients remained disabled. Thus, clinicians must determine how they can best enhance plasticity and improve the functional capacity of patients with neurobehavioral deficits. In addition to advising patients to discontinue medications that may impair neuroplasticity and treating patients with medications and procedures (e.g., transcranial magnetic stimulation and transcranial direct current stimulation) that can enhance plasticity, clinicians may also have patients engage in activities that will allow them to relearn the cognitive skills they have lost. In addition, clinicians may help patients develop compensatory neurobehavioral procedures, including prosthetic devices that can reduce these patients' disability.

In this book, experts discuss many of the diseases and disorders that induce neurobehavioral deficits; however, rather than just focusing on the familiar signs, symptoms, and the pathophysiology of these diseases and disorders, emphasis is placed on describing the neuroplastic responses and cognitive mechanisms of reorganization related to both spontaneous recovery and successful intervention. There are many disorders in which both spontaneous recovery and intervention fail, and these suffering patients remain disabled. The reasons for these failures, as well as the future research that is needed to develop successful interventions, are also discussed in this important book. A particularly interesting feature of this book is its examination of neurobehavioral plasticity from a number of different perspectives: specific neurologic diseases (e.g., stroke, epilepsy), particular neurobehavioral conditions (e.g., aphasia, amnesia), and emerging technologies. The chapter authors focus on the dynamic changes that occur over time in each condition or with specific clinical interventions. The volume as a whole offers interesting and innovative insights at the level of neural networks. The book makes clear that an emphasis on dynamic change in neural networks is increasingly relevant to behavioral neurology and cognitive neurorehabilitation, and will yield great progress in these fields. The editors are to be commended for putting together a fine team of experts and creating a book that focuses on broadly applicable principles related to cognitive and behavioral plasticity, one that will be of much interest to a wide readership, including both clinicians and scientists.

Kenneth M. Heilman, MD
Department of Neurology, the University of Florida College of Medicine,
and the Malcom Randall Veteran's Affairs Hospital,
Gainesville, Florida

Contributors

Anthony Angwin, PhD
School of Health and Rehabilitation
Sciences,
The University of Queensland,
Queensland, Australia

Paolo Bartolomeo, MD, PhD
Brain and Spine Institute, Groupe,
Hospitalier Pitié-Salpêtrière,
Paris, France

Niels Birbaumer, PhD
Institute of Medical Psychology and
Behavioral Neurobiology & German
Center for Diabetes Research,
(DZD e.V.), University of Tübingen,
Tübingen, Germany
Ospedale San Camillo, Istituto di
Ricovero e Cura a Carattere Scientifico
(IRCCS),
Venezia, Italy

Anthony J. W. Chen, MD
University of California, San Francisco,
VA Northern California Health Care
System,
Martinez, California

Leonardo G. Cohen, MD
Human Cortical Physiology and Stroke
Neurorehabilitation Section,
National Institute of Neurological,
Disorders and Stroke, NIH,
Bethesda, Maryland

David A. Copland, PhD
School of Health & Rehabilitation,
Sciences & Centre for Clinical
Research,
The University of Queensland,
Queensland, Australia

Mar Cortes, MD
Weill Cornell Medical College,
Non-invasive Brain Stimulation and
Human Motor Control Laboratory
The Burke Medical Research Institute
of Cornell University,
White Plains, New York

Bruce Crosson, PhD
Center for Visual and Neurocognitive
Rehabilitation,
Atlanta VA Medical Center,
Atlanta, Georgia

Mark D'Esposito, MD
Henry H. Wheeler, Jr. Brain Imaging
Center,
University of California,
Berkeley and Department of Psychology,
Helen Wills Neuroscience Institute,
Berkeley, California

John DeLuca, PhD
Senior Vice President for Research
Kessler Foundation,
West Orange, New Jersey
Department of Physical Medicine and
Rehabilitation,
Department of Neurology and
Neurosciences,
Rutgers, New Jersey Medical School,
Newark, New Jersey

Gaelle Doucet, PhD
Department of Neurosurgery,
Thomas Jefferson University/Jefferson
Medical College,
Philadelphia, Pennsylvania

Hugues Duffau, MD, PhD
Department of Neurosurgery,
Gui de Chauliac Hospital,
Montpellier University Medical Center,
Montpellier, France

Dylan J. Edwards, PT, PhD
Weill Cornell Medical College,
Non-invasive Brain Stimulation and
Human Motor,
Control Laboratory,
The Burke Medical Research,
Institute of Cornell University,
White Plains, New York

**Benjamin M. Hampstead, PhD,
ABPP/CN**
Atlanta VAMC RR&D Center of
Excellence for Visual and
Neurocognitive Rehabilitation,
Decatur, Georgia
Department of Rehabilitation Medicine,
Emory University,
Atlanta, Georgia

Frank G. Hillary, PhD
Department of Psychology,
Social Life and Engineering Sciences
Imaging Center,
Pennsylvania State University,
University Park, Pennsylvania

Andrew Mayes, PhD
School of Psychological Sciences and
Centre for Clinical and Cognitive
Neuroscience,
University of Manchester,
Manchester, United Kingdom

Keith M. McGregor, PhD
Center for Visual and Neurocognitive
Rehabilitation,
Atlanta VA Medical Center,
Department of Neurology,
Emory University,
Atlanta, Georgia

Ana H. Medeiros, PT, PhD
Conselho Nacional de Pesquisa e
Desenvolvimento, CNPq—Brazil,
Non-invasive Brain Stimulation and
Human Motor Control Laboratory,
The Burke Medical Research Institute
of Cornell University,
White Plains, New York

Jesper Mogensen, PhD
The Unit for Cognitive Neuroscience,
Department of Psychology,
University of Copenhagen,
Copenhagen, Denmark

Stephen E. Nadeau, MD
Research Service, Malcom Randall VA
Medical Center,
Department of Neurology,
University of Florida College of Medicine,
Gainesville, Florida

Lindsay M. Oberman, PhD
Neuroplasticity and Autism
Spectrum Disorder Program,
Department of Psychiatry
and Human Behavior,

E. P. Bradley Hospital and Warren Alpert
Medical School of Brown University,
East Providence, Rhode Island
and
Berenson-Allen Center for Noninvasive
Brain Stimulation,
Beth Israel Deaconess Medical Center
Division of Epilepsy and Clinical
Neurophysiology,
Boston Children's Hospital,
Boston, Massachusetts

Karol Osipowicz, PhD
Department of Psychology,
Drexel University,
Philadelphia, Pennsylvania

Alvaro Pascual-Leone, MD, PhD
Associate Dean for Clinical and
Translational Research,
Harvard Medical School,
Berenson-Allen Center for
Noninvasive Brain Stimulation,
Department of Neurology,
Beth Israel Deaconess
Medical Center,
Harvard Medical School,
Boston, Massachusetts

Dorian Pustina, PhD
Department of Neurology,
Thomas Jefferson University/Jefferson
Medical College,
Philadelphia, Pennsylvania

Sarah M. Rajtmajer, PhD
Department of Mathematics,
Pennsylvania State University,
University Park, Pennsylvania

Alexander Rotenberg, MD, PhD
Berenson-Allen Center for Noninvasive
Brain Stimulation,
Department of Neurology,
Beth Israel Deaconess Medical Center
and Harvard Medical School,
Division of Epilepsy and Clinical

Neurophysiology,
Children's Hospital,
Boston, Massachusetts

K. Sathian, MD, PhD, FANA
Departments of Neurology,
Rehabilitation Medicine and Psychology,
Emory University,
Atlanta, Georgia
Atlanta VAMC RR&D Center of
Excellence for Visual and Neurocognitive
Rehabilitation,
Decatur, Georgia

Surjo R. Soekadar, MD
Department of Psychiatry and
Psychotherapy & Institute of Medical
Psychology and
Behavioral Neurobiology
University Hospital of Tübingen
Tübingen, Germany

Jelena Stojanovic-Radic, PhD
Kessler Foundation, West Orange,
New Jersey
Department of Physical medicine and
Rehabilitation Rutgers,
University-New Jersey Medical School,
New Jersey

Joseph I. Tracy, PhD, ABPP/CN
Jefferson Hospital for Neuroscience,
Department of Neurology,
Thomas Jefferson University/Jefferson
Medical College,
Philadelphia, Pennsylvania

Umesh M. Venkatesan, MS
Department of Psychology,
Pennsylvania State University,
University Park, Pennsylvania

Lewis A. Wheaton, PhD
Cognitive Motor Control Laboratory,
School of Applied Physiology,
Georgia Tech,
Atlanta, Georgia

PART ONE

Plasticity of Cognition in Neurologic Disorders

Recovery, Compensation, and Reorganization in Neuropathology

Levels of Conceptual and Methodological Challenges

Jesper Mogensen

Introduction

If an individual loses one of the extremities—for example, a front leg, or in case of humans, an arm—to injury or disease, the subsequent process is species-dependent. If the affected individual is a salamander, the limb is likely to regenerate, and eventually the result of this regrowth will be an organism with a full complement of extremities (e.g., Brockes & Kumar, 2005). But in the case of most other species, such a regeneration is not going to happen. In humans suffering the loss of an arm, the subsequent course of events is likely to include a lengthy process in which the preserved arm will play a more prominent role than it had pretraumatically. A right-handed person losing the right arm is, for instance, likely to develop a higher dexterity using the left arm and hand—and potentially even the ability to write with the left hand. The one-armed individual may also be helped by the fitting of a prosthetic arm, which may become a useful replacement of the lost arm. While the salamander can recover fully—via its ability to regenerate the lost limb—the human patient is forced to undergo a lifelong process of compensation—be it via the use of the preserved arm and/or via the application of a prosthesis.

A distinction between recovery processes and their compensational counterparts is clear as long as we are considering the fate of an individual losing one of the extremities. Recovery returns an injured individual to normality. And in the case of compensation, the original situation is not re-created, but a level of proficiency is achieved via the use of alternative or prosthetic devices. This straightforward distinction, as well as most of the clarity, is lost if the organ under consideration is the brain. The purpose of this chapter is to present some methodological and conceptual issues relevant to the distinction (or lack thereof) between compensational and recovery processes related to neurological diseases. Due to the focus of most of the research explicitly dealing with such issues, the focus here will primarily be on the post-traumatic processes after focal brain injury. The discussed issues are, however, relevant to most, if not all, of the neurological diseases affecting the brain.

Recovery Versus Compensation

In case of traumatic brain injury (TBI) or vascular brain injury, the term "recovery" is in some instances (e.g., Levin et al., 2009) being used to indicate a true re-creation of what has been lost to one or another type of trauma. If the injured patient in the absence of re-creation of the lost neural structure is still able to return to at least a measure of normality within the affected domain, the process is seen as one of "compensation." Other authors (e.g., Mogensen, 2011a, 2011c, 2012a, 2012b; Mogensen & Malá, 2009) apply the term "recovery" in a broader manner—speaking about "functional recovery" as a general description of any reduction or elimination of trauma-associated symptoms. In the present chapter, the term "recovery" may—if stated in isolation—be used in this general sense. In contrast, the terminology "re-creational recovery" will be used to describe situations in which something lost to injury or disease is fully re-established.

Wilson (2000) deals with the concept and methods of compensation within neurorehabilitation after brain injury. Addressing compensational methods in the case of amnesia, Wilson (2000) mentions the support of memory by diaries, tape recorders, and alarm-watches. In the same context, compensation for speech and language deficits are discussed in terms of voice synthesizers and alternative communication systems, as well as mime and gesture. Clearly, these types of compensation are of a "prosthetic" nature. But does this mean that if a brain-injured patient regains, for instance, memory or speech in the absence of external prosthetic devices, then the process represents a full re-creation of the pretraumatic situation—re-creational recovery?

Concerning the motor systems, Levin et al. (2009) have emphasized the need for a more thorough conceptual clarification regarding recovery and compensation, respectively. While such conceptual progress is clearly important regarding post-traumatic processes related to motor performance, a similar clarification is even more difficult and needed within the cognitive domains. Although most of the discussions regarding such issues have occurred in the context of traumatic and vascular acquired brain injury, the neural and cognitive processes—and thereby the conceptual and methodological challenges—are likely to be similar within most, if not all, neurological diseases.

A seductively simple way of defining recovery and compensation, respectively, is to reserve the term "recovery" for situations in which a process re-creates exactly what has been lost to injury or disease, while any other process that allows some type of preservation of or return to normality is defined as "compensation." But if such a definition is adopted, one must realize that the investigation of whether or not "the same" has been re-created (or preserved) has to be conducted at a variety of levels of analysis, and that in any given situation, the answer may not be identical at all levels. An additional and far from trivial problem is technically how to establish whether—at a given level—something is, indeed, "the same" (e.g., Wilms & Mogensen, 2011).

Levels of Analysis

One of the major goals of cognitive neuroscience is to relate the neural processes—as they can be measured in terms of action potentials, production and release of neurochemical substances, changes in regional metabolism of the brain, and so on—to the surface phenomena at the mental/behavioral level. These surface phenomena include recordable behavior measured in terms of muscular contractions, movement of limbs, verbal output, scores on cognitive tests, and so on—as well as the conscious manifestations, which are of a subjective nature and thereby inaccessible to direct, external observation. The fact that manifestations of consciousness cannot be measured directly by an external observer does not, however, mean that they are inaccessible to scientifically valid scrutiny. It has, for instance, been possible to develop methods that allow a graded and reliable test of the level of consciousness related to a particular observation (e.g., Overgaard, 2006; Overgaard & Timmermans, 2010).

At both the neural level and the level of behavioral/mental phenomena, the recent decades have seen an unprecedented accumulation of data. At both the cellular and macroscopic levels, we are constantly gaining new insight into the intricacies of the brain. And at the "surface" level of behavioral and mental phenomena, an almost similar explosion of understanding has been achieved—even reaching a deeper understanding of something as complex as conscious experience. But how are the processes of these two levels to be related to each other?

Within the philosophical disciplines attempting to relate especially conscious manifestations to their neural substrates, one of the dominating trends is known as type identity theory; it predicts that conscious experiences relate to neural processes in a "1:1" fashion. This means that for any mental state there can be only one corresponding neural state. The major, contrasting, standpoint is functionalism, which predicts "1:many" relations—meaning that the same mental state can be mediated by different neural substrates (Overgaard & Mogensen, 2011).

But to relate the phenomena of the "surface" level directly to those of the neural level may be trying to bridge too wide a gap. Instead, it has been suggested that a third, intermediate level is introduced. Such suggestions have been made on many occasions. The perhaps best-known model in which an intermediate level is imposed is the one proposed by Marr (e.g., 1982). More recently, Carandini (2012) has made suggestions along the same lines. An important difference between the intermediate levels of Marr (1982) and Carandini (2012) is that the algorithmic ("computational") level of Marr primarily consists of computational steps deduced from what is observed at the level of mental states. In contrast, the more recent suggestions of Carandini primarily assume the (intermediate) level of computational states to be constructed on the basis of direct neural experimentation (primarily recordings). As pointed out by, for instance, Overgaard and Mogensen (2011), the introduction of an intermediate computational level increases the number of possible interlevel relationships—including "1:1:1," "1:1:many," "1:many:1," and so on.

The final part of this chapter will deal with a model including such a three-layered analysis. But first, the focus will be on issues of re-creation of what has been lost versus compensation. Initially, this will be done at the neural level. Subsequently, similar issues will be considered at the behavioral/cognitive level.

Re-creation of the Neural Substrate?

Addressing whether or not what has been preserved or re-created is "the same" at the neural level is in some instances extremely easy—but it may also pose some of the greatest challenges. In cases of vascular or traumatic brain injury, it can in most instances easily be established that there is, in a strict sense, no post-traumatic re-establishment of "the same." An injured part of the brain will at a later point in time normally be found to be either missing (as is the case if a cortical region has experimentally been ablated) or replaced by scar tissue. One never finds a re-creation of the neural structure that existed pretraumatically.

In cases of neurodegenerative conditions, the situation may, however, be slightly more complicated. If a rather homogeneous projection system suffers a neurodegenerative process eliminating part of that projection, sprouting and/or upregulation of, for instance, post-synaptic receptors, the level of release of neurotransmitters, and so on, may occur. And such changes may allow the remaining parts of that projection to fulfill a neural function that is essentially identical to what was seen in the premorbid situation.

Another factor to consider is the fact that neurogenesis is a lifelong process that, even in the adult brain, constantly provides newborn neurons that are able to migrate into various parts of the brain (e.g., Ming & Song, 2005; Suh et al., 2009). Such newly created neurons may participate in a re-establishment of the neural networks partially lost to either degeneration or injury. In cases of experimental brain injury, it has been demonstrated that immature neurons may at least under certain circumstances migrate toward the site of injury (Hicks et al., 2007). Also, in animal models, it appears that at least in case of lesions to the infant brain there may be a process at least resembling a re-creation. A traumatized part of the brain does not regain anything like the original structure, but there is still within that region cellular elements that participate in the mediation of the post-traumatic functional recovery (e.g., Dallison & Kolb, 2003). Robertson and Murre (1999) have provided a theoretical model demonstrating that if neural networks are partially lesioned, they may be able to reorganize in ways that can at least theoretically subserve a functional performance more or less identical to what was present pretraumatically.

While such examples point to at least a certain level of re-creation of the neural machinery lost to injury or degeneration, it is still clear that in most cases the neural changes found during various rehabilitative processes do not (re)produce a neural structure similar to what was seen premorbidly—at least not if addressed in terms of the cytoarchitecture and connectivity of the normal brain (see further discussions in Mogensen, 2011a).

But even if such a literal re-creation of the neural structures is not occurring, there may be other ways to re-create "the same" neural substrate. It may be possible to establish neural networks, which are processing information in ways that are identical to those achieved by the neural circuits lost to injury or degeneration. Theoretically, reorganizational processes elsewhere in the brain could establish neural processes offering information processing identical to those originally provided by the lost structure. This may be achieved in two different ways.

The first of these ways is by the de novo creation of networks distal to the site of injury. In principle, the creation of "replacement" networks may follow the same steps as those encountered during the original development of the brain. During maturation, neurons undergo changes that reduce their similarity to the developing neurons present during the original establishment of the circuitry of the brain (e.g., D. F. Chen et al., 1995; Fawcett et al., 1989; Goldberg et al., 2002). Such changes, however, should not discourage the idea that loss of neural tissue may be followed by de novo creation of circuitry. Neurogenesis continues throughout life (e.g., Ming & Song, 2005; Suh et al., 2009), and injury to the central nervous system further enhances such neurogenesis (e.g., Arvidsson et al., 2002; J. Chen et al., 2004; Magavi et al., 2000; Nakatomi et al., 2002; Scharff et al., 2000). These newly created neurons are essentially similar to the newborn neurons present during original development. Furthermore, mature astrocytes are able to transform themselves into radial glial cells that can guide the migration of immature neurons within the adult brain (in ways similar to the migration processes seen during original development) (e.g., Leavitt et al., 1999). Most, if not all, of the substances (neuroattractants and neurorepellants, respectively) that during original development guide the outgrowth of dendrites and axons are still present in the adult brain (e.g., Koeberle & Bahr, 2004). A less encouraging aspect—with respect to the possibility of de novo circuitry creation—is that such substances are distributed in a different manner in the adult brain when compared to what was the case during original development (e.g., Harel & Strittmatter, 2006). While such a changed distribution within the adult brain may be a limiting factor, the perhaps most crucial limitation stems from the fact that the production of a number of inhibitory factors associated with glial cells and myelin is important in achieving the termination of the various "critical periods" during development (e.g., Berry, 1982; Schäfer et al., 2008; Schwab & Thoenen, 1985). The especially high openness to environmentally driven reorganization of networks seen during developmentally "critical periods" is at least partly terminated by such substances. These substances apparently stabilize basic networks throughout the remaining life of the individual. A family of substances of special importance in this context seems to be the astrocyte-produced CSPGs (chondroitin sulfate proteoglycans) (e.g., Berardi et al., 2004; McGee et al., 2005; Pizzorusso et al., 2002). Studies addressing the CSPGs have demonstrated that these substances contribute to the prevention of adult re-creation of circuitry lost to acquired brain injury (Del Rio & Soriano, 2007; Schäfer et al., 2008). Pharmacological inhibition of CSPGs (e.g., Del Rio & Soriano, 2007)—and especially local application of such pharmacological inhibitors within the affected region of the brain (e.g., Lin et al., 2008)—is associated with an improved recovery after brain injury. Such improvements may be achieved via a level of circuitry re-creation.

Now we turn to the second mechanism that may provide—within parts of the brain distal or proximal to the site of injury—a "re-establishment" of what has been lost. This mechanism is to engage networks that were premorbidly able to perform the same type of information processing—but that did so on other types of neural input. If such a "redundancy" exists, a rerouting of the input/output originally related to the lost part of the brain may be sufficient to re-create essentially the original type of neural information processing.

Such a shift to similar neural processing on a novel input may be what we see in a multitude of examples related to the processing of sensory information. Within both the somatosensory and auditory systems of the brain, sensory representations at both cortical and subcortical levels are arranged in the form of a "map." Within the somatosensory system, the map consists of a somatotopic representation of the body, while auditory representations are arranged tonotopically. One encounters all parts of the body, represented one after another, when moving from one end to the other of the somatotopic representation. The tonotopic map represents one tonal frequency after another in an ascending order of frequencies. There is, however, a substantial plasticity involved in the way various body parts and tonal frequencies, respectively, are represented within these "maps."

If part of the somatosensory map lacks its input, the "vacant" part of the map is gradually taken over by the neighboring representations. If, for instance, a hand is amputated, the contralateral somatosensory representation of that hand will obviously lack a sensory input. Under such circumstances, the representation of the two body parts normally found on either side of the now missing hand representation—the representations of the face and arm, respectively—will "grow" and eventually completely cannibalize the area previously representing the amputated hand (e.g., Karl et al., 2001; Weiss et al., 2000; Yang et al., 1994). In animal models, similar results have been obtained—for instance, in studies of monkeys after amputation of a finger (Merzenich & Jenkins, 1993). In a parallel to these results, it has been found that if the brain no longer receives auditory input representing particular tonal bands—thereby leaving part of the tonotopic representation vacant—the representations of the "neighboring" tones are expanding to fill out the part of the tonotopic map left vacant due to the lack of input (e.g., Irvine, 2007; Robertson & Irvine, 1989; Scheich, 1991; Thai-Van et al., 2007). The selective lesions within the ear causing such a lack of tonal input can thus provoke reorganizations with many similarities to those seen in case of amputation of body parts.

When a missing sensory input provokes such reorganizations, one result will be that what is represented next to the "vacant" area will eventually gain a larger than normal representation within the map. It has been demonstrated that the tones which have thus gained a larger than normal representation within the tonotopic map can subsequently be discriminated more easily (Thai-Van et al., 2007). Apparently, the reorganization provides a certain sensory aspect (tone) both a larger representation and improved information processing.

Changing the relative demands for information processing within the tonotopic or somatotopic representation in the intact individual can also change these sensory maps. When the discrimination of particular tonal frequencies is needed in order to solve a behavioral task, training on such a task is associated with a relative growth of the representation of those tones within the tonotopic map (e.g., Irvine, 2007; Recanzone et al., 1993; Scheich, 1991). And there is a positive correlation between the obtained proficiency of task solution and the degree of expansion of the relevant tonal areas within the tonotopic representation (e.g., Recanzone et al., 1993). Within the somatosensory domain, Merzenich and Jenkins (1993) studied the consequences of a training procedure in which monkeys were to solve a task that required somatosensory information processing related to the tip of two of the digits of the hand. Under such circumstances, the somatotopic representation of the two "trained" digits exhibited a relative growth compared to the representation of the untrained digits (Merzenich & Jenkins, 1993). A number of additional studies (e.g., Elbert et al., 1995; Münte et al., 2002; Xerri et al., 1996) have confirmed that when a training procedure emphasizes somatosensory information processing related to a particular part of the body, the representation of that body part exhibits a relative growth within the somatotopic representation.

It appears that within the somatotopic and tonotopic representations, the neural mechanisms involved in information processing relative to particular body parts or tonal frequencies are relatively "interchangeable" within a given modality. Processing mechanisms originally related to one body part or tonal frequency may also subserve information related to a different body part or tonal band. Such a flexibility can most easily be explained by the assumption that the neural apparatus of such a map consists of a huge number of more or less identical processing "modules," which intrinsically perform a particular type of information processing relevant to the modality in question (e.g., Mogensen, 2012b). That processing is, in principle, independent of the body region or tonal frequency to which the processing is related. Thereby, a processing module is in principle "omnipotent" relative to information within that modality. It is only the input/output relationship of the module that determines its specific association with a body region or tonal frequency. Modules can change their input/output relationship and thereby shift from an association with one body part or tonal frequency, respectively, to another.

"Modules" that are able to perform a particular type of information processing, on input which is different from what is normally seen, may not exclusively be a feature of various parts of the primary sensory "maps." Some data indicate that even across modalities, certain networks may provide more or less identical information processing to input that they do not receive in the normal brain. Studies of intermodal plasticity have, for instance, addressed the possibility of providing blind individuals with a "prosthetic vision" in which somatosensory pathways are utilized in order to provide at least a crude representation of the visual world (e.g., Bach-y-Rita et al., 1969, 1998; Kaczmarek et al., 1991; Ptito et al., 2005). Information regarding the visual world is delivered to "early blind" individuals via a somatosensory input. And in such a situation, spatial orientation discrimination tasks are partly mediated by a cortical region that in individuals with normal vision is associated with performance of visual tasks requiring discrimination of the spatial orientation of figures (Ptito et al., 2005). In contrast, blindfolded but otherwise normally sighted individuals performing the same task (based on the same somatosensory input) did not demonstrate a similar activation of the "visual" area in question (Ptito et al., 2005). Apparently, the cortical region in question mediates information processing relevant to the analysis of spatial orientation of figures. Under normal circumstances, it performs such operations on the basis of visual input. But in the case of at least "early blind" individuals, a more or less similar form of information processing is achieved on somatosensory information representing the visual world.

Thus, "modules" within at least some sensory systems appear to be "omnipotent" in the sense that they may perform similar or closely related information processing on "atypical" input (as in the examples discussed earlier). This may open a broader possibility of processes that in a certain manner can be considered a re-creational recovery. Such processes would "replace" the lost neural circuitry with pre-existing basic circuitry elsewhere in the brain—and would do so by a rerouting of input/output connections. Such possibilities need to be taken into account when interpreting the neural substrate found to mediate cognitive recovery processes after brain injury or other neuropathological processes.

Studies of the Neural Substrate of Rehabilitation After Brain Injury

In brain-injured patients, attempts are being made to identify the neural substrate of post-traumatic recovery within various cognitive functions. For instance, patients suffering aphasias (normally after injury to the left hemisphere) have been studied. Ipsilateral (left hemisphere) contributions to mediation of reacquisition of linguistic functions have been demonstrated by, for instance, Meinzer et al. (2008), Perani et al. (2003), Specht et al. (2009), and Szaflarski et al. (2011). In the study by Meinzer et al. (2008), it was found that post-traumatic treatment induced reintegration of various perilesional areas into the mediation of linguistic recovery. A dominating issue within such studies is whether the contralateral (right) hemisphere contributes significantly to the mediation of post-traumatic recovery. Many studies appear to provide a positive answer to this question. For instance, involvement of structures within the right hemisphere has been demonstrated by Ansaldo and Arguin (2003), Ansaldo et al. (2002), Baumgaertner et al. (2005), Perani et al. (2003), Specht et al. (2009), Thomas et al. (1997), and Thulborn et al. (1999). The pattern of shift toward right hemisphere mediation of linguistic performance appears to differ between types of aphasia (e.g., Thomas et al., 1997). Also, shifts toward right hemisphere mediation of language may be accompanied by reorganizations within the left hemisphere—recruiting uninjured regions within the injured left hemisphere (e.g., Thompson et al., 2010). In most cases, the apparent shift toward a right hemisphere mediation is seen after general rehabilitative training of linguistic functions—but without deliberate attempts at achieving a left-to-right shift. There are, however, cases in which training has more specifically aimed at achieving a right hemisphere mediation of linguistic tasks (e.g., Crosson et al., 2009). Crosson et al. (2009) required the patients to initiate each naming trial by a manipulation task using the left hand—thereby activating at least some right hemisphere structures. These procedures were developed specifically to ensure that an independent right hemisphere activation occurred concurrently with the initiation of the linguistic task. And the procedure appeared to be at least somewhat successful in improving the performance of the naming task—the rehabilitative process (Crosson et al., 2009).

Attempts to identify the neural substrate of cognitive rehabilitation after focal brain injury mostly rely on changes in local metabolism visualized by neuroimaging techniques such as functional magnetic resonance imaging (fMRI) or positron emission tomography (PET). Much may be learned from such studies. But it must be remembered that unless independently demonstrated to be so, changed levels of activity revealed by, for instance, fMRI are not necessarily a sign that the structure in question is participating in mediation of the functional recovery. The changed activation may be the result of any one of a number of trauma-related neural changes—for example, "disinhibition." To demonstrate that a structure is, indeed, participating in mediation of the recovering function(s), additional data are required. An example of such data within the field of aphasia has been published by Meinzer et al. (2007) in their study of a bilingual aphasic patient. Activation of part of the superior temporal lobe of the right hemisphere was exclusively associated with the use of the post-traumatically trained language—while such a pattern of right hemisphere activation was absent using the untrained language. It is, however, only in rare cases that a cognitive recovery can be studied in the presence of such an "internal control."

In most cases, the potential neural substrate of the functional recovery needs to be addressed in other ways. It has been argued (e.g., Mogensen, 2011b; Mogensen & Malá, 2009) that in order to "map" the neural substrate of cognitive recovery in animal models, one needs to perform a number of "organic challenges" and study the degree to which such challenges modify the behavioral/cognitive performance of the animal. Organic challenges include temporary inhibition of neurochemical systems (e.g., a neurotransmitter system being partially or totally "inactivated" by systemic administration of an antagonist), regional application of pharmacological agents within parts of the brain, as well as the infliction of additional focal lesions of neural structures or substructures. By performing such manipulations after a full level of post-traumatic recovery has been achieved, the relative importance of various neural systems in mediation of that recovery can be estimated (e.g., Mogensen, 2011b; Mogensen & Malá, 2009). In humans, however, there are obviously major restrictions regarding the degree to which similar challenges can be applied. A promising tool in this context is transcranial magnetic stimulation (TMS). At least for cortical regions, TMS may be used to selectively inactivate areas that have been identified as candidates for the mediation of a cognitive recovery process. By applying inhibiting TMS while conducting a cognitive evaluation of the patient, one may achieve valuable information regarding the degree to which that structure contributes to the mediation of the recovered cognitive processes.

In animal models and patients alike, a level of understanding has been achieved regarding the changed pattern of neural activities accompanying some of the cognitive recovery processes. But in spite of this partial solution of some of the problems associated with such research, we need to return to the original question of this chapter: When do such reorganizational processes represent a re-creational recovery—re-creation of what has been lost—and when is the process of a compensatory nature?

With the presently available methods, it is not realistic to establish the details of the neural information processing at a scale necessary to judge whether or not an "alternative neural substrate" represents information processing that is identical to what was lost to injury elsewhere in the brain. Progress has recently been made in analyzing information processing within structures relevant to the mediation of advanced cognitive levels (e.g., Jeewajee et al., 2008; Moser et al., 2014; Poucet et al., 2014; Yoon et al., 2013). And Carandini (2012) has expressed optimism regarding the possibility of constructing a conceptual level of "computational states" on the basis of direct neural experimentation (primarily single unit recordings). It is, however, striking that the examples stressed by Carandini (2012) all tend to be recordings performed in structures close to the input or output pathways of the brain. Even within these brain structures, it is highly challenging to analyze the intricacies of neural information processing. But it is in such cases possible to perform the analysis coordinated with controlled sensory input or to examine the activity of an output system coordinated with the performance of a particular motor act. If, however, the brain regions addressed are mediating the cognitive functions more distal to input and output pathways of the brain, it becomes far more challenging (and presently akin to impossible) to identify the relevant circuitry and the exact circumstances under which to perform the recordings. Thus, it is unlikely that one can identify—on a purely neural level of experimentation—whether or not the recruitment of alternative brain regions represents a re-creational recovery or a compensational process in which something truly different (in terms of information processing) substitutes for what has been lost.

Studies of the Cognitive Mechanisms of Rehabilitation After Brain Injury

In order to come closer to such conceptual clarification (should such a clarification be possible), one needs to address the actual cognitive and behavioral performance of the individual. What is required is a detailed behavioral/cognitive analysis of the recovered patient (or experimental subject in an animal model).

To establish on a behavioral/cognitive level whether or not what has been (re)gained is, indeed, "the same" or something of a more compensatory nature is frequently not as simple as it may seem. If a "recovered" aphasic patient, instead of the statement "I saw a bird," utters the sentence "I saw the thing in trees and up in the air," one may safely conclude that the patient has not fully regained the linguistic abilities—but has developed a compensatory strategy. Such obvious signs are, however, often not available. And what is required is an evaluation utilizing tests of various kinds. But such tests are not always able to reveal all relevant aspects of the performance and ability of an individual.

Frequently, one encounters the situation that a cognitive test, despite its widespread use and acceptance as a clinical tool, is able to provide only rather limited information. Clinical tests of hemispatial neglect may, in the initial phases of a (usually right hemisphere) injury-induced neglect, be able clearly to demonstrate this condition. Nevertheless, during later phases of the process, the standardized neglect tests may demonstrate an absence of neglect, while the behavioral performance and general clinical impression of the patient testify to the fact that a significant level of neglect is still present (e.g., Azouvi et al., 2002). Using a standard test of hemispatial neglect, the patient may appear to be fully recovered, but may still fail to dress the left side of the body and fail to reserve adequate space for the left shoulder when attempting to pass through a doorway.

Another example of the need for a more detailed analysis of cognitive symptoms in brain-injured patients is provided by studies of the deficits demonstrated by the patient D. F. (e.g., Milner et al., 1991). Initial results indicated perceptual disturbances agreeing with the interpretation of visual processing that the "dorsal stream" can be characterized as the "where" stream, while the ventral stream can be characterized as the "what" stream (e.g., Ungerleider et al., 1998). However, subsequent and more detailed studies (e.g., Schenk, 2006) have modified this characterization and thereby have brought significant doubts to the perhaps overly simplified interpretation of the two "streams of visual perceptual analysis."

In animal models, one may find a corresponding list of examples demonstrating that, if taken at face value without further refinement, various behavioral tests are unable to reveal the true mechanisms of a particular condition. For instance, standard testing apparently shows that neither the hippocampal formation nor the cholinergic systems of the brain contribute significantly to the mediation of a non-mapping type place-learning task administered in a water maze (e.g., Mogensen et al., 2002; Wörtwein et al., 1995). Nevertheless, additional scrutiny demonstrated such a conclusion to be in error (Mogensen et al., 1995,

2002; Wörtwein et al., 1995). Furthermore, behavioral tests utilized in animal models may have a striking degree of "method dependency" regarding whether or not a particular neural manipulation can reflect itself in behavioral performance. For instance, Lepore et al. (1985) studied in cats whether or not a "split-brain" operation (accompanied by transection of the optic clasm) prevents the interhemispheric transfer of monocularly acquired visual information. The animals acquired a visual discrimination task using one eye (thereby receiving the discrimination-relevant information only within one hemisphere) and were subsequently tested using exclusively the other eye—thereby being required to use mechanisms within the contralateral hemisphere. No interhemispheric information transfer was found when the animals were tested in a classical "two-choice discrimination box" in which food was offered as reinforcement. When, however, trained and tested in a "Lashley-type" jumping stand, the animals demonstrated a rather high level of interhemispheric transfer of information (Lepore et al., 1985). A related example of the importance of the apparatus in which a cognitive test is administered was published by Mogensen et al. (1987). The experimental animals (rats) suffered a massive destruction of prefrontal structures and were subsequently subjected to a spatial delayed alternation task that is frequently considered the "Babinski sign" of the prefrontal system—it is seen as the test that is the most sensitive to injury within the prefrontal system. When the spatial delayed alternation task was encountered in an operant chamber, the rats performed at a normal level of proficiency in spite of their injury. But their performance of the spatial delayed alternation task was severely impaired if the test was administered in a T-maze (Mogensen et al., 1987).

As mentioned earlier, it has been argued that in order to reach a better understanding of the neural processes involved in post-traumatic cognitive recovery in animal models, such studies need to include the use of "organic challenges" (e.g., Mogensen, 2011b; Mogensen & Malá, 2009). In parallel to the need for such "organic challenges"—and as a consequence of the mentioned shortcomings of many standardized behavioral tests—the animal models scrutinizing post-traumatic processes also must include behavioral/cognitive challenges (e.g., Mogensen, 2011b; Mogensen & Malá, 2009). These challenges are behavioral methods that can reveal not only to what extent but also how a given cognitive task is being solved. Traditionally, the focus has been on the degree of behavioral impairment seen in, for instance, a brain-injured group of animals. What has been stressed has been exclusively the number of errors, the speed of task acquisition, or similar measures reflecting the "proficiency" of task performance. The "challenge" methods are designed to step beyond the proficiency to address the underlying cognitive mechanisms. Like the "organic" challenges, the behavioral/cognitive challenges are not a standard repertoire but are pragmatically selected according to the issues of the study in question. Examples of such behavioral/cognitive challenges are the removal of the target platform in a water maze–based spatial task (e.g., Mogensen et al., 2004), the removal and/or manipulation of visual cues in spatial orientation tasks (e.g., Malá et al., 2007; Mogensen et al., 2002), and the introduction of various types of retention pauses within or between test sessions (e.g., Malá et al., 2007, 2012; Mogensen et al., 2007).

An example of the use of behavioral challenges is a study in which one of the issues was to what extent the prefrontal cortex participates in the mediation of post-traumatic recovery of allocentric place learning in a water maze after lesions of the hippocampus (Mogensen et al., 2004). In that study the participating rats were subjected to either hippocampal lesions, lesions of the prefrontal cortex, or a combined (simultaneous) lesion including both the hippocampus and the prefrontal cortex. Additionally, a group subjected to "sham" (control) surgery without brain injury was included. When the postoperative performance of the allocentric place-learning task was studied, the results indicated that while the prefrontally lesioned animals were marginally (but significantly) impaired, the task performance of the hippocampally lesioned group demonstrated a severe impairment of task solution. Both of these individually lesioned groups did, however, eventually undergo a complete behavioral recovery, and by the end of the rehabilitative training process both hippocampally lesioned and prefrontally lesioned animals performed at the same level of proficiency as the group subjected to the control procedure. A crucial question was, however, whether or not the addition of a prefrontal lesion to the hippocampal lesion would prevent the recovery after hippocampal lesions. Since there is a substantial overlap among the behavioral tasks that are impaired by lesions of the hippocampus and the prefrontal cortex, respectively (see, e.g., Mogensen et al., 2004), one may speculate that the prefrontal cortex plays a significant role in mediation of the behavioral recovery after hippocampal lesions. If this is the case, one would expect the animals subjected to combined lesions of the prefrontal cortex and the hippocampus either to show no recovery or at least to be severely impaired relative to the animals undergoing hippocampal lesions in isolation. The performance of the animals did, however, demonstrate that the two hippocampally lesioned groups (with and without an additional lesion of the prefrontal cortex, respectively) performed at equal levels of proficiency. The two groups were equally impaired and eventually reached the same level of (perfect) proficiency of task performance. Furthermore, the number of rehabilitative sessions required to reach this level of perfection did not differ between the groups (in fact, the animals given combined lesions performed insignificantly better than the animals subjected to isolated lesions of the hippocampus). An obvious conclusion from these results seems to be that the prefrontal cortex does not play any role in the mediation of the recovery process after hippocampal lesions—at least in rats performing the task in question. Subsequent administration of challenges did, however, negate such a conclusion. When a level of perfect task solution had been acquired by all subjects, they were given a session in which the goal platform was removed and it was measured to what extent the animals under such circumstances performed their search at the (previous) goal position. Thus, it could be established not only whether or not the animals could quickly and directly reach the goal platform (as they did in the normal administration of the task) but also whether or not they possessed a "cognitive representation" of the spatial position of the (submerged and thereby invisible) goal platform. The two individually lesioned groups (hippocampal or prefrontal lesions in isolation) revealed a fully normal level of representation of the spatial position of the goal. In contrast, the animals subjected to the combined lesion of the hippocampus and the prefrontal cortex were significantly inferior to the other groups in searching at the adequate position (Mogensen et al., 2004). Contrary to the incorrect conclusion that would have been reached without the administration of the behavioral challenge, the prefrontal cortex does, in fact, normally participate in mediation of the cognitive recovery processes related to this task. If present, the prefrontal cortex allows hippocampally lesioned animals to establish a "cognitive representation" of the spatial position that the animal is to reach during task performance. But when both the hippocampus and the prefrontal cortex were absent, the utilization of a cognitive strategy not requiring such a cognitive representation of the goal position still enables the animal to reach a perfect proficiency of task solution—and to do so as quickly as the animals that were subjected to hippocampal lesions but were allowed the benefits of the presence of the prefrontal cortex. Administration of "organic challenges" in this and other studies (e.g., Mogensen et al., 2004) indicated that in the absence of both the hippocampus and the prefrontal cortex, the parietal "association" cortex (e.g., Wörtwein et al., 1993) participates significantly in mediation of the recovery of this allocentric place-learning task.

Neural and Cognitive Mechanisms of Functional Rehabilitation After Brain Injury

An extensive animal model–based research program (e.g., Mogensen et al., 1995, 2002, 2003, 2004, 2005, 2007; Wörtwein et al., 1995) has addressed the neural and cognitive mechanisms of post-traumatic cognitive recovery after various types of brain injury. The studies have utilized a spectrum of behavioral/cognitive tasks reflecting a variety of cognitive dimensions as well as a spectrum of types of brain injury. The present chapter cannot be a forum for a more detailed description of the outcome of individual studies, but in general the results can be summarized as pointing to three principles describing the situation after the completion of a post-traumatic recovery/rehabilitative process of cognitive functions. These three principles of the neurocognitive mechanisms of cognitive recovery are:

A. Modification of the degree of contribution to task mediation by individual brain structures

Mapping the neural substrate of task performance after a successful cognitive recovery, one finds that the pattern of structures participating in task mediation—as well as the degree of participation of individual structures—is different in recovered, brain-injured individuals and normal individuals performing the same task, respectively. Individual structures exhibit an increased or decreased level of contribution to task mediation—and in some instances an unchanged level (decreased levels of task mediation are not restricted to the injured structure or structures).

B. Task-dependent and dissimilar neural substrates

After a given lesion (defined in terms of the structure being lesioned as well as the degree to which that structure has been injured), the functional recovery of various cognitive tasks is mediated by unique and dissimilar neural substrates. In other words, a question such as "which structure mediates cognitive recovery after hippocampal injury?" cannot be answered in a universal manner. Various cognitive tasks (in spite of all of these tasks being impaired by hippocampal injury) are, after a successful recovery process, mediated by different neural substrates.

C. Application of new cognitive strategies

The fully recovered individuals solve a given task by applying cognitive/behavioral strategies that are dissimilar to those applied pretraumatically. Furthermore, dissimilar cognitive/behavioral strategies are found in individuals subjected to and recovered after dissimilar types of brain injury (defined in terms of localization and extent of lesion).

These three principles have implications regarding whether or not the rehabilitative processes establish something "similar" to what has been lost or something that is of a more "compensational" nature. Principle A, if taken alone, cannot testify to such a differentiation. This principle (A) is a statement that the recovery process establishes a novel substrate of task mediation within preserved parts of the brain. In itself, such a statement is rather trivial—although it does contradict the possibility that recovery is exclusively mediated by mechanisms within the perilesional part of the brain. If, however, principle A is combined with principle B, a theoretically more telling pattern emerges. Not only does the recovery process establish a novel pattern of structures participating in task mediation, that pattern is dissimilar when compared across tasks. After the loss of a given structure (e.g., the hippocampus), the recovery process does not universally upgrade the participation of one specific part of the brain. Instead, the rehabilitative process forms a spectrum of different structural patterns, each mediating the recovery of a particular task after the same initial injury. If the cognitive recovery after a given type of brain injury led to the recruitment or creation of a "copy" of the structure that was lost to injury, that "backup" part of the brain would act as a universal substitute of the lost structure. In the case of the hippocampus, there could theoretically be a "redundant" "backup hippocampus" available within, for instance, the prefrontal cortex. Or plastic processes may create such a "copy-of-hippocampus" within, for instance, the prefrontal cortex. But in either case one would expect that "substitute hippocampus" to step in whenever the lost hippocampus would have been required to play its role. In other words, if such processes were prominent, the neural substrate of functional recovery after hippocampal injury (or injury to any other brain structure) would universially engage that "backup" region of the brain whenever the individual faces a task normally dependent on the lost structure. Combining principles A and B, one is led to the conclusion that the neural processes mediating cognitive recovery after focal brain injury represent compensational mechanisms rather than the re-creation of networks similar to those lost to injury. Turning to principle C, the indication once again is that the processes in question are of compensational rather than re-creational nature. Although the task solution within a given domain may at the end of the recovery process be at the same proficiency as that of normal individuals, the underlying cognitive strategies appear to be dissimilar from the normal situation.

Jointly, the research summarized within principles A, B, and C uniformly points to compensational neurocognitive processes rather than to the re-establishment of the pre-traumatic neural networks and cognitive mechanisms.

But what are the reorganizational processes that seem to be of a "compensational" nature and still are able to achieve a potentially "full recovery" (defined as the achievement of a fully normal level of task proficiency)? The framework that has been proposed to account for these and other findings regarding such mechanisms (e.g., Mogensen, 2011a, 2011c, 2012a, 2012b; Mogensen & Malá, 2009) not only suggests organizational principles and mechanisms for functional recovery, it also suggests a partial reconceptualization of the spectrum ranging from compensation to re-creational recovery.

The REF Model

This framework—known as the REF model (the reorganization of elementary functions model)—was originally developed as an attempt to reconcile two apparently contradictive principles of cognitive neuroscience: (1) the "functional localization" of cognitive functions (the well-established fact that various cognitive functions appear to be associated with specific brain structures); and (2) the "functional recovery" seen after focal brain injury (e.g., Mogensen, 2011c; Mogensen & Malá, 2009).

The REF model resolves the apparent contradiction between localization and recovery of functions partly by re-conceptualizing what is considered to be a cognitive "function" and by analyzing the functional processes within a three-level structure (e.g., Mogensen, 2011a, 2011c, 2012a, 2012b; Mogensen & Malá, 2009) (see Figure 1.1, panel A). The three levels of the REF model resemble, but are not identical, to the levels proposed by Marr (e.g., 1982).

The level at which the psychologically defined functions, such as "expressive language," "allocentric spatial orientation," "episodic memory," and the like, are encountered is the "upper" level of surface phenomena. The surface phenomena include the solution of specific tasks and performance on psychological tests, as well as the "inner phenomena" of mental states, such as conscious awareness. It is at the level of surface phenomena that we diagnose the loss or impairment of various cognitive functions. At the level of surface phenomena, formalized tests or clinical observations evaluate what has been affected by a pathological process and to what extent this has happened.

It is also at the level of surface phenomena that we evaluate the degree of "recovery," defined as return to a pretraumatic level of cognitive proficiency. If the patient suffering expressive aphasia is again able to score at a normal level in a naming test, express herself or himself verbally, and function at a level of verbal proficiency similar to that of uninjured

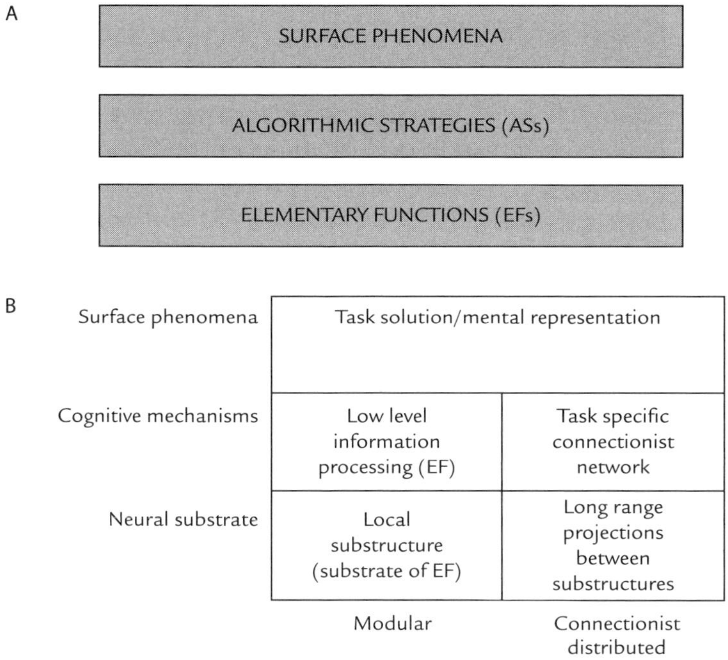

A

SURFACE PHENOMENA

ALGORITHMIC STRATEGIES (ASs)

ELEMENTARY FUNCTIONS (EFs)

B

	Modular	Connectionist distributed
Surface phenomena	Task solution/mental representation	
Cognitive mechanisms	Low level information processing (EF)	Task specific connectionist network
Neural substrate	Local substructure (substrate of EF)	Long range projections between substructures

FIGURE 1.1 Panel A: The three levels of the REF model: surface phenomena, algorithmic strategies, and elementary functions. Panel B: Illustration of the subdivision of the cognitive mechanisms and neural substrate, respectively, into modular and connectionist distributed subdivisions (according to the REF model).

individuals, we would consider the patient to be "fully recovered." According to the REF model, the phenomenon of "functional recovery" (as traditionally defined) is to be found at the level of surface phenomena.

In contrast, the phenomenon of a "functional localization" is found at the lowermost of the three levels—the level of elementary functions (EFs). Each EF performs a "modular" type of information processing. The functional properties of individual EFs are presently poorly characterized. But there is a significant conceptual difference between the EFs and the traditionally defined cognitive ("psychological") functions. While the "functions" of the level of surface phenomena are best characterized in the language of cognitive psychology, EFs are best described in mathematical terms. To illustrate the level at which the information processing of an EF is expressed, one may turn to models of visual perception. In the visual perceptual model of Marr and Hildreth (1980), the "zero-crossing" algorithm proposed to explain visual edge-detection cannot be considered an EF. Rather, the individual calculation steps within that algorithm may be at the level of individual EFs. The EFs are truly localized—in the sense that each EF is mediated by a specific substructure of a brain region. The traditionally defined brain structures (e.g., the hippocampus, the prefrontal cortex, or a region of the neostriatum) contain the neural substrates of an immense number of EFs. And when a brain structure or substructure is lost to injury, all EFs mediated by that part of the brain are irreversibly lost. At the level of the EFs, functional localization is fully present, and recovery of function is absent.

The bridge between the level of EFs and the level of surface phenomena is the level of algorithmic strategies (ASs). An AS consists of numerous interacting EFs. The ASs are primarily established through experience and learning (although it cannot be ruled out that a minority may be genetically preprogrammed). An AS is the "cognitive mechanism" or "program" of a specific surface phenomenon (e.g., a specific task solution or mental representation). The neural substrate of an AS consists of the neural substrates of all its constituent EFs plus the interconnections between the neural substrates of these EFs. In most cases, the constituent EFs of an AS are found within a multitude of traditionally defined brain structures. While an EF is strictly localized to a specific subregion of a brain structure, most ASs are thus distributed across many regions of the brain. While the information processing of an AS is the mechanism mediating a specific surface phenomenon (e.g., a specific solution of a specific task), most surface phenomena (e.g., the solution of a particular type of task such as an allocentric place-learning task) can be realized via the activity of a multitude of ASs. Task solutions achieved via activation of various ASs may provide outcomes of equal proficiency. And unless special analytical techniques (e.g., some of the above-mentioned challenge methods) are employed, it is normally not possible at the level of surface phenomena to discriminate between behavioral or mental phenomena reflecting two related but different ASs. When injury destroys the neural substrate of one or more of the constituent EFs within an AS, that AS is lost, and post-traumatically the surface phenomenon relying on that AS is impaired.

Whenever an individual encounters a situation calling for a broadly defined problem-solving process, two possibilities exist. The situation may already be associated (through experience) with a specific task solution and thereby routine-based activation of an AS. Or the situation may be novel in the sense that it has not yet been associated with a specific AS activation. In the latter case, a selector/evaluator mechanism activates an existing AS, and the behavior/mental process (surface phenomenon) associated with that AS is brought to action. The outcome of that behavioral/mental process is then evaluated by the evaluator mechanism (relative to the desired outcome). If the outcome is appropriate, that AS will in the future be associated with that problem-solving situation. If not, the selector mechanism will activate another AS—and the surface phenomenon associated with that AS is brought to bear upon the situation.

Such a process may lead to a successful solution of the task. But, alternatively, it may be that no pre-existing AS is able to lead to a sucessful task solution. If so, what is required is the creation of a novel AS and thereby a novel surface phenomenon. The process through which ASs are modified or created de novo is the actual REF process—the reorganization of elementary functions into new interactions and "programs"/ASs.

Whenever the success or failure of a surface phenomenon (and thereby activation of an AS) takes place, one of the results is a "back-propagation" process through which the internal connectivity of activated as well as non-activated ASs is modified (modifications reflecting the success or failure). Through such back-propagation mechanisms, the cognitive "program" of an AS may be modified and novel ASs created. The interactions between

EFs within an AS may be modified, new EFs may be incorporated into an AS—or EFs within an AS may be removed from its network. These back-propagation mechanisms are the main mechanism of establishment and modification of ASs.

In a brain-injured individual, behavioral and mental activities constantly achieve such reorganizational changes in her or his repertoire of ASs. These activities include—but are not restricted to—formalized rehabilitative training. Also the "daily activities" (which may, at least immediately after a trauma-provoking event, be somewhat restricted and atypical of normality) contribute to the reorganizational processes—something that should be taken into account when evaluating so-called "spontaneous recovery" (e.g., León-Carrión & Machuca-Murga, 2001). Such a "spontaneous" recovery is defined as any cognitive normalization that takes place in the absence of formalized training and is mostly seen as the expression of "automatic" neural processes, which are independent of both the environment and the activities of the individual. The resolution of a "penumbra" after stroke (e.g., Choi et al., 2007) and similar changes may, indeed, be the mechanism of some types of spontaneous recovery. But there can be no doubt that reorganizational plastic processes guided by the more or less restricted life activities of the brain-injured patient also contribute significantly. Some may argue that such a differentiation is of only theoretical interest. It should, however, be remembered that the "life situation" of the brain-injured patient (for instance during hospitalization) contributes to reorganization processes. And it may do so in positive as well as negative ways. If the patient is not challenged and guided in adequate ways, the plastic processes may achieve the development of maladaptive strategies rather than promoting results conducive to future independent living.

If the activity-provoked reorganizational processes (at the neural level, modified connectivity in short- as well as long-range projections) achieve establishment of an AS which—when activated—mediates an adequate surface phenomenon, one will clinically evaluate the performance of the task in question to have "fully recovered." Such a formulation, however, begs the question: What is an adequate surface phenomenon? As mentioned earlier, a patient is normally deemed to be "fully recovered" if the surface phenomena of daily activities—and potentially the performance on cognitive tests—reveal no inferiority to the pretraumatic, "normal" level of proficiency. Therefore, an AS leading to a surface phenomenon of such proficiency is the mechanism of a "full" cognitive recovery.

Recovery and Compensation in the Context of the REF Model

Returning to the main question of this chapter—the differentiation between compensation and re-creational recovery—the mechanisms described by the REF model are (at least when viewed superficially) of a purely compensational nature. At the level of the EFs, the EFs lost to injury are not replaced. And whatever EFs are subsequently recruited are different from those lost due to the destruction of their neural substrate. At the level of the

ASs, the "cognitive strategies" potentially achieving a normal proficiency of task solution are different from those achieving similar results pretraumatically. And finally, at the level of surface phenomena, one may argue that although neither clinical observation nor the use of standard cognitive tests may be able to demonstrate any difference from the pretraumatic situation, this is an expression of methodological shortcomings rather than a case of full re-establishment of the pretraumatic task solution.

Additional implications of the REF model may, however, need to be taken into account when evaluating to what extent this "completely compensational" evaluation means that only something inferior to the normal situation is achieved.

The REF model has been developed in the context of post-traumatic cognitive recovery after brain injury, but it is a model of general neurocognitive organization and reorganization in the intact as well as injured brain (e.g., Mogensen, 2012b). Models of the functional organization of the brain are traditionally divided into, on the one hand, models emphasizing a "modular" organization of the brain (e.g., Barrett & Kurzban, 2006; Fodor, 2000; Pinker, 1999) and, on the other hand, models emphasizing organization in connectionist networks (e.g., McClelland et al., 1986; McLeod et al., 1998; Rumelhart & McClelland, 1986). The REF model represents a combination of or compromise between these two types of models. It can best be described as modularity within connectionist networks (e.g., Mogensen, 2012b).

Modular theories (e.g., Barrett & Kurzban, 2006; Fodor, 2000; Pinker, 1999) emphasize localized and specialized "modules" performing specific information processing. The REF model is modular in the sense that the EFs fit such a "modular" description. The more traditional modular theories, however, operate with modules at a much higher level and higher degree of association to specific cognitive domains. Traditionally, one would include, for instance, a "language module"—for example, in the form of "the language faculty" of Chomsky (e.g., Hauser et al., 2002). In contrast, the modules (EFs) of the REF model are specific for a much lower level type of information processing—while having no specific association to any cognitive domain. Most EFs are simultaneously (via different ASs) associated with participation in a multitude of task solutions and, for that matter, a multitude of traditionally defined cognitive domains.

Connectionist models (e.g., McClelland et al., 1986; McLeod et al., 1998; Rumelhart & McClelland, 1986) emphasize connectionist networks within which the "unit" is a functionally completely neutral "neuron." The connections within these networks are shaped by experience—via back-propagation mechanisms. Due to the connectionist nature of the ASs, the REF model partially falls within the domains of connectionist models. But since the "unit" of the connectionist networks of the ASs are the EFs—which in themselves mediate a rather advanced information processing—the REF model is in sharp contrast to the rather diffuse and "localization-indifferent" connectionist networks of traditional versions of such models.

One may describe the REF model as being "modular" and as dominated by functional localization at the lower level (of the EFs), while being connectionist and dominated by the potential of functional reorganization (and thereby post-traumatic functional recovery) at the intermediate level of the ASs (see Figure 1.1, panel B). And such a situation has implications for the understanding of the baseline from which concepts such as compensation and re-creational recovery are to be evaluated.

What we consider cognitive functions in the normal, intact individual are defined, as has been mentioned, at the level of surface phenomena. And while such surface phenomena may appear rather similar across individuals, they are the reflection of ASs. Such ASs are (at least partly) organized and potentially reorganized as a reflection of individual experiences. Methodological limitations, under most circumstances, may prevent an understanding of individual differences in how a given surface phenomenon is neurally and cognitively mediated. But at least in some instances we are beginning to see glimpses of the ways in which specific experiences result in neurocognitive differences among normal individuals. The Broca area within the left frontal lobe is in practically all individuals associated with the mediation of expressive language. In professional musicians, however, this brain region (in contrast to what is the case in musically naïve individuals) also participates in the mediation of mental rotation (Sluming et al., 2007).

If the neurocognitive organization is experience-dependent to such an extent, it may be surprising to find a reasonable degree of similarity regarding the neural substrates of task mediation across normal individuals. However, it must be remembered that many tasks and behavioral challenges are highly common to practically all human beings, and that, additionally, many of these tasks can most easily be solved by application of ASs including certain populations of EFs (at least under normal circumstances). Only when the individual is exposed to the challenges of being a professional musician, or in other ways is subjected to special "training" circumstances, will such circumstances push the ASs and thereby the neurocognitive processes in more unusual directions.

But in spite of such similarities between most "normal" individuals, it has to be remembered that a given surface phenomenon (and thereby traditionally defined "function") does not necessarily have either the same neural substrate or identical cognitive mechanisms as its mediating processes across individuals. And such a fact argues against at least some of the implications of the concept of "compensation." As discussed above, the REF model points in the direction of practically all trauma-associated recovery processes being of a "compensational" rather than re-creational nature. But is the "compensational" aspect of such a neurocognitive reorganization to be seen as "compensational" in its more traditional sense? Compensation is often interpreted as something inferior taking the place of the normal and optimal mechanism. Many of the described reorganizational processes may, indeed, create a useful but still inferior level of task solution in a brain-injured individual. But the mere fact that something is the result of a neurocognitive reorganization does not in itself speak to the direction in which this moves the quality of cognition. We do, for instance—perhaps optimistically—assume that the neurocognitive reorganizational processes that we provoke in our university students result in reorganized but not inferior ASs.

Many of the conceptual and methodological challenges facing our understanding of the dynamic brain processes provoked by pathological processes within the brain will only be resolved in the future. We are just beginning to scratch the surface of issues that, without doubt, will prove to be much more complicated than what we presently imagine them to be. Technology and improved research methods will eliminate many of the methodological shortcomings we are presently suffering. And conceptually we need to remain open to novel ways of understanding both the outcome of our experiments and the brain in general. Even the relatively new REF model is presently undergoing a substantial expansion in the form of the REFCON (reorganization of elementary functions and consciousness) model, which addresses not only problem-solving but also perceptual analysis and conscious awareness (e.g., Mogensen & Overgaard, submitted; Overgaard & Mogensen, 2014). Without constant reorganization, the brains of neuroscientists will not be able to grasp their own complexity.

Acknowledgment

The present study was supported by a grant from the Danish Council for Independent Research.

References

Ansaldo, A. I., & Arguin, M. (2003). The recovery from aphasia depends on both the left and right hemispheres: Three longitudinal case studies on the dynamics of language function after aphasia. *Brain Lang, 87,* 177–178.

Ansaldo, A. I., Arguin, M., & Lecours, A. R. (2002). The contribution of the right cerebral hemisphere to the recovery from aphasia: A single longitudinal case study. *Brain Lang, 82,* 206–222.

Arvidsson, A., Collin, T., Kirik, D., Kokaia, Z., & Lindvall, O. (2002). Neuronal replacement from endogenous precursors in the adult brain after stroke. *Nature Med, 8,* 963–970.

Azouvi, P., Samuel, C., Louis-Dreyfus, A., Bernati, T., Bartolomeo, P., Beis, J-M., Chokron, S., Leclercq, M., Marchal, F., Martin, Y., de Montety, G., Olivier, S., Perennou, D., Pradat-Diehl, P., Prairial, C., Rode, G., Siéroff, E., Wiart, L., & Rousseaux, M. (2002). Sensitivity of clinical and behavioural tests of spatial neglect after right hemisphere stroke. *J Neurol Neurosur Ps, 73,* 160–166.

Bach-y-Rita, P., Collins, C.C., Saunders, F. A., White, B., & Scadden, L. (1969). Vision substitution by tactile image projection. *Nature, 221,* 963–964.

Bach-y-Rita, P., Kaczmarek, K. A., Tyler, M. E., & Garcia-Lara, J. (1998). Form perception with a 49-point electrotactile stimulus array on the tongue: A technical note. *J Rehabil Res Dev, 35,* 1–7.

Barrett, H. C., & Kurzban, R. (2006). Modularity in cognition: Framing the debate. *Psychol Rev, 113,* 628–647.

Baumgaertner, A., Schraknepper, V. & Saur, D. (2005). Differential recovery of aphasia and apraxia of speech in an adolescent after infarction of the left frontal lobe: Longitudinal behavioral and fMRI data. *Brain Lang, 95,* 211–212.

Berardi, N., Pizzorusso, T., & Maffei, L. (2004). Extracellular matrix and visual cortical plasticity: Freeing the synapse. *Neuron, 44,* 905–908.

Berry, M. (1982). Post-injury myelin-breakdown products inhibit axonal growth: An hypothesis to explain the failure of axonal regeneration in the mammalian central nervous system. *Bibl Anat, 23,* 1–11.

Brockes, J. P., & Kumar, A. (2005). Appendage regeneration in adult vertebrates and implications for regenerative medicine. *Science, 310,* 1919–1923.

Carandini, M. (2012). From circuits to behavior: A bridge too far? *Nat Neurosci, 15*, 507–509.

Chen, D. F., Jhaveri, S., & Schneider, G. E. (1995). Intrinsic changes in developing retinal neurons result in regenerative failure of their axons. *P Natl Acad Sci USA, 92*, 7287–7291.

Chen, J., Magavi, S. S., & Macklis, J. D. (2004). Neurogenesis of corticospinal motor neurons extending spinal projections in adult mice. *P Natl Acad Sci USA, 101*, 16357–16362.

Choi, J. Y., Lee, K. H., Na, D. L., Byun, H. S., Lee, S. J., Kim, H., Kwon, M., Lee, K-H., & Kim, B-T. (2007). Subcortical aphasia after striatocapsular infarction: Quantitative analysis of brain perfusion SPECT using statistical parametric mapping and a statistical probabilistic anatomic map. *J Nucl Med, 48*, 194–200.

Crosson, B., Moore, A. B., McGregor, K. M., Chang, Y-L., Benjamin, M., Gopinath, K., Sherod, M. E., Wierenga, C. E., Peck, K. K., Briggs, R. W., Rothi, L. J. G., & White, K. D. (2009). Regional changes in word-production laterality after a naming treatment designed to produce a rightward shift in frontal activity. *Brain Lang, 111*, 73–85.

Dallison, A., & Kolb, B. (2003). Recovery from infant medial frontal cortical lesions in rats is reversed by cortical lesions in adulthood. *Behav Brain Res, 146*, 57–63.

Del Rio, J. A., & Soriano, E. (2007). Overcoming chondroitin sulphate proteoglycan inhibition of axon growth in the injured brain: Lessons from chondroitinase ABC. *Curr Pharm Des, 13*, 2485–2492.

Elbert, T., Pantev, C., Weinbruch, C., Rockstroh, B., & Taub, E. (1995). Increased cortical representation of the fingers of the left hand in string players. *Science, 270*, 305–307.

Fawcett, J. W., Housden, E., Smith-Thomas, L., & Meyer, R. L. (1989). The growth of axons in three-dimensional astrocyte cultures. *Dev Biol, 135*, 449–458.

Fodor, J. (2000). *The mind doesn't work that way: The scope and limits of computational psychology.* Cambridge, MA: MIT Press.

Goldberg, J. L., Klassen, M. P., Hua, Y., & Barres, B. A. (2002). Amacrine-signaled loss of intrinsic axon growth ability by retinal ganglion cells. *Science, 296*, 1860–1864.

Harel, N. Y., & Strittmatter, S. M. (2006). Can regenerating axons recapitulate developmental guidance during recovery from spinal cord injury? *Nature Rev Neurosci, 7*, 603–616.

Hauser, M. D., Chomsky, N., & Fitch, W. C. (2002). The language faculty: What is it, who has it, and how did it evolve? *Science, 298*, 1569–1579.

Hicks, A. U., Hewlett, K., Windle, V., Chernenko, G., Ploughman, M., Jolkkonen, J., Weiss, S., & Corbett, D. (2007). Enriched environment enhances transplanted subventricular zone stem cell migration and functional recovery after stroke. *Neuroscience, 146*, 31–40.

Irvine, D. R. F. (2007). Auditory cortical plasticity: Does it provide evidence for cognitive processing in the auditory cortex? *Hearing Res, 229*, 158–170.

Jeewajee, A., Barry, C., O'Keefe, J., & Burgess, N. (2008). Grid cells and theta as oscillatory interference: Electrophysiological data from freely moving rats. *Hippocampus, 18*, 1175–1185.

Kaczmarek, K. A., Webster, J. G., Bach-y-Rita, P., & Tompkins, W. J. (1991). Electrotactile and vibrotactile displays for sensory substitutionsystems. *Biomed Eng, 38*, 1–16.

Karl, A., Birbaumer, N., Lutzenberger, W., Cohen, L. G., & Flor, H. (2001). Reorganization of motor and somatosensory cortex in upper extremity amputees with phantom limb pain. *J Neurosci, 15*, 3609–3618.

Koeberle, P. D., & Bahr, M. (2004). Growth and guidance cues for regenerating axons: Where have they gone? *J Neurobiol, 59*, 162–180.

Leavitt, B. R., Hernit-Grant, C. S., & Macklis, J. D. (1999). Mature astrocytes transform into transitional radial glia within adult mouse neocortex that supports directed migration of transplanted immature neurons. *Exp Neurol, 157*, 43–57.

León-Carrión, J., & Machuca-Murga, F. (2001). Spontaneous recovery of cognitive functions after severe brain injury: When are neurocognitive sequelae established? *Rev Esp Neur, 3*, 58–67.

Lepore, F., Ptito, M., Provencal, C., Bedard, S., & Guillemot, J-P. (1985). Interhemispheric transfer of visual training in the split-brain cat: Effects of the experimental set-up. *Can J Psychol, 39*, 527–528.

Levin, M. F., Kleim, J. A., & Wolf, S. L. (2009). What do motor "recovery" and "compensation" mean in patients following stroke? *Neurorehab Neural Re, 23*, 313–319.

Lin, R., Kwok, J. C. F., Crespo, D., & Fawcett, J. W. (2008). Chondroitinase ABC has a long-lasting effect on chondroitin sulphate glycosaminoglycan content in the injured rat brain. *J Neurochem, 104*, 400–408.

Magavi, S. S., Leavitt, B. R., & Macklis, J. D. (2000). Induction of neurogenesis in the neocortex of adult mice. *Nature, 405*, 951–955.

Malá, H., Castro, M. R., Jørgensen, K. D., & Mogensen, J. (2007). Effects of erythropoietin on posttraumatic place learning in fimbria-fornix transected rats after a 30-day postoperative pause. *J Neurotraum, 24*, 1647–1657.

Malá, H., Castro, M. R., Pearce, H., Kingod, S. C., Nedergaard, S. K., Scharff, Z., Zandersen, M., & Mogensen, J. (2012). Delayed intensive acquisition training alleviates the lesion-induced place learning deficits after fimbria-fornix transection in the rat. *Brain Res, 1445*, 40–51.

Marr, D. (1982). *Vision: A computational investigation into the human representation and processing of visual information*. San Francisco, CA: W. H. Freeman.

Marr, D., & Hildreth, E. (1980). Theory of edge detection. *P Roy Soc London B, 207*, 187–217.

McClelland, J. L., Rumelhart, D. E., & The PDP Research Group (1986). *Parallel distributed processing: Vol. 2, Psychological and biological models*. Cambridge, MA: MIT Press.

McGee, A. W., Yang, Y., Fischer, Q. S., Daw, N. W., & Strittmatter, S. M. (2005). Experience-driven plasticity of visual cortex limited by myelin and Nogo receptor. *Science, 309*, 2222–2226.

McLeod, P., Plunkett, K., & Rolls, E.T. (1998). *Introduction to connectionist modelling of cognitive processes*. Oxford: Oxford University Press.

Meinzer, M., Obleser, J., Flaisch, T., Eulitz, C., & Rockstroh, B. (2007). Recovery from aphasia as a function of language therapy in an early bilingual patient demonstrated by fMRI. *Neuropsychologia, 45*, 1247–1256.

Meinzer, M., Flaisch, T., Breitenstein, C., Wienbruch, C., Elbert, T., & Rockstroh, B. (2008). Functional re-recruitment of dysfunctional brain areas predicts language recovery in chronic aphasia. *NeuroImage, 39*, 2038–2046.

Merzenich, M. M., & Jenkins, W. M. (1993). Reorganization of cortical representations of the hand following alterations of skin inputs induced by nerve injury, skin island transfers, and experience. *J Hand Ther, 6*, 89–104.

Milner, A. D., Perrett, D. I., Johnston, R. S., Benson, P. J., Jordan, T. R., Heeley, D. W., Bettucci, D., Mortara, F., Mutani, R., Terazzi, E., & Davidson, D. L. W. (1991). Perception and action in "visual form agnosia." *Brain, 114*, 405–428.

Ming, G-L., & Song, H. (2005). Adult neurogenesis in the mammalian central nervous system. *Ann Rev Neurosci, 28*, 223–250.

Mogensen, J. (2011a). Almost unlimited potentials of a limited neural plasticity: Levels of plasticity in development and reorganization of the injured brain. *J Consciousness Stud, 18*, 13–45.

Mogensen, J. (2011b). Animal models in neuroscience. In J. Hau & S. J. Schapiro (Eds.), *Handbook of laboratory animal science*, 3rd ed., Vol. II, *Animal models* (pp. 47–73). Boca Raton, FL: CRC Press LLC.

Mogensen, J. (2011c). Reorganization in the injured brain: Implications for studies of the neural substrate of cognition. *Front Psychol, 2*(7), 1–10.

Mogensen, J. (2012a). Cognitive recovery and rehabilitation after brain injury: Mechanisms, challenges and support. In A. Agrawal (Ed.), *Brain injury: Functional aspects, rehabilitation and prevention* (pp. 121–150). Rijeka, Croatia: InTech.

Mogensen, J. (2012b). Reorganization of elementary functions (REF) after brain injury: Implications for the therapeutic interventions and prognosis of brain injured patients suffering cognitive impairments. In A. J. Schäfer & J. Müller (Eds.), *Brain damage: Causes, management and prognosis* (pp. 1–40). Hauppauge, NY: Nova Science Publishers.

Mogensen, J., & Malá, H. (2009). Post-traumatic functional recovery and reorganization in animal models: A theoretical and methodological challenge. *Scand J Psychol, 50*, 561–573.

Mogensen, J., Iversen, I. H., & Divac, I. (1987). Neostriatal lesions impaired rats' delayed alternation performance in a T maze but not in a two-key operant chamber. *Acta Neurobiol Exp, 47*, 45–54.

Mogensen, J., Pedersen, T. K., Holm, S., & Bang, L. E. (1995). Prefrontal cortical mediation of rats' place learning in a modified water maze. *Brain Res Bull, 38*, 425–434.

Mogensen, J., Christensen, L. H., Johansson, A., Wörtwein, G., Bang, L. E., & Holm, S. (2002). Place learning in scopolamine treated rats: The roles of distal cues and catecholaminergic mediation. *Neurobiol Learn Mem, 78*, 139–166.

Mogensen, J., Wörtwein, G., Plenge, P., & Mellerup, E. T. (2003). Serotonin, locomotion, exploration, and place recall in the rat. *Pharmacol Biochem Be, 75*, 381–395.

Mogensen, J., Lauritsen, K. T., Elvertorp, S., Hasman, A., Moustgaard, A., & Wörtwein, G. (2004). Place learning and object recognition by rats subjected to transection of the fimbria-fornix and/or ablation of the prefrontal cortex. *Brain Res Bull, 63*, 217–236.

Mogensen, J., Moustgaard, A., Khan, U., Wörtwein, G., & Nielsen, K. S. (2005). Egocentric spatial orientation in a water maze by rats subjected to transection of the fimbria-fornix and/or ablation of the prefrontal cortex. *Brain Res Bull, 65,* 41–58.

Mogensen, J., Hjortkjær, J., Ibervang, K. L., Stedal, K., & Malá, H. (2007). Prefrontal cortex and hippocampus in posttraumatic functional recovery: Spatial delayed alternation by rats subjected to transection of the fimbria-fornix and/or ablation of the prefrontal cortex. *Brain Res Bull, 73,* 86–95.

Moser, E. I., Moser, M-B., & Roudi, Y. (2014). Network mechanisms of grid cells. *Philos T Roy Soc B, 369,* 20120511.

Münte, T. F., Altenmüller, E., & Jäncke, L. (2002). The musician's brain as a model of neuroplasticity. *Nat Rev Neurosci, 3,* 473–478.

Nakatomi, H., Kuriu, T., Okabe, S., Yamamoto, S-C., Hatano, O., Kawahara, N., Tamura, A., Kirino, T., & Nakafuku, M. (2002). Regeneration of hipppocampal pyramidal neurons after ischemic brain injury by recruitment of endogenous neural progenitors. *Cell, 110,* 429–441.

Overgaard, M. (2006). Introspection in science. *Conscious Cogn, 15,* 629–633.

Overgaard, M., & Mogensen, J. (2011). A framework for the study of multiple realizations: The importance of levels of analysis. *Front Psychol, 2:79,* 1–10.

Overgaard, M., & Mogensen, J. (2014). Visual perception from the perspective of a representational, non-reductionistic, level-dependent account of perception and conscious awareness. *Philos T Roy Soc London B, 369,* 20130209.

Overgaard, M., & Timmermans, B. (2010). How unconscious is subliminal perception? In D. Schmicking & S. Gallagher (Eds.), *Handbook of phenomenology and cognitive science* (pp. 501–519). Heidelberg: Springer Verlag.

Perani, D., Cappa, S. F., Tettamanti, M., Rosa, M., Scifo, P., Miozzo, A., Basso, A., & Fazio, F. (2003). A fMRI study of word retrieval in aphasia. *Brain Lang, 85,* 357–368.

Pinker, S. (1999). *How the mind works.* London: Penguin Books.

Pizzorusso, T., Medini, P., Berardi, N., Chierzi, S., Fawcett, J. W., & Maffei, L. (2002). Reactivation of ocular dominance plasticity in the adult visual cortex. *Science, 298,* 1248–1251.

Poucet, B., Sargolini, F., Song, E. Y., Hangya, B., Fox, S., & Muller, R. U. (2014). Independence of landmark and self-motion-guided navigation: A different role for grid cells. *Philos T Roy Soc B, 369,* 20130370.

Ptito, M., Moesgaard, S. M., Gjedde, A., & Kupers, R. (2005). Cross-modal plasticity revealed by electrotactile stimulation of the tongue in the congenitally blind. *Brain, 128,* 606–614.

Recanzone, G. H., Schreiner, C. E., & Merzenich, M. M. (1993). Plasticity in the frequency representation of primary auditory cortex following discrimination training in adult owl monkeys. *J Neurosci, 13,* 87–103.

Robertson, D., & Irvine, D. R. F. (1989). Plasticity of frequency organization in auditory cortex of guinea pigs with partial unilateral deafness. *J Comp Neurol, 282,* 456–471.

Robertson, I. H., & Murre, J. M. J. (1999). Rehabilitation of brain damage: Brain plasticity and principles of guided recovery. *Psychol Bull, 125,* 544–575.

Rumelhart, D., & McClelland, J. (1986). *Parallel distributed processing.* Cambridge, MA: MIT Press.

Schäfer, R., Dehn, D., Burbach, G. J., & Deller, T. (2008). Differential regulation of chondroitin sulfate proteoglycan mRNAs in the denervated rat fascia dentata after unilateral entorhinal cortex lesion. *Neurosci Lett, 439,* 61–69.

Scharff, C., Kirn, J. R., Grossman, M., Macklis, J. D., & Nottebohm, G. (2000). Targeted neuronal death affects neuronal replacement and vocal behavior in adult songbirds. *Neuron, 25,* 481–492.

Scheich, H. (1991). Auditory cortex: Comparative aspects of maps and plasticity. *Curr Opin Neurobiol, 1,* 236–247.

Schenk, T. (2006). An allocentric rather than perceptual deficit in patient D.F. *Nature Neurosci, 9,* 1369–1370.

Schwab, M. E., & Thoenen, H. (1985). Dissociated neurons regenerate into sciatic but not optic nerve explants in culture irrespective of neurotrophic factors. *J Neurosci, 5,* 2415–2423.

Sluming, V., Brooks, J., Howard, M., Downes, J. J., & Roberts, N. (2007). Broca's area supports enhanced visuospatial cognition in orchestral musicians. *J Neurosci, 27,* 3799–3806.

Specht, K., Zahn, R., Willmes, K., Weis, S., Holtel, C., Krause, B. J., Herzog, H., & Huber, W. (2009). Joint independent component analysis of structural and functional images reveals complex patterns of functional reorganisation in stroke aphasia. *NeuroImage, 47,* 2057–2063.

Suh, H., Deng, W., & Gage, F. H. (2009). Signaling in adult neurogenesis. *Annu Rev Cell Dev Biol, 25,* 253–275.

Szaflarski, J. P., Eaton, K., Ball, A. L., Banks, C., Vannest, J., Allendorfer, J. B., Page, S., & Holland, S. K. (2011). Poststroke aphasia recovery assessed with functional magnetic resonance imaging and a picture identification task. *J Stroke Cerebrovasc Dis, 20*, 336–345.

Thai-Van, H., Micheyl, C., Norena, A., Veuillet, E., Gabriel, D., & Collet, L. (2007). Enhanced frequency discrimination in hearing-impaired individuals: A review of perceptual correlates of central neural plasticity induced by cochlear damage. *Hearing Res, 233*, 14–22.

Thomas, C., Altenmüller, E., Marckmann, G., Kahrs, J., & Dichgans, J. (1997). Language processing in aphasia: changes in lateralization patterns during recovery reflect cerebral plasticity in adults. *Electroen Clin Neuro, 102*, 86–97.

Thompson, C. K., den Ouden, D-B., Bonakdarpour, B., Garibaldi, K., & Parrish, T. B. (2010). Neural plasticity and treatment-induced recovery of sentence processing in agrammatism. *Neuropsychologia, 48*, 3211–3227.

Thulborn, K. R., Carpenter, P. A., & Just, M. A. (1999). Plasticity of language-related brain function during recovery from stroke. *Stroke, 30*, 749–754.

Ungerleider, L. G., Courtney, S. M., & Haxby, J. V. (1998). A neural system for human visual working memory. *P Natl Acad Sci USA, 95*, 883–890.

Weiss, T., Miltner, W. H. R., Huonker, R., Friedel, R., Schmidt, I., & Taub, E. (2000). Rapid functional plasticity of the somatosensory cortex after finger amputation. *Exp Brain Res, 134*, 199–203.

Wilms, I., & Mogensen, J. (2011). Dissimilar outcomes of apparently similar procedures as a challenge to clinical neurorehabilitation and basic research: When the same is not the same. *NeuroRehabilitation, 29*, 221–227.

Wilson, B. A. (2000). Compensating for cognitive deficits following brain injury. *Neuropsychol Rev, 10*, 233–243.

Wörtwein, G., Mogensen, J., & Divac, I. (1993). Retention and relearning of spatial delayed alternation in rats after combined or sequential lesions of the prefrontal and parietal cortex. *Acta Neurobiol Exp, 53*, 357–366.

Wörtwein, G., Saerup, L. H., Charlottenfeld-Starpov, D., & Mogensen, J. (1995). Place learning by fimbria-fornix transected rats in a modified water maze. *Int J Neurosci, 82*, 71–81.

Xerri, C., Coq, J., Merzenich, M., & Jenkins, W. (1996). Experience-induced plasticity of cutaneous maps in the primary somatosensory cortex of adult monkeys and rats. *J Physiol, 90*, 277–287.

Yang, T. T., Gallen, C. C., Ramachandran, V. S., Cobb, S., Schwartz, B. J., & Bloom, F. E. (1994). Noninvasive detection of cerebral plasticity in adult human somatosensory cortex. *Neuroreport, 5*, 701–704.

Yoon, K., Buice, M. A., Barry, C., Hayman, R., Burgess, N., & Fiete, I. R. (2013). Specifric evidence of low-dimensional continuous attractor dynamics in grid cells. *Nature Neurosci, 16*, 1077–1087.

2

Seizure-Induced Neuroplasticity and Cognitive Network Reorganization in Epilepsy

Joseph I. Tracy, Dorian Pustina, Gaelle Doucet, and Karol Osipowicz

Introduction

In this chapter we will argue that epilepsy is a network disorder in which the brain's representations of cognitive functions, and their related circuitry, are prone to reorganize. While seizures are the final common pathway of a whole host of pathophysiologic processes (viral, fungal, parasitic, metabolic, toxic, congenital, traumatic) and form a variety of epilepsy subtypes, we will focus on temporal lobe epilepsy (TLE), and will present evidence to suggest that even focal lesional TLE (e.g., identified as a focal pathology through techniques such as magnetic resonance imaging [MRI]), disrupts a wide array of neurocognitive networks. We will demonstrate how seizure networks by their very nature are disposed to plasticity, altering cognitive networks over the course of the disease, with a particular eye on the cognitive network alterations that occur after key clinical interventions, most notably, anterior temporal lobectomy (ATL). We will describe the growing literature on functional connectivity (FC), defined as a neurophysiologic index reflecting the observed temporal correlation between separate brain regions (Friston, Frith, Liddle, & Frackowiak, 1993), and its role in clarifying the effects of seizure propagation on neuronal communication and networks. We argue that only by understanding and measuring the potential for neuroplasticity will we be able to effectively predict cognitive outcomes in epilepsy, as it is these neuroplastic responses that govern the status of both neurocognitive and epileptogenic networks postsurgery. Finally, multimodal imaging will be discussed as a potentially effective means of understanding the mechanisms that might be at work to implement neuroplasticity after procedures such as resective surgery.

Neuroplastic Processes Inherent to Seizures and the Development of Epileptiform Networks

The brain is not fixed in its representation of cognitive skill. Indeed, brain plasticity occurs with normal learning (May, 2011; Tracy et al., 2003), in response to chronic disease (Haut, Lim, & MacDonald, 2010; Lefaucheur, 2009), acute injury (Demirtas-Tatlidede, Vahabzadeh-Hagh, Bernabeu, Tormos, & Pascual-Leone, 2011; Meinzer, Harnish, Conway, & Crosson, 2011; Xiong, Mahmood, & Chopp, 2010), and resective brain surgery (McCormick, Quraan, Cohn, Valiante, & McAndrews, 2013). The neuroplastic ramifications of epileptic activity in the brain include (1) intracellular changes (i.e., expression of cellular proteins, alterations of neurotransmitters such as gamma-amino butyric acid [GABA], calcium channels, or signaling molecules); (2) injury to cortical pyramidal neurons, making membrane ion channels more amenable to excitatory input; (3) mossy fiber and axonal sprouting within pyramidal cells that enhances excitatory connections; (4) hyper-innervation; (5) failure to prune immature connections when occurring early in life; and (6) changes in glial cells and in the organization of axons and dendrites to favor hypersynchrony (Ben-Ari, Crepel, & Represa, 2008; Jacobs, Graber, Kharazia, Parada, & Prince, 2000; Somera-Molina et al., 2007; Sutula & Dudek, 2007).[1] All constitute mechanisms of neuroplasticity at different levels of organization, working in a single or combined way to restructure surviving synapses, leading to the reorganization of surviving neuronal networks.

These modifications dispose cells in remote sites to seize (i.e., display abnormal spiking patterns) following initial activity in the original epileptic focus, intensifying epileptic dynamics by forcing the abnormal integration of new cells into the epileptogenic network (Schneider-Mizell et al., 2010). Eventually the remote cells, after joining the hypersynchronous activity of the ictal focus, may come to initiate seizures independently (e.g., mirror focus; Morrell & deToledo-Morrell, 1999), forcing both functional and structural connectivity changes. The ictal focus of a seizure can be seen as initiating a neural circuit—a circuit that, if instantiated repeatedly by ongoing seizures, leads to frequent aberrant neural "communication" with other regions of the brain. Cells downstream from the seizure generator will respond to the excitation of seizures as if learning occurred.[2] Thus, epileptogenesis can be seen as involving a process similar to long-term potentiation (LTP) (Shimizu et al., 2000; Tracy et al., 2009), with these aberrant networks active not just during ictal stimulation, but also during cognitive stimulation of one or more network nodes, ultimately disrupting the underlying cognition. Eventually, through a process that

1. Such neuroplastic changes are best established within the hippocampus, but have been observed in neocortex as well; see review by Schwartzkroin (2001).
2. The main neurotransmitters involved in seizures such as GABA and NMDA are crucial to the capacity to learning. NMDA receptor density is high in regions prone to seizures such as hippocampal CA1 and CA2 fields. To some degree, NMDA receptor density predicts both the probability of Hebbian learning and epileptogenicity (McClelland, 2001). The factors that upregulate plasticity for learning also set the stage for seizures.

reduces action potential thresholds similar to neural kindling (Goddard, 1967; Wada & Mizoguchi, 1984), these epileptogenic pathways create a biased, favored network that is both maladaptive to cognition, and pathologic to otherwise healthy neural tissue, as it now has to bear the burden of periodic epileptiform activity. In this way, seizures produce a dysfunctional, maladaptive cognitive network by linking brain areas randomly through seizure propagations and secondary epileptogenesis, rather than through normal adaptive learning and experience-driven plasticity and connectivity. Accordingly, the development of normal neural networks, through the LTP or long-term depression associated with normal learning, appears to bear a striking resemblance to epileptogenesis. Figure 2.1 depicts a pathway for the development of seizure networks, maladaptive to cognition but triggering reorganization, carried through to intervention by ATL.

The Development of Cognitive Deficits Outside the Epileptogenic Zone

While it is readily known that generalized tonic-clonic (Wang et al., 2011) and absence seizures (Luo et al., 2011) can cause widespread disruptions of neural connectivity patterns and can lead to diffuse cognitive dysfunction, well beyond the regions considered most likely to be the ictal generator (i.e., the thalamus), there is also evidence that such remote effects emerge from focal epilepsies such as temporal lobe epilepsy (Liao et al., 2010; Waites, Briellmann, Saling, Abbott, & Jackson, 2006), with both ictal and interictal activity playing a role (Fahoum, Lopes, Pittau, Dubeau, & Gotman, 2012). Several studies have documented that cognitive dysfunction in mesial TLE can extend to other cognitive domains, including language and executive functions, that are not ordinarily considered to be affected by strictly mesial temporal lobe pathology (Corcoran & Thompson, 1993; Grant, Henry, Fernandez, Hill, & Sathian, 2005; B. P. Hermann, Wyler, & Richey,

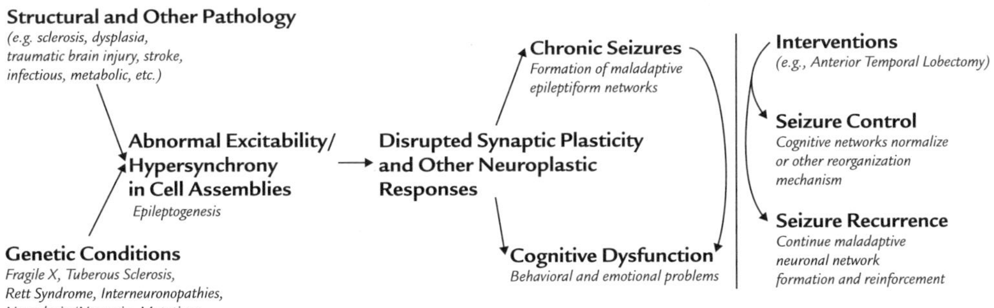

FIGURE 2.1 Pathway depicting the development of seizure networks, maladaptive to cognition but triggering reorganization, carried through to intervention by ATL. More specifically, pathology or genetically driven abnormal excitability induces neuronal neuroplastic responses, causing cognitive network dysfunction both directly and indirectly through the formation of seizure/epileptiform networks. Interventions such as ATL can also trigger cognitive reorganization adaptively through seizure control, or maladaptively through seizure recurrence.

1988; R. Martin, Sawrie, Edwards, Roth, Kuzniecky, et al., 2000; Shulman, 2000; Strauss, Hunter, & Wada, 1993; Trenerry, Jack, & Ivnik, 1993). Several mechanisms appear to offer explanation for these extratemporal deficits. These include undiagnosed seizure activity elsewhere in the brain, in addition to processes such as diaschisis, seizure propagation, and secondary epileptogenesis (see Tracy et al., 2010, for further exploration of these processes).

Accordingly, the cellular and structural changes associated with intractable seizures, particularly frequent seizures, have the potential to adversely affect cognitive representations, not just in the ictal region and the symptomatogenic zone (areas that produce observable clinical symptoms during the seizure), but also in remote regions. To understand this impact outside the epileptogenic zone, we must account both for the new neural connections built up by epileptogenesis and the burden that accrues from seizure spread (e.g., secondary generalization, interictal activity). These effects are not considered truly random, as they likely take advantage of relative differences in the breakdown of inhibitory neuronal processes in other brain areas. For instance, ipsilateral frontal cortex seems to be a common dispersion pathway for temporal lobe seizures, spreading through the uncinate fasciculus, with the contralateral temporal lobe (Morrell & deToledo-Morrell, 1999) being another common spread path.

Evidence of the extratemporal seizure impact can be found in remote non-ictal gray matter. For instance, structural neuroimaging studies have consistently shown atrophy in an extensive bilateral extratemporal network in unilateral TLE patients, most reliably in thalami, parietal, cerebellar, and contralateral temporal cortex, including the contralateral hippocampus and parahippocampal gyrus (Bonilha et al., 2007; see review of Keller & Roberts, 2008; Riederer et al., 2008; Staba et al., 2012). Interestingly, there is some indication that this type of gray matter extratemporal damage is more widespread in left- compared to right-sided TLE (Riederer et al., 2008), raising the possibility that regional seizure network growth may be influenced by brain function properties such as the presence of language dominance. This extratemporal seizure burden also appears in white matter, with diffusivity abnormalities in TLE patients not restricted to the known epileptogenic temporal lobe (Gross, 2011), but extending to regions such as the posterior corpus callosum (Arfanakis et al., 2002), cerebellum, and the contralateral white matter near the healthy (e.g., non-sclerotic) hippocampus, amygdala, and temporal pole (Thivard et al., 2005). Additionally, metabolic compromise appears to emerge both in the ipsilateral (ictal) and contralateral hemisphere in TLE patients, consisting in abnormal N-acetyl aspartate/choline ratios as derived from magnetic resonance spectroscopy. Finally, from yet another level of analysis, resting state FC work from our lab (Tracy et al., 2014) has shown that highly focal, unilateral TLE, with no evidence of interictal activity outside the ictal temporal lobe, is associated with a strong inhibitory surround (i.e., anti-correlated activity) in the contralateral hemisphere. In contrast, TLE patients who display extratemporal interictal activity lack this surrounding anti-correlated activity. Thus, large regions of healthy cortex seem to respond, through contralateral anti-correlated activity, even to focal seizures, representing a form of protective and adaptive inhibition, helping to constrain epileptiform activity to the pathologic temporal lobe (see Figure 2.2). In summary,

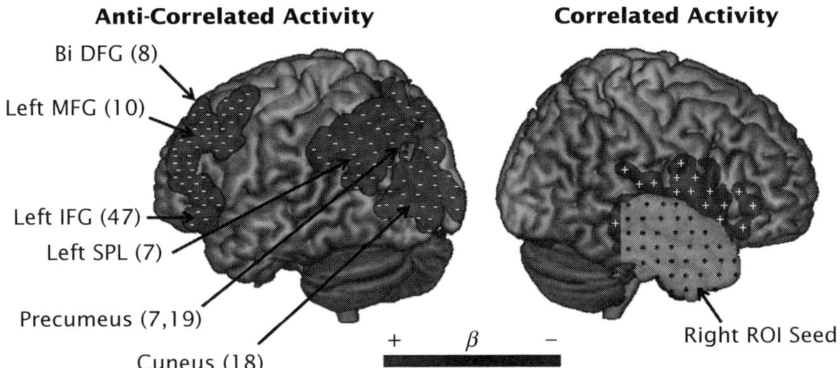

FIGURE 2.2 Positive (+) and negative (–) functional connectivity with the right temporal lobe ROI (*) in right unilateral TLE patients. DFG = medial part of superior frontal gyrus; MFG = middle frontal gyrus; IFG = inferior frontal gyrus; SPL = superior parietal lobule. Brodmann areas are in parentheses. Modified and reprinted with permission from *Human Brain Mapping*, Tracy et al. (2014), John Wiley and Sons.

all the above evidence is consistent with the likelihood that even lesional epilepsy with focal seizures causes reactions throughout large regions of the brain, potentially impacting multiple cognitive functions and networks.

Seizure-Induced Reorganization of Cognitive Networks

Neuropsychological studies of patients with focal, lesional TLE have consistently demonstrated neurocognitive impairments in intelligence, language, visuospatial, executive, or motor function—impairments that cannot be solely explained by the underlying focal neuropathology (B. Hermann, Seidenberg, & Jones, 2008). In this sense, studies of the famous epilepsy and amnesia patient (i.e., H. M.), which helped show that episodic memory relies on the hippocampi, also slant our view of TLE and its cognitive impact to a single brain region.

Neuropsychological, intracarotid amobarbital (popularly known as the Wada test), functional magnetic resonance imaging (fMRI), and FC studies have all provided evidence that the brain representation of cognitive functions in patients with TLE, for a variety of tasks, can reorganize to regions not seen in matched control samples. Neuropsychological and intracarotid amobarbital studies, particularly in early onset left TLE, provided evidence for reorganization of verbal memory and expressive language skills, with indications of either a left-to-right inter-hemispheric or anterior-to-posterior intra-hemispheric reorganization pattern (Jokeit, Ebner, Holthausen, Markowitsch, & Tuxhorn, 1996; Seidenberg et al., 1997). The best-substantiated cases of cognitive reorganization involve individuals with early onset epilepsy (Springer et al., 1999). While seizures at an early age put individuals at risk for the effects of chronicity, the young brain exhibits greater plasticity, making it both more hyperexcitable and prone to seizures (Raol, Budreck, & Brooks-Kayal, 2003), but also better suited for cognitive reorganization. It is also interesting to note that early life neural repair may be a double-edged sword, as there is work indicating that it may deplete neural progenitor cells, which have a finite number of divisions in their lifetime. For instance, Dallison and Kolb (2003) found that when rats suffered early brain damage, hippocampal neurogenesis in adulthood was far below that of controls. It is important to note that the implication of much of the literature in cognitive network reorganization is that it is not a transient phenomenon; however, longitudinal studies verifying the stability or permanency of these network changes have not been undertaken.

Language Reorganization

Left-sided hemispherectomy patients can display reorganization of language to the right side, with some reports claiming that this can occur up to age 9, though these children still have deficits (Hertz-Pannier et al., 2002; Vargha-Khadem et al., 1997). The phenomenon of "crowding" makes clear that while language can reorganize to the right hemisphere in left hemisphere epilepsy, there is a cost often in terms of material-specific memory loss or conflicts in information processing, disabling, for instance, simultaneous verbal and visual-spatial processing (Helmstaedter, Kurthen, Linke, & Elger, 1994). In an intracarotid amobarbital study of TLE from our lab (Tracy et al., 2009), we found that 40.3% of left TLE patients (n = 124) displayed atypical language organization (i.e., stronger right hemisphere representation) on at least one language skill (n.b., the skills measured were repetition, naming, comprehension, reading, and speech quality/dysarthria). While the majority (60%) of patients showing atypical language representation do so on more than one language skill, the proportion showing atypicality on all five skills was low, only 5.6% of the left TLE sample. These data clearly show atypical hemispheric dominance is not an "all-or-nothing" phenomenon, with all aspects of language reorganizing together in a monolithic fashion. Thus, hemispheric language dominance and its reorganization are heterogeneous, complex processes, with distinct language systems showing independence, making clear that the pressures compelling atypical reorganization in TLE do not work with equal force on all language functions.

Task-driven fMRI studies have also verified that TLE patients show altered organization of major cognitive networks such as those involved in expressive language. Several studies are noteworthy. For instance, an fMRI study by Wilke et al. (2011), using narrative and letter sound processing tasks in epileptic children and matched controls, found a high rate of atypical language organization, with the homotopic contralateral region the most common site of reorganization, though the distribution of left hemisphere representations (frontal and temporal regions) also showed alterations from normative locations (e.g., classical Broca's and Wernicke's areas). Cousin et al. (2008) found that the asymmetry of typical language lateralization was significantly lower in left TLE patients than controls, with early onset patients showing stronger signs of right temporal and parietal reorganization than late onset patients, in addition to a tendency toward intra-hemispheric reorganization involving the frontal lobe. They also found that hippocampal sclerosis increased the probability of inter-hemispheric shift of the temporal lobe activation. Rosenberger and colleagues (2009) looked at fMRI language activation patterns in left TLE patients during a lexical decision task (e.g., correct/incorrect definitions provided auditorily) and found an increased frequency of atypical language representations involving right hemisphere language areas, homologs of left hemisphere Broca and Wernicke's areas. Interestingly, they found little evidence for intra-hemispheric reorganization in patients with left hemisphere epilepsy who remained left language dominant by fMRI, and these effects did not vary by age at epilepsy onset, duration of epilepsy, or pathology. Hamberger and Cole (2011) reviewed the area of language reorganization and found that preserved naming ability in the setting of hippocampal sclerosis was associated with intra-hemispheric (i.e., more posterior temporal) reorganization in response to early disease in the mesial temporal region. They noted that this pattern makes sense, given the known bias of TLE seizure discharges to proceed anteriorly. The authors concluded that in TLE contralateral reorganization, often homotopic, is common, but ipsilateral, perilesional language reorganization can also occur. It is worth noting that it is unclear how large the epileptogenic region (or lesion) has to be to force contralateral language reorganization. Also unclear is the degree to which inter-hemispheric reorganization is dependent on the particular brain region housing the pathology. There is, however, some evidence that damage to the hippocampus may be the crucial structure compelling contralateral, as opposed to ipsilateral, language reorganization (for review, see Tracy & Boswell, 2008). If this is the case, it may suggest that the inputs and computations of the contralateral hippocampus are sought out when unavailable in the ipsilateral hemisphere.

Memory Reorganization

In terms of memory, Figueiredo et al. (2008) utilized a visual episodic memory fMRI task, and found that, relative to controls, right TLE patients with hippocampal sclerosis demonstrated functional reorganization through the transfer of function from the right to the left hemisphere, with preserved visual memory performance. Richardson et al. (2003) utilized a verbal encoding fMRI task and found that successful encoding was associated with activation of the left hippocampus in normal individuals, but the right hippocampus and parahippocampal gyrus in left TLE patients. A study of verbal semantic memory by Koylu et al. (2006) showed that, compared to controls, left TLE patients showed a shift in activation from the typical left frontal and medial temporal areas to homologs in the right hemisphere. The left TLE patients also recruited subcortical structures, such as the thalamus and putamen, to accomplish the task. In contrast, the right TLE patients more closely resembled normal controls, though they did exhibit bilateral frontal hypoactivation. Alessio et al. (2013) studied verbal and visual memory in patients with hippocampal sclerosis (HS), and found left hippocampal sclerosis patients produced more bilateral or right-lateralized verbal encoding-related activations, suggesting reorganization in reaction to a dysfunctional mesial temporal lobe. For the visual memory-encoding task in this study, the left and right HS groups, in addition to the controls, recruited widespread cortical bilaterally. The right HS group was the only group recruiting the left inferior temporal cortex, interpreted by the authors to reflect material-specific memory compensation of right mesial temporal dysfunction.

Interestingly, there is evidence from task-based fMRI studies of memory that reorganization may not always be adaptive. For instance, a study by Vannest et al. (2008) demonstrated that intractable epilepsy (mixed pathology, some mesial temporal sclerosis, MTS) influenced the functional neuroanatomy of a scene-encoding task, with both left and right epilepsy patients showing a pattern of increased contralateral medial temporal activation, within the setting of broader bilateral activation compared to healthy controls. This contralateral activation was associated with decreased memory performance, potentially providing evidence that not all reorganization is necessarily adaptive. However, it is important to note that when unique (non-normative) fMRI activation patterns are associated with lower cognitive performance, this could still represent adaptive compensation, emerging from incomplete or flawed compensation efforts. A similar pattern of findings was observed by Powell et al. (2007), who found that reorganization to the contralateral undamaged hippocampus (in either right or left TLE) was associated with worse material-specific memory performance. In fact, greater activation in the damaged left hippocampus was correlated with better verbal memory performance in left TLE patients, and greater right hippocampal activation was associated with better nonverbal memory in right TLE patients.

Functional Connectivity Evidence of Reorganization

While the above studies demonstrate the impact of seizures on the spatial distribution of task-driven activation, there is emerging evidence from resting state fMRI of altered network organization and connectivity patterns, with the bulk of the data again involving TLE. Whole-brain network alterations have been observed in TLE relative to healthy controls in several specific functional networks including the well-known default-mode network (DMN),[3] in addition to attention, perceptual, and language networks (Liao et al., 2010; Waites et al., 2006; Zhang, Lu, Zhong, Tan, Liao, et al., 2009; Zhang, Lu, Zhong, Tan, Yang, et al., 2009; Zhang et al., 2010). These studies provide strong evidence that epileptic activity causes functional changes in complex and widespread resting state networks (RSNs), putting at risk a wide range of neurocognitive and affective functions.

---

3. The "default-mode network" (DMN) includes the medial prefrontal cortex, the precuneus/posterior cingulum, the inferior parietal cortex, the mesial temporal lobes, and the lateral temporal cortex. Previous investigations have provided rich insights into its major role in internally focused tasks, most notably, episodic memory processing, but also in theory of mind and mind wandering (Buckner, Andrews-Hanna, & Schacter, 2008).

Most studies of resting state FC in mesial TLE have focused on FC emerging from the ictal hippocampus (Doucet, Osipowicz, Sharan, Sperling, & Tracy, 2013a; Morgan, Rogers, Sonmezturk, Gore, & Abou-Khalil, 2011; Pereira et al., 2010; Zhang et al., 2010). The findings suggest that, compared to controls, there is increased connectivity with the contralateral hippocampus, as well as other contralateral limbic structures, with this interpreted as a form of compensatory connectivity (Bettus et al., 2009; Bettus et al., 2010; Doucet, Osipowicz, et al., 2013a; Pittau, Grova, Moeller, Dubeau, & Gotman, 2012). However, there is counter-evidence, as Pereira et al. (2010) detected reduced resting state FC between hippocampi in patients with unilateral TLE and HS. They demonstrated that this effect was more pronounced for the left than the right TLE group, implying that these connectivity differences may be mediated by factors such as left hemispheric dominance for language.

Importantly, these changes in network organization and FC appear related to actual cognitive performance, raising the possibility that episodic memory deficits in TLE are associated with changes in neocortical-hippocampal communication or interactions (i.e., changes in the excitatory/inhibitory balance) (Bartolomei et al., 2004; Liao et al., 2010; Tracy et al., 2014; Waites et al., 2006). For instance, Wagner and colleagues (2007) showed that stronger FC between the hippocampus and neocortical regions (e.g., inferior frontal and superior temporal cortices) was associated with better performance in right and left TLE patients during a verbal encoding and recognition memory task composed of concrete and highly imaginable word-pairs. Bettus et al. (2009) showed that increased FC between the posterior and anterior parts of the right (healthy) hippocampus are correlated with working memory scores in left TLE, with the authors suggesting that increased FC in regions of the contralateral, healthy hemisphere provide an efficient means of cognitive (i.e., working memory) compensation. Lastly, work from our lab (Doucet, Osipowicz, et al., 2013a) has found the FC between the left non-pathologic mesial TL and the medial frontal cortex was positively correlated with delayed recall scores on a nonverbal memory task in right TLE patients, suggesting that adaptive connectivity changes took place to preserve this memory function (see Figure 2.3). In contrast, we observed a negative correlation between verbal memory performance and the level of FC between the left pathologic mesial TL and posterior cingulate cortex in left TLE patients, suggesting potential maladaptive changes in the pathologic hemisphere.

What is particularly interesting about FC-based methods is that they can show different networks to be active in distinct patient groups, even when the groups do not differ in cognitive performance (Doucet, Osipowicz, Sharan, Sperling, & Tracy, 2013b; Ranganath, Heller, Cohen, Brozinsky, & Rissman, 2005; Rodrigo et al., 2007). For instance, in our lab we demonstrated that right and left TLE groups show distinct patterns of hippocampal FC during visuospatial working memory tasks even when overall recall accuracy was the same in each group (Doucet, Osipowicz, et al., 2013b). More specifically, we observed a positive relationship between performance and FC between the left hippocampus and the precuneus in the right TLE group; whereas

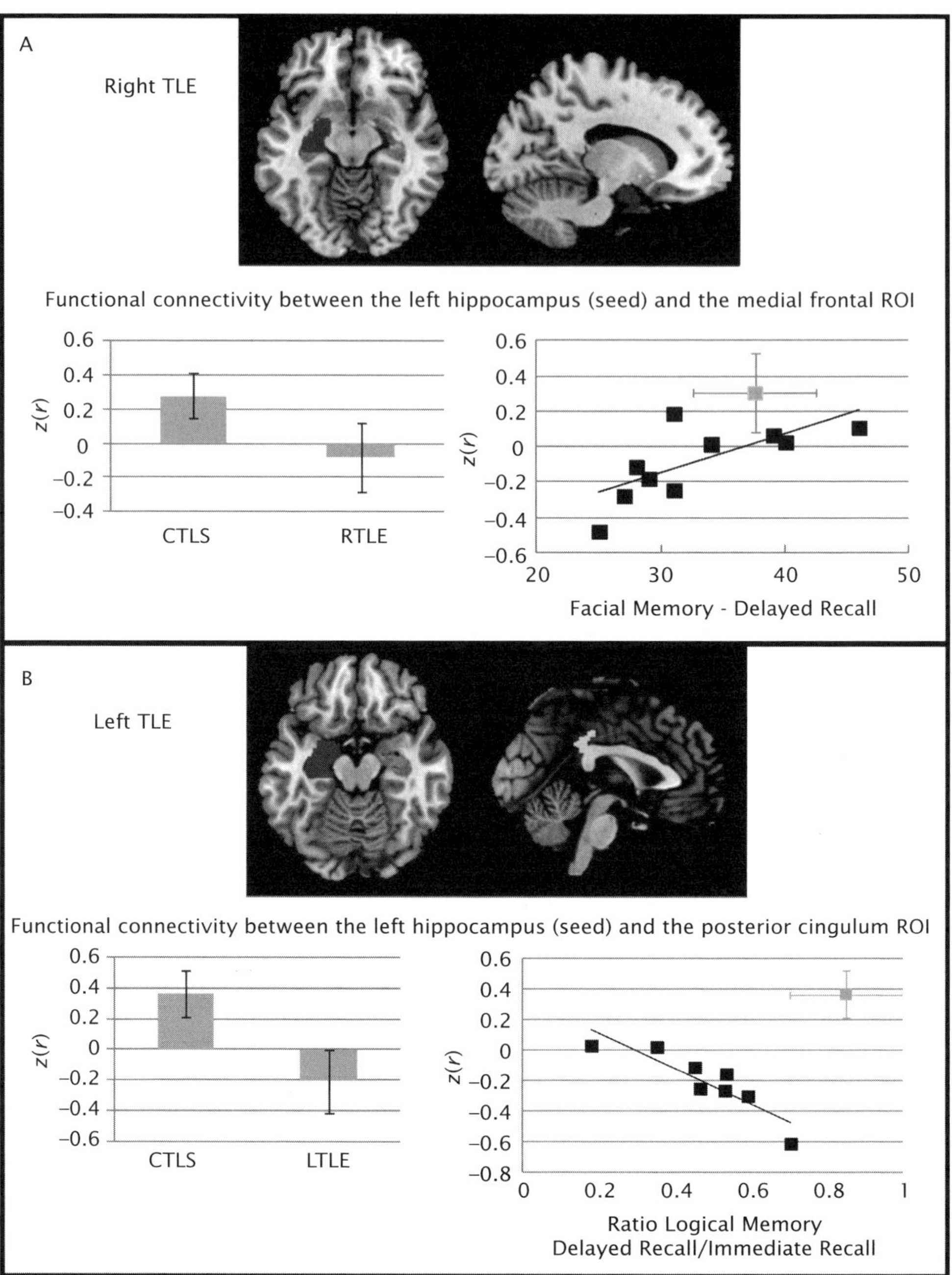

FIGURE 2.3 Correlation between FC values with the left hippocampal seed in right mesial TLE (RTLE), panel A, and in left mesial TLE (LTLE), panel B, with episodic memory scores. A: Reduced FC between the left hippocampal seed (blue) and medial frontal cortex (green, x = −14, y = 56, z = −10) in right mesial TLE patients compared with controls (*left bottom plot*); positive correlation between FC values between these two regions and the Facial Memory II Delayed Recall scores (*right bottom plot*, Spearman correlation, r = 0.78; p = 0.0045). The normative values of the controls on the right bottom plot are shown by the green data point where the *y axis* indicates the average FC value of the controls' data and the *x axis* is the normative value of age-matched healthy controls of the Facial Memory II Delayed Recall scores (Wechsler, 1997). Bars indicate standard deviation.B: Reduced FC between the left seed (blue) and posterior cingulate cortex (green, x = 2, y = −36, z = 32) in left mesial TLE patients compared with controls (*left bottom plot*); negative correlation between the FC values between these two regions and the ratio Logical Memory II Delayed Recall scores/Logical memory I Immediate Recall scores (*right bottom plot*, Spearman correlation, r = −0.93; p = 0.001). The normative values of the controls are shown through the green data point where the *y axis* indicates the average FC value of the controls' data and the *x axis* is the normative value of age-matched healthy controls of the Logical Memory ration (II/I) score (Wechsler, 1997). Bars indicate standard deviation. Modified and reprinted with permission from *Human Brain Mapping*, Doucet et al. (2013a), John Wiley and Sons. (see color insert)

the left TLE group demonstrated a negative relationship between performance and FC between both hippocampi and ipsilateral cerebellar clusters. While these data show that unilateral TLE can cause distinct patterns of functional network responses according to the side of seizures, it also indicates that, in the setting of identical performance, distinct brain connectivity responses can be observed. Accordingly, FC may be a means of identifying abnormal or unique brain networks implementing a task, information that cannot be discerned at the level of behavior through such techniques as neuropsychological testing.

Diffusion Tensor/White Matter Evidence of Reorganization

White matter (WM) connectivity, of course, can also be used to address issues of network reorganization. Fractional anisotropy (FA), which reflects microstructural integrity of white matter, has shown that tracts proximal to the ictal focus have reduced FA in chronic TLE patients, that is, the uncinate, the parahippocampal fasciculus, and the inferior longitudinal fasciculus (Ahmadi et al., 2009; Concha, Beaulieu, Collins, & Gross, 2009; Liacu, Idy-Peretti, Ducreux, Bouilleret, & de Marco, 2012). In addition, there is evidence that WM tracts in areas remote from the pathology have reduced FA as well, that is, the corpus callosum, the internal/external capsules, and the arcuate fasciculus (Arfanakis et al., 2002; Otte et al., 2012). FA reductions, at least in part, appear to depend on the side of epilepsy, with left TLE associated with more extensive FA reductions bilaterally, whereas those with right TLE have more limited reductions, often restricted to ipsilateral tracts (Kemmotsu et al., 2011; Pustina et al., in press; Voets et al., 2009). These FA reductions in some instances correlate with diminished memory performance (Diehl et al., 2008; Yogarajah et al., 2008). Recent work from our lab, however, suggests that the relationship between FA and seizures is mediated by other factors. We compared healthy controls with unilateral (ictal) TLE patients who had either bilateral or unilateral interictal spikes on electroencephalography (EEG).[4] Unexpectedly, patients with bilateral interictal spikes had more normative FA values in tracts connecting the two hemispheres, suggesting that the spread of epileptic pathology occurs in the context of better WM structural connectivity (Osipowicz, Pajor, et al., under review). Thus, impaired WM connectivity indexed by an FA decrease may have the benefit of isolating the ictal focus from the rest of the brain, thus mitigating or delaying the effect of epileptic activity on remote healthy areas.

---

4. A majority of unilateral TLE patients show not just ictal, but also interictal, activity, in the epileptogenic temporal lobe. A smaller proportion of these unilateral patients also show contralateral interictal activity in the non-ictal temporal lobe. The prevalence of TLE patients with bilateral spikes in a sample from our center (n = 40, 35%, unpublished) is similar to other reports of patients with bilateral epileptiform activity: 27% in McCarthy, O'Connor, & Sperling (1997); 38% in Sampaio, Yacubian, & Manreza (2004); 33% in Janszky et al. (2003); 35% in Morrell, Rasmussen, Gloor, & De Toledo-Morrell (1983); 40% in Hughes (1985) The study we refer to from our laboratory compared unilateral TLE patients with and without this contralateral interictal activity.

Based on all the work reviewed earlier on cognitive network reorganization in TLE, it is tempting to conclude that recruiting regions of the healthy hemisphere into the network is an adaptive response to seizures, perhaps following the logic of material specificity (e.g., verbal memory shows a left-to-right hemisphere shift and recruitment in the setting of left temporal pathology and left language dominance). The evidence, however, is still too mixed, and other influential factors in terms of seizure type, strength of hemispheric dominance, education, chronological age, and variations in brain reserve have yet to be adequately explored. Indeed, when altered networks in TLE are discovered, it is very difficult to know whether the pattern is innate and premorbid, or one that initially organized normally and then reorganized in response to emergent and ongoing seizures, with the latter being the working assumption of most studies. One particular mediating factor that has been investigated involves the high potential for perturbing cognitive network architecture that comes with the accumulating effects of seizures, that is, seizure chronicity and age of seizure onset.

Time-Related Factors Mediating Cognitive Reorganization in Epilepsy

When seizures remain intractable, epilepsy can be viewed as a progressive condition with accumulating adverse effects (Bernhardt, Chen, He, Evans, & Bernasconi, 2011; Sutula, 2004). In fact, some studies suggest that the duration of active epilepsy is actually a better predictor of the severity of cognitive deficits than the type or location of the seizures (Farwell, Dodrill, & Batzel, 1985). Studies confirm at least a mild accumulating and deteriorative effect on IQ in TLE (Dodrill, 2004), with some cross-sectional studies suggesting that IQ declines after about three decades (Jokeit & Ebner, 2002). Other longitudinal studies make clear that TLE causes a slow and steady decline in episodic memory that cannot strictly be accounted for by age (Hamberger & Cole, 2011; Jokeit & Ebner, 1999; Rausch et al., 2003). However, there are some data that have suggested that memory decline in epilepsy can be stopped, even reversed, if seizures are fully controlled (Helmstaedter, Kurthen, Lux, Reuber, & Elger, 2003).

Factors such as the temporal pattern of the brain insult (slow versus rapid) change the likelihood of both reorganization and the restoration of function, with "slow growing" pathologies, such as intractable seizures, increasing the probability and efficiency of reorganization processes (Braun et al., 2008), particularly in regions more remote from the "at risk" skill or function. Interestingly, the initial brain insult that might produce a seizure is often followed by a long latency period of epileptogenesis (i.e., years), before a clinically observable seizure occurs. Likewise, cognitive problems are often not demonstrated until after this latency period. Yet, once seizures begin, the disease and cognitive problems can progress even during the non-symptomatic interictal state, although very little is known about the potentially unique cognitive impact of this interictal period.

Resting State Studies of Connectivity Change Over Time

With this in mind, understanding the cognitive impact of seizures becomes quite elusive, as there is an inherent tendency for the representation of cognitive networks in TLE patients to change in response to intractable seizures, with chronicity, of course, interacting with the effects of advancing age. Resting state FC is proving to be informative in this regard. For instance, a resting state study by Morgan et al. (2011) showed that cross-hippocampal connectivity may vary with TLE duration. In the first 10 years of seizures, connectivity was variable and often diminished, but beyond that point interhemispheric connectivity appeared to increase. Wang et al. (2011) investigated generalized tonic-clonic seizure (GTCS) patients at rest, and found that the degree of FC within key regions of either the DMN (the right medial prefrontal cortex), or the dorsal attention network (e.g., left intraparietal sulcus) were negatively correlated with epilepsy duration, suggesting that damage accrues to these networks in association with more chronic GTCS. McGill et al. (2012) extended these results by investigating the DMN in idiopathic generalized epilepsy (IGE) patients at rest, and found that seizure duration was negatively correlated with FC between the posterior cingulate cortex and medial frontal cortex. The authors suggested that the chronic effects of epileptiform activity and its underlying abnormalities disrupt functional integration between medial posterior and frontal regions. Zhang and colleagues (2011) found that the degree of coupling between functional (resting state) and structural (DTI) connectivity networks exhibited a negative correlation with epilepsy duration in IGE patients, suggesting a decoupling of functional and structural connectivity with longer illness history. Using electroencephalography (EEG) data, van Dellen et al. (2009) found that longer epilepsy duration was associated with both lower temporal lobe FC and more random network configuration in TLE. FC data from our lab (Doucet et al., in press; Doucet, Skidmore, et al., 2013) suggest that the characteristics of whole brain organization (e.g., measures of segregation, such as clustering coefficient, CC) vary as an interaction between age of seizure onset and lesional status in TLE (see Figure 2.4). For instance, when TLE onset comes early in life, the impact of MTS (the most common etiology for TLE) on whole brain organization may be mitigated. Such data is concordant with the notion that early onset epilepsies are associated with compensatory mechanisms as the younger brain is more plastic and can adapt more easily than an adult mature brain (Helmstaedter, Sonntag-Dillender, Hoppe, & Elger, 2004). In our data the late onset MTS group had an illness duration three times shorter than the early onset group, suggesting that the adult injured brain may need more time to develop compensatory responses to adult MTS pathology. Interestingly, we found very few differences between the late and early onset groups in non-lesional TLE (i.e., no evidence of a structural lesion), suggesting that age of onset has little progressive impact on FC when no focal lesion is detectable.

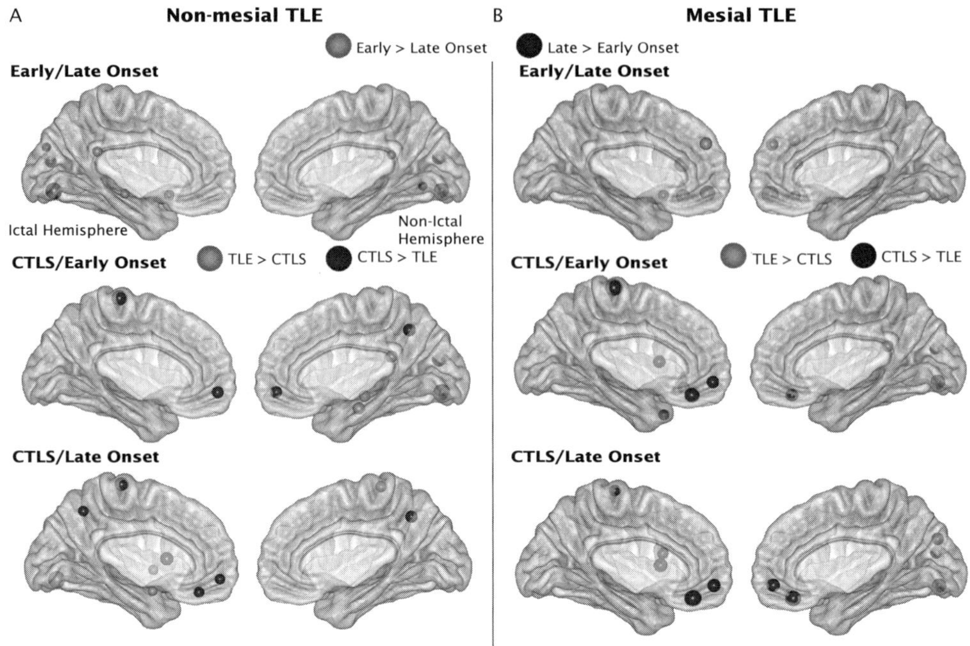

FIGURE 2.4 Depiction of the sites of the 10 largest clustering coefficient differences between early and late seizure onset groups and normal controls (CTL) within the non-lesional TLE (nTLE, panel A) or the mesial TLE (mTLE, panel B) groups. Modified and reprinted with permission from *Brain Topography*, Doucet et al. (in press).

EEG and Electrocorticography Studies of Connectivity Dynamics

From the above macroscopic time perspective involving years of seizure activity, it is clear that epilepsy can perturb functional architecture. But we know that seizure activity also causes neuronal synchronization changes that operate on a smaller, microscopic scale. Kindling is known to arise from post-synaptic brain stimulation on the order of tenths of seconds to seconds in length. This makes it likely that even short duration seizure events cause alterations in synaptic networks of the dentate gyrus of the hippocampus, for instance (Hannesson & Corcoran, 2000). Synapses along the dendritic spines were once thought to be relatively stable, but recent imaging experiments have shown that synapse turnover can actually occur on a timescale of minutes, particularly in response to deprivation or enrichment (Holtmaat, De Paola, Wilbrecht, & Knott, 2008).

EEG and electrocorticography (eCOG) studies have begun to unravel the FC effects of seizures at finer timescales. In an EEG study, Kramer et al. (2010) showed that as a seizure moves from onset to termination, "a large subnetwork of connected nodes emerges . . . with this dominant component fracturing [. . .] then approaching seizure termination these subnetworks rejoin to again establish a dominant network component" (p. 9). Thus, synchrony and connectivity are not uniform across a seizure, with the onset and termination phases showing the strongest hypersynchrony. Research by Rubinov et al. (2009) makes clear that spike-timing dependent changes in FC can be observed, but will vary by the time window of the activity measured (Honey, Kotter, Breakspear, & Sporns, 2007). For instance, functional networks observed during long windows of neural activity (minutes) appear to correspond to underlying anatomical/structural networks, with hubs in these functional networks corresponding to structural hubs. Analysis of shorter time windows (seconds), however, yields fluctuations in underlying network organization (i.e., typology), with a loss of connections, and unstable hub dynamics, including fluctuations in the locations of central nodes (hubs) over time (Honey et al., 2007). Schindler and colleagues (2008) demonstrated that intense neuronal firing at the onset of a seizure may saturate "hub" neurons (i.e., those neurons with both strong local connections and strong distal connections with other neural modules), suggesting that seizures may shut down these hubs, causing functional disconnection, that is, decreased coupling, between both local and more distant connections (Schindler et al., 2008). These data make clear that hypersynchrony and resultant FC vary across the time interval of a seizure. Even accounting for this variability, however, several authors have argued that small-world properties generally remain evident and heightened during the ictal period of seizures (Netoff, Clewley, Arno, Keck, & White, 2004; Ponten, Bartolomei, & Stam, 2007).

This point about different timescales is important, as it makes clear there will not necessarily be a correspondence in the FC findings emerging from blood oxygen level dependent fMRI, surface EEG, and single cell recordings. Said differently, the ways in which neural synchrony on a microscopic scale translates into large-scale changes in eCOG rhythms and macroscopic connectivity changes between brain regions during a seizure are unclear. There is a building body of work using eCOG data, which shows that specific cortical oscillations may provide a marker for specific circuit-level cognitive mechanisms (Donner & Siegel, 2011). For instance, the local excitatory-inhibitory interactions that shape neuronal sensory, motor, and cognitive systems produce local gamma band oscillations. Higher integrative functions such as decision-making are mediated by long-range cortical interactions, producing more diverse local oscillation patterns involving the beta range. Such work has shown that regional global hubs residing in areas such as the medial temporal, parietal, and sensorimotor regions form unique regional correlation patterns depending on the oscillation frequency. This suggests that the large-scale organization of the brain consists of interacting (and hierarchical) frequency-specific and region-specific correlation structures, each providing unique signatures for different components of cognitive processing (Hipp, Hawellek, Corbetta, Siegel, & Engel, 2012). No doubt, by integrating neuronal coupling information at these different time scales (EEG/eCOG and BOLD resting state data), we will come closer to capturing the impact of FC dynamics on both the acute/transient and more permanent patterns of cognitive reorganization set in motion by seizures.

Cognitive Plasticity in Response to Surgical Treatment

Despite efforts to only remove pathologic tissue, we know that clinical interventions such as resective surgery can modify cognitive networks (Doucet et al., 2014; Johnston et al., 2008). The adaptive or maladaptive cognitive mechanisms that might be triggered by this type of acute network disruption have yet to be determined. The size of the resection appears to matter in terms of postoperative cognitive status (the larger the resection, the greater the decline) and seizure outcome, leading to the possibility that this mediates the level of functional reorganization (Helmstaedter, 2004; Helmstaedter, Petzold, & Bien, 2011; Quigg et al., 2011; Wong et al., 2009). In addition, there is evidence to suggest that cognitive plasticity in response to surgery varies as a function of seizure control (Helmstaedter et al., 2003).

Following ATL, about 60% of patients are seizure-free (Engel, 1992; Englot, Ouyang, Garcia, Barbaro, & Chang, 2012). Overall, the most reliable current predictors of postsurgical cognitive outcome remain baseline neurocognitive testing, the surgical hemisphere (dominant or non-dominant, as defined by the intracarotid amobarbital exam or task-based fMRI), and age of onset of epilepsy (Baxendale, 2002; Baxendale, Thompson, & Duncan, 2008; Binder, Swanson, Hammeke, & Sabsevitz, 2008; Chelune, Naugle, Luders, Sedlak, & Awad, 1993; Davies, Risse, & Gates, 2005; Lineweaver et al., 2006; Loring et al., 1990; Powell et al., 2008; Potter et al., 2009). As an example of neuropsychological outcome, a recent review by Ives-Deliperi and Butler (2012) suggested that the absence of hippocampal pathology and late-age onset epilepsy were the strongest predictors of naming decline. Unfortunately, there have been no studies comparing these more established predictors to the more recent neuroimaging techniques (resting state FC, task fMRI, and structural data, e.g., DTI) for their ability to predict cognitive outcome following surgery.

fMRI Studies of Cognitive Outcome

fMRI studies have mostly suggested that the functional adequacy of the cortex ipsilateral to the ictal focus is predictive of adverse cognitive outcome. For instance, Powell et al. (2008) found that patients with greater ipsilateral fMRI activation had greater memory decline following surgery, and this occurred in a material-specific fashion for dominant and non-dominant ATL patients, as activation in the dominant hippocampus predicted verbal memory change, whereas activity in the non-dominant hippocampus did not. Bonelli et al. (2013), who studied outcome 4 months after ATL, found that good memory outcome was associated with preoperative reorganization of verbal memory to the ipsilateral posterior medial temporal lobe, indicating that the functional adequacy of the posterior remnant of the ipsilateral hippocampus is crucial for maintaining verbal memory after left ATL. In contrast, postoperative reorganization to the ipsilateral posterior or contralateral medial temporal lobe structures did not appear to support better memory performance.

In a study of language network changes following ATL (Bonelli et al., 2012), individuals with left TLE had greater bilateral middle/inferior frontal fMRI activation and stronger FC with the contralateral frontal lobe than preoperatively, and this was not observed in individuals with right TLE. However, a decline in naming scores correlated with contralateral activation, while correlation of performance with the remaining left posterior hippocampus was associated with no decline, suggesting that the latter region remained important for maintaining language. In contrast, an fMRI study by Kim et al. (2010) showed that movement toward a more bilateral semantic network following surgery in left TLE patients is associated with cognitive recovery. Using a word-generation task, the authors found that semantic-specific activations in the inferior prefrontal region became more bilateral in left TLE patients with HS, but more left-lateralized in right TLE/HS patients after ATL. These results indicate that the best functional recovery in a language semantic network in both left and right TLE was associated with recruitment of inferior prefrontal cortex contralateral to the epileptogenic side.

The above data seem to suggest that cognitive reserve in the contralateral hemisphere is more important than ipsilateral integrity in terms of predicting cognitive outcome (see Chelune et al., 1993).

Resting State and Diffusion Tensor Imaging (DTI) Studies of Cognitive or Seizure Outcome

McCormick et al. (2013) found that stronger presurgical resting state FC involving the bilateral posterior cingulate cortex (seed) to the pathologic hippocampus was associated with better presurgical memory and greater postsurgical memory decline. However, stronger posterior cingulate connectivity (same bilateral seed) with the contralateral hippocampus was associated with better postsurgical memory outcome. Negishi et al. (2011) utilized both whole brain resting state fMRI and surface EEG data to examine FC presurgery (mixed sample of resective surgeries). The results suggested that seizure recurrence was associated with a less lateralized FC pattern than seizure freedom, suggesting that high laterality (i.e., stronger FC in the ictal hemisphere) predicted better seizure outcome. In contrast, Antony et al. (2013) utilized intracranial electrode data to compute FC statistics, presurgery, and found that 90% of TLE patients with weak and homogenous FC within the ictal temporal lobe were seizure-free one year after surgery. In contrast, 85% of patients with recurrent seizures experienced stronger and more heterogenous FC within the temporal lobe. Thus, these studies differ in terms of what strong FC in the ictal hemisphere implies in terms of seizure outcome, but it is worth noting that they used very different methods (i.e., Negishi et al., 2011, utilized whole brain coverage in a mixed group of focal epilepsies; Antony et al., 2013, utilized intracranial EEG with coverage only of the ictal hemisphere in a solely unilateral TLE sample). Note, both studies lacked correlation with indices of cognitive outcome. Nonetheless, these studies do suggest that resting state FC has promise as a predictor of postsurgical seizure control.

It is important to note that better cognitive outcome has also been associated with changes in white matter structural connectivity. In a study of postsurgery changes in white matter and language network integrity, Yogarajah et al. (2010) investigated 26 left and 20 right TLE patients both pre- and post-ATL resection, and found a mean 8% increase in FA after left ATL resection in the ipsilateral external capsule and posterior internal capsule/corona radiata, a region considered part of a ventromedial language network; this increase in FA correlated positively with confrontation naming performance. The authors suggested that the existence of an active ventrolateral language network presurgery increased the capacity for further structural reorganization along this pathway, perhaps as a compensatory response. A problem with DTI studies of surgical outcome such as the above is that they do not take into account the degree to which Wallerian degeneration and the "crossing fiber" problem in DTI can significantly confound depictions of outcome. In a study from our laboratory, we used FA to distinguish between genuine plasticity and artifactual changes in white matter (Pustina et al., in press). Though we found similar FA increase to Yogarajah et al. (2010), several comparisons indicated that this was caused by fiber degeneration in areas with crossing fibers. Instead, we demonstrated that genuine reorganization occurs in the non-dominant language tracts after dominant hemisphere resection, a process that may help implement the inter-hemispheric shift of language activation found in fMRI or resting state studies from our lab as well as others (Bonelli et al., 2012; Kim et al., 2010; Noppeney, Price, Duncan, & Koepp, 2005; Osipowicz, Sharan, Sperling, & Tracy, under review; Wong et al., 2009). In sum, results indicate that left TLE patients, despite showing presurgical white matter deficits in the contralateral hemisphere, have the potential for greater adaptive change.

Cognitive Rehabilitation Studies

In a study of memory rehabilitation, Koorenhof et al. (2012) demonstrated postsurgical improvement in episodic verbal memory following external (e.g., memory aid devices) and internal (e.g., mnemonics) memory support strategies. Improvement was observed after a month of rehabilitation, whether the rehabilitation took place before or after (3–6 months) surgery. The positive memory improvements, however, were associated with improvements in mood, making it unclear what types of psychological processes mediated improvement. Helmstaedter et al. (2008) analyzed pre- and post-ATL (3 months) memory performance in matched left and right TLE groups, with half of each group undergoing memory training. The risk of performance declines on verbal learning and recognition memory measures (n.b., not recall) was about four times higher without memory rehabilitation, with the gains in verbal learning higher for the right TLE group. Seizure outcomes were good in both TLE groups, and this factor did not alter the above risk level. The rehabilitation involved metacognitive training of compensatory strategies and computer-based cognitive exercises of several types. The authors interpret the data to suggest that rehabilitation can counteract the negative effects of ATL on lateral/neocortical–associated aspects of memory (i.e., learning/acquisition) as compared to more mesial-temporal aspects (i.e., retention). The implication is that right ATL patients benefit more than the left, perhaps suggesting that left-sided surgery may injure the capacities needed to respond to verbal memory training. An alternative, though somewhat counterintuitive, possibility is that the right ATL group also sustained damage to verbal memory processing, but were able to use visuospatial strategies to compensate. It is important to note that the long-term effects of rehabilitation training, verifying permanent cognitive reorganization effects, have not yet been examined.

Predicting outcome following resective brain surgery remains a high-priority goal. If, as we have tried to show, epilepsy displays an inherent cognitive plasticity, then predicting cognitive outcome depends on a proper understanding of the principles and patterns that govern the brain's neuroplastic response to seizures and subsequent surgery. Toward this goal, neuroimaging can be of help in identifying the relevant structural and functional networks before surgery and then determining how these networks are likely to change after surgery.

Modeling Neurocognitive Plasticity Following ATL

Few longitudinal studies of cognitive outcome with pre- and postsurgical imaging data in epilepsy exist, and those that do involve only one imaging modality, most commonly fMRI (Bonelli et al., 2010; Kim et al., 2010; Powell et al., 2008; Rabin et al., 2004). When cognitive outcomes from ATL are discussed in the literature, these renderings are quite general and, most important, do not link the recovery to specific cognitive mechanisms, nor to the specific changes on neuroimaging modalities that might be observed to help distinguish the mechanisms (Haut et al., 2010; Poldrack, 2000; Stein & Hoffman, 2003). For instance, the Kim et al. (2010) study, demonstrating postsurgical right hemisphere recruitment to help maintain expressive language in left TLE, lacked a means of verifying the cognitive mechanism driving the apparent reorganization.

We argue that the three major MRI neuroimaging modalities (task-driven fMRI, resting state fMRI, and DTI, or newer renditions of white matter imaging such as high angular resolution diffusion imaging) can be conceptually combined to obtain a more complete view of the neural modules and connectivity networks implementing cognitive reorganization, driving the adaptive or maladaptive neuroplasticity responses in the brain after ATL.[5] For instance, fMRI can be used to define an active network implementing a key cognitive function that might be "at risk" with temporal lobe surgery (e.g., episodic memory). Resting state fMRI can be used to capture correlated neuronal signaling, identifying gray matter networks that are biased toward neuronal communication either toward the formation of cognitive or seizure networks. Finally, DTI can be used to evaluate white

---

5. Our focus here is on these three neuroimaging modalities. Other methods of measuring functional connectivity and cognitive network integrity are important (e.g., anatomical MRI, EEG, eCOG), and will have great value in capturing cognitive reorganization and neuroplastic responses following ATL.

matter integrity and specify anatomical connectivity between the relevant gray matter regions emerging from the other two modalities. In short, resting state fMRI can identify the cortical regions communicating within a network, DTI can verify that these regions are, indeed, anatomically connected, and fMRI can define/verify the specific cognitive function(s) the network may be communicating about. In practical terms, all three can be gathered during one MRI scanning session with minimal increase in scanning time, and no increase in patient discomfort.

In the first paper of its kind, we recently published data combining these three major MRI modalities (task-driven fMRI, rsfMRI, and DTI) to yield a statistical model predictive of postsurgical verbal fluency status following ATL for intractable TLE (Osipowicz, Sperling, Sharan, & Tracy, 2014). Specifically, we showed that a model combining three change variables, each mapping out change in the patients' verbal fluency network, reliably predicted postsurgical verbal fluency scores, outperforming the three presurgical baseline neuroimaging measures (one from each modality) and established predictors of cognitive outcome (e.g., baseline neuropsychological performance). The regional nature of the change primarily involved postsurgical recruitment of a right inferior frontal region (homologous to Broca's area). Figure 2.5 shows the predictive probability of this three-variable model, displaying the strong separation between the good and poor outcome groups when plotting classification accuracy. The model explained 52% of the variance in verbal fluency outcome, correctly classifying 87% of the patients. The direction of change scores indicated that for the good outcome patients, all three imaging modalities displayed a better match to the normative brain maps postsurgery, with FA (from DTI) being the strongest predictor of this convergence to normal. These data suggest that achieving a good outcome involves engaging normative regions to complete the task—regions that were previously less involved (n.b., in the case of this verbal fluency task, the right inferior frontal gyrus was present in age-matched normals, all native English speakers). In contrast, for the poor outcome patients the pattern of change was mixed, deviating more from normal for all three modalities. While the change scores for each imaging modality

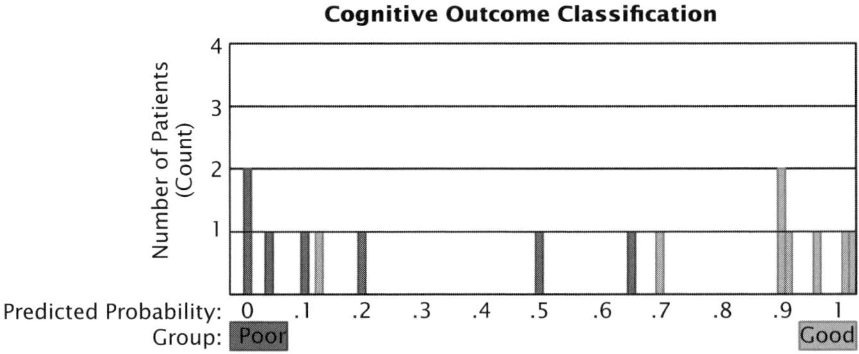

FIGURE 2.5 Classification plot with patient frequency counts, for a three-imaging modality logistical regression model predicting verbal fluency outcome. Modified and reprinted with permission from *Journal of Neurosurgery*, Osipowicz et al. (2014), JNS Publishing Group.

were superior in predictive power compared to baseline imaging values, there was still a statistical trend suggesting that with larger samples baseline neuroimaging characteristics may also become a reliable predictor of cognitive status. Such data demonstrate that presurgical deviation from normal (i.e., a measure of reorganization in response to pathology) has the potential to become an important predictor of cognitive outcome.

In a previous study from our laboratory (Tracy & Osipowicz, 2011), we articulated several mechanisms of neuroplasticity, graphically depicted and distinguished in Figure 2.6 (see also Table 2.1), linking each to a particular pattern of change seen on task-based fMRI, resting state fMRI, and DTI, demonstrating that on an individual basis these modalities can be used to determine if cognitive network reorganization has occurred and, if so, the nature of the underlying cognitive mechanism. The mechanisms we defined were functional redundancy, functional substitution, cognitive control, and cognitive reserve. We should note that we view these types of reorganization as occurring in the setting of a complex network, with the particular task function or cognitive component that is redundant, substituted, and so on, varying not just with the nature of task, but in accord with the clinical pathology, disease duration, chronological age, and a host of other factors. We define functional redundancy as the presence of duplicate representation of a function, which gets unmasked and recruited into a network, and is then used to successfully implement the task following acquired injury (i.e., resective surgery). Functional substitution utilizes a new, previously unincorporated neural region to substitute for the function of a lost node, which lacked redundant representation in the brain. Cognitive control utilizes supervisory systems to alter the affected or impaired network by increasing attentional resources, facilitating information exchange, improving sensory filtering/suppression, or increasing executive monitoring. Cognitive reserve[6] is a general mechanism of resiliency, utilizing the remaining healthy brain to withstand injury and protect against a loss of function. Finally, a fifth mechanism, normalization (though not included in the list of Figure 2.6 or Table 2.1), is defined based on evidence that patients with surgically relieved seizure burden can undergo cognitive reorganization of language function or other cognitive functions that returns functional neuroanatomical representations to their more normative locations (Lutz, Clusmann, Elger, Schramm, & Helmstaedter, 2004; R. C. Martin, Sawrie, Edwards, Roth, Faught, et al., 2000; Takaya et al., 2009). Importantly, normalization, which takes into account the potential abnormal functional organization presurgery, highlights the fact that the new area(s) recruited may be normative for the task. In the context of neuroimaging, normalization involves the reorganization of cognitive networks not through the formation of atypical, compensatory networks, as is the case with the other mechanisms noted earlier, but by the emergence of a network that better resembles the normative, age-appropriate network implementing a task. In this sense,

---

6. Cognitive reserve appears to increase in association with high IQ, extended education, and general brain health (for a review, see Stern (2007)).

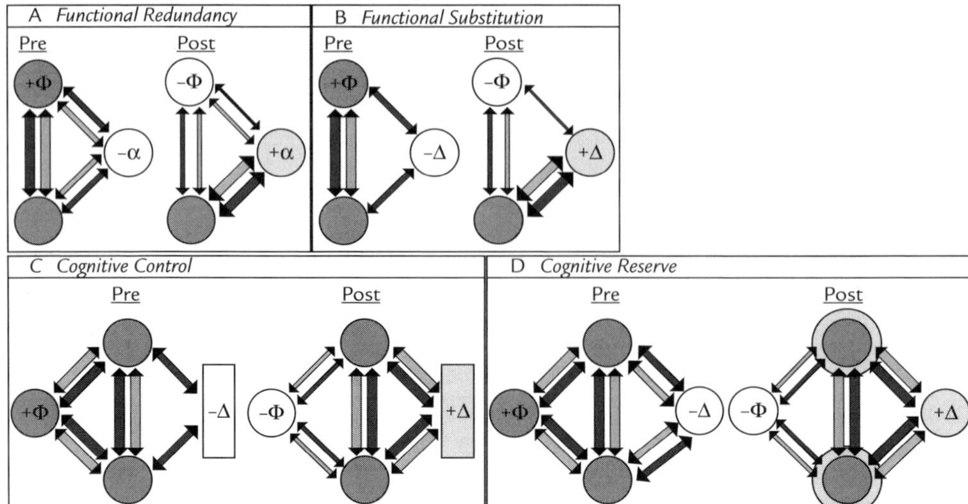

FIGURE 2.6 Graphical depiction of multimodal neuroimaging frameworks. *Panel A*: Functional redundancy. *Panel B*: Functional substitution. *Panel C*: Cognitive control. *Panel D*: Cognitive reserve. Legend: White indicates no fMRI activity in the region. Red circles indicate an area of cognitive functionality as revealed by fMRI. Yellow indicates a new region of fMRI activity, and in the case of cognitive reserve also reflects a change in the spatial extent or intensity of activation within the network (n.b., the yellow halo around the red circles of the network). Arrows indicate connectivity, with green lines depicting the rsfMRI findings and blue lines depicting the DTI findings; the arrows indicate the specific brain areas connected. The strength of connectivity is indicated by the thickness of the line, with thicker lines indicating stronger connectivity. The + and − indicate the presence or absence of fMRI activity in cases where a change in fMRI occurs across the two time points measured. The Greek letter α indicates a brain area that becomes unmasked at the second scan (e.g., after intervening event such as lesion, brain injury, or surgery); Δ marks and highlights an area that becomes newly active on the second scan; Φ indicates a brain area where fMRI activation is lost or drops out of the second scan. From Tracy & Osipowicz (2011). Copyright permission from *Journal of NeuroRehabilitation*, IOS Press. (see color insert)

the first four cognitive mechanisms appear more suited to explaining neuroplastic compensation following acute injury, such as traumatic brain injury or stroke. One must be careful in applying them to chronic disorders, such as epilepsy, which may have the propensity to disrupt functional neuroanatomy early on, altering or perhaps never even allowing for normative patterns to develop (for a review, see Cadotte et al., 2009; Elger, Helmstaedter, & Kurthen, 2004). Much of the work cited earlier in the chapter showing cognitive reorganization argues that such reorganization is a compensatory correction to previously intact network. This may be the case with lateonset epilepsy with previously healthy adults. However, based on our earlier work investigating a verbal fluency network pre- and postsurgery in TLE patients with varying onset age (Osipowicz et al., 2014), we found a pattern better described as "normalization," a term more accurate for capturing the emergence of improved cognitive functioning when the presence of prior normative organization cannot be presumed. This notion of normalization is orthogonal to the other reorganization mechanisms, which refer more strictly to the restoration and compensation of function. Yet, it is an important concept to consider when trying to fully characterize the set of possible neuroplastic responses. In the setting of epilepsy,

TABLE 2.1 List and Definition of Cognitive Mechanisms, With Associated Changes Observed on Task fMRI, Resting State fMRI (rsfMRI), and Diffusion Weighting Imaging (DTI)

Cognitive Mechanism	Definition	fMRI Changes	rsfMRI Changes	DTI Changes
Functional Redundancy *(See Figure 2.6, Panel a)*	Lost function/skill has duplicate representation elsewhere in the brain, and this representation is unmasked and utilized by the network.	Lost region not evident on post-IE scan. New region, not evident previously, is unmasked on post-IE scan.	Latent connectivity to the new, unmasked fMRI region is evident on pre-IE scan. Connectivity to lost region deteriorated on post-IE scan.	Latent connectivity to the new, unmasked fMRI region is evident on pre-IE scan. Connectivity to lost region deteriorated on post-IE scan.
Functional Substitution *(See Figure 2.6, Panel b)*	Lost skill no longer represented. Incorporation of a new cognitive component into the network.	Lost region not evident on post-IE scan, with emergence of new, substituted region.	No latent connection to the new, substituted fMRI region evident on pre-IE scan. New connectivity to the substituted region on the post-IE scan.	Deterioration of WM track integrity to lost fMRI region. Increase in WM track integrity/ density to new, substituted fMRI region at post-IE scan.
Cognitive Control *(See Figure 2.6, Panel c)*	Incorporation of monitoring and supervisory systems that control subroutines for (1) allocation of specific or general attentional resource pools, (2) information exchange, (3) sensory filtering/suppression, (4) executive or non-executive (automatic) error monitoring and correction, and performance control.	Lost region not evident on post-IE scan, with emergence of new area implementing cognitive control.	Deterioration of connectivity to the lost fMRI region evident on post-IE scan, with new connectivity to area for cognitive control, an area with no latent connectivity at the pre-IE scan.	Deterioration of WM integrity to lost fMRI region evident on post-IE scan, with increase in WM track integrity/ density to area for cognitive control.
Cognitive Reserve *(See Figure 2.6, Panel d)*	Reflects general brain reserve and resilience. Indexes the strength of cognitive resources above and beyond control functions noted above, which involve compensation through a more specific cognitive component or mechanism. Reserve captures the general protective resources of the brain to withstand injury, and initiate a recovery response.	Lost region not evident on post-IE scan, with evidence of increased spatial extent or intensity in pre-existing regions of network. New regional activation reflecting new resources brought to bear, may appear on post-IE scan.	Deterioration of connectivity to lost fMRI region evident on post-IE scan, with increased connectivity to areas of expanded fMRI activation, or to any new fMRI region bringing resources. Latent connectivity to these expanded or new fMRI activations is evident on pre-IE scan.	Deterioration of connectivity to lost fMRI region evident on post-IE scan, with increased WM connectivity to areas of expanded fMRI activation, or to any new fMRI region bringing resources. Latent WM connectivity to these expanded or new fMRI activations is evident on pre-IE scan.

IE = Intervening event such as brain lesion, injury, or brain surgery.

Modified and reprinted with permission from Tracy & Osipowicz (2011), IOS Press.

longitudinal studies capturing both the early pre- and later postsurgical changes in network organization will be needed to understand all the patterns behind the considerable inter-individual variation that is at work when studying neuroplastic responses following surgery. Clearly, much more work needs to be done to understand the demographic, clinical (both neurologic and neuropsychological), and baseline imaging characteristics that might estimate on a presurgical basis the probability of "good" versus "poor" cognitive outcome. Of foremost importance, however, is to specify the cognitive mechanisms and principles driving such adaptive or maladaptive reorganization, as it is these that will guide rehabilitation treatment.

Conclusions

In this chapter, we have shown that cognitive networks in the setting of epilepsy show altered organization and plasticity over the course of the disease and in response to key interventions such as resective surgery. Data verifying the brain representations of cognitive activity following the chronic effects of seizures, or the more acute impact of surgical resection, clearly demonstrate that these cognitive representations are not static. Epilepsy induces a variety of cellular, electrophysiologic, and structural changes that create a set of biased, favored seizure networks that are maladaptive to cognition. Our primary message is that large portions of the brain respond to even focal epilepsy, and understanding neurocognitive status requires accounting for the formation and influence of seizure networks, realizing that their impact extends well beyond the epileptogenic (ictal origin) or symptomatogenic (overt symptom generating) zone. The common patterns from task-based fMRI, DTI, and resting state FC suggest that when cognitive reorganization does occur, it often involves recruitment of the contralateral hemisphere, especially homologous regions, to compensate and preserve function. Yet, such patterns are by no means settled and the variety of factors (e.g., disease duration, hemispheric dominance) or structures that may mediate such reorganization effects (i.e., contralateral hippocampal recruitment prompted by damage to hippocampus ipsilateral to ictal focus) have yet to be worked out and fully explored. Resting state FC and EEG/eCOG analyses in TLE have yielded valuable information about broad network changes involving mesial and neocortical interactions, providing examples of both adaptive compensations and a cost to epileptic activity in terms of neural network organization. Understanding the cognitive impacts of these network changes will be necessary before it is possible to capture accurately the cognitive effects of seizures, particularly over the course of chronic seizure disorders.

Multimodal neuroimaging holds promise in terms of going beyond more standard predictors of cognitive outcome, as it can help specify the cognitive mechanisms that implement cognitive reorganization and neuroplasticity. Ultimately, understanding the principles that govern the altered network organization initiated by seizures, and the neuroplastic responses engendered through the chronic seizure burden (or the acute resection of epileptogenic tissue) is the only means of effectively predicting postsurgical neurocognitive outcomes. Initial work in our lab suggests that TLE patients with a good cognitive outcome after ATL may not recruit regions to compensate for lost functions, as these patients may never have formed a normal network. Instead, a process of normalization may best characterize their postsurgical neuroplastic response, engendering positive outcomes. Identifying the spatial location/extent and network properties of current seizure activity in relation to the localization of functionally intact cognitive networks (even further, identifying the postsurgical networks to which the cognitive networks are likely to reorganize) will provide the ability to tailor surgical resections to avoid functionally intact brain networks. This will improve postsurgical cognitive outcomes, and will open the benefits of epilepsy surgery to a wider range of patients who might have been excluded because of concerns about cognitive morbidity. Such network information will provide clues as to where seizures are placing their most significant burden on the brain, and where rehabilitation interventions are most needed to facilitate adaptive reorganization. From a neuroscience perspective, characterizing the different patterns of reorganization and abnormal connectivity in epilepsy will have implications for our understanding of maladaptive neural circuit formation and development, and will provide a viable means of predicting the recovery potential of an individual brain.

References

Ahmadi, M. E., Hagler, D. J., Jr., McDonald, C. R., Tecoma, E. S., Iragui, V. J., Dale, A. M., & Halgren, E. (2009). Side matters: Diffusion tensor imaging tractography in left and right temporal lobe epilepsy. *AJNR Am J Neuroradiol, 30*(9), 1740–1747. doi: 10.3174/ajnr.A1650

Alessio, A., Pereira, F. R., Sercheli, M. S., Rondina, J. M., Ozelo, H. B., Bilevicius, E., . . . Cendes, F. (2013). Brain plasticity for verbal and visual memories in patients with mesial temporal lobe epilepsy and hippocampal sclerosis: An fMRI study. *Hum Brain Mapp, 34*(1), 186–199. doi: 10.1002/hbm.21432

Antony, A. R., Alexopoulos, A. V., Gonzalez-Martinez, J. A., Mosher, J. C., Jehi, L., Burgess, R. C., . . . Galan, R. F. (2013). Functional connectivity estimated from intracranial EEG predicts surgical outcome in intractable temporal lobe epilepsy. *PLoS One, 8*(10), e77916. doi: 10.1371/journal.pone.0077916

Arfanakis, K., Hermann, B. P., Rogers, B. P., Carew, J. D., Seidenberg, M., & Meyerand, M. E. (2002). Diffusion tensor MRI in temporal lobe epilepsy. *Magn Reson Imaging, 20*(7), 511–519.

Bartolomei, F., Wendling, F., Regis, J., Gavaret, M., Guye, M., & Chauvel, P. (2004). Pre-ictal synchronicity in limbic networks of mesial temporal lobe epilepsy. *Epilepsy Res, 61*(1–3), 89–104. doi: 10.1016/j.eplepsyres.2004.06.006

Baxendale, S. (2002). The role of functional MRI in the presurgical investigation of temporal lobe epilepsy patients: A clinical perspective and review. *J Clin Exp Neuropsychol, 24*(5), 664–676. doi: 10.1076/jcen.24.5.664.1005

Baxendale, S., Thompson, P. J., & Duncan, J. S. (2008). Evidence-based practice: A reevaluation of the intracarotid amobarbital procedure (Wada test). *Arch Neurol, 65*(6), 841–845. doi: 10.1001/archneur.65.6.841

Ben-Ari, Y., Crepel, V., & Represa, A. (2008). Seizures beget seizures in temporal lobe epilepsies: The boomerang effects of newly formed aberrant kainatergic synapses. *Epilepsy Curr, 8*(3), 68–72. doi: 10.1111/j.1535-7511.2008.00241.x

Bernhardt, B. C., Chen, Z., He, Y., Evans, A. C., & Bernasconi, N. (2011). Graph-theoretical analysis reveals disrupted small-world organization of cortical thickness correlation networks in temporal lobe epilepsy. *Cereb Cortex, 21*(9), 2147–2157. doi: 10.1093/cercor/bhq291

Bettus, G., Bartolomei, F., Confort-Gouny, S., Guedj, E., Chauvel, P., Cozzone, P. J., . . . Guye, M. (2010). Role of resting state functional connectivity MRI in presurgical investigation of mesial temporal lobe epilepsy. *J Neurol Neurosurg Ps, 81*(10), 1147–1154. doi: 10.1136/jnnp.2009.191460

Bettus, G., Guedj, E., Joyeux, F., Confort-Gouny, S., Soulier, E., Laguitton, V., . . . Guye, M. (2009). Decreased basal fMRI functional connectivity in epileptogenic networks and contralateral compensatory mechanisms. *Hum Brain Mapp, 30*(5), 1580–1591. doi: 10.1002/hbm.20625

Binder, J. R., Swanson, S. J., Hammeke, T. A., & Sabsevitz, D. S. (2008). A comparison of five fMRI protocols for mapping speech comprehension systems. *Epilepsia, 49*(12), 1980–1997. doi: 10.1111/j.1528-1167.2008.01683.x

Bonelli, S. B., Powell, R. H., Yogarajah, M., Samson, R. S., Symms, M. R., Thompson, P. J., . . . Duncan, J. S. (2010). Imaging memory in temporal lobe epilepsy: Predicting the effects of temporal lobe resection. *Brain, 133*(Pt 4), 1186–1199. doi: 10.1093/brain/awq006

Bonelli, S. B., Thompson, P. J., Yogarajah, M., Powell, R. H., Samson, R. S., McEvoy, A. W., . . . Duncan, J. S. (2013). Memory reorganization following anterior temporal lobe resection: a longitudinal functional MRI study. *Brain, 136*(Pt 6), 1889–1900. doi: 10.1093/brain/awt105

Bonelli, S. B., Thompson, P. J., Yogarajah, M., Vollmar, C., Powell, R. H., Symms, M. R., . . . Duncan, J. S. (2012). Imaging language networks before and after anterior temporal lobe resection: Results of a longitudinal fMRI study. *Epilepsia, 53*(4), 639–650. doi: 10.1111/j.1528-1167.2012.03433.x

Bonilha, L., Rorden, C., Halford, J. J., Eckert, M., Appenzeller, S., Cendes, F., & Li, L. M. (2007). Asymmetrical extra-hippocampal grey matter loss related to hippocampal atrophy in patients with medial temporal lobe epilepsy. *J Neurol Neurosurg Ps, 78*(3), 286.

Braun, M., Finke, C., Ostendorf, F., Lehmann, T. N., Hoffmann, K. T., & Ploner, C. J. (2008). Reorganization of associative memory in humans with long-standing hippocampal damage. *Brain, 131*(Pt 10), 2742–2750.

Buckner, R. L., Andrews-Hanna, J. R., & Schacter, D. L. (2008). The brain's default network: Anatomy, function, and relevance to disease. *Ann N Y Acad Sci., 1124*, 1–38. doi: 10.1196/annals.1440.011

Cadotte, A. J., Mareci, T. H., DeMarse, T. B., Parekh, M. B., Rajagovindan, R., Ditto, W. L., . . . Carney, P. R. (2009). Temporal lobe epilepsy: Anatomical and effective connectivity. *IEEE T Neur Sys Reh Engineering, 17*(3), 214–223.

Chelune, G. J., Naugle, R. I., Luders, H. O., Sedlak, J., & Awad, I. A. (1993). Individual change after epilepsy surgery: Practice effects and base-rate information. *Neuropsychology, 7*(1), 41–52.

Concha, L., Beaulieu, C., Collins, D. L., & Gross, D. W. (2009). White-matter diffusion abnormalities in temporal-lobe epilepsy with and without mesial temporal sclerosis. *J Neurol Neurosurg Ps, 80*(3), 312–319. doi: 10.1136/jnnp.2007.139287

Corcoran, R., & Thompson, P. (1993). Epilepsy and poor memory: Who complains and what do they mean? *Brit J Clin Psychol, 32*, 199–208.

Cousin, E., Baciu, M., Pichat, C., Kahane, P., & Le Bas, J. F. (2008). Functional MRI evidence for language plasticity in adult epileptic patients: Preliminary results. *Neuropsychiatr Dis Treat, 4*(1), 235–246.

Dallison, A., & Kolb, B. (2003). Recovery from infant medial frontal cortical lesions in rats is reversed by cortical lesions in adulthood. *Behav Brain Res, 146*(1–2), 57–63.

Davies, K. G., Risse, G. L., & Gates, J. R. (2005). Naming ability after tailored left temporal resection with extraoperative language mapping: Increased risk of decline with later epilepsy onset age. *Epilepsy Behav, 7*(2), 273–278. doi: 10.1016/j.yebeh.2005.05.016

Demirtas-Tatlidede, A., Vahabzadeh-Hagh, A. M., Bernabeu, M., Tormos, J. M., & Pascual-Leone, A. (2011). Noninvasive brain stimulation in traumatic brain injury. *J Head Trauma Rehab, 27*(4), 274–292.

Diehl, B., Busch, R. M., Duncan, J. S., Piao, Z., Tkach, J., & Luders, H. O. (2008). Abnormalities in diffusion tensor imaging of the uncinate fasciculus relate to reduced memory in temporal lobe epilepsy. *Epilepsia, 49*(8), 1409–1418. doi: 10.1111/j.1528-1167.2008.01596.x

Dodrill, C. B. (2004). Neuropsychological effects of seizures. *Epilepsy Behav, 5*(Suppl 1), S21–24.

Donner, T. H., & Siegel, M. (2011). A framework for local cortical oscillation patterns. *Trends Cogn Sci, 15*(5), 191–199. doi: 10.1016/j.tics.2011.03.007

Doucet, G., Osipowicz, K., Sharan, A., Sperling, M. R., & Tracy, J. I. (2013a). Extratemporal functional connectivity impairments at rest are related to memory performance in mesial temporal epilepsy. *Hum Brain Mapp, 34*(9), 2202–2216. doi: 10.1002/hbm.22059

Doucet, G., Osipowicz, K., Sharan, A., Sperling, M. R., & Tracy, J. I. (2013b). Hippocampal functional connectivity patterns during spatial working memory differ in right versus left temporal lobe epilepsy. *Brain Connect, 3*(4), 398–406. doi: 10.1089/brain.2013.0158

Doucet, G., Sharan, A., Pustina, D., Skidmore, C., Sperling, M., & Tracy, J. (in press). Early and late age of seizure onset have a differential impact on brain resting-state organization in temporal lobe epilepsy. *Brain Topogr*. doi: 10.1007/s10548-014-0366-6.

Doucet, G., Skidmore, C., Evans, A., Sharan, A., Sperling, M., Pustina, D., & Tracy, J. (2014). Temporal lobe epilepsy and surgery selectively alter the dorsal, not the ventral, default-mode network. *Front Neurol, 5*, 23. doi: 10.3389/fneur.2014.00023

Doucet, G., Skidmore, C., Pustina, D., Sharan, A., Sperling, M., & Tracy, J. (2013). *Effect of age of seizure onset and mesial temporal sclerosis on brain functional organization in temporal lobe epilepsy.* Paper presented at the American Epilepsy Society, Washington, DC.

Elger, C. E., Helmstaedter, C., & Kurthen, M. (2004). Chronic epilepsy and cognition. *Lancet Neurol, 3*(11), 663–672.

Engel, J., Jr. (1992). Recent advances in surgical treatment of temporal lobe epilepsy. *Acta Neurol Scand Suppl, 140*, 71–80.

Englot, D. J., Ouyang, D., Garcia, P. A., Barbaro, N. M., & Chang, E. F. (2012). Epilepsy surgery trends in the United States, 1990–2008. *Neurology, 78*(16), 1200–1206. doi: 10.1212/WNL.0b013e318250d7ea

Fahoum, F., Lopes, R., Pittau, F., Dubeau, F., & Gotman, J. (2012). Widespread epileptic networks in focal epilepsies: EEG-fMRI study. *Epilepsia, 53*(9), 1618–1627. doi: 10.1111/j.1528-1167.2012.03533.x

Farwell, J. R., Dodrill, C. B., & Batzel, L. W. (1985). Neuropsychological abilities of children with epilepsy. *Epilepsia, 26*(5), 395–400.

Figueiredo, P., Santana, I., Teixeira, J., Cunha, C., Machado, E., Sales, F., . . . Castelo-Branco, M. (2008). Adaptive visual memory reorganization in right medial temporal lobe epilepsy. *Epilepsia, 49*(8), 1395–1408. doi: 10.1111/j.1528-1167.2008.01629.x

Friston, K. J., Frith, C. D., Liddle, P. F., & Frackowiak, R. S. (1993). Functional connectivity: The principal-component analysis of large (PET) data sets. *J Cereb Blood Flow Metab, 13*(1), 5–14. doi: 10.1038/jcbfm.1993.4

Goddard, G. V. (1967). Development of epileptic seizures through brain stimulation at low intensity. *Nature, 214*(5092), 1020–1021.

Grant, A. C., Henry, T. R., Fernandez, R., Hill, M. A., & Sathian, K. (2005). Somatosensory processing is impaired in temporal lobe epilepsy. *Epilepsia, 46*(4), 534–539. doi: 10.1111/j.0013-9580.2005.54604.x

Gross, D. W. (2011). Diffusion tensor imaging in temporal lobe epilepsy. *Epilepsia, 52 Suppl 4*, 32–34. doi: 10.1111/j.1528-1167.2011.03149.x

Hamberger, M. J., & Cole, J. (2011). Language organization and reorganization in epilepsy. *Neuropsychol Rev, 21*(3), 240–251. doi: 10.1007/s11065-011-9180-z

Hannesson, D. K., & Corcoran, M. E. (2000). The mnemonic effects of kindling. *Neurosci Biobehav Rev, 24*(7), 725–751.

Haut, K. M., Lim, K. O., & MacDonald, A., III. (2010). Prefrontal cortical changes following cognitive training in patients with chronic schizophrenia: Effects of practice, generalization, and specificity. *Neuropsychopharmacology, 35*(9), 1850–1859. doi: 10.1038/npp.2010.52

Helmstaedter, C. (2004). Neuropsychological aspects of epilepsy surgery. *Epilepsy Behav, 5*(Suppl 1), S45–55.

Helmstaedter, C., Kurthen, M., Linke, D. B., & Elger, C. E. (1994). Right hemisphere restitution of language and memory functions in right hemisphere language-dominant patients with left temporal lobe epilepsy. *Brain, 117*(Pt 4), 729–737.

Helmstaedter, C., Kurthen, M., Lux, S., Reuber, M., & Elger, C. E. (2003). Chronic epilepsy and cognition: A longitudinal study in temporal lobe epilepsy. *Ann Neurol, 54*(4), 425–432. doi: 10.1002/ana.10692

Helmstaedter, C., Loer, B., Wohlfahrt, R., Hammen, A., Saar, J., Steinhoff, B. J., . . . Schulze-Bonhage, A. (2008). The effects of cognitive rehabilitation on memory outcome after temporal lobe epilepsy surgery. *Epilepsy Behav, 12*(3), 402–409. doi: 10.1016/j.yebeh.2007.11.010

Helmstaedter, C., Petzold, I., & Bien, C. G. (2011). The cognitive consequence of resecting nonlesional tissues in epilepsy surgery: Results from MRI- and histopathology-negative patients with temporal lobe epilepsy. *Epilepsia, 52*(8), 1402–1408. doi: 10.1111/j.1528-1167.2011.03157.x

Helmstaedter, C., Sonntag-Dillender, M., Hoppe, C., & Elger, C. E. (2004). Depressed mood and memory impairment in temporal lobe epilepsy as a function of focus lateralization and localization. *Epilepsy Behav, 5*(5), 696 701. doi: 10.1016/j.yebeh.2004.06.008

Hermann, B., Seidenberg, M., & Jones, J. (2008). The neurobehavioural comorbidities of epilepsy: Can a natural history be developed? *Lancet Neurol, 7*(2), 151–160. doi: 10.1016/S1474-4422(08)70018-8

Hermann, B. P., Wyler, A. R., & Richey, E. T. (1988). Wisconsin Card Sorting Test performance in patients with complex partial seizures of temporal-lobe origin. *J Clin Exp Neuropsyc, 10*(4), 467–476.

Hertz-Pannier, L., Chiron, C., Jambaque, I., Renaux-Kieffer, V., Van de Moortele, P. F., Delalande, O., . . . Le Bihan, D. (2002). Late plasticity for language in a child's non-dominant hemisphere: A pre- and post-surgery fMRI study. *Brain, 125*(Pt 2), 361–372.

Hipp, J. F., Hawellek, D. J., Corbetta, M., Siegel, M., & Engel, A. K. (2012). Large-scale cortical correlation structure of spontaneous oscillatory activity. *Nat Neurosci, 15*(6), 884–890. doi: 10.1038/nn.3101

Holtmaat, A., De Paola, V., Wilbrecht, L., & Knott, G. W. (2008). Imaging of experience-dependent structural plasticity in the mouse neocortex in vivo. *Behav Brain Res, 192*(1), 20–25.

Honey, C. J., Kotter, R., Breakspear, M., & Sporns, O. (2007). Network structure of cerebral cortex shapes functional connectivity on multiple time scales. *Proc Natl Acad Sci U S A, 104*(24), 10240–10245. doi: 10.1073/pnas.0701519104

Hughes, J. R. (1985). Long-term clinical and EEG changes in patients with epilepsy. *Arch Neurol, 42*(3), 213–223.

Ives-Deliperi, V. L., & Butler, J. T. (2012). Naming outcomes of anterior temporal lobectomy in epilepsy patients: A systematic review of the literature. *Epilepsy Behav, 24*(2), 194–198. doi: 10.1016/j.yebeh.2012.04.115

Jacobs, K. M., Graber, K. D., Kharazia, V. N., Parada, I., & Prince, D. A. (2000). Postlesional epilepsy: The ultimate brain plasticity. *EPILEPSIA, 41*(Suppl 6), S153–161.

Janszky, J., Rasonyi, G., Clement, Z., Schulz, R., Hoppe, M., Barsi, P., . . . Ebner, A. (2003). Clinical differences in patients with unilateral hippocampal sclerosis and unitemporal or bitemporal epileptiform discharges. *Seizure, 12*(8), 550–554.

Johnston, J. M., Vaishnavi, S. N., Smyth, M. D., Zhang, D., He, B. J., Zempel, J. M., . . . Raichle, M. E. (2008). Loss of resting interhemispheric functional connectivity after complete section of the corpus callosum. *J Neurosci, 28*(25), 6453–6458. doi: 10.1523/JNEUROSCI.0573-08.2008

Jokeit, H., & Ebner, A. (1999). Long term effects of refractory temporal lobe epilepsy on cognitive abilities: A cross sectional study. *J Neurol Neurosurg Ps, 67*(1), 44–50.

Jokeit, H., & Ebner, A. (2002). Effects of chronic epilepsy on intellectual functions. *Prog Brain Res, 135*, 455–463. doi: 10.1016/S0079-6123(02)35042-8

Jokeit, H., Ebner, A., Holthausen, H., Markowitsch, H. J., & Tuxhorn, I. (1996). Reorganization of memory functions after human temporal lobe damage. *Neuroreport, 7*(10), 1627–1630.

Keller, S. S., & Roberts, N. (2008). Voxel-based morphometry of temporal lobe epilepsy: an introduction and review of the literature. *EPILEPSIA, 49*(5), 741–757. doi: 10.1111/j.1528-1167.2007.01485.x

Kemmotsu, N., Girard, H. M., Bernhardt, B. C., Bonilha, L., Lin, J. J., Tecoma, E. S., . . . McDonald, C. R. (2011). MRI analysis in temporal lobe epilepsy: Cortical thinning and white matter disruptions are related to side of seizure onset. *Epilepsia, 52*(12), 2257–2266. doi: 10.1111/j.1528-1167.2011.03278.x

Kim, J. H., Lee, J. M., Kang, E., Kim, J. S., Song, I. C., & Chung, C. K. (2010). Functional reorganization associated with semantic language processing in temporal lobe epilepsy patients after anterior temporal lobectomy: A longitudinal functional magnetic resonance image study. *J Korean Neurosurg Soc, 47*(1), 17–25. doi: 10.3340/jkns.2010.47.1.17

Koorenhof, L., Baxendale, S., Smith, N., & Thompson, P. (2012). Memory rehabilitation and brain training for surgical temporal lobe epilepsy patients: A preliminary report. *Seizure, 21*(3), 178–182. doi: 10.1016/j.seizure.2011.12.001

Koylu, B., Trinka, E., Ischebeck, A., Visani, P., Trieb, T., Kremser, C., . . . Benke, T. (2006). Neural correlates of verbal semantic memory in patients with temporal lobe epilepsy. *Epilepsy Res, 72*(2–3), 178–191. doi: 10.1016/j.eplepsyres.2006.08.002

Kramer, M. A., Eden, U. T., Kolaczyk, E. D., Zepeda, R., Eskandar, E. N., & Cash, S. S. (2010). Coalescence and fragmentation of cortical networks during focal seizures. *J Neurosci, 30*(30), 10076–10085. doi: 10.1523/JNEUROSCI.6309-09.2010

Lefaucheur, J. P. (2009). Treatment of Parkinson's disease by cortical stimulation. *Expert Rev Neurother, 9*(12), 1755–1771.

Liacu, D., Idy-Peretti, I., Ducreux, D., Bouilleret, V., & de Marco, G. (2012). Diffusion tensor imaging tractography parameters of limbic system bundles in temporal lobe epilepsy patients. *J Magn Reson Imaging, 36*(3), 561–568. doi: 10.1002/jmri.23678

Liao, W., Zhang, Z., Pan, Z., Mantini, D., Ding, J., Duan, X., . . . Chen, H. (2010). Altered functional connectivity and small-world in mesial temporal lobe epilepsy. *PloS One, 5*(1), e8525. doi: 10.1371/journal.pone.0008525

Lineweaver, T. T., Morris, H. H., Naugle, R. I., Najm, I. M., Diehl, B., & Bingaman, W. (2006). Evaluating the contributions of state-of-the-art assessment techniques to predicting memory outcome after unilateral anterior temporal lobectomy. *Epilepsia, 47*(11), 1895–1903. doi: 10.1111/j.1528-1167.2006.00807.x

Loring, D. W., Meador, K. J., Lee, G. P., Murro, A. M., Smith, J. R., Flanigin, H. F., . . . King, D. W. (1990). Cerebral language lateralization: evidence from intracarotid amobarbital testing. *Neuropsychologia, 28*(8), 831–838.

Luo, C., Li, Q., Lai, Y., Xia, Y., Qin, Y., Liao, W., . . . Gong, Q. (2011). Altered functional connectivity in default mode network in absence epilepsy: A resting state fMRI study. *Hum Brain Mapp, 32*(3), 438–439.

Lutz, M. T., Clusmann, H., Elger, C. E., Schramm, J., & Helmstaedter, C. (2004). Neuropsychological outcome after selective amygdalohippocampectomy with transsylvian versus transcortical approach: A randomized prospective clinical trial of surgery for temporal lobe epilepsy. *Epilepsia, 45*(7), 809–816. doi: 10.1111/j.0013-9580.2004.54003.x

Martin, R., Sawrie, S., Edwards, R., Roth, D., Kuzniecky, R., Morawetz, R., & Gilliam, F. (2000). Investigation of executive function change following anterior temporal lobectomy: Selective normalization of verbal fluency. *Neuropsychology, 14*(4), 501–508.

Martin, R. C., Sawrie, S. M., Edwards, R., Roth, D. L., Faught, E., Kuzniecky, R. I., . . . Gilliam, F. G. (2000). Investigation of executive function change following anterior temporal lobectomy: Selective normalization of verbal fluency. *Neuropsychology, 14*(4), 501–508.

May, A. (2011). Experience-dependent structural plasticity in the adult human brain. *Trends Cogn Sci, 15*(10), 475–482.

McCarthy, R. J., O'Connor, M. J., & Sperling, M. R. (1997). The mirror focus phenomenon and secondary epileptogenesis in human epilepsy. *J Epilepsy, 10*(2), 78–85.

McClelland, J. L. (2001). Failures to learn and their remediation: A Hebbian account. In J. L. McClelland & R. S. Siegler (Eds.), *Mechanisms of cognitive development: Behavioral and neural perspectives* (pp. 97–121). Mahwah, NJ: Lawrence Erlbaum Associates.

McCormick, C., Quraan, M., Cohn, M., Valiante, T. A., & McAndrews, M. P. (2013). Default mode network connectivity indicates episodic memory capacity in mesial temporal lobe epilepsy. *Epilepsia, 54*(5), 809–818. doi: 10.1111/epi.12098

McGill, M. L., Devinsky, O., Kelly, C., Milham, M., Castellanos, F. X., Quinn, B. T., . . . Thesen, T. (2012). Default mode network abnormalities in idiopathic generalized epilepsy. *Epilepsy Behav, 23*(3), 353–359. doi: 10.1016/j.yebeh.2012.01.013

Meinzer, M., Harnish, S., Conway, T., & Crosson, B. (2011). Recent developments in functional and structural imaging of aphasia recovery after stroke. *Aphasiology, 25*(3), 271–290.

Morgan, V. L., Rogers, B. P., Sonmezturk, H. H., Gore, J. C., & Abou-Khalil, B. (2011). Cross hippocampal influence in mesial temporal lobe epilepsy measured with high temporal resolution functional magnetic resonance imaging. *Epilepsia, 52*(9), 1741–1749. doi: 10.1111/j.1528-1167.2011.03196.x

Morrell, F., & deToledo-Morrell, L. (1999). From mirror focus to secondary epileptogenesis in man: An historical review. *Adv Neurol, 81*, 11–23.

Morrell, F., Rasmussen, T., Gloor, P., & De Toledo-Morrell, L. (1983). Secondary epileptogenic foci in patients with verified temporal lobe tumors. *Eletroencephalogr Clin Neurophysiol, 54*, 26.

Negishi, M., Martuzzi, R., Novotny, E. J., Spencer, D. D., & Constable, R. T. (2011). Functional MRI connectivity as a predictor of the surgical outcome of epilepsy. *Epilepsia, 52*(9), 1733–1740. doi: 10.1111/j.1528-1167.2011.03191.x

Netoff, T. I., Clewley, R., Arno, S., Keck, T., & White, J. A. (2004). Epilepsy in small-world networks. *J Neurosci, 24*(37), 8075–8083. doi: 10.1523/JNEUROSCI.1509-04.2004

Noppeney, U., Price, C. J., Duncan, J. S., & Koepp, M. J. (2005). Reading skills after left anterior temporal lobe resection: An fMRI study. *Brain, 128*(Pt 6), 1377–1385. doi: 10.1093/brain/awh414

Osipowicz, K., Pajor, N., Sharan, A., Skidmore, C., Sperling, M., & Tracy, J. (under review). The effects of interictal seizure burden on white matter in temporal lobe epilepsy.

Osipowicz, K., Sharan, A., Sperling, M., & Tracy, J. (under review). Combined fMRI, rsfMRI, and DTI analysis of language recovery and neuroplasticity following anterior temporal lobectomy.

Osipowicz, K., Sperling, M., Sharan, A., & Tracy, J. (2014). fMRI, resting-state, and DTI changes predict verbal fluency outcome following resective surgery for temporal lobe epilepsy. *J Neurosurg*, in press.

Otte, W. M., van Eijsden, P., Sander, J. W., Duncan, J. S., Dijkhuizen, R. M., & Braun, K. P. (2012). A meta-analysis of white matter changes in temporal lobe epilepsy as studied with diffusion tensor imaging. *Epilepsia, 53*(4), 659–667. doi: 10.1111/j.1528-1167.2012.03426.x

Pereira, F. R., Alessio, A., Sercheli, M. S., Pedro, T., Bilevicius, E., Rondina, J. M., . . . Cendes, F. (2010). Asymmetrical hippocampal connectivity in mesial temporal lobe epilepsy: Evidence from resting state fMRI. *BMC Neurosci, 11*, 66. doi: 10.1186/1471-2202-11-66

Pittau, F., Grova, C., Moeller, F., Dubeau, F., & Gotman, J. (2012). Patterns of altered functional connectivity in mesial temporal lobe epilepsy. *Epilepsia, 53*(6), 1013–1023. doi: 10.1111/j.1528-1167.2012.03464.x

Poldrack, R. A. (2000). Imaging brain plasticity: Conceptual and methodological issues—a theoretical review. *NeuroImage, 12*(1), 1–13. doi: 10.1006/nimg.2000.0596

Ponten, S. C., Bartolomei, F., & Stam, C. J. (2007). Small-world networks and epilepsy: Graph theoretical analysis of intracerebrally recorded mesial temporal lobe seizures. *Clin Neurophysiol, 118*(4), 918–927. doi: 10.1016/j.clinph.2006.12.002

Potter, J. L., Schefft, B. K., Beebe, D. W., Howe, S. R., Yeh, H. S., & Privitera, M. D. (2009). Presurgical neuropsychological testing predicts cognitive and seizure outcomes after anterior temporal lobectomy. *Epilepsy Behav, 16*(2), 246–253. doi: 10.1016/j.yebeh.2009.07.007

Powell, H. W., Richardson, M. P., Symms, M. R., Boulby, P. A., Thompson, P. J., Duncan, J. S., & Koepp, M. J. (2007). Reorganization of verbal and nonverbal memory in temporal lobe epilepsy due to unilateral hippocampal sclerosis. *Epilepsia, 48*(8), 1512–1525. doi: 10.1111/j.1528-1167.2007.01053.x

Powell, H. W., Richardson, M. P., Symms, M. R., Boulby, P. A., Thompson, P. J., Duncan, J. S., & Koepp, M. J. (2008). Preoperative fMRI predicts memory decline following anterior temporal lobe resection. *J Neurol Neurosurg Ps, 79*(6), 686–693. doi: 10.1136/jnnp.2007.115139

Pustina, D., Doucet, G., Evans, J., Sharan, A., Skidmore, C., Sperling, M., & Tracy, J. (in press). Genuine and artifactual white matter plasticity following anterior temporal lobectomy in epilepsy, *PlosONE* D-13-48548R3, doi: 10.1371/journal.pone.0104211

Quigg, M., Broshek, D. K., Barbaro, N. M., Ward, M. M., Laxer, K. D., Yan, G., & Lamborn, K. (2011). Neuropsychological outcomes after Gamma Knife radiosurgery for mesial temporal lobe epilepsy: A prospective multicenter study. *Epilepsia, 52*(5), 909–916. doi: 10.1111/j.1528-1167.2011.02987.x

Rabin, M. L., Narayan, V. M., Kimberg, D. Y., Casasanto, D. J., Glosser, G., Tracy, J. I., . . . Detre, J. A. (2004). Functional MRI predicts post-surgical memory following temporal lobectomy. *Brain, 127*(Pt 10), 2286–2298. doi: 10.1093/brain/awh281

Ranganath, C., Heller, A., Cohen, M. X., Brozinsky, C. J., & Rissman, J. (2005). Functional connectivity with the hippocampus during successful memory formation. *Hippocampus, 15*(8), 997–1005. doi: 10.1002/hipo.20141

Raol, Y. S., Budreck, E. C., & Brooks-Kayal, A. R. (2003). Epilepsy after early-life seizures can be independent of hippocampal injury. *Ann Neurol, 53*(4), 503–511. doi: 10.1002/ana.10490

Rausch, R., Kraemer, S., Pietras, C. J., Le, M., Vickrey, B. G., & Passaro, E. A. (2003). Early and late cognitive changes following temporal lobe surgery for epilepsy. *Neurology, 60*(6), 951–959.

Richardson, M. P., Strange, B. A., Duncan, J. S., & Dolan, R. J. (2003). Preserved verbal memory function in left medial temporal pathology involves reorganisation of function to right medial temporal lobe. *Neuroimage, 20*(Suppl 1), S112–119.

Riederer, F., Lanzenberger, R., Kaya, M., Prayer, D., Serles, W., & Baumgartner, C. (2008). Network atrophy in temporal lobe epilepsy. *Neurology, 71*(6), 419.

Rodrigo, S., Oppenheim, C., Chassoux, F., Golestani, N., Cointepas, Y., Poupon, C., . . . Meder, J. F. (2007). Uncinate fasciculus fiber tracking in mesial temporal lobe epilepsy: Initial findings. *Eur Radiol, 17*(7), 1663–1668. doi: 10.1007/s00330-006-0558-x

Rosenberger, L. R., Zeck, J., Berl, M. M., Moore, E. N., Ritzl, E. K., Shamim, S., . . . Gaillard, W. D. (2009). Interhemispheric and intrahemispheric language reorganization in complex partial epilepsy. *Neurology, 72*(21), 1830–1836. doi: 10.1212/WNL.0b013e3181a7114b

Rubinov, M., Sporns, O., van Leeuwen, C., & Breakspear, M. (2009). Symbiotic relationship between brain structure and dynamics. *BMC Neurosci, 10*, 55. doi: 10.1186/1471-2202-10-55

Sampaio, L., Yacubian, E. M., & Manreza, M. L. (2004). The role of mirror focus in the surgical outcome of patients with indolent temporal lobe tumors. *Arq Neuro-Psiquiat, 62*(1), 9–14.

Schindler, K. A., Bialonski, S., Horstmann, M. T., Elger, C. E., & Lehnertz, K. (2008). Evolving functional network properties and synchronizability during human epileptic seizures. *Chaos, 18*(3), 033119. doi: 10.1063/1.2966112

Schneider-Mizell, C. M., Caboclo, L. O., Parent, J. M., Ben-Jacob, E., Zochowski, M. R., & Sander, L. M. (2010). From network structure to network reorganization: Implications for adult neurogenesis. *Phys Biol, 7*(4), 046008. doi: 10.1088/1478-3975/7/4/046008

Schwartzkroin, P. A. (2001). Mechanisms of brain plasticity: From normal brain function to pathology. In J. Engel, P. A. Schwartzkroin, S. L. Moshe, & D. H. Lowenstein (Eds.), *Brain plasticity and epilepsy* (pp. 1–15). San Diego, CA: Academic Press.

Seidenberg, M., Hermann, B. P., Schoenfeld, J., Davies, K., Wyler, A., & Dohan, F. C. (1997). Reorganization of verbal memory function in early onset left temporal lobe epilepsy. *Brain Cogn, 35*(1), 132–148. doi: 10.1006/brcg.1997.0931

Shimizu, T., Nariai, T., Maehara, T., Hino, T., Komori, T., Shimizu, H., . . . Senda, M. (2000). Enhanced motor cortical excitability in the unaffected hemisphere after hemispherectomy. *Neuroreport, 11*(14), 3077–3084.

Shulman, M. B. (2000). The frontal lobes, epilepsy, and behavior. *Epilepsy Behav, 1*(6), 384–395.

Somera-Molina, K. C., Robin, B., Somera, C. A., Anderson, C., Stine, C., Koh, S., . . . Wainwright, M. S. (2007). Glial activation links early-life seizures and long-term neurologic dysfunction: Evidence using a small molecule inhibitor of proinflammatory cytokine upregulation. *Epilepsia, 48*(9), 1785–1800. doi: 10.1111/j.1528-1167.2007.01135.x

Springer, J. A., Binder, J. R., Hammeke, T. A., Swanson, S. J., Frost, J. A., Bellgowan, P. S., . . . Mueller, W. M. (1999). Language dominance in neurologically normal and epilepsy subjects: A functional MRI study. *Brain, 122 (Pt 11)*, 2033–2046.

Staba, R. J., Ekstrom, A. D., Suthana, N. A., Burggren, A., Fried, I., Engel, J., Jr., & Bookheimer, S. Y. (2012). Gray matter loss correlates with mesial temporal lobe neuronal hyperexcitability inside the human seizure-onset zone. *Epilepsia, 53*(1), 25–34. doi: 10.1111/j.1528-1167.2011.03333.x

Stein, D. G., & Hoffman, S. W. (2003). Concepts of CNS plasticity in the context of brain damage and repair. *J Head Trauma Rehab, 18*(4), 317–341.

Stern, Y. (2007). *Cognitive reserve, theory and application.* New York: Taylor & Francis.

Strauss, E., Hunter, M., & Wada, J. (1993). Wisconsin card sorting performance: Effects of age of onset of damage and laterality of dysfunction. *J Clin Exp Neuropsyc, 15*, 896–902.

Sutula, T. P. (2004). Mechanisms of epilepsy progression: Current theories and perspectives from neuroplasticity in adulthood and development. *Epilepsy Res, 60*(2–3), 161–171. doi: 10.1016/j.eplepsyres.2004.07.001

Sutula, T. P., & Dudek, F. E. (2007). Unmasking recurrent excitation generated by mossy fiber sprouting in the epileptic dentate gyrus: An emergent property of a complex system. *Prog Brain Res, 163*, 541–563. doi: 10.1016/S0079-6123(07)63029-5

Takaya, S., Mikuni, N., Mitsueda, T., Satow, T., Taki, J., Kinoshita, M., . . . Fukuyama, H. (2009). Improved cerebral function in mesial temporal lobe epilepsy after subtemporal amygdalohippocampectomy. *Brain, 132*(Pt 1), 185–194. doi: 10.1093/brain/awn218

Thivard, L., Lehericy, S., Krainik, A., Adam, C., Dormont, D., Chiras, J., . . . Dupont, S. (2005). Diffusion tensor imaging in medical temporal lobe epilepsy with hippocampal sclerosis. *NeuroImage, 28*(3), 682–690.

Tracy, J. I., & Boswell, S. (2008). Modeling the interaction between language and memory: The case of temporal lobe epilepsy. In B. S. H. Whitaker (Ed.), *Handbook of the neuroscience of language* (pp. 319–328). San Diego, CA: Academic Press.

Tracy, J. I., Flanders, A., Madi, S., Laskas, J., Stoddard, E., Pyrros, A., . . . DelVecchio, N. (2003). Regional brain activation associated with different performance patterns during learning of a complex motor skill. *Cereb Cortex, 13*(9), 904–910.

Tracy, J. I., Osipowicz, K., Spechler, P., Sharan, A., Skidmore, C., Doucet, G., & Sperling, M. R. (2014). Functional connectivity evidence of cortico-cortico inhibition in temporal lobe epilepsy. *Hum Brain Mapp, 35*(1), 353–366. doi: 10.1002/hbm.22181

Tracy, J. I., Osipowicz, K., Stamos, C., & Berman, A. (2010). Epilepsy and cognitive plasticity. In C. Amstrong & L. Morrow (Eds.), *The neuropsychology of medical disorders* (pp. 3–16). New York: Springer.

Tracy, J. I., & Osipowicz, K. Z. (2011). A conceptual framework for interpreting neuroimaging studies of brain neuroplasticity and cognitive recovery. *NeuroRehabilitation, 29*(4), 331–338. doi: 10.3233/NRE-2011-0709

Tracy, J. I., Waldron, B., Glosser, D., Sharan, A., Mintzer, S., Zangaladze, A., . . . Sperling, M. R. (2009). Hemispheric lateralization and language skill coherence in temporal lobe epilepsy. *Cortex, 45*(10), 1178–1189. doi: 10.1016/j.cortex.2009.01.007

Trenerry, M., Jack, C., & Ivnik, R. (1993). MRI hippocampal volumes and memory function before and after temporal lobectomy. *Neurology, 43*, 1800–1805.

van Dellen, E., Douw, L., Baayen, J. C., Heimans, J. J., Ponten, S. C., Vandertop, W. P., . . . Reijneveld, J. C. (2009). Long-term effects of temporal lobe epilepsy on local neural networks: A graph theoretical analysis of corticography recordings. *PLoS One, 4*(11), e8081. doi: 10.1371/journal.pone.0008081

Vannest, J., Szaflarski, J. P., Privitera, M. D., Schefft, B. K., & Holland, S. K. (2008). Medial temporal fMRI activation reflects memory lateralization and memory performance in patients with epilepsy. *Epilepsy Behav, 12*(3), 410–418. doi: 10.1016/j.yebeh.2007.11.012

Vargha-Khadem, F., Carr, L. J., Isaacs, E., Brett, E., Adams, C., & Mishkin, M. (1997). Onset of speech after left hemispherectomy in a nine-year-old boy. *Brain, 120 (Pt 1)*, 159–182.

Voets, N. L., Adcock, J. E., Stacey, R., Hart, Y., Carpenter, K., Matthews, P. M., & Beckmann, C. F. (2009). Functional and structural changes in the memory network associated with left temporal lobe epilepsy. *Hum Brain Mapp, 30*(12), 4070–4081. doi: 10.1002/hbm.20830

Wada, J. A., & Mizoguchi, T. (1984). Limbic kindling in the forebrain-bisected photosensitive baboon, Papio papio. *Epilepsia, 25*(3), 278–287.

Wagner, K., Frings, L., Halsband, U., Everts, R., Buller, A., Spreer, J., . . . Schulze-Bonhage, A. (2007). Hippocampal functional connectivity reflects verbal episodic memory network integrity. *Neuroreport, 18*(16), 1719–1723. doi: 10.1097/WNR.0b013e3282f0d3c5

Waites, A. B., Briellmann, R. S., Saling, M. M., Abbott, D. F., & Jackson, G. D. (2006). Functional connectivity networks are disrupted in left temporal lobe epilepsy. *Ann Neurol, 59*(2), 335–343.

Wang, Z., Lu, G., Zhang, Z., Zhong, Y., Jiao, Q., Tan, Q., . . . Liu, Y. (2011). Altered resting state networks in epileptic patients with generalized tonic-conic seizures. *Brain Research, 1374*, 134–141.

Wechsler, D. (1997). *Wechsler Memory Scale, third edition.* San Antonio, TX: The Psychological Corporation.

Wilke, M., Pieper, T., Lindner, K., Dushe, T., Staudt, M., Grodd, W., . . . Krageloh-Mann, I. (2011). Clinical functional MRI of the language domain in children with epilepsy. *Hum Brain Mapp, 32*(11), 1882–1893. doi: 10.1002/hbm.21156

Wong, S. W., Jong, L., Bandur, D., Bihari, F., Yen, Y. F., Takahashi, A. M., . . . Mirsattari, S. M. (2009). Cortical reorganization following anterior temporal lobectomy in patients with temporal lobe epilepsy. *Neurology, 73*(7), 518–525. doi: 10.1212/WNL.0b013e3181b2a48e

Xiong, Y., Mahmood, A., & Chopp, M. (2010). Neurorestorative treatments for traumatic brain injury. *Discovery medicine, 10*(54), 434–442.

Yogarajah, M., Focke, N. K., Bonelli, S. B., Thompson, P., Vollmar, C., McEvoy, A. W., . . . Duncan, J. S. (2010). The structural plasticity of white matter networks following anterior temporal lobe resection. *Brain, 133*(Pt 8), 2348–2364. doi: 10.1093/brain/awq175

Yogarajah, M., Powell, H. W., Parker, G. J., Alexander, D. C., Thompson, P. J., Symms, M. R., . . . Duncan, J. S. (2008). Tractography of the parahippocampal gyrus and material specific memory impairment in unilateral temporal lobe epilepsy. *Neuroimage, 40*(4), 1755–1764. doi: 10.1016/j.neuroimage.2007.12.046

Zhang, Z., Liao, W., Chen, H., Mantini, D., Ding, J. R., Xu, Q., . . . Lu, G. (2011). Altered functional-structural coupling of large-scale brain networks in idiopathic generalized epilepsy. *Brain, 134*(Pt 10), 2912–2928. doi: 10.1093/brain/awr223

Zhang, Z., Lu, G., Zhong, Y., Tan, Q., Liao, W., Chen, Z., . . . Liu, Y. (2009). Impaired perceptual networks in temporal lobe epilepsy revealed by resting fMRI. *J Neurol, 256*(10), 1705–1713. doi: 10.1007/s00415-009-5187-2

Zhang, Z., Lu, G., Zhong, Y., Tan, Q., Liao, W., Wang, Z., . . . Liu, Y. (2010). Altered spontaneous neuronal activity of the default-mode network in mesial temporal lobe epilepsy. *Brain Res, 1323*, 152–160. doi: 10.1016/j.brainres.2010.01.042

Zhang, Z., Lu, G., Zhong, Y., Tan, Q., Yang, Z., Liao, W., . . . Liu, Y. (2009). Impaired attention network in temporal lobe epilepsy: A resting fMRI study. *Neurosci Lett, 458*(3), 97–101. doi: 10.1016/j.neulet.2009.04.040

3

Neuroplastic Mechanisms of Language Recovery After Stroke

Stephen E. Nadeau

Introduction

Language recovery after stroke depends on (1) mechanisms underlying spontaneous recovery, subsumable under the rubric of reactive neuroplasticity, and (2) normal learning mechanisms engaged not only by the speech-language therapist but also by family and friends who help to drive the long-term therapeutic process—processes definable as experience-dependent neuroplasticity. This chapter begins with a brief consideration of mechanisms underlying reactive and experience-dependent neuroplasticity. In ensuing sections, I review evidence of the amount of language recovery that is attributable to reactivity neuroplasticity and the amount that has been achievable with current techniques engaging experience-dependent neuroplasticity. This leads inevitably to the therapeutic challenge of achieving generalization of speech-language therapy—generalization not just to untrained exemplars but also to daily verbal communicative life. To understand the potential opportunities for generalization requires an understanding of neural network processes supporting language function. With this background in mind, I then consider two highly innovative therapies for anomia (the most common and disabling component of aphasia) that are leveraged on intrinsic mechanisms and that offer the potential for broad generalization, one phonologic and one semantic. I conclude with a consideration of potential brain mechanisms for generalization, taking the broadest possible perspective.

This journey serves to delineate in a more precise way the opportunities that lie before us for achieving greater language recovery after stroke. To take advantage of these opportunities, two things are essential: (1) a better understanding of the neurobiology of recovery from stroke, and (2) a wedding of speech-language therapy development to brain mechanisms, particularly those expressed at the neural network level.

Reactive and Experience-Dependent Neuroplasticity

Reactive neuroplasticity consists of reduction in necrotic and apoptotic cell death, angiogenesis, neurogenesis, neural migration, axonal growth, remyelination, expansion of dendritic spines, and synaptogenesis (Iadecola & Anrather, 2011; Wieloch & Nikolich, 2006). Several of these processes likely underlie the resolution of diaschisis—the transient loss of function of brain regions connected to the area of injury. Reactive neuroplasticity is maximal in the weeks following brain injury. It is likely responsible for most of what we commonly refer to as spontaneous recovery from stroke, though of course, during the time that reactive plasticity is maximal, patients are also engaging mechanisms of experience-dependent neuroplasticity, both in formal speech therapy and in therapy associated with attempted conversation with family and friends (McClung, Rothi, & Nadeau, 2010).

Experience-dependent neuroplasticity involves normal learning mechanisms, including non-declarative memory acquisition (e.g., procedural memory), which takes place directly in the neural structures supporting the functions involved, and declarative memory acquisition, which depends upon the hippocampus and associated mesial temporal structures. It predominantly involves the genesis of dendritic spines, synaptogenesis, and modification of existing synapses (Dancause & Nudo, 2011). Neurorehabilitation most explicitly targets experience-dependent neuroplasticity. Its impact on reactive neuroplasticity is largely unknown.

Both reactive and experience-dependent neuroplasticity involved in language recovery also reflect the degree to which neural networks unaffected by the stroke (most notably those in the right hemisphere) contain redundant language knowledge. This knowledge may become manifest during spontaneous recovery in the process of resolution of diaschisis (Feeney & Baron, 1986; Finger, Koehler, & Jagella, 2004; von Monakow, 1914; Weber et al., 2008; Witte, Bidmon, Schiene, Redecker, & Hagemann, 2000), but the neural networks supporting it also provide the substrate for language relearning during the engagement of mechanisms of experience-dependent neuroplasticity. The mechanisms underlying diaschisis are not well understood, but one prime candidate that is fully consonant with von Monakow's (1914) ideas derives from the fact that cortical neurons normally enjoy steady input that drives a low-level background-firing rate ("noise"). Only modest increases in input are then needed to elicit the higher firing rates that constitute signal. However, for neurons deprived of major sources of input because of acute or subacute stroke, much greater input firing rates are needed to elicit signal. This is also likely the case for right hemisphere neurons that are the recipients of transcallosal afferents from left hemisphere language regions. However, eventually, with synaptic modification, the mechanisms of which are largely unknown, the loss of input is compensated, and surviving neurons in both hemispheres regain their normal sensitivity to input. Resolution of diaschisis is emerging as a major, and perhaps the most important, factor underlying early recovery of cognitive function following stroke (Weber et al., 2008).

The Extent of Language Recovery That Can Be Attributed to Reactive Neuroplasticity

Studies providing data on spontaneous recovery of language function after stroke are detailed in Table 3.1. With few exceptions, the patients in these studies were right-handed, and most had experienced a single left hemisphere ischemic stroke. The outcome measures used often reflected not just verbal language production and auditory verbal comprehension but also other linguistic functions such as reading and writing. Many patients had undergone speech-language therapy. However, because none of these studies employed therapy that was likely to generalize to untrained stimuli, and in particular to performance on the outcome measures used, I will assume that these data reflect predominantly, if not exclusively, spontaneous recovery. Notably, none of the patients in the study by Mazzoni et al. (1992) had undergone speech-language therapy, yet the gains in function they exhibited were not obviously different from those observed in other studies in which some (Kertesz & McCabe, 1977) or nearly all (Demeurisse et al., 1980; Lazar, Speizer, Festa, Krakauer, & Marshall, 2008; Nicholas, Helm-Estabrooks, Ward-Longergan, & Morgan, 1993) had received such therapy.

The heterogeneity of the patients in these studies and in the outcome measures used, and the variability in time of assessment, particularly in the days and weeks immediately following stroke, when rapid changes are occurring, preclude detailed analysis. However, several things are apparent. First, gains in function over the first 6 months are dramatic, in many studies yielding close to a doubling of performance. The study by Nicholas et al. (1993) shows that even among patients with severe aphasia, substantial further recovery occurs between 6 and 24 months (see also Hanson, Metter, & Riege, 1989). Thus, there is a great danger of misinterpreting gains in function during aphasia treatment trials as reflecting solely the effects of treatment. Only randomized controlled trials (RCTs) or trials conducted with very chronic patients can transcend this problem. A recent RCT of the treatment of 170 subjects completed within 6 months of acute stroke failed to demonstrate any difference in outcome with communication therapy (mainly impairment focused) compared with similarly resourced social contact (Bowen et al., 2012; see also Brady, Kelly, Godwin, & Enderby, 2012). Conflation of early gains in function due to reactive neuroplasticity with gains due to treatment has no doubt contributed to the widespread perception that behavioral therapy is best administered early. The effect of the timing of speech-language therapy in relation to stroke has never been adequately tested. Recent phase III trials of upper extremity therapy (3–9 months versus 15–21 months) (Wolf et al., 2006, 2010) and lower extremity therapy (2–5 months versus 6–9 months) (Duncan et al., 2011), directed at improving motor function, have shown that long-term outcome is the same, regardless of the timing of therapy. On the other hand, in the meta-analyses conducted by Robey (1994, 1998), the difference in effect size between treated and untreated individuals was somewhat greater for treatment conducted during the first 3–4 months than for treatment conducted in more chronic phases of stroke.

TABLE 3.1 Spontaneous Language Recovery Following Acute Left Hemisphere Stroke

Study	Outcome metric	Aphasia type	N	<3 d	<2 wks.	<45 d	3 mos.	6 mos.	12 mos.	18 mos.	24 mos.
								Mean outcome score			
Kertesz & McCabe (1977)	WAB[1]	Global	10			22.8	33.7	31.6			
		Broca's	4			35.6	72.4	73.3			
		Conduction	4			60.5	95.4				
		Wernicke's	4			34	48.9				
		Anomic	14			76.9	84.8				
Demeurisse et al. (1980)	Study specific[2]	Global	9		0		3	3			
		Expression			0		6.7	7			
		Comprehension									
		Broca's	46		12.5		25	30.4			
		Expression			43.2		59	61.2			
		Comprehension									
		Wernicke's	20		19.2		42.7	47.3			
		Expression			35.1		56.5	60.5			
		Comprehension									
Mazzoni et al. (1992)	Basso scale (Basso, Capitani, & Vignolo, 1979)[3]	Fluent	23		1.0		1.9	2.2			
		Expression			2.2		3.5	3.6			
		Comprehension									
		Non-fluent	22		0.7		1.2	1.3			
		Expression			1.8		3.4	3.5			
		Comprehension									
		Moderate	21		1.8		2.9	3.2			
		Expression			3.5		4	4			
		Comprehension									
		Severe	24		0		0.3	0.5			
		Expression			0.7		30	3.3			
		Comprehension									
Nicholas et al. (1993)	Boston Assessment of Severe Aphasia[4]	Severe aphasia (nearly all global)	24			22.9		29.6	36.6		40.0

Study	Test	Subgroup							
Laska et al. (2001)	ANELT[5]	All	70		2.0		4.6	4.6	4.6
		Conduction	15		4.2		4.9	5.0	5.0
		Wernicke's	19		1.0		4.2	4.1	4.0
		Global	8		0		1.2	1.1	1.3
Lazar et al. (2008)	BDAE/WAB[6]	Total	22	19.6			25.2		
		Comprehension		6.6			8.6		
		Naming		6.8			8.2		
		Repetition		6.3			8.4		
El Hachioui et al. (2013)	Token Test[7]		147	17	20	25	27	27	27

[1] Western Aphasia Battery (Kertesz, 1982).

[2] Expression: two 7-point Likert scales, one for Broca's, one for Wernicke's; comprehension: one 5-point Likert scale; total score possible for each functional domain = 100.

[3] 4-point Likert scale for expression and comprehension.

[4] Helm-Estabrooks (Helm-Estabrooks, Ramsberger, Morgan, & Nicholas, 1989).

[5] Amsterdam-Nijmegen Everyday Language Test of verbal communication: 5-point Likert scale (Blomert, Kean, Koster, & Schokker, 1994).

[6] Boston Diagnostic Aphasia Exam/Western Aphasia Battery (Goodglass & Kaplan, 2000; Kertesz, 1982). Each domain score scaled to 10 points; maximum total score (summed over three domains) = 30.

[7] Token Test (De Renzi & Faglioni, 1978): Maximum score 36.

Robey's results notwithstanding, it is also worth considering the fact that allowing spontaneous recovery to occur and diaschisis to resolve before initiating treatment may substantially expand the linguistic substrate for treatment.

Second, it is evident that comprehension is always better preserved than production. This may reflect the fact that comprehension is intrinsically easier: context may aid comprehension and a near miss may suffice, whereas any deviation in production is likely to constitute an error. It may also reflect the likelihood that networks unaffected by a perisylvian lesion in the left hemisphere (e.g., those supporting semantic function) and in the intact right hemisphere may rapidly become available to subserve comprehension. Studies of patients who have undergone corpus callosotomy or complete commissurotomy have shown that although the isolated right hemisphere consistently demonstrates impoverished phonology and grammar (at least in English; see Nadeau, 2012), it supports a rich lexical semantic system. It also supports substantial capacity for auditory comprehension and, to a lesser extent, visual word recognition. Finally, it supports competence in comprehension of affective prosody and facial expression accompanying verbal communication (Zaidel, Iacoboni, Berman, Zaidel, & Bogen, 2012; see also Nadeau, 2010). The inverse relationship between language recovery and lesion size is a measure of the degree to which spontaneous recovery depends on left hemisphere mechanisms (Cherney & Robey, 2008).

Third, expression and comprehension improve more or less in parallel. Given the substantial differences in mechanisms supporting language comprehension and expression, this suggests that mechanisms most active in spontaneous language recovery are largely nonspecific (e.g., resolution of diaschisis). Given the magnitude of change in language function attributable to spontaneous recovery, neurobiological measures that only modestly enhance reactive neuroplasticity could provide major benefits to patients.

Experience-Dependent Neuroplasticity: Conventional Speech-Language Therapy

One of the most common and debilitating features of aphasia is impairment in the ability to retrieve words, whether it involves naming seen objects or producing nouns, verbs, and other words conveying meaning in spontaneous propositional language (Goodglass, 1993). Consequently, treatment of anomia will be the singular focus of this chapter. There have been over 160 trials of treatment for anomia following stroke (see www.u.arizona.edu/~pelagie/ancds/index.html). These have employed a variety of strategies but most have focused on training object naming in conjunction with further development of semantic or phonological feature knowledge, sometimes both (see Nickels, 2002, for a landmark review of single subject trials). The effectiveness of these approaches has been quantitatively assessed in a recent meta-analysis of 44 studies involving two or more subjects, most of whom were treated more than 6 months after stroke (Wisenburn &

Mahoney, 2009). The unbiased effect size for the entire corpus of treated words was 2.66 (SD 3.23).[1] However, the effect size for items to which the subjects had never been exposed was only 0.44 (SD 0.33), *whether or not these items were related semantically or phonologically to trained exemplars*. The effect sizes for exposed items were 1.73 (SD 1.06) for related words and 1.78 (SD 2.02) for unrelated words, indicating that mere repeated exposure to picture-word pairs through the course of extended treatment can improve the naming of these words, regardless of the relationship to the target words. The effect size for trained words did not decline much over 3 months of follow-up, but the effect size for untrained items fell sharply, leading to a global 3-month effect size of 0.48 (SD 0.33). Time elapsed from stroke did not exert a discernible effect. No treatment, whether semantic, phonological, or mixed, clearly emerged as superior. Thus, we have strong empirical evidence that currently used therapies do not yield enduring generalization to untrained stimuli. Studies that have provided evidence of generalization have suggested that, to the extent that it occurs, it is limited to words that are semantically closely related to those in the training corpus (Edmonds & Babb, 2011; Kiran & Thompson, 2003; McNeil, 1997; Nickels, 2002). Treatment effects from training atypical exemplars in a domain generalize to typical exemplars but not vice versa because atypical exemplars are characterized by both core domain features and atypical features, whereas typical exemplars are characterized only by core domain features (Kiran, 2007; Plaut, 1996; Thompson, Shapiro, Kiran, & Sobecks, 2003). Naming treatments that target words used in functional contexts that are particularly important to a specific patient's daily life can certainly have some value (Hillis, 1998). However, only broadly generalizing treatments can enhance the ability of the patient to flexibly communicate verbally regardless of context—the true measure of rehabilitative success.

We address these questions in the next two sections: Why have conventional speech-language therapies achieved such poor generalization? And are there alternative therapies that could achieve broad generalization?

Experience-Dependent Neuroplasticity and the Matter of Generalization

Speech-language therapy leverages experience-dependent neuroplasticity. This section will address the following questions: How can we design speech-language therapies in such a way that the effects of therapy generalize to untrained stimuli and to daily verbal

---

1. For trials employing repeated measures analysis of variance, the benchmarks for ranking statistical effects are higher than those set by Cohen (1988). From Robey (1994), d(repeated measures) = d(independent measures)/Sqrt[1 rho(pre post)], yielding effect size thresholds of 0.63, 1.58, and 2.53 for small, medium, and large, respectively (assuming rho = 0.9). When effect sizes are calculated as mean $(\Delta X)/SD(\Delta X)$, these figures must be divided by Sqrt 2, because SD(change) = SD(common at pre and post)(Sqrt[2*(1-rho)]). This yields thresholds of <0.45 for small, 0.46–1.12 for medium, and >1.12 for large effect sizes (Samuel S. Wu, personal communication, May 28, 2013).

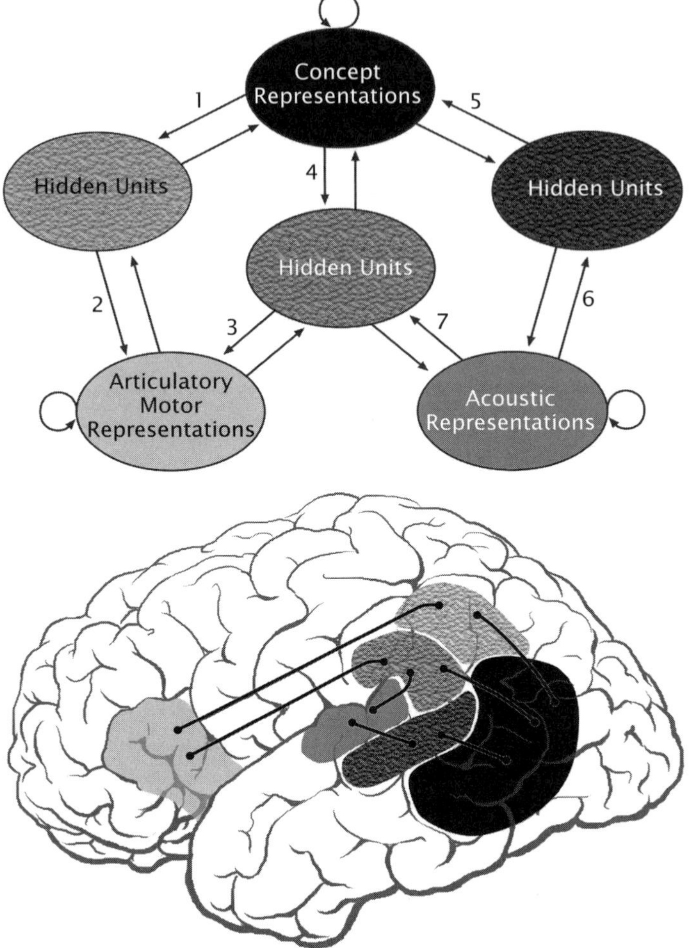

FIGURE 3.1 Top. Proposed parallel distributed processing model of language. Connectivity within the substrate for concept representations defines semantic knowledge. Connectivity within the perisylvian acoustic-articulatory motor network defines phonologic sequence knowledge. Connectivity between the substrate for concept representations and the acoustic-articulatory motor pattern associator defines lexical knowledge (see text for details). Bottom. Illustration depicting the network of Figure 3.1 mapped onto the brain. Shade coding is as in 3.1. Concept representations are assumed to be widely distributed across association cortices throughout the brain. In this illustration, only the region of presumed interface between concept representations and the remainder of the model is depicted. Source: Roth, H. L., Nadeau, S. E., Hollingsworth, A. L., Cimino-Knight, A. M. & Heilman, K. M. (2006). "Naming Concepts: Evidence of Two Routes." *Neurocase, 12*, 61–70.

communication, which is, after all, the ultimate goal of such therapy? Are there ways of designing therapies such that language function will continue to grow after formal speech therapy is completed? How can we know the answers to these questions? In this section I will focus on the basis for intrinsic generalization, that is, generalization related to neural mechanisms of language per se. The best clues come from what we understand about neural network structure and function.

Linguists have mapped the topography of language behavior in many languages in immaculate detail. However, to understand how the brain supports language function, it is necessary to bring the principles and regularities of neural function to the table. Mechanisms of neurolinguistic function cannot be inferred solely from observations of normal and impaired language. Our understanding of principles and regularities of neural function relevant to language stems predominantly from two sources: (1) knowledge of neuroanatomy and the neural systems that are based upon this anatomy; and (2) knowledge of the patterns of behavior of neural networks composed of large numbers of highly interconnected units, which support population-based (distributed) representations. The science of parallel distributed processing (PDP) provides the basis for understanding the latter source (McClelland, Rumelhart, & PDP Research Group, 1986; Nadeau, 2000).

The Wernicke-Lichtheim (W-L) information-processing model of language function has played a dominant role in understanding aphasic syndromes (Lichtheim, 1885) and has stood the test of time in defining the topographical relationship between the modular domains (acoustic representations, articulatory motor representations, and concept representations) underlying spoken language function. Unfortunately, the W-L information-processing model does not specify the characteristics of the representations within these domains and how they might be stored in the brain. It also does not address the means by which these domains might interact. I have proposed a PDP model that uses the same general topography as the W-L model (Nadeau, 2001, 2012; Nadeau & Kendall, 2012; Roth, Nadeau, Hollingsworth, Cimino-Knight, & Heilman, 2006), but also specifies how representations are generated in the modular domains and how knowledge is represented in the links between these domains (see Figure 3.1). Although not tested in simulations, this model is neurally plausible and provides a cogent explanation for a broad range of psycholinguistic phenomena in normal subjects and subjects with aphasia.

Readers can refer to the references cited in the foregoing for a detailed discussion of the model and its principles of operation. Here I will focus on the central topic of this section: mechanisms of treatment generalization founded in neural network structure and function.

Most treatments of aphasic anomia today can be characterized as lexical, as they seek to remodel connectivity between the substrates for semantics (concept representations in Figure 3.1) and phonological representations (the acoustic-articulatory motor network in Figure 3.1)—in linguistic terms, the substrate for the phonologic output lexicon. Unfortunately, because the relationship between word meaning and word sound is largely arbitrary (except for onomatopoeic words and derivational forms), there is little opportunity for the networks connecting these two substrates to acquire knowledge of regularities in the relationships between semantics and phonology. If one has learned the names of 100 objects, this provides no assistance in naming the 101st. Contrast this with a network that captures extensive regularities in the course of its experience: the network linking orthographic representations to phonologic representations, which enables reading aloud. For example, if one learns that "ust" of "must" is pronounced /ʌst/, then one has also learned the pronunciation of trust, bust, lust, crust, gust, just, and rust. However, to train the semantic-phonologic network, one would have to train every single word a patient is likely to use in everyday life, something that Anna Basso (2003) actually succeeded in doing with an extraordinarily determined patient, but that is not feasible in routine practice.

Are there any networks relevant to the problem of treating anomia that encode sufficient regularities to leverage a treatment that intrinsically generalizes? The answer is yes: (1) the substrate for phonologic sequence knowledge, and (2) the substrate for semantics.

The perisylvian acoustic-articulatory motor network, through its extensive experience with the relationship between acoustic and articulatory motor sequences, acquires extensive knowledge of the phonologic sequence regularities of a language, no less than the network linking the substrates for orthographic and articulatory motor representations. If the substrate for the acoustic-articulatory motor network is damaged, retraining of the limited repertoire of phonemes and phonemic sequences (whether in the damaged left hemisphere network or the underdeveloped right hemisphere networks) has the potential for facilitating the production of all words, since all words employ this repertoire. The task of training can be reduced by training atypical sequence exemplars, thereby training the substrate for both atypical and typical exemplars, as I noted in the case of semantics (Kiran & Thompson, 2003; Plaut, 1996). Training phonologic sequence knowledge also has the potential for enabling continued growth of vocabulary after completion of therapy because it re-establishes the basis for phonological neighborhoods—provided there are some remnants of connections between the substrates for semantics and phonology. A phonologic neighborhood is the corpus of words that share a given phonologic sequence (Vitevitch, 1997)—most important, the initial 1–3 phonemes of a word. Phonologic neighborhoods are based upon the presumptive long white matter connections that reciprocally link the perisylvian substrate for phonologic sequence knowledge and the association cortices throughout the brain that instantiate semantic knowledge. These connections support such things as the phonologic input and output lexicons, the orthographic input lexicon, and the inscriptional output lexicon. I have dubbed these the "fan arrays" because they consist of white matter pathways of diverse origin throughout association cortices that converge upon the perisylvian regions (Nadeau, 2012). Re-establishing the network connectivity underlying a precise phonologic sequence representation of a word provides the phonologic sequence target to which the semantic exemplars of the phonologic neighborhood can reconnect, via Hebbian learning processes, in post-therapy language efforts. Training phonological sequence knowledge that lays the foundation for subsequent expansion of vocabulary recapitulates the process of language acquisition in children (Gathercole, 1995; Gathercole & Martin, 1996).

The substrate for semantics—association cortices throughout the brain—also encodes many regularities, which also potentially can be leveraged in the treatment process to achieve generalization. For example, mammals share an enormous number of features. If one acquires knowledge about one mammal, one knows a great deal about the rest. Unfortunately, despite the substantial potential for the generalization of semantic knowledge, this generalization will be limited to the domains explicitly treated (enhancing one's knowledge of animals does nothing to enhance one's knowledge of birds) unless techniques can be developed to efficiently train semantic knowledge across many domains.

Intrinsically Generalizing Language Therapies

In this section, I will discuss two language therapies that engage mechanisms of experience-dependent neuroplasticity to treat anomia in aphasia. Both are directed at components of the language network, phonologic sequence and semantics, that instantiate extensive regularities and therefore are capable of yielding broad generalization from the training experience.

Phonologic Sequence Therapy

Kendall and colleagues are currently developing and testing a phonological therapy that, by targeting phonologic sequence knowledge, could potentially achieve broad generalization and could pave the way for continued growth of vocabulary after completion of therapy. The initial results have been reported (D. L. Kendall et al., 2008) and a trial of 30 subjects of a revised version is underway. The operational goal of the treatment is to develop phonologic sequence knowledge, but one cannot hope to develop knowledge of sequences until there is neural instantiation of individual phonemes. The first phase of treatment therefore consists of developing the neural substrate for linked distributed representations of individual phonemes. If treatment were completely successful, insertion of any form of a phoneme into any given domain of the network would instantly generate distributed representations of all corresponding forms in all domains (conceptual, articulatory, acoustic, and orthographic). For example, at the end of completely successful training, insertion of the acoustic form of /b/ into the acoustic domain (by saying /b/ to the subject) would instantly lead to generation of distributed representations of the articulatory form of /b/, a concept of /b/, the sound of /b/, and an orthographic representation corresponding to the letter *b*. The concept of /b/ is formed in a variety of ways: labeling it as a "lip-popper"; the tactile feel of the patient's larynx during phonation; a picture of a sagittal section through the head, with mouth and oropharynx positioned for the production of /b/; and the patient's recalled image of her own mouth, reflected in a mirror, as she produces the phoneme. The second phase of treatment consists of training in the regularities of English phonological sequences, first by inserting single syllables into the network, later by inserting 2- or 3-syllable non-words into the network. Distributed representations are presumably generated in all domains and pathways of the network by this phonological sequence input. However, one network, the perisylvian acoustic-articulatory network (see Figure 3.1), is uniquely equipped for accumulating knowledge of the regularities of phonological sequences because it is uniquely exposed to sequential input paired with sequential output. Thus, the second phase of treatment primarily involves building up phonological sequence knowledge in the acoustic-articulatory networks on the two sides of the brain. In the current (second) phase of treatment development, phonological sequence training is limited to atypical exemplars.

Preliminary results of the current trial (in progress) are depicted in Table 3.2 (D. Kendall, Brookshire, Oelke, & Nadeau, 2012). The effect sizes are in the small range by Robey's benchmarks (Robey, 1994) (see footnote 1). In part, this reflects the fact that, although on average the effect of the therapy was substantial, there was also considerable variability in response to treatment. It also suggests that in group trials of a treatment marked by considerable heterogeneity of response (the rule with neurorehabilitation studies), omnibus effect size calculations may be somewhat misleading by virtue of the large standard deviations. Therefore, it might be of value to calculate effect sizes separately for responders. Most crucially, the treatment of Kendall and colleagues generalized to untrained words, and both

TABLE 3.2 Preliminary Results of Phonological Treatment of Anomia (D. Kendall et al., 2012)

	Research aim	Outcome measure	Acquisition (pre- versus immediately post-)	3-month maintenance (pre- versus 3-month post-)	1-year maintenance (pre- versus 1-year post-)
N			20	16	8
Primary outcome	Generalization to lexical	Untrained real word confrontation naming	Pre 64% (SD 25%) Post 70% (SD 25%) p = 0.001 ES = 0.21	Pre 66% (SD 25%) Post 71% (SD 26%) p = 0.033 ES = 0.28	Pre 68% (SD 20%) Post 81% (SD 19%) p = 0.033 ES = 0.68
Secondary outcomes	Acquisition	Trained non-word repetition	p = 0.000	p = 0.000	p = 0.000
		Trained real word confrontation naming	Pre 64% (SD 26%) Post 82% (SD 17%) p = 0.000 ES = 0.69	Pre 66% (SD 25%) Post 79% (SD 22%) p = 0.000 ES = 0.59	Pre 70% (SD 18%) Post 86% (SD 7%) p = 0.016 ES = 0.88
	Generalization to phonological processes	SAPA (maximum score 151)	Pre 97 (SD 25) Post 106 (SD 24) p = 0.000	Pre 97 (SD 25) Post 106 (SD 26) p = 0.000	Pre 100 (SD 23) Post 115 (SD 15) p = 0.010
		Untrained non-word repetition	Pre 69% (SD 21%) Post 82% (SD 15%) p = 0.000	Pre 68% (SD 22%) Post 83% (SD 16%) p = 0.000	Pre 75% (SD 17%) Post 84% (SD 14%) p = 0.069
	Ecological validity	FOQ-A	Pre 3.93 (SD 0.62) Post 4.24 (SD 0.54) p = 0.025	Pre 3.98 (SD 0.58) Post 4.36 (SD 0.83) p = 0.115	Not available
		SALQOL	Pre 3.37 (SD 0.76) Post 3.81 (SD 0.85) p = 0.011	Pre 3.50 (SD 0.77) Post 3.75 (SD 0.73) p = 0.182	Pre 3.43 (SD 0.66) Post 4 (SD 0.66) p = 0.085

ES: Effect size; SAPA: Standardized Assessment of Phonology in Aphasia (D. Kendall et al., 2010); FOQ-A: Functional Outcomes Questionnaire for Aphasia (Glueckauf et al., 2003); SALQOL: Stroke and Aphasia Quality of Life Scale (Hilari, Byng, Lamping, & Smith, 2003).

magnitude of gain and effect size for untrained words grew with time, reaching a maximum at 1 year after completion of therapy. Thus, the treatment appears to be achieving both the effects predicted by the theory that inspires it: (1) training perisylvian phonologic sequence knowledge in both the dominant and non-dominant hemispheres, and (2) thereby facilitating the development of phonologic neighborhoods—reflecting renewed connectivity between association cortices supporting semantics and the substrate for phonologic sequence knowledge. Furthermore, the fact that treatment of non-words composed of atypical phonological sequences shows incipient evidence of generalizing to non-words composed of typical sequences that were not trained (with an N of 8 the result is not statistically significant) constitutes early evidence that a principle noted repeatedly in this chapter also holds true for phonological sequences: training atypical exemplars generalizes to typical exemplars.

Semantic Impairment

In a PDP conceptualization, anomia, to the extent that it is due to semantic impairment, reflects insufficient engagement of representations of the critical features that distinguish concepts from each other. The goal of therapy is to alter network connectivity within association cortices such that these distinguishing features are more reliably engaged at the same time that features shared with other items are relatively disengaged. The left hemisphere perisylvian lesions that are commonly responsible for aphasia and its associated anomia frequently do not involve a substantial portion of the association cortices that provide the basis for semantic representations. They may, however, damage Brodmann's area 37 and surrounding regions in the posterior temporal cortex, which appear to provide the interface between cortices supporting semantic representations and the dominant perisylvian language cortex (producing anomia as a disconnection syndrome; Geschwind, 1965). Semantic therapy might aid anomia by retraining damaged left hemisphere semantic substrates and by training up inadequately trained right brain cortices supporting semantic representations.

Various approaches to semantic therapy have been employed with some success (Raymer & Rothi, 2000). These have included (1) word-picture matching tasks using semantically related foils, (2) answering yes-no questions about semantic features of pictured objects, (3) semantic sorting of objects, (4) variously cued matching of semantic associates as the number and relatedness of semantic foils are increased, (5) correction of naming errors by provision of additional semantic information that distinguishes the erroneous response from the correct response, and (6) systematic training in the semantic features of objects. Unlike naming therapy directed to lexical deficits, therapy directed to semantic deficits might be expected to intrinsically generalize to a substantial degree, as refining the featural relationships of trained items (the regularities in the knowledge implicit in the network) will benefit the naming of untrained items to the extent that they share some of these featural relationships (Plaut, 1996). Even a damaged network still contains a great deal of information, so that the task of therapy is to refine network knowledge, rather than to re-establish it (Plaut, 1996).

However, the potential for generalization using current semantic therapy techniques is doomed to be modest unless the scope of intrinsic generalization can be expanded, thereby impacting a significant portion of the semantic domain used in daily life. Broad intrinsic generalization is difficult to achieve for most semantic therapies because their principal aim is to enlarge knowledge of the semantic attributes of single items, one item at a time. The extent to which this leads to incorporation of semantic features shared with other entities is largely a matter of chance. Knowledge of particular semantic domains (e.g., animals) might usefully be fleshed out in this way, but semantic knowledge that spans the breadth of daily life is difficult to achieve with this approach. Recently, Edmonds and colleagues (Edmonds & Babb, 2011; Edmonds, Nadeau, & Kiran, 2009) have developed an innovative and fundamentally broader approach. This therapy focuses on verbs. It takes advantage of the fact that many verbs admit of a very broad range of possibilities for both agent and patient (aka goal), thereby providing an opportunity for highly diverse modifications of the distributed concept representations of agent and patient, and engagement of atypical exemplars of agent and patient. Verbs prime commonly associated agents and patients (Ferretti, McRae, & Hatherell, 2001) and nouns prime commonly associated verbs (McRae, Hare, Elman, & Ferretti, 2005). Verbs, no less than nouns, prime other verbs with which they share features (Rössler, Streb, & Haan, 2001). By centering the therapy on verbs, the spectrum of semantic features that are incorporated in the training is vastly expanded. The therapy also provides subjects the opportunity to draw exemplars from daily life, so long as they are acceptable agents or patients for the verb being presented (thereby facilitating generalization to daily life).

In the first phase of therapy, subjects are presented with 10 individual verbs (e.g., "write"), one at a time, and are tasked with producing three agents for each verb (e.g., author, journalist, mother) or three patients for each verb (e.g., story, articles, to-do list), while being cued with "who" or "what" questions. They then have to create suitable agent/patient pairs (e.g., author/story). If necessary, subjects are semantically cued through provision of appropriate targets mixed with foils. Subjects are also asked to produce one personal response (e.g., husband/songs). In the second phase of therapy, subjects are tasked with answering "when," "where," and "why" questions about particular agent/patient pairs. In the third phase of treatment, subjects are read 12 sentences containing the target verb: three semantically correct, three containing an inappropriate agent, three containing an inappropriate patient, and three semantically correct but with agent and patient reversed. They are asked to judge the correctness of these sentences and, with cueing as needed, to explain their choice. A fourth phase replicates the first phase, but without cueing. Six subjects, two with transcortical motor aphasia, two with conduction aphasia, and two with Broca's aphasia, received 2 hours of therapy/week for 4–8 weeks in a single-subject, multiple baseline design.

All subjects demonstrated clinically meaningful gains pre- to post-treatment, not just with sentences employing trained verbs but also with sentences employing semantically related untrained verbs and their untrained agents and patients (Edmonds & Babb, 2011;

TABLE 3.3 Results of VNest Semantic Treatment of Anomia in Aphasia (Edmonds & Babb, 2011; Edmonds et al., 2009)

Subject #	WAB (AQ)		BNT (%)		Connected speech (%)*		NVPB	
	Pre-	Post-	Pre-	Post-	Pre-	Post-	Pre-	Post-
1	76.4	82.5	71.7	83	52	82.1	54.5	86.4
2	78.5	86.4	81.7	90	50.9	67.8	59.1	81.8
3	73.8	81.6	45	55	64.6	90.8	72.7	86.4
4	70.6	82.3	45	68.3	50.4	52.8	31.8	63.6
5	45.2	55.5	35	36.6			25	25
6	36.4	48.1	8.3	26.6			0	22.2

WAB (AQ): Western Aphasia Battery Aphasia Quotient (Kertesz, 1982); BNT: Boston Naming Test (Goodglass & Kaplan, 2000); NVPB: Northwestern Verb Production Battery/Northwestern Assessment of Verbs and Sentences (Thompson, 2012).

* Percentage of sentences that contained subject and verb, with or without object, and were relevant to the topic. Connected speech was generated in response to the picture description task of the WAB, the cookie theft picture of the Boston Diagnostic Aphasia Examination, and the Cinderella story.

Edmonds et al., 2009). In addition, subjects improved on general measures of language function (see Table 3.3), which is further evidence of broad generalization of the treatment.

Generalization in a Broader Context

In this section I briefly consider the full spectrum of mechanisms that might support broad generalization (see Nadeau, Rothi, & Rosenbek, 2008, for greater detail). Many of these mechanisms could account for the modest generalization effects that are irregularly reported in speech-language therapy studies.

1. *Intrinsic*: Application of knowledge acquired in therapy (e.g., semantic features, phonological sequences, phonetic sounds, syntactic techniques) to other knowledge that shares these features or sequences, or to situations that allow application of the acquired techniques.

In the preceding section, we discussed two intrinsically generalizing language therapies, one phonologic and one semantic. The phonologic therapy generalizes because it trains the phonological sequence knowledge that underlies all words. The semantic therapy generalizes only because of its unique engagement of verbs to drive the treatment process. Broad intrinsic generalization has been reported with other therapies. Thompson and colleagues reported a syntactic therapy in which improvements in syntactic function were limited to the structures actually trained and to linguistically closely related forms. For example, training to produce "who" questions from simple declarative sentences generalized to "what" questions (in both cases, there is an agent and a patient) but not to "when" and "where" questions (which involve an agent, verb, and adjunctive phrase), and vice versa (Thompson, Shapiro, & Roberts, 1993). Training of object-relative sentences generalized to object-cleft and "who" questions, but not the other way around, because for syntax, as for semantics, training of atypical exemplars (in the case of syntax, an atypical sequence) also trains the production of typical exemplars, but not the other way around (Thompson et al., 2003; see also Nadeau, 2012, for a broader discussion of these issues).[2] In any event, re-acquired capability to produce a certain syntactic structure generalizes to all concepts and words that can be entrained to that structure. In this respect, syntactic therapies have the potential for broad generalization.

2. *Cross-Function*: Development of knowledge during therapy that can be applied to multiple tasks. For example, semantic therapy could benefit oral word production, written word production, oral word comprehension, and written word comprehension because all four capacities involve networks linked to association cortices supporting concept representations (in traditional terms, all four capacities depend on the integrity of the semantic field).

3. *Extrinsic*: Development during therapy of a knowledge-acquisition/skill-learning technique that subjects with motivation, and capable of engaging motivation to employ the technique, can use during and outside therapy to rebuild language function (e.g., semantic therapy, phonological sequence therapy, syntactic therapy). Here, it is not the substantive material learned in therapy that is crucial to ongoing progress outside therapy (although a critical mass of substantive knowledge may be necessary)—it is the acquisition of a therapeutic technique that the subject, perhaps with help from family, can continue to apply in the months and years outside therapy. For example, a subject who has received the semantic therapy of Edmonds and colleagues (Edmonds & Babb, 2011; Edmonds et al., 2009) could continue to use the techniques acquired during therapy, thereby continuing to develop the semantic field long after the conclusion of therapy. Indeed, this may account to a substantial degree for the large gains they reported. Even lexical therapy can make use of this generalization mechanism, as demonstrated by Basso (2003): exceptionally capable subjects can be given the guidance and techniques to practice naming the thousands of words needed to communicate in daily life. We have preliminary evidence from a study of semantic therapy that only subjects who demonstrate intact frontal function show widespread generalization that also impacts daily communicative behavior (Nadeau & Kendall, 2006).

4. *Mechanistic*: Training of a key brain resource, essential to language processing but not fundamentally linguistic, that enables improvement in language function. Three subtypes can be postulated:

A. Development of working memory capacity needed for language. This is likely to be particularly important for normal grammatic function, in which multiple distributed concept representations need to be maintained simultaneously, sufficiently long for appropriate modifications to be made and language to be spoken—at the least, representations corresponding to agent, verb, and patient, possibly theme, possibly referents (in the case of articles, auxiliary verbs, and pronouns), and possibly corresponding representations

---

2. An example of an object-relative sentence would be "The police arrested the man she had recommended." An example of an object-cleft sentence would be "It was the lamp that the cat knocked down."

within embedded clauses (Nadeau, 2012). In support of this concept, Thompson and colleagues (Thompson, Riley, den Ouden, Meltzer-Asscher, & Lukic, 2013) reported, in a group of patients with Broca's aphasia, the generalization of training of three-argument verbs (e.g., *give*: "He gives the flowers to Mary") to one- and two-argument verbs, thereby augmenting their production.

B. Development of the ability to endogenously generate distributed concept representations. This ability, which is most impaired in adynamic aphasia (Gold et al., 1997), may be the same as that in 4A. However, the differences between adynamic aphasia (in which there is difficulty self-generating concept representations) and Broca's aphasia, in which there appears to be particular difficulty in modifying and manipulating representations, suggest that this is not the case.

C. Development of a new intentional bias that favors language use over either nonuse or gestural communication, the cardinal example being constraint induced language therapy (CILT) (Faroqi-Shah & Virion, 2009; Maher et al., 2003; Meinzer, Djundja, Barthel, Elbert, & Rockstroh, 2005; Meinzer, Streiftau, & Rockstroh, 2007; Pulvermüller et al., 2001). In one version, CILT involves a small group of subjects with aphasia and a therapist in a game in which each subject is dealt a set of cards, all different, and must communicate verbally with other subjects to find the one duplicate of a given card. The complexity of required verbalization can be gradually shaped by increasing the complexity of the card stimuli and increasing demands on the complexity of the required verbalization.

The idea here is that because of frustration with language impairment, which is particularly severe in the months immediately following a stroke, stroke victims develop an intentional habit of minimal effort to communicate verbally, or a habit that leads to alternative communicative modes such as gesture. This intentional bias then persists, despite substantial improvement in the capacity for language, and thereby actually inhibits linguistic communication and further retraining of language substrates over the long run. Training that alters this bias can enable the subject to take full advantage of partially recovered language function. There may be other mechanisms at play in mediating the effects of CILT (e.g., generalization mechanism #7) but this particular one, modification of intentional bias, is the one that has motivated the development of this therapy and appears to be most responsible for the gains associated with the previously developed constraint induced movement therapy (CIMT). Studies of CILT in patients with chronic stroke have demonstrated rather modest effects—for example, approximately 0.2 SD improvement on the Aachen Aphasie Battery (AAB), but effect sizes, defined by the AAB, which are indicative of broad generalization, have been in the 1.4–2.3 range (i.e., medium to large) and have been shown to be sustained 6 months after treatment (Meinzer et al., 2005). Barthel and colleagues (Barthel, Meinzer, Djundja, & Rockstroh, 2008) achieved similar results with a completely different therapy, model-oriented aphasia therapy (MOAT), which is comparable in intensity to CILT. MOAT is a therapist-directed, domain-oriented therapy inspired by Lyndsey Nickels's work (Nickels, 2002) that focuses on specific impediments to language production stemming from impairment in semantics, phonology, or the phonological lexicons. It includes training of verbs, refinement of semantic knowledge, developing strategies to deal with anomia, role-playing, and involvement of relatives.

Neither CILT nor MOAT incorporates components likely to support significant intrinsic generalization. Their comparable efficacy suggests that intentional bias not to speak can be overcome in a variety of ways, so long as the aphasia treatment is sufficiently intensive and places a high demand on the patient to produce propositional language. In principle, the effective treatment of negative intentional bias might make it possible for the patient to achieve greater gain from the ambient language environment, particularly if family members are recruited to the treatment team, thereby enabling long-term growth of language capacity. However, so far, such long-term growth has not been demonstrated.

5. *Substrate mediated*: Development of the critical mass of language skill needed to enable conversation at home and elsewhere, and thereby further the therapeutic process. This is probably necessary to enable both intrinsic and extrinsic generalization mechanisms to operate. If, however effective the language therapy, the patient is still left with such severe impairment that she finds most attempts at verbal communication very frustrating, she is not likely to continue to speak sufficiently to further develop language facility over time. To some extent, this problem might be mitigated by explicitly recruiting relatives for the ongoing, long-term, post-therapist treatment process.

Furthermore, for therapies seeking to leverage intrinsic mechanisms to achieve broad generalization, a substantial portion of the critical underlying substrate must be trained. For example, for a phonological therapy to broadly generalize, a substantial portion of the phonologic sequence repertoire of the language must be trained.

6. *Contextual*: Acquisition of knowledge, predominantly contextual, during speech-language therapy, that aids retrieval of knowledge outside therapy (see Nadeau et al., 2008, for more detailed discussion). In essence, the principle is that when we learn, the knowledge that is acquired includes not only the intended material but also knowledge about the context. This knowledge may include attributes of other stimuli introduced during a treatment session. It may also include more general attributes of the situation, for example, where the treatment was provided, characteristics of the treatment room and the therapist, who else was present, the mood of the participant, participant attitudes toward the stroke experience and the associated disability, and the strategies that the participant brings to therapy. The greater the resemblance between context in the learning environment and context in the retrieval environment, the higher the likelihood of success in retrieval (Glenberg, 1979; Glenberg & Lehmann, 1980). This principle suggests that the conduct of speech-language therapy in the patient's home might be considerably more effective.

Most studies of language rehabilitation after stroke have focused on the difference between performance at baseline and performance at the end of treatment. However, most would agree that the truest measure of treatment effectiveness is the knowledge and skills acquired during treatment that are retained by the subject through the months and years after the conclusion of treatment. Only changes retained by the brain over the long run can have a lasting impact on daily performance, activity, participation, and quality of life. Contextual generalization does not involve the generalization of trained to untrained stimuli. Rather, it involves the generalization of trained stimuli (and exemplars to which they generalize by other generalization mechanisms) to daily conversational life, long after the conclusion of therapy.

The principle that the greater the resemblance between context in the learning environment and context in the retrieval environment, the greater the likelihood of success in retrieval, accounts for the "spacing effect," at least in part. The term "spacing effect" refers to the observation that long-term retention of acquired knowledge or skills is greater if a given amount of training is delivered over an extended period of time, rather than concentrated as massed practice (Nadeau et al., 2008). This phenomenon was first reported by Ebbinghaus (1885) in a declarative learning task in which he himself was the subject. Since then, literally hundreds of investigations involving a wide range of knowledge and skill types have shown that, with very few exceptions, distributed practice is superior to massed practice in its effects on knowledge and skill retention, whether the training involves factual knowledge, simple motor skills, or more complex tasks. Of particular potential relevance to rehabilitation are the small number of studies that have tested the impact of the distribution of practice over extended periods of time (e.g., weeks or months). These have included training of addition skills in third graders (Pyle, 1913); training of 2-year-olds on novel nouns and verbs (Childers & Tomasello, 2002); training left-handed javelin throw in schoolgirls (Murphy, 1916); training of adults on dynamic balance and calibrated sequential key-press timing tasks (Shea, Lai, Black, & Park, 2000); training on Space Fortress, a complex task involving acquisition of factual knowledge, motor skills, and strategy (Shebilske, Goettl, Corrington, & Day, 1999); training English-Spanish word pairs (Bahrick & Phelps, 1987); and training British postal workers to type (Baddeley & Longman, 1978). In each of these studies, greater distribution of training was associated with greater long-term retention.

Many theories have been offered to account for the spacing effect (Greene, 1989; Hintzman, 1974; Shebilske et al., 1999). Although no theory has been shown to account for all experimental results, including both declarative and procedural knowledge, or to fully accommodate our current understanding of the neurobiological basis of memory, the component levels theory of Glenberg comes closest (Glenberg, 1979; Glenberg & Lehmann, 1980). It was Glenberg who suggested that the spacing effect is based on the principle that more distributed training, by virtue of the greater variety of training contexts incorporated, offers a greater opportunity for the achievement of conditions at the time of retrieval that resemble those at the time of learning.

Greater distribution of training also allows greater time for the consolidation of memory, both declarative and procedural. This appears to predominantly occur during sleep, which is emerging as a major engine of neuroplasticity in species ranging from fruit flies to zebra fish to rodents to humans (Dudai, 2012; Saletin & Walker, 2012; Wang, Grone, Colas, Appelbaum, & Mourrain, 2011).

Unfortunately, to date, although the potential superiority of massed rehabilitation is widely touted, few neurorehabilitation studies have tested the spacing effect. The results of these have been promising but inconclusive (Goverover, Arango-Lasprilla, Hillary, Chiaravalloti, & DeLuca, 2009; Goverover, Hillary, Chiaravalloti, Arango-Lasprilla, & DeLuca, 2009; Hillary et al., 2003; Hochhalter, Overmier, Gasper, Bakke, & Holub, 2005). In our own recent RCT comparing the effect of CIMT delivered over 2 weeks with that of an equal amount of CIMT delivered over 10 weeks, we found no difference in retention 3 months after treatment (Nadeau, Davis, Wu, Dai, & Richards, 2014). While this study failed to provide evidence of a spacing effect, perhaps because of errors in its parameters, it did cast doubt on the idea of the particular efficacy of massed practice. Because therapies involving declarative learning (like speech-language therapy), which depend on the medial temporal lobe, are more likely than those largely engaging (medial temporal lobe-independent) procedural learning (like CIMT) to benefit from general context effects on retention, studies of the spacing effect on long-term outcome from speech-language therapy are warranted.

7. *Socially mediated*: Change in the perception of the subject and her family regarding her role in the family unit, with the adoption of a new/revised role that subsumes more expectation of speech, more pressure to speak, and greater language production (Blonder, 2000). As Blonder has shown, the alterations in lives produced by aphasia may be profound and, even if stroke victims do not become socially isolated, the value of language facility may be fundamentally reduced. Thus, to varying degrees, the restoration of daily communicative ability may require some restoration of a social context that will promote language use as an instrumental device.

Conclusion

Progress in advancing the treatment of aphasia after stroke has been painfully slow. In part this can be attributed to our primitive understanding of the mechanisms of reactive neuroplasticity underlying spontaneous recovery and the complete absence of proven adjuvants to reactive neuroplasticity. Unfortunately, the field of stroke is still largely focused on the first 3 hours and only a few neuroscientists are doing work that will lead to neuro-biologic adjuvants.

Progress in advancing the experience-dependent neuroplasticity engaged by speech-language therapy has also been painfully slow. This can be attributed to a failure to prioritize generalizability and a substantial failure to take into account the strengths and limitations of the specific brain mechanisms involved in language function (e.g., the intrinsic non-generalizability of lexical knowledge). In this chapter I have focused on the specifics of neural networks involved in language function and the implications of their structure for intrinsic generalization. I have sought to make clear that the essential attribute of intrinsically generalizing therapy is engagement and further development of regularities instantiated in neural network connectivity that can be leveraged to benefit untrained elements (phonemic sequences, morphemes, words, and sentences) and, hence, daily communicative life. I have also sketched out hypotheses on broader mechanisms of widespread generalization, most fundamentally nonlinguistic, that might be usefully engaged by speech-language therapists, pending further empirical validation.

References

Baddeley, A. D., & Longman, D. J. A. (1978). The influence of length and frequency of training session on the rate of learning to type. *Ergonomics, 21,* 627–635.

Bahrick, H. P., & Phelps, E. (1987). Retention of Spanish vocabulary over 8 years. *J Exp Psychol: Learn Mem Cogn, 13,* 344–349.

Barthel, G., Meinzer, M., Djundja, D., & Rockstroh, B. (2008). Intensive language therapy in chronic aphasia: Which aspects contribute most? *Aphasiology, 22,* 408–421.

Basso, A. (2003). *Aphasia and its therapy.* New York: Oxford University Press.

Basso, A., Capitani, E., & Vignolo, L. A. (1979). Influence of rehabilitation on language skills in aphasic patients. *Arch Neurol, 36,* 190–196.

Blomert, L., Kean, M.-L., Koster, C., & Schokker, J. (1994). Amsterdam-Nijmegen-Everyday-Language-Test: Construction, reliability and validity. *Aphasiology, 8,* 381–407.

Blonder, L. X. (2000). Language use. In S. E. Nadeau, L. J. Gonzalez Rothi, & B. Crosson (Eds.), *Aphasia and language: Theory to practice* (pp. 284–295). New York: Guilford Press.

Bowen, A., Hesketh, A., Patchick, E., Young, A. W., Davies, L., Vail, A., . . . Tyrrell, P. J. (2012). Effectiveness of enhanced communication therapy in the first four months after stroke for aphasia and dysarthria: A randomised controlled trial. *BMJ, 345,* e4407. doi:10.1136/bmj.e4407.

Brady, M. C., Kelly, H., Godwin, J., & Enderby, P. (2012). Speech and language therapy for aphasia following stroke. *Cochrane Database Syst Rev, 5,* CD000425.

Cherney, L. R., & Robey, R. R. (2008). Aphasia treatment: Recovery, prognosis, and clinical effectiveness. In R. Chapey (Ed.), *Language intervention strategies in aphasia and related neurogenic communication disorders* (5th ed., pp. 186–202). Philadelphia: Wolters Kluwer.

Childers, J. B., & Tomasello, M. (2002). Two-year-olds learn novel nouns, verbs, and conventional actions from massed or distributed exposures. *Develop Psychol, 38,* 967–978.

Cohen, J. (1988). *Statistical power analysis for the behavioral sciences* (2nd ed.). Hillsdale, NJ: Lawrence Erlbaum Associates.

Dancause, N., & Nudo, R. J. (2011). Shaping plasticity to enhance recovery after injury. *Prog Brain Res, 192,* 273–295.

De Renzi, E., & Faglioni, P. (1978). Normative data and screening power of a shortened version of the Token test. *Cortex, 14,* 41–49.

Demeurisse, G., Demol, O., Derouck, M., de Beuckelaer, R., Coekaerts, M.-J., & Capon, A. (1980). Quantitative study of the rate of recovery from aphasia due to ischemic stroke. *Stroke, 11,* 455–458.

Dudai, Y. (2012). The restless engram: Consolidations never end. *Annu Rev Neurosci, 35,* 227–247.

Duncan, P. W., Sullivan, K. J., Behrman, A. L., Azen, S. P., Wu, S. S., Nadeau, S. E., . . . for the LEAPS Investigative Team. (2011). Body-weight–supported treadmill rehabilitation after stroke. *N Engl J Med, 364,* 2026–2036.

Ebbinghaus, H. (1885). *Memory: A contribution to experimental psychology.* Berlin: Privat Docent in Philosophy at the University of Berlin. Reprint, New York: Dover, 1964.

Edmonds, L. A., & Babb, M. (2011). Effect of verb network strengthening treatment in moderate-to-severe aphasia. *Am J Speech-Lang Pathol, 20,* 131–145.

Edmonds, L. A., Nadeau, S. E., & Kiran, S. (2009). Effect of verb network strengthening treatment (VNeST) on lexical retrieval of content words in sentences in persons with aphasia. *Aphasiology, 23,* 402–424.

El Hachioui, H., Lingsma, H. F., van de Sandt-Koenderman, M. E., Dippel, D. W. J., Koudstaal, P. J., & Visch-Brink, E. G. (2013). Recovery of aphasia after stroke: A 1-year follow-up study. *J Neurol, 260,* 166–171.

Faroqi-Shah, Y., & Virion, C. R. (2009). Constraint-induced language therapy for agrammatism: Role of grammaticality constraints. *Aphasiology, 23,* 977–988.

Feeney, D. M., & Baron, J.-C. (1986). Diaschisis. *Stroke, 17,* 817–830.

Ferretti, T. R., McRae, K., & Hatherell, A. (2001). Integrating verbs, situation schemas, and thematic role concepts. *J Mem Language, 44,* 516–547.

Finger, S., Koehler, P. J., & Jagella, C. (2004). The Monakow concept of diaschisis. *Arch Neurol, 61,* 283–288.

Gathercole, S. E. (1995). Is nonword repetition a test of phonological memory or long-term knowledge? It all depends on the nonwords. *Memory and Cognition, 23,* 83–94.

Gathercole, S. E., & Martin, A. J. (1996). Interactive processes in phonological memory. In S. E. Gathercole (Ed.), *Models of short term memory* (pp. 71–100). Hove, East Sussex, UK: Psychology Press.

Geschwind, N. (1965). Disconnexion syndromes in animals and man. *Brain, 88,* 237–294, 585–644.

Glenberg, A. M. (1979). Component-levels theory of the effects of spacing of repetitions on recall and recognition. *Memory and Cognition, 7,* 95–112.

Glenberg, A. M., & Lehmann, T. S. (1980). Spacing repetitions over 1 week. *Memory and Cognition, 8,* 528–538.

Glueckauf, R. L., Blonder, L. X., Ecklund-Johnson, E., Crosson, B., Maher, L. M., & Rothi, L. J. G. (2003). Functional Outcomes Questionnaire for Aphasia: Overview and preliminary psychometric evaluation. *Neurorehabilitation, 18,* 281–290.

Gold, M., Nadeau, S. E., Jacobs, D. H., Adair, J. C., Gonzalez-Rothi, L. J., & Heilman, K. M. (1997). Adynamic aphasia: A transcortical motor aphasia with defective semantic strategy formation. *Brain Lang, 57,* 374–393.

Goodglass, H. (1993). *Understanding aphasia.* San Diego, CA: Academic Press.

Goodglass, H., & Kaplan, E. (2000). *Boston Diagnostic Aphasia Examination* (3rd ed.). East Moline, IL: LinguiSystems.

Goverover, Y., Arango-Lasprilla, J. C., Hillary, F. G., Chiaravalloti, N., & DeLuca, J. (2009). Application of the spacing effect to improve learning and memory for functional tasks in traumatic brain injury: A pilot study. *Am J Occup Ther, 63,* 543–548.

Goverover, Y., Hillary, F. G., Chiaravalloti, N., Arango-Lasprilla, J. C., & DeLuca, J. (2009). A functional application of the spacing effect to improve learning aand memory in persons with multiple sclerosis. *J Clin Exp Neuropsychol, 31,* 513–522.

Greene, R. L. (1989). Spacing effects in memory: Evidence for a two-process account. *J Exp Psychol: Learn Mem Cogn, 15,* 371–377.

Hanson, W. R., Metter, E. J., & Riege, W. H. (1989). The course of chronic aphasia. *Aphasiology, 3,* 19–29.

Helm-Estabrooks, N., Ramsberger, G., Morgan, A. R., & Nicholas, M. (1989). *Boston assessment of severe aphasia.* Chicago: Riverside.

Hilari, K., Byng, S., Lamping, D. L., & Smith, S. C. (2003). Stroke and Aphasia Quality of Life Scale-39 (SAQOL-39): Evaluation of acceptability, reliability, and validity. *Stroke, 34,* 1944–1950.

Hillary, F. G., Schultheis, M. T., Challis, B. H., Carnevale, G. J., Galshi, T., & DeLuca, J. (2003). Spacing of repetitions improves learning and memory after moderate and severe TBI. *J Clin Exp Neuropsychol, 25,* 49–58.

Hillis, A. E. (1998). Treatment of naming disorders: New issues regarding old therapies. *J Int Neuropsychol Soc, 4,* 648–660.

Hintzman, D. L. (1974). Theoretical implications of the spacing effect. In R. L. Solso (Ed.), *Theories in cognitive psychology: The Loyola Symposium* (pp. 77–99). Potomac, MD: Lawrence Erlbaum.

Hochhalter, A. K., Overmier, J. B., Gasper, S. M., Bakke, B. L., & Holub, R. J. (2005). A comparison of spaced retrieval to other schedules of practice for people with dementia. *Exp Aging Res, 31,* 101–118.

Iadecola, C., & Anrather, J. (2011). Stroke research at a crossroad: Asking the brain for directions. *Nature Neuroscience, 14,* 1363–1368.

Kendall, D., Brookshire, L., Oelke, M., & Nadeau, S. (2012). *Intensive phonomotor rehabiitation of anomia in seventeen individuals with aphasia.* Paper presented at the Clinical Aphasiology Conference, Lake Tahoe, CA.

Kendall, D., del Toro, C., Nadeau, S., Johnson, J., Rosenbek, J., & Velozo, C. (2010). *The development of a standardized assessment of phonology in aphasia.* Paper presented at the Clinical Aphasiology Conference, Isle of Palm, SC.

Kendall, D. L., Rosenbek, J. C., Heilman, K. M., Conway, T. W., Klenberg, K., Gonzalez Rothi, L. J., & Nadeau, S. E. (2008). Phoneme-based rehabilitation of anomia in aphasia. *Brain & Lang, 105,* 1–17.

Kertesz, A. (1982). *Western Aphasia Battery.* New York: Grune and Stratton.

Kertesz, A., & McCabe, P. (1977). Recovery patterns and prognosis in aphasia. *Brain, 100,* 1–18.

Kiran, S. (2007). Complexity in the treatment of naming disorders. *Am J Speech-Lang Pathol, 16*, 18–29.

Kiran, S., & Thompson, C. K. (2003). The role of semantic complexity in treatment of naming deficits: Training semantic categories in fluent aphasia by controlling exemplar typicality. *J Speech Lang Hearing Res, 46*, 773–787.

Laska, A. C., Hellblom, A., Murray, V., Kahan, T., & von Arbin, M. (2001). Aphasia in acute stroke and relation to outcome. *J Internal Med, 249*, 413–422.

Lazar, R. M., Speizer, A. E., Festa, J. R., Krakauer, J. W., & Marshall, R. S. (2008). Variability in language recovery after first-time stroke. *J Neurol Neurosurg Psychiatry, 79*, 530–534.

Lichtheim, L. (1885). On aphasia. *Brain, 7*, 433–484.

Maher, L. M., Kendall, D., Swearengin, J. A., Pingel, K., Holland, A., & Roth, L. J. G. (2003). Constraint induced language therapy for chronic aphasia: Preliminary findings. *J Int Neuropsychol Soc, 9*, 192.

Mazzoni, M., Vista, M., Pardossi, L., Avila, L., Bianchi, F., & Moretti, P. (1992). Spontaneous evolution of aphasia after ischaemic stroke. *Aphasiology, 4*, 387–396.

McClelland, J. L., Rumelhart, D. E., & PDP Research Group. (1986). *Parallel distributed processing.* Cambridge, MA: MIT Press.

McClung, J. S., Rothi, L. J. G., & Nadeau, S. E. (2010). Ambient experience in restitutive treatment of aphasia. *Frontiers Human Neurosci, 4*, 1–19.

McNeil, M. R. (1997). *Clinical management of sensorimotor speech disorders.* New York: Thieme.

McRae, K., Hare, M., Elman, J. L., & Ferretti, T. R. (2005). A basis for generating expectancies for verbs from nouns. *Memory and Cognition, 33*, 1174–1184.

Meinzer, M., Djundja, D., Barthel, G., Elbert, T. R., & Rockstroh, B. (2005). Long-term stability of improved language functions in chronic aphasia after constraint-induced aphasia therapy. *Stroke, 36*, 1462–1466.

Meinzer, M., Streiftau, S., & Rockstroh, B. (2007). Intensive language training in the rehabilitation of chronic aphasia: efficient training by laypersons. *J Int Neuropsychol Soc, 13*, 846–853.

Murphy, H. H. (1916). Distribution of practice periods in learning. *J Educ Psychol, 7*, 150–162.

Nadeau, S. E. (2000). Connectionist models and language. In S. E. Nadeau, L. J. Gonzalez Rothi, & B. Crosson (Eds.), *Aphasia and language: Theory to practice* (pp. 299–347). New York: Guilford Press.

Nadeau, S. E. (2001). Phonology: A review and proposals from a connectionist perspective. *Brain Lang, 79*, 511–579.

Nadeau, S. E. (2010). Hemispheric asymmetry: What, why, and at what cost? *J Int Neuropsychol Soc, 27*, 1–3.

Nadeau, S. E. (2012). *The Neural architecture of grammar.* Cambridge, MA: MIT Press.

Nadeau, S. E., Davis, S. E., Wu, S. S., Dai, Y., & Richards, L. G. (2014). A pilot randomized controlled trial of d-cycloserine and distributed practice as adjuvants to constraint induced movement therapy after stroke. *Neurorehabil Neural Repair*, Epub PMID: 24769437.

Nadeau, S. E., & Kendall, D. L. (2006). Significance and possible mechanisms underlying generalization in aphasia therapy: Semantic treatment of anomia. *Brain Lang, 99*, 10–11.

Nadeau, S. E., & Kendall, D. L. (2012). Phonology, semantics, and lexical semantics. In K. M. Heilman & E. Valenstein (Eds.), *Clinical neuropsychology* (5th ed., pp. 42–85). New York: Oxford University Press.

Nadeau, S. E., Rothi, L. J. G., & Rosenbek, J. C. (2008). Language rehabilitation from a neural perspective. In R. Chapey (Ed.), *Language intervention strategies in aphasia and related neurogenic communication disorders* (5th ed., pp. 689–734). Philadelphia, PA: Lippincot Williams & Wilkins.

Nicholas, M. L., Helm-Estabrooks, N., Ward-Longergan, J., & Morgan, A. R. (1993). Evolution of severe aphasia in the first two years post onset. *Arch Phys Med Rehab, 74*, 830–836.

Nickels, L. (2002). Therapy for naming disorders. *Aphasiology, 16*, 935–979.

Plaut, D. C. (1996). Relearning after damage in connectionist networks: Toward a theory of rehabilitation. *Brain Lang, 52*, 25–82.

Pulvermüller, F., Neininger, B., Elbert, T., Mohr, B., Rockstroh, B., Koebbel, P., & Taub, E. (2001). Constraint-induced therapy of chronic aphasia after stroke. *Stroke, 32*, 1621–1626.

Pyle, W. H. (1913). Economical learning. *J Educ Psychol, 4*, 148–158.

Raymer, A. M., & Rothi, L. J. G. (2000). The semantic system. In S. E. Nadeau, L. J. G. Rothi, & B. Crosson (Eds.), *Aphasia and language: Theory to practice* (pp. 108–132). New York: Guilford.

Robey, R. R. (1994). The efficacy of treatment for aphasic persons: A meta-analysis. *Brain Lang, 47*, 582–608.

Robey, R. R. (1998). A meta-analysis of clinical outcomes in the treatment of aphasia. *J Speech Lang Hearing Res, 41*, 172–187.

Rössler, F., Streb, J., & Haan, H. (2001). Event-related brain potentials evoked by verbs and nouns in primed lexical decision. *Psychophysiology, 38,* 694–703.

Roth, H. L., Nadeau, S. E., Hollingsworth, A. L., Cimino-Knight, A. M., & Heilman, K. M. (2006). Naming concepts: Evidence of two routes. *Neurocase, 12,* 61–70.

Saletin, J. M., & Walker, M. P. (2012). Nocturnal mnemonics: Sleep and hippocampal memory processing. *Frontiers in Neurology, 3,* 1–12.

Shea, C. H., Lai, Q., Black, C., & Park, J.-H. (2000). Spacing practice sessions across days benefits the learning of motor skills. *Hum Movement Sci, 19,* 737–760.

Shebilske, W. L., Goettl, B. P., Corrington, K., & Day, E. A. (1999). Interlesson spacing and task-related processing during complex skill acquisition. *J Exp Psychol: Appl, 5,* 413–437.

Thompson, C. K. (2012). Northwestern Assessment of Verbs and Sentences (NAVS). Chicago: Wellspring Worldwide. http://flintbox.com/public/project/9299/.

Thompson, C. K., Riley, E. A., den Ouden, D.-B., Meltzer-Asscher, A., & Lukic, S. (2013). Training verb argument structure production in agrammatic aphasia: Behavioral and neural recovery patterns. *Cortex, 49,* 2358–2376.

Thompson, C. K., Shapiro, L. P., Kiran, S., & Sobecks, J. (2003). The role of syntactic complexity in treatment of sentence deficits in agrammatic aphasia: The complexity account of treatment efficacy (CATE). *J Speech Lang Hearing Res, 46,* 591–607.

Thompson, C. K., Shapiro, L. P., & Roberts, M. M. (1993). Treatment of sentence production deficits in aphasia: A linguistic-specific approach to wh- interrogative training and generalization. *Aphasiology, 7,* 111–133.

Vitevitch, M. S. (1997). The neighborhood characteristics of malapropisms. *Lang and Speech, 40,* 211–228.

von Monakow, C. (1914). *Die Lokalisation im Grosshirn.* Wiesbaden: Bergmann.

Wang, G., Grone, B., Colas, D., Appelbaum, L., & Mourrain, P. (2011). Synaptic plasticity in sleep: Learning, homeostasis and disease. *TINS, 34,* 452–463.

Weber, R., Ramos-Cabrer, P., Justicia, C., Wiedermann, D., Strecker, C., Sprenger, C., & Hoehn, M. (2008). Early prediction of functional recovery after experimental stroke: Functional magnetic resonance imaging, electrophysiology, and berhavioral testing in rats. *J Neurosci, 28,* 1022–1029.

Wieloch, T., & Nikolich, K. (2006). Mechanisms of neural plasticity following brain injury. *Curr Opin Neurol, 16,* 258–264.

Wisenburn, B., & Mahoney, K. (2009). A meta-analysis of word-finding treatments for aphasia. *Aphasiology, 23,* 1338–1352.

Witte, O. W., Bidmon, H.-J., Schiene, K., Redecker, C., & Hagemann, G. (2000). Functional differentiation of multiple perilesional zones after focal cerebral ischemia. *J Cereb Blood Flow Metab, 20,* 1149–1165.

Wolf, S. L., Thompson, P. A., Winstein, C. J., Miller, J. P., Blanton, S. R., Nichols-Larsen, D. S., . . . Sawaki, L. (2010). The EXCITE stroke trial: Comparing early and delayed constraint-induced movement therapy. *Stroke, 41,* 2309–2315.

Wolf, S. L., Winstein, C. J., Miller, J. P., Taub, E., Uswatte, G., Morris, D., . . . the EXCITE Investigators. (2006). Effect of constraint-induced movement therapy on upper extremity function 3 to 9 months after stroke: The EXCITE randomized clinical trial. *JAMA, 296,* 2095–2104.

Zaidel, E., Iacoboni, M., Berman, S. M., Zaidel, D. W., & Bogen, J. E. (2012). Callosal syndromes. In K. M. Heilman & E. Valenstein (Eds.), *Clinical neuropsychology* (5th ed., pp. 349–416). New York: Oxford University Press.

4

Cognitive Plasticity in Parkinson's Disease

David A. Copland and Anthony Angwin

Introduction

Parkinson's disease (PD) is a neurodegenerative condition associated primarily with degeneration of the nigrostriatal system and subsequent altered striatal output (Gerfen, 1992), although it is increasingly acknowledged that non-dopaminergic pathology across a wide range of structures is implicated in PD, particularly with disease progression (see Braak & Del Tredici, 2008). Though the most recognized clinical manifestations of the disease are motor symptoms such as tremor, bradykinesia, and rigidity, a decline in cognitive function is also a well-recognized feature of the disease. Dopaminergic dysregulation is often assumed to underlie such symptoms; however, the precise neurobiological basis of cognitive deficits and the neuroplastic mechanisms underlying changes in cognition are a matter of debate.

Parkinson's disease and its treatment provide a unique window into synaptic plasticity in the striatum. Both long-term potentiation (LTP) and long-term depression (LTD) have been observed in corticostriatal synapses and broader circuits, with striatal LTD requiring endogenous dopamine and failures in striatal LTD following dopaminergic denervation being restored with exogenous dopamine (see Calabresi et al., 2007). These findings in animals may be related to cognitive function in PD, given that one of the hallmark treatments of the disease is dopaminergic medications, which act to increase exogenous dopamine. The more recent treatment approaches using deep brain stimulation provide a further window into cognitive plasticity in PD by helping to isolate the effects of specific types of neuromodulation on cognitive function. In addition to the improvements in motor function offered by such treatments, research has increasingly demonstrated that such treatments may have both beneficial and detrimental impacts on cognitive function. This chapter will outline the cognitive effects of these treatments in the context of PD and will consider the underlying neuroplastic mechanisms that these treatments help initiate.

Different cognitive impairments in PD may arise from nigrostriatal pathology, limbic or cortical Lewy body-type pathology, or concurrent Alzheimer's pathology (Calabresi et al., 2007); however, it is widely recognized that even in the absence of overt dementia, the integrity of various cognitive functions is often compromised in PD. Such impairments encompass a wide range of domains of cognitive skills, including attention, planning (e.g., Tower of London), working memory, cognitive flexibility and inhibition, and use of rules and feedback (see Kehagia et al., 2010, for a review). It is also clear, however, that substantial heterogeneity exists with respect to the nature and extent of cognitive decline in PD. This heterogeneity may be explained in part by differing underlying pathologies and disease progression. For instance, it has been proposed that executive deficits and mild cognitive impairment in early PD most likely relate to fronto-striatal dysfunction (particularly involving dorsolateral circuitry), while noradrenergic deficits may underlie attentional set shifting, and cholinergic deficits may contribute to visuospatial and mnemonic impairments and play a key role in the development of dementia in PD (Kehagia et al., 2010).

Dopaminergic Influences on Cognition in Parkinson's Disease

One of the most prominent factors known to influence cognitive variability in PD is the manner in which dopaminergic medication, used to treat motor symptoms of the disease, interacts with the underlying neuropathology of the disease. Several anatomically segregated and possibly functionally distinct components of circuitry link the basal ganglia and cerebral cortex (Alexander, Crutcher, & DeLong, 1990; Alexander, DeLong, & Strick, 1986; Middleton & Strick, 2000), and in the early stages of PD, dopamine depletion is restricted primarily to the dorsal striatum, while the ventral striatum remains relatively spared by comparison (Kish et al., 1988) (see Figure 4.1). Accordingly, it is well recognized that this differential progression of dopamine loss can result in more impaired performance on cognitive tasks that recruit the dorsal striatum and dorsolateral prefrontal cortex circuitry, relative to tasks that recruit the ventral striatum and the orbitofrontal cortex.

More important, researchers have also illustrated that while dopaminergic medication in PD has the capacity to remediate cognitive performance deficits on dorsal striatal tasks, such medication can simultaneously impair performance on ventral striatal tasks as a result of overdosing this circuitry (e.g., Cools et al., 2001, 2003; Swainson et al., 2000). A task commonly used to investigate the impact of dopaminergic medication on cognition in PD is the probabilistic reversal learning task. In such tasks, participants can be presented with two visual stimuli and are asked to choose which stimulus is correct. The participants' selections are then reinforced according to a set contingency (e.g., an 80/20 ratio of positive and negative feedback for selection of the correct stimulus; a 20/80 ratio for the incorrect stimulus). Periodically during the experiment, a reversal in feedback occurs, such that the previously correct stimulus is now reinforced as the incorrect response. Consequently, participants must utilize this negative feedback to inhibit their learned

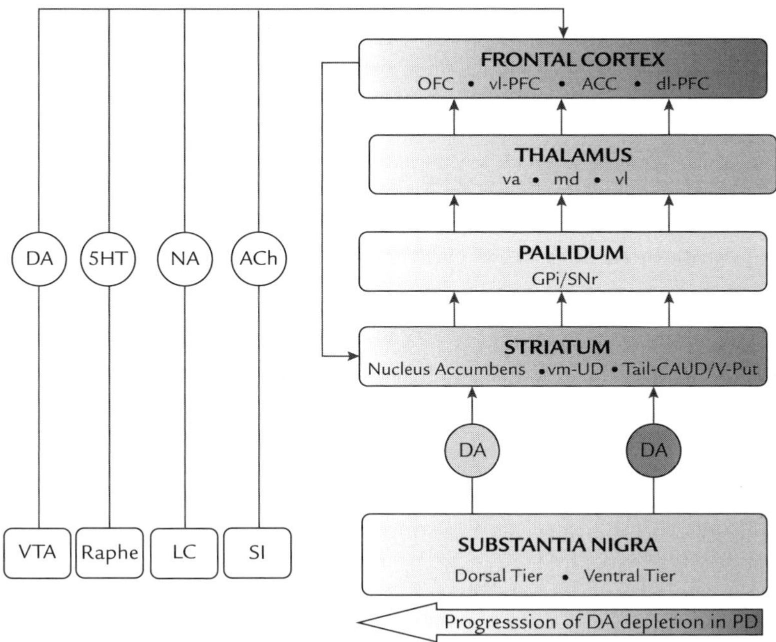

FIGURE 4.1 Chemical neuropathology in PD. This involves cell degeneration of dopamine (DA), where color gradients represent the progression of the pathology and different colors represent different components of frontal-subcortical circuits. Degeneration progresses from the ventral to the dorsal tier of the midbrain, including the ventral tegmental area (VTA). The ventral midbrain tier primarily projects DA to the dorsal striatum, and to more dorsal and lateral portions of the prefrontal cortex (PFC). The dorsal midbrain tier primarily projects DA to the ventral striatum and, via the output nuclei of the basal ganglia and the thalamus, to medial and lateral orbitofrontal cortex (ventrolateral and ventromedial PFC). Abbreviations: VTA, ventral tegmental area; DA, dopamine; Raphe, dorsal and medial raphe nuclei; 5HT, serotonin; LC, locus coeruleus; NA, noradrenaline; SI, substantia innominata; ACh, acetylcholine; vm-CAUD, ventromedial caudate nucleus; Tail-CAUD, tail of the caudate nucleus; V-Put, ventral putamen; DL-Put dorsolateral putamen; GPi, internal segment of the globus pallidus; SNr, substantia nigra pars reticulata; va, ventral anterior nucleus; md, dorsomedial nucleus; vl, ventrolateral nucleus; OFC, orbitofrontal cortex; vl-PFC, ventrolateral PFC; ACC, anterior cingulate nucleus; dl-PFC, dorsolateral PFC; SMA, supplementary motor area; PMC, premotor cortex. Modified and reprinted with permission from Elsevier Publishers; Cools, R., Lewis, S. J. G., Clark, L., Barker, R. A., & Robbins, T. W. (2007). L-DOPA disrupts activity in the nucleus accumbens during reversal learning in Parkinson's disease. *Neuropsychopharmacology, 32,* 180–189.

responses and begin selecting the alternative stimulus as the correct response instead. Utilizing functional magnetic resonance imaging (fMRI), Cools et al. (2002) confirmed the role of ventral striatal circuitry in the performance of such tasks, demonstrating that recruitment of the ventrolateral prefrontal cortex and ventral striatal region is associated with the final reversal error on the task. This error type represents the point at which participants stop responding to the previously learned stimulus and shift their responses to the newly learned stimulus pattern instead.

Consistent with the role of ventral striatal circuitry in probabilistic reversal learning, research has provided substantial evidence to suggest that dopaminergic medication in PD can overdose this circuitry and can alter performance on such tasks. For instance,

Cools et al. (2001) found that reversal learning performance was more impaired for PD patients on medication compared to off medication. Utilizing fMRI, Cools et al. (2007) also demonstrated increased activity in the nucleus accumbens during reversal learning in PD patients off levodopa medication, but not when they were on levodopa medication. In contrast, Cools et al. (2007) observed no such medication effects on activity within the dorsal striatum or prefrontal cortex, confirming the deleterious cognitive effects of selective overdosing of ventral striatal circuitry through dopaminergic medication. Moreover, there is evidence to suggest that patients medicated with the dopamine agonist pramipexole may be particularly impaired on reversal learning (Cools et al., 2006). As noted by Cools et al. (2006), such findings strengthen the notion of dopaminergic overdosing of ventral striatal circuitry, as pramipexole is highly selective for dopaminergic D3 receptors (Gerlach et al., 2003), which are predominantly located in the ventral, but not the dorsal, striatum (Murray et al., 1994).

Providing a critical extension of the dopamine overdose hypothesis is Frank's (2005) mechanistic account for how dopamine modulates learning through differential components of basal ganglia circuitry. Each frontal-subcortical circuit contains a direct pathway and an indirect pathway, which exert opposing effects on the thalamic nuclei and cortical output. The direct pathway governs the execution of responses (i.e., via a "Go" signal), whereas the indirect pathway inhibits them (via a "NoGo" signal) (see Figure 4.2). Frank's model suggests that these direct and indirect pathways control basal ganglia output in a competitive fashion via the action of bursts and dips in dopamine. Within the context of learning from positive and negative feedback, Frank (2005) suggests that bursts of dopamine in response to positive feedback support "Go" learning of the correct response, by increasing synaptic plasticity within the direct pathway and suppressing the indirect pathway. By contrast, decreases in dopamine in response to negative feedback have the opposite effect, such that the indirect pathway is released from suppression, thereby supporting "NoGo" learning to avoid the incorrect response.

This mechanistic account explains findings that patients off medication learned from negative outcomes more effectively than positive outcomes on procedural learning tasks—an effect that was reversed when the patients were medicated (Frank et al., 2004). Specifically, within the context of Frank's (2005) neuro-computational model, the dopamine dips that are essential to learning from negative outcomes via the indirect pathway are blocked by dopaminergic medication, leading to impaired learning from such negative feedback while medicated. Frank's (2005) model also provides a crucial framework for the interpretation of other studies that have shown a detrimental impact of medication on learning from punishment, but not reward, in PD (e.g., Bódi et al., 2009; Cools et al., 2006).

It is important to consider that changes to performance on probabilistic learning tasks such as that used by Frank et al. (2004) following dopaminergic medication may not solely be mediated by changes to the learning process itself, but may be at least partially mediated by application of the learned associations to novel contexts (Shiner et al., 2012;

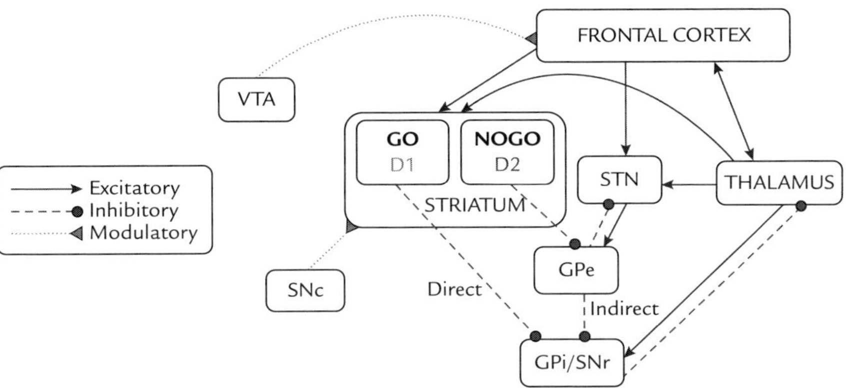

FIGURE 4.2 Schematic of the basal ganglia circuitry. Striatal "Go" cells project directly to the GPi to disinhibit the thalamus and facilitate the execution of actions in the frontal cortex. Striatal "NoGo" cells project indirectly to the GPi via the GPe, and suppress the execution of actions. Dopamine from the SNc differentially modulates activity in the direct and indirect pathways by activating different receptors in the striatum: D1 receptors expressed by the "Go" cells, and D2 receptors expressed by the "NoGo" cells. The STN is involved in a hyperdirect pathway receiving inputs from the frontal cortex and directly projecting to both the GPe and GPi. Abbreviations: GPi, internal segment of the globus pallidus; GPe, external segment of the globus pallidus; SNc, substantia nigra pars compacta; SNr, substantia nigra pars reticulata; STN, subthalamic nucleus; VTA, ventral tegmental area. Modified and reprinted with permission from MIT Press; Frank, M. J. (2005). Dynamic dopamine modulation in the basal ganglia: A neurocomputational account of cognitive deficits in medicated and nonmedicated Parkinsonism. *Journal of Cognitive Neuroscience, 17*(1), 51–72.

Smittenaar et al., 2012). Dopaminergic medication has also been shown to impair the learning of stimulus associations in PD patients even in the absence of explicit feedback or reward during task performance (MacDonald et al., 2011). Given the clear impact of dopaminergic therapy on cognition, it can be anticipated that performance on cognitive tasks should be affected not just by medication in PD, but also by individual baseline levels of dopamine in the striatum. Consistent with this notion, Cools et al. (2009) demonstrated that inter-individual variability in dopamine synthesis capacity in healthy adults modulated learning capacity from positive and negative outcomes. Specifically, when on placebo, healthy adults with higher baseline dopamine synthesis capacity demonstrated better reversal learning from unexpected rewards than punishments. Moreover, reward-based reversal learning was improved by a D2 receptor agonist (bromocriptine) in those with low baseline dopamine synthesis capacity, while the reverse pattern was observed in those with high baseline dopamine. Such findings highlight the need for further research in PD to determine the impact of baseline dopamine synthesis capacity on cognitive symptoms and their response to treatment.

Dopamine and Language Processing

Studies of language processing have also provided critical insight into the neuromodulation of cognition in PD. Some of the most common aspects of language processing observed to be impaired in PD include deficits in verbal fluency (Henry & Crawford, 2004), semantic processing (Arnott et al., 2010; Portin et al., 2000), and sentence processing (Angwin et al., 2006a; Colman et al., 2011; Grossman et al., 2000; Kemmerer, 1999; Lee et al., 2003; Ye et al., 2012). Importantly, the impairments to these components of language processing are directly impacted by the magnitude of dopamine depletion in PD, and these functions have been linked to frontostriatal circuits or components implicated in PD.

Deficits in PD have been observed on action/verb processing tasks such as verb generation and action naming (Bertella et al., 2002; Cotelli et al., 2007; Péran et al., 2003; Rodríguez-Ferreiro et al., 2009), with emerging evidence suggesting that such deficits are modulated by dopamine depletion. For instance, research has found that priming of concrete nouns does not differ between PD patients on and off levodopa. In contrast, priming of action verbs is directly impacted, with an absence of priming in PD patients off levodopa, which is normalized by medication (Boulenger et al., 2008). Reductions in action verbal fluency have also been observed in patients off medication relative to those on medication (Herrera et al., 2012), together with longer reaction times during naming of pictures, with a high degree of motor content in patients off medication relative to those on medication (Herrera & Cuetos, 2012). While the relationship between verb processing and the motor system remains a point of contention, a recent fMRI study of action and object naming have shown increased activation within the premotor cortex for PD patients on relative to off levodopa (Péran et al., 2013) identifying a potential neural basis for this cognitive deficit in PD.

Semantic priming, most often assessed using lexical decision tasks, has been used extensively to explore neuromodulatory changes to semantic processing in PD. These tasks often involve the presentation of word pairs (i.e., a prime word and a target word), with a participant required to make a lexical decision to the target word. Semantic priming refers to the widely demonstrated phenomenon that lexical decisions to the target word are faster when preceded by a related prime word (e.g., tiger-stripe) compared to an unrelated word (e.g., table-stripe).

These semantic priming effects can be a result of automatic spreading activation (Collins & Loftus, 1975; Neely, 1977). The notion of spreading activation relies on the assumption that concepts are stored within an interconnected semantic network, and when one node becomes activated, a spreading of activation occurs to other semantically or associatively related nodes. The presentation of a related prime word in a semantic priming task will partially activate the target word, thereby facilitating lexical access and speeding the lexical decision reaction time. Hence, manipulation of the stimulus onset asynchrony (SOA; i.e., the amount of time between presentation of the prime and the target word) makes it possible to investigate the time course of automatic semantic activation. It must be noted, however, that semantic priming can also be induced by conscious, attention-based processes. Specifically, semantic priming effects can be induced by the creation of pre-lexical expectancies or by the use of post-lexical semantic matching strategies (see Neely, 1991, for a review), and experiments are typically designed to encourage either automatic or controlled processes.

To date, research on semantic priming in healthy adults has provided convincing evidence for dopaminergic modulation of semantic activation. The nature of this neuro-modulatory effect, however, varies across studies. Some research has documented dopaminergic changes to the temporal dynamics of semantic activation, with observations suggesting that the onset and decay of semantic activation occurs earlier in healthy adults on levodopa relative to placebo (Angwin et al., 2004). In contrast, other research has suggested that hyperdopaminergic states in healthy adults lead to a focusing of semantic activation within semantic networks (Copland et al., 2003, 2009; Kischka et al., 1996; Roesch-Ely et al., 2006). The functional consequence of such focused activation is typically a loss or reduction of semantic priming for distantly related word pairs (e.g., a reduction in priming for "lion-stripe," a word pair that is only related via the intervening word "tiger"). This focusing of activation has been explained within the context of dopamine's proposed impact on the signal to noise ratio (SNR) of information processing, such that increased dopamine levels have the capacity to enhance salient signals and dampen weaker signals within neural networks (Cepeda & Levine, 1998; Servan-Schreiber et al., 1990).

Overall, research in healthy adults suggests that dopamine exerts a dual neuromodulatory influence on semantic activation, impacting not only the temporal availability of semantic information but also modulating the saliency of information within semantic networks. Based on such findings, it would be expected that dopamine depletion in PD will result in opposite changes to those observed in healthy adults in a hyperdopaminergic state. Comparisons of semantic priming in PD patients on versus off medication provide some degree of support for this assumption.

Some research has shown an absence of semantic priming in PD patients off levodopa medication, with semantic priming emerging in these same patients once optimally medicated (Angwin et al., 2007). Such findings are consistent with delays to semantic activation under conditions of increased dopamine depletion in PD, leading to an absence of priming during medication withdrawal. Of note, however, is the finding that priming effects were only partially restored by levodopa medication, as evidenced by the fact that control participants showed priming at short SOAs, whereas PD patients on medication only showed priming at longer SOAs. However, other semantic priming research in PD patients on medication has produced inconsistent results. Some studies have been able to induce semantic priming at short SOAs in PD patients tested on medication (Copland, 2003; Filoteo et al., 2003), suggesting intact automatic semantic activation, while others have found delayed automatic semantic activation in medicated PD patients (Arnott et al., 2001). As suggested by Grossman et al. (2002), it is likely that the extent to which semantic activation is delayed in PD is dependent on the magnitude of endogenous dopamine depletion and subsequent fronto-striatal dysfunction for individual patients. Indeed, positron emission tomography (PET) research has shown that cognitive slowing in PD is linked to dopaminergic dysfunction in fronto-striatal circuitry (Jokinen et al., 2013). Taken together, the results of such research suggest that changes to automatic semantic activation may only become apparent on behavioral testing once dopamine depletion and frontal-striatal dysfunction have reached a certain threshold. Thus, for some patients, the magnitude of dopamine depletion at the time of testing may not be sufficient to induce a measurable change in semantic activation. Instead, such deficits may only become apparent after further disease progression.

Research has also found results consistent with the impact of dopamine depletion on the SNR of semantic processing. Angwin et al. (2006b) utilized a multi-priming paradigm involving the presentation of two prime words, such that the first, second, or both prime words could be related to the target. At a short SOA, both control participants and PD patients (tested while optimally medicated) demonstrated priming for each related prime condition. In contrast, when these same PD patients were tested while off levodopa medication, they exhibited an absence of priming when the second prime word was unrelated to the target. These findings are potentially consistent with the impact of dopamine on SNRs, with increased dopamine depletion leading to a reduced salience of related words and increased salience of unrelated words within semantic networks. As a result, priming is more prone to disruption when an unrelated word is presented between the first related prime word and the target. Changes to prime salience also potentially explain findings of faster RTs to unrelated relative to related targets in PD patients off, but not on, medication (Angwin et al., 2009).

The impact of reduced SNRs on language processing is not restricted to semantic priming tasks. Righi et al. (2007) presented PD participants with an object identification task for tools and animals. Pictures were spatially filtered, ranging from entirely blurred to an optimal resolution. Drug-naïve PD participants required a greater spatial resolution than control and medicated PD participants to correctly identify animals, but not tools. When these drug-naïve PD participants were retested when medicated at a later time point, their performance was similar to that of the control participants. The authors suggested that the findings were consistent with dopamine's capacity to enhance task-relevant signals and inhibit irrelevant information through cortical-striatal circuitry. Specifically, increased dopamine depletion in the drug-naïve patients may lead to impaired bottom-up processing of the visual-perceptual attributes of the pictures, together with impaired top-down processing that produces increased semantic activation whereby multiple conflicting hypotheses about the identity of the stimulus become activated. This overload of semantic activation can be viewed as similar to the increased salience of unrelated semantic information that becomes activated during semantic priming tasks in PD patients off medication (Angwin et al., 2006b).

It appears that dopamine depletion in PD can disrupt both the timing and saliency of semantic activation within semantic networks, and that these effects can be ameliorated, at least partially, by dopaminergic medication. Importantly, the evidence also indicates that such effects are dissociable. For instance, even in those patients with a spared time course of semantic activation, disruptions to the SNR of semantic processing or other disruptions to controlled semantic activation have been evident (Angwin et al., 2005; 2006b; Arnott et al., 2011). Accordingly, while mild levels of dopamine depletion may be enough to alter the SNR of information processing, a greater magnitude of depletion appears necessary before measurable changes in the speed of semantic activation occur.

The dopaminergic changes to cognition and semantic processing in PD can also be expected to have functional, downstream consequences on other aspects of language processing. In particular, the comprehension of syntactically complex sentences is reliant on various cognitive resources, including working memory and speed of semantic activation. Although research has conclusively demonstrated impaired sentence comprehension for some patients with PD (e.g., Angwin et al., 2006a; Grossman et al., 2000; Kemmerer, 1999; Lee et al., 2003; Ye et al., 2012), studies of sentence comprehension in PD patients on and off levodopa have been surprisingly limited to date and the results have been equivocal. Grossman et al. (2001) found that sentence-processing impairments evident in PD patients off medication were normalized by levodopa medication, whereas Skeel et al. (2001) observed sentence-comprehension impairments in PD patients both on and off medication. Despite these conflicting findings, there is still much evidence to suggest that dopaminergic alterations to cognitive resources such as working memory and semantic activation contribute to sentence-processing difficulties in PD.

A number of researchers have explored the time course of lexical access in PD patients with good versus poor comprehension of complex sentences. Grossman et al. (2002) observed that semantic priming effects were delayed only in a subgroup of PD patients with poor comprehension of complex sentences, suggesting that comprehension impairments become manifest in those patients whose dopamine depletion is sufficient to delay semantic activation. Similarly, other studies have also found increased delays to semantic activation in PD patients with poor sentence comprehension, although of interest is the observation of mild delays to semantic activation, even in those with good sentence comprehension (Angwin et al., 2005, 2007). The maintenance of good sentence comprehension skills despite minor delays to semantic activation indicates that the depletion of dopamine, and the resultant delays to semantic activation, must reach a critical threshold before sentence comprehension impairments become evident.

Compensatory neural mechanisms may also contribute to the maintenance of sentence-comprehension skills in PD. During sentence processing in people with mild PD, Grossman et al. (2003) observed reduced activation of a broad neural network important for cognitive resources, including the striatum, the left anteromedial prefrontal cortex, and the right posterolateral temporal cortex. Of further interest, however, is their observation of increased activation of the right inferior frontal cortex and left posterolateral temporo-parietal areas in PD patients relative to controls. As the authors noted, these regions may support verbal working memory and linguistic aspects involved in sentence comprehension, and the increased activation in these regions may reflect a compensatory mechanism that allows patients in the early stages of PD to maintain an adequate level of sentence comprehension accuracy.

Symptom Influences on Cognition

Symptomatic variables in PD have also been shown to have a significant impact on cognitive performance in PD. For instance, the predominant type of motor symptom can potentially influence the nature of cognitive dysfunction, with patients presenting with akinesia and rigidity symptoms performing more poorly on demanding working memory tasks relative to those patients with tremor (Moustafa et al., 2013). A recent review of the literature has also demonstrated that the side of motor symptom predominance can influence some aspects of cognition in PD (Verreyt et al., 2011). The review indicates that PD patients with left side motor symptom predominance often exhibit more difficulties on tasks involving spatial attention, visuospatial orientation, and mental imagery, whereas patients with a predominance of right-sided motor symptoms more frequently exhibit difficulties on language-related tasks and verbal memory. In contrast, however, the majority of studies have found no difference in attention or executive function between those with right and left motor symptoms (Verreyt et al., 2011).

Interestingly, although recent research suggests that the lateralization of motor symptoms may have little impact on cognition in the early, unmedicated stages of PD (Poletti et al., 2013), there is emerging evidence to suggest that dopaminergic medication can overdose the less affected hemisphere and thereby impact cognition in some patients. For instance, Maril et al. (2013) found that during performance of a probabilistic feedback task, patients with right onset motor symptoms (and hence left hemisphere dominance of dopamine depletion) performed better at attempting to minimize losses rather than gain rewards when off medication, a pattern that was reversed in these patients once medicated. In accordance with the dopamine overdose hypothesis, the findings were linked to the impact of dopaminergic medication on the asymmetric pathology in these PD patients. Specifically, medication has the capacity to reduce left hemisphere impairments to reward-based learning, while simultaneously having a detrimental impact on punishment-based learning by overdosing the less affected right hemisphere.

Disease Progression

Some key predictors of cognitive decline have been identified in PD. Specifically, clinical predictors of cognitive decline include a non-tremor dominant phenotype, impaired semantic but not phonemic fluency, and impaired pentagon copying at presentation (Williams-Gray et al., 2007). Interestingly, Williams-Gray et al. (2007) argued that impaired semantic fluency was more likely to reflect non-dopaminergic pathology in posterior cortical (temporal) regions rather than frontostriatal circuitry. However, this interpretation is still a matter of debate, given other evidence linking frontostriatal dysfunction to semantic fluency deficits. Others have reported progressive changes in a neurocognitive network in PD involving reductions in metabolism of the dorsolateral prefrontal cortex, pre-supplementary motor area (pre-SMA), and superior parietal cortex, and increased metabolism in the cerebellum (Huang et al., 2007). Consideration must also be given to how the neurodegenerative nature of PD influences the impact of dopaminergic medication on cognition. While ventral striatal circuitry may remain relatively spared in the early stages of the disease, this circuitry will become increasingly disrupted with progression of the disease and increases in dopamine depletion. MacDonald et al. (2013) found that PD patients in the early stage of the disease (duration <5 years) had normal reward-based learning when off medication, which was impaired by dopaminergic medication, consistent with the dopamine overdose hypothesis. In contrast, later stage PD patients (duration >5 years) demonstrated impaired reward-based learning when off medication, although surprisingly this was not ameliorated by medication. These findings highlight that the differential impact of dopaminergic medications on frontal-striatal circuitry is a dynamic process, subject to substantial change during progression of the disease. Similarly, disease progression will also be expected to alter hemispheric asymmetry of dopamine depletion, such that the impact of medication on such cognitive variability will change over time. Accordingly, ongoing research is still required to delineate the multifaceted interaction of cognitive impairment and disease progression in PD, also considering the increasing prevalence of non-dopaminergic pathology over time (Braak et al., 2003). With regard to the influence of disease progression on subcortical circuitry in the long term, it has been suggested that loss of dendritic spines may occur as a protective or neuroplastic mechanism in order to reduce excessive cortical output from the indirect pathway, with this loss of spines possibly due to Lewy body pathology in corticostriatal projections, particularly in later stages (see Braak & Del Tredici, 2008).

Long-Term Effects of Dopamine Depletion

Dopamine is also critical to long-term synaptic changes within striatal circuitry. Specifically, dopamine has been shown to modulate long-term potentiation, depression, and depotentiation, all key aspects of long-term synaptic plasticity (Calabresi et al., 2007, for a review). Indeed, it is suggested that changes, induced by dopamine depletion, to these forms of synaptic plasticity within frontostriatal circuitry can lead to both motor and cognitive symptoms in PD (Calabresi et al., 2006, 2007). In a recent review, Zhuang et al. (2013) illustrated how dopamine influences cortical-striatal plasticity in the direct and indirect pathways to impact motor impairments in PD. Specifically, reduced dopamine can lead to "learned" motor inhibition (e.g., akinesia) via long-term potentiation of cortical-striatal circuitry in the indirect pathway. Importantly, while the acute effects of dopaminergic medication only partially remediate this aberrant pattern of activation, repeated dopaminergic therapy can facilitate long-term depression within the indirect pathway, thereby normalizing function. Despite the plethora of studies confirming the short-term, acute effects of dopamine replacement therapy on cognition, very little is currently known about the longer term impact of dopamine replacement on cognition and its effects on synaptic plasticity. Accordingly, future research needs to explore how such neuroplastic changes in response to dopamine loss and long-term administration of dopaminergic medication can influence cognitive performance in PD. Another avenue that requires further research is the role of other neurotransmitter systems in cognitive plasticity in PD (see Figure 4.1), particularly given proposals that cognitive deficits in PD may arise in part from an imbalance in cholinergic to dopaminergic neurotransmitters at the cortical level (Calabresi et al., 2007). The importance of this balance is further highlighted by observations that cholinergic agents can provide modest improvements in PD patients for aspects of cognition, including attention (Kehagia et al., 2010).

Modulation of Cognition in PD with Deep Brain Stimulation

The last decade has seen increased use of deep brain stimulation (DBS) to treat movement disorders in Parkinson's disease, which provides another aspect of treatment-induced cognitive plasticity to consider. While this treatment (usually involving targeting of the subthalamic nucleus [STN] or the internal segment of the globus pallidus [GPi]) generally has significant benefits for motor dysfunction, its effects on non-motor function, including cognition, are less clear. A meta-analysis by Parsons et al. (2006) showed that compared to presurgery, DBS of the STN has a small, but significant, negative impact on executive function and verbal learning and memory, and is associated with a moderate decline in verbal fluency. Importantly, the effect of DBS on verbal fluency was not associated with dopaminergic medication, disease duration, or stimulation parameters and appears to persist in the long term (Fasano et al., 2010).

It is challenging to tease apart what neurocognitive mechanisms may underlie this phenomenon, in part because verbal fluency performance involves a number of distinct cognitive operations and motor-speech, which are often not controlled for. Producing a word list based on a category involves (1) immediate verbal attention to initiate the word generation, (2) an intact lexical-semantic system from which to select words, (3) retrieval from verbal declarative memory, (4) switching between subcategories, (5) inhibition of previous productions, and (6) executive coordination of the process, including working memory, in order to monitor performance and adhere to the rules (Ruff et al., 1997). While lexical-semantic representations are assumed to be intact in PD, controlled retrieval of lexical-semantic representations can be impaired in PD, which may relate to frontostriatal dysfunction (Copland et al., 2003) and cognitive functions, including attention, verbal memory, executive function, and working memory; these are all implicated in PD and likewise have been linked to subcortical-frontal circuitry, although not exclusively (see previous discussion in this chapter). The notion that DBS of the STN could alter subcortical-frontal mechanisms supporting lexical-semantic retrieval is further supported by electrical stimulation and electrode recording studies suggesting that the caudate plays a role in cognitive control, word retrieval, and semantic processing (Abdullaev et al 1998; Gil Robles et al., 2005). The influence of the STN on word retrieval is also consistent with evidence of caudate-thalamic-pre-SMA activity during category member generation in healthy individuals (Crosson et al., 2003).

One difficulty with the proposal that STN stimulation modifies activity within these relevant frontal-subcortical circuits is that placement of electrodes is often assumed to be in the motor portion of the STN, which may therefore not modulate relevant striato-thalamo-cortical circuitry. However, placement may not always be confined to this region; the field of stimulation may extend beyond the sensorimotor region of the STN (e.g., McIntyre et al., 2004), and these conclusions are based on the assumption that these circuits remain segregated (Parsons et al., 2006). More direct evidence for the role of the STN in these DBS-induced changes has been obtained with local field potential recordings showing that verbal fluency is associated with changes in the STN local field potential power, which correlates with behavioral fluency performance and switching (Anzak et al., 2011). Similar techniques have shown modulation of STN activity during inhibition in a verbal Stroop task (Brittain et al., 2012) and response inhibition (Alegre et al., 2013), which may also account for observations of impaired verbal fluency post-DBS of the STN. Based on such findings, Anzak et al. (2011) proposed that the STN may serve to modulate dorsolateral prefrontal cortex–driven selection and inhibition during verbal fluency by inhibiting thalamic output to the temporal cortex such that only appropriate words are selected, or it may receive a frontal signal resulting in a switch from automatic to controlled processing during the task (see also Schroeder et al., 2003, for PET evidence that DBS of the STN modulates frontotemporal activity).

The other challenge in explaining the underlying mechanism of these post-DBS changes in cognition and understanding the underlying neuroplasticity involved is the influence of surgery on symptoms, with some suggesting that microlesions in the cortical structures involved in word fluency may account for DBS-related deficits (De Gaspari et al., 2006). Another factor to consider is that patients may have reduced dopaminergic treatment post-DBS. Studies investigating on versus off DBS postsurgery may provide a clearer picture regarding stimulation-induced short-term plasticity of cognition. Indeed, observed behavioral changes on versus off DBS confirm that the effects of DBS are not solely due to surgical effects; however, it appears that the acute effects of DBS of the STN on cognition vary depending on the operations engaged, with improvement, declines, and no change in function being reported. For instance, in a series of studies on language-related processes in the same cohort of PD patients, Castner et al. (2007a) observed that attention-based semantic priming and the ability to suppress prepotent words in a sentence-completion task was improved in PD patients on versus off stimulation of the STN, while initiation of sentence completion was slowed (Castner et al., 2007b) and impairments in semantic switching during word production were heightened (Castner et al., 2008). Meanwhile, performance on a variation of the Stroop (picture-word interference task) with semantic distractors showed no effect of STN stimulation (Castner et al., 2007b). Taken together, these studies suggest that acute stimulation of the STN improves efficiency of lexical-semantic processing in comprehension and the ability to suppress verbal production when requiring internal generation of alternative responses; however, aspects of verbal production related to initiation, selection, and switching may be compromised with STN stimulation (see also Castner et al., 2008). The differential influence of DBS of the STN on these different cognitive processes may reflect the modulation of activity in different frontostriatal circuits. For instance, controlled semantic priming, which is improved, is associated with anterior cingulate circuitry, whereas suppression and switching, which is impaired, is associated with dorsolateral prefrontal cortex. In sum, these studies highlight the complexity of cognitive plasticity in response to DBS, highlight a number of circuits that may be implicated, and underscore the need to more directly examine the neural mechanisms underpinning the numerous cognitive changes observed with this treatment.

Functional neuroimaging during DBS provides such an opportunity, although challenges exist regarding fMRI during DBS stimulation, and as a consequence only a limited number of other imaging modalities have been employed to address this issue. For instance, Schroeder et al. (2002) observed decreased regional cerebral blood flow (rCBF) in the right anterior cingulate and ventral striatum on STN stimulation, which was associated which poorer Stroop performance. In a subsequent study, Schroeder et al. (2003) observed that decreased verbal fluency on DBS of the STN was associated with decreased rCBF in the left inferior frontal gyrus and inferior temporal gyrus, suggesting that stimulation of the STN modulates activity beyond frontostriatal circuitry. Cilia et al. (2007) used single photon emission computed tomography to demonstrate that decreased verbal fluency on DBS of the STN was associated with decreased left dorsolateral prefrontal, anterior cingulate, and caudate perfusion.

Further imaging work may also provide much-needed insights into the longer-term neuroplastic mechanisms underlying DBS in PD. A range of mechanisms has been proposed to underlie the short- and long-term effects of DBS in PD. These include changing neuronal firing pattern and rate in the basal ganglia, effects on synaptic function triggering neurotransmitter release (e.g., glutamate and adenosine), and increasing blood flow and neurogenesis, with more recent proposals suggesting that local neuronal cell inhibition and excitation of surrounding axons may account for DBS actions (Okun, 2012). Mueller et al. (2012) recently provided resting state fMRI data supporting the view that DBS modulates and normalizes connectivity between STN and the premotor hub, with PD connectivity directly relating to clinical symptoms; however, the influence of such DBS-induced changes in connectivity on cognitive function remains to be examined. The timing of DBS implantation may also be critical, with earlier DBS resulting in greater neuroplastic change in the context of disease progression (see Fasano & Deuschl, 2012). This discussion has focused on DBS of the STN, as the majority of work on cognition and DBS has been done with STN implantation. There is some evidence to suggest that DBS of the STN is more likely to impact verbal fluency than DBS of the globus pallidus interna, although overall cognitive outcomes may not differ (Okun et al., 2009).

Cognitive Plasticity Induced by Behavioral Interventions

Despite evidence of frequent cognitive deficits in PD, there are surprisingly few adequately controlled studies of cognitive interventions (see Hindle et al., 2013), and the structural or functional plasticity underlying such interventions is not well established. In a small sample randomized controlled trial (RCT), Sammer et al. (2006) found that 10 sessions of training focused on working memory abilities that require executive function significantly improved performance in a group of PD patients compared to a control group receiving standard treatment; however, significant improvements were limited to a standard test of rule-shifting. More widespread benefits were observed in an RCT of 4 weeks of computer-assisted training addressing a number of cognitive domains, including working memory, attention, executive function, and visuospatial function (Paris et al., 2011). Improved performance was noted across a range of cognitive functions (including attention and executive function) compared to participants receiving an active control of speech therapy. In the largest study to date, Naismith et al. (2013) recently conducted a single-blind wait list controlled trial combining computer-based cognitive training (focused on memory) with a psychoeducational package, demonstrating significant improvements on tests of learning and memory.

These aforementioned studies demonstrate that a range of cognitive deficits may be improved by training in PD, but they do not provide insights into structural or functional brain changes associated with treatment-related improvements in cognition, and this may be premature given the scarcity of large studies demonstrating behavioral benefits. Preliminary work on this question was conducted in a small sample, nonrandomized fMRI study of PD patients before and after 6 months of voluntary Sudoku, revealing greater activity on the second scan in the untrained than the trained group in a large number of regions, including frontal, temporal, and parietal areas. The attenuation of this extensive activity in the trained group was interpreted as reflecting training-related changes in cortical activity, although the differences between the scan task and the training, the dispersed brain activity observed, and the potential for bias in more capable subjects choosing the Sudoku training limit the interpretation of this study.

Other work examining brain changes in brain activity associated with motor interventions may also provide insight into potential brain mechanisms involved in cognitive treatments in PD. For instance, PET studies of speech treatments in PD have demonstrated normalization of motor-premotor activation, a shift to right hemisphere activity, and recruitment of alternative frontostriatal circuitry involving the dorsolateral prefrontal cortex (Narayana, 2010). Sehm et al. (2013) observed changes in gray matter volume following 6 weeks of training in a balance task, which suggested possible learning-dependent structural plasticity in PD patients that was distinct from structural changes observed in controls performing the same training. In the initial stages of training, controls showed changes in hippocampal gray matter associated with learning, whereas PD patients demonstrated transient learning-related changes in a range of regions, including premotor and inferior parietal cortex, which was interpreted as arising from an early reliance on task-relevant sensory processing during the learning task in compensation for reduced striato-mesial frontal input. In the long term, PD subjects showed increased right cerebellar gray matter volume post-training, while controls showed decreased volume in this region (which in itself is difficult to interpret). While these data are intriguing, such findings should be viewed with caution given questions regarding the ability of such techniques to reliably detect changes in gray matter (see Thomas & Baker, 2013). Overall, these studies in motor training demonstrate neuroplasticity mechanisms and principles in PD that may also underpin cognitive interventions, including normalization of brain activity, right hemisphere upregulation for left hemisphere functions, and compensatory recruitment of related fronto-striatal, parietal, premotor, or cerebellar mechanisms, which may result in structural plasticity that varies as a function of the nature and phase of the training. Recruitment of such mechanisms may account for why some PD patients maintain relatively intact cognitive function.

Evidence that cardiovascular fitness is associated with superior cognitive performance in PD (Uc et al., 2008) and that exercise interventions may improve certain cognitive domains, particularly executive function (e.g., Cruise et al., 2011) also suggests possible neuroplastic mechanisms that may modify cognitive changes in PD. The influence of exercise, and combined exercise and cognitive training, on cognitive function in PD requires further well-controlled studies identifying the type and dose of exercise required, and it is still unclear whether exercise influences cognition in persons with PD in a substantially different way from its effect on cognition in healthy older adults. Regardless, the potential role of brain derived neurotrophic factor (BDNF) in mediating exercise-induced plasticity and cognitive improvement in PD has been proposed, based on supporting but indirect evidence that BDNF is expressed in neurons affected in PD and protects dopaminergic cells (Ahlskog, 2011) and that post-exercise increases in BDNF are associated with enhanced cognitive performance in humans (e.g., Winter et al., 2007). Finally, the influence of cognitive or cognitive plus exercise interventions on PD has not been considered in the context of disease duration or severity, cognitive symptoms, or pharmacological or neurostimulation treatments, which would further inform regarding the form of neural plasticity that drives enhanced cognition in PD.

Conclusions

There is mounting evidence of cognitive plasticity in PD in response to neuromodulation via deep brain stimulation and pharmacological interventions, in addition to more preliminary work regarding behavioral interventions. However, elucidating the neurobiological basis of such changes is challenging in this heterogeneous neurodegenerative disorder, which includes non-dopaminergic and non-subcortical pathology. While functional plasticity and upregulation within frontostriatal circuits are likely, the clearest indications to date have been derived from studies looking at more acute effects of neuromodulation (either dopaminergic or via deep brain stimulation) on cognition; however, much work needs to be done to understand longer-term neural plasticity occurring as a consequence of these treatments in the context of disease progression, behavioral interventions, and other pathophysiological mechanisms inherent to this disease. Certain aspects of cognition are modulated most likely through frontal-subcortical circuit-specific mechanisms; however, the role of specific components within these circuits may be further defined with exciting advances in electrical recordings from selective subcortical components, as recently demonstrated with the STN. Non-invasive brain stimulation (e.g., rTMS and tDCS) will provide further avenues for exploring cognitive plasticity in this population, with tDCS in PD modulating working memory (Boggio et al., 2006). While cognition has traditionally been neglected in PD, current efforts to understand cognitive plasticity and its underlying mechanisms will provide unprecedented insights into human frontal-subcortical organization, cognitive function, and plastic potential. This knowledge has considerable implications for understanding cognitive plasticity in other populations with subcortical dysfunction (e.g. Huntington's disease, autism spectrum disorders, subcortical stroke) and dopaminergic dysregulation (e.g. schizophrenia, ADHD) and has the potential to drive new treatments targeting cognition, such as dopaminergic pharmacotherapy and brain stimulation.

References

Abdullaev, Y. G., Bechtereva, N. P., & Melnichuk, K. V. (1998). Neuronal activity of human caudate nucleus and prefrontal cortex in cognitive tasks. *Behav Brain Res, 97*, 159–177.

Ahlskog, J. (2011). Does vigorous exercise have a neuroprotective effect in Parkinson disease? *Neurology, 77*, 288–294.

Alegre, M., Lopez-Azcarate, J., Obeso, I., Wilkinson, L., Rodriguez-Oroz, M. C., Valencia, M., . . . Obeso, J. A. (2013). The subthalamic nucleus is involved in successful inhibition in the stop-signal task: a local field potential study in Parkinson's disease. *Exp Neurol, 239*, 1–12.

Alexander, G. E., Crutcher, M. D., & DeLong, M. R. (1990). Basal ganglia-thalamocortical circuits: parallel substrates for motor, oculomotor, "prefrontal" and "limbic" functions. *Prog Brain Res, 85*, 119–146.

Alexander, G. E., DeLong, M. R., & Strick, P. L. (1986). Parallel organization of functionally segregated circuits linking basal ganglia and cortex. *Annual Review of Neurosci, 9*, 357–381.

Angwin, A. J., Arnott, W. L., Copland, D. A., Haire, M. P. L., Murdoch, B. E., Silburn, P. A., & Chenery, H. J. (2009). Semantic activation in Parkinson's disease patients on and off levodopa. *Cortex, 45*, 950–959.

Angwin, A. J., Chenery, H. J., Copland, D. A., Arnott, W. L., Murdoch, B. E., & Silburn, P. A. (2004). Dopamine and semantic activation: An investigation of masked direct and indirect priming. *J Int Neuropsych Soc, 10*, 15–25.

Angwin, A. J., Chenery, H. J., Copland, D. A., Murdoch, B. E., & Silburn, P. A. (2005). Summation of semantic priming and complex sentence comprehension in Parkinson's disease. *Cognitive Brain Res, 25*, 78–89.

Angwin, A. J., Chenery, H. J., Copland, D. A., Murdoch, B. E., & Silburn, P. A. (2006a). Self-paced reading and sentence comprehension in Parkinson's disease. *J Neurolinguist, 19*, 239–252.

Angwin, A. J., Chenery, H. J., Copland, D. A., Murdoch, B. E., & Silburn, P. A. (2006b). The influence of dopamine on semantic activation in Parkinson's disease: Evidence from a multi-priming task. *Neuropsychology, 20*, 299–306.

Angwin, A. J., Chenery, H. J., Copland, D. A., Murdoch, B. E., & Silburn, P. A. (2007). The speed of lexical activation is altered in Parkinson's disease. *J Clin Exp Neuropsyc, 29*, 73–85.

Anzak, A., Gaynor, L., Beigi, M., Limousin, P., Hariz, M., Zrinzo, L., . . . Jahanshahi, M. (2011) A gamma band specific role of the sub-thalamic nucleus in switching during verbal fluency tasks in Parkinson's disease. *Exp Neurol, 232*, 136–142.

Arnott, W. A., Chenery, H. J., Angwin, A. J., Murdoch, B. E., Silburn, P. A., & Copland, D. A. (2010). Decreased semantic competitive inhibition in Parkinson's disease: Evidence from an investigation of word search performance. *Int J Speech Lang Pathol, 12*(5), 437–445.

Arnott, W. L., Chenery, H. J., Murdoch, B. E., & Silburn, P. A. (2001). Semantic priming in Parkinson's disease: Evidence for delayed spreading activation. *J Clin Exp Neuropsyc, 23*(4), 502–519.

Arnott, W. A., Copland, D. A., Chenery, H. J., Murdoch, B. E., Silburn, P. A., & Angwin, A. J. (2011). The influence of dopamine on automatic and controlled semantic activation in Parkinson's disease. *Parkinson's Disease, 2011*, 157072.

Bertella, L., Albani, G., Greco, E., Priano, L., Mauro, A., Marchi, S., Bulla, D., & Semenza, C. (2002). Noun verb dissociation in Parkinson's disease. *Brain Cognition, 48*, 277–280.

Bódi, N., Kéri, S., Nagy, H., Moustafa, A., Myers, C. E., Daw, N., Dibó, G., Takáts, A., Bereczki, D., & Gluck, M. A. (2009). Reward-learning and the novelty-seeking personality: A between and within subjects study of the effects of dopamine agonists on young Parkinson's patients. *Brain, 132*, 2385–2395.

Boggio, P. S., Ferrucci, R., Rigonatti, S. P., et al. (2006). Effects of transcranial direct current stimulation on working memory in patients with Parkinson's disease. *J Neurol Sci, 249*, 31–38.

Boulenger, V., Mechtouff, L., Thobois, S., Broussolle, E., Jeannerod, M., & Nazir, T. A. (2008). Word processing in Parkinson's disease is impaired for action verbs but not for concrete nouns. *Neuropsychologia, 46*, 743–756.

Braak, H., & Del Tredici, K. (2008). Cortico-basal ganglia-cortical circuitry in Parkinson's disease reconsidered. *Exp Neurol, 212*, 226–229.

Braak, H., Del Tredici, K., Rüb, U., de Vos, R. A. I., Jansen Steur, E. N. H., Braak, E., (2003). Staging of brain pathology related to sporadic Parkinson's disease. *Neurobiol Aging, 24*, 197–211.

Brittain, J. S., Watkins, K. E., Joundi, R. A., Ray, N. J., Holland, P., Green, A. L., . . . Jenkinson, N. (2012). A role for the subthalamic nucleus in response in- hibition during conflict. *J Neurosci, 32*, 13396–13401.

Calabresi, P., Picconi, B., Parnetti, L., & Di Filippo, M. (2006). A convergent model for cognitive dysfunctions in Parkinson's disease: the critical dopamine-acetylcholine synaptic balance. *Lancet Neurol, 5*, 974–983.

Calabresi, P., Picconi, B., Tozzi, A., & Di Filippo, M. (2007). Dopamine-mediated regulation of corticostriatal synaptic plasticity. *Trends Neurosci, 30*, 211–219.

Castner, J. E., Chenery, H. J., Copland, D. A., Coyne, T. J., Sinclair, F., & Silburn, P. A. (2007a). Semantic and affective priming as a function of stimulation of the subthalamic nucleus in Parkinson's disease. *Brain, 130*, 1395–1407.

Castner, J., Copland, D. A., Silburn, P. A., Coyne, T. J., Sinclair, F., & Chenery, H. J. (2007b). Lexical-semantic inhibitory mechanisms in Parkinson's disease as a function of subthalamic stimulation. *Neuropsychologia, 45*, 3167–3177.

Castner, J. E., Copland, D. A., Silburn, P. A., Coyne, T. J., Sinclair, F., & Chenery, H. J. (2008). Subthalamic stimulation affects homophone meaning generation in Parkinson's disease. *J Int Neuropsychological Society, 14*, 890–894.

Cepeda, C., & Levine, M. S. (1998). Dopamine and N-Methyl-D-Aspartate receptor interactions in the neostriatum. *Dev Neurosci, 20*, 1–18.

Cilia, R., Siri, C., Marotta, G., De Gaspari, D., Landi, A., Mariani, C. B., . . . Antonini A. (2007). Brain networks underlining verbal fluency decline during STN-DBS in Parkinson's disease: an ECD-SPECT study. *Parkinsonism Relat Disord, 13*, 290–294.

Collins, A. M., & Loftus, E. F. (1975). A spreading activation theory of semantic processing. *Psychol Rev, 82*, 407–428.

Colman, K. S. F., Koerts, J., Stowe, L. A., Leenders, K. L., & Bastiaanse, R. (2011). Sentence comprehension and its association with executive functions in patients with Parkinson's disease. *Parkinson's Disease, 2011*, 213983.

Cools, R. (2006). Dopaminergic modulation of cognitive function: Implications for l-dopa treatment in Parkinson's disease. *Neurosci Biobehav R, 30*, 1–23.

Cools, R., Altamirano, L., & D'Esposito, M. (2006). Reversal learning in Parkinson's disease depends on medication status and outcome valence. *Neuropsychologia, 44*, 1663–1673.

Cools, R., Barker, R. A., Sahakian, B. J., & Robbins, T. W. (2001). Enhanced or impaired cognitive function in Parkinson's disease as a function of dopaminergic medication and task demands. *Cereb Cortex, 11*, 1136–1143.

Cools, R., Barker, R. A., Sahakian, B. J., & Robbins, T. W. (2003). L-dopa medication remediates cognitive inflexibility, but increases impulsivity in patients with Parkinson's disease. *Neuropsychologia, 41*, 1431–1441.

Cools, R., Clark, L., Owens, A. M., & Robbins, T. W. (2002). Defining the neural mechanisms of probabilistic reversal learning using event-related functional magnetic resonance imaging. *J Neurosci, 22*(11), 4563–4567.

Cools, R., Frank, M. J., Gibbs, S. E., Miyakawa, A., Jagust, W., & D'Esposito, M. (2009). Striatal dopamine predicts outcome-specific reversal learning and its sensitivity to dopaminergic drug administration. *J Neurosci, 29*(5), 1538–1543.

Cools, R., Lewis, S. J. G., Clark, L., Barker, R. A., & Robbins, T. W. (2007). L-DOPA disrupts activity in the nucleus accumbens during reversal learning in Parkinson's disease. *Neuropsychopharmacol, 32*, 180–189.

Copland, D. A. (2003). The basal ganglia and semantic engagement: Potential insights from semantic priming in individuals with subcortical vascular lesions, Parkinson's disease, and cortical lesions. *J Int Neuropsych Soc, 9*(7), 1041–1052.

Copland, D. A., Chenery, H. J., Murdoch, B. E., Arnott, W. L., & Silburn, P. A. (2003). Dopamine enhances semantic salience: Semantic priming evidence from healthy individuals. *Brain Lang, 87*(1), 103–104.

Copland, D. A., McMahon, K. L., Silburn, P. A., & de Zubicaray, G. I. (2009). Dopaminergic neuromodulation of semantic processing: A 4-T fMRI study with levodopa. *Cereb Cortex, 19*, 2651–2658.

Cotelli, M., Borroni, B., Manenti, R., Zanetti, M., Arévalo, A., Cappa, S. F., & Padovani, A. (2007). Action and object naming in Parkinson's disease without dementia. *Eur J Neurol, 14*, 632–637.

Crosson, B., Benefield, H., Cato, M., Sadek, J., Moore, A., et al. (2003). Left and right basal ganglia and frontal activity during language generation: Contributions to lexical, semantic, and phonological processes. *J International Neuropsychological Society, 9*, 1061–1077.

Cruise, K. E., Bucks, R. S., Loftus, A. M., Newton, R. U., Pegoraro, R., & Thomas, M. G. (2011). Exercise and Parkinson's: benefits for cognition and quality of life. *Acta Neurol Scand, 123*, 13–19.

De Gaspari, D., Siri, C., Di Gioia, M., et al. (2006). Clinical correlates and cognitive underpinnings of verbal fluency impairment after chronic subthalamic stimulation in Parkinson's disease. *Parkinsonism Relat Disord, 12*, 289–295.

Fasano, A., & Deuschl, G. (2012). Patients and DBS targets: Is there any rationale for selecting them. *Basal Ganglia, 2*, 211–219.

Fasano, A., Romito, L. M., Daniele, A., Piano, C., Zinno, M., Bentivoglio, A. R., & Albanese, A. (2010). Motor and cognitive outcome in patients with Parkinson's disease 8 years after subthalamic implants. *Brain, 133*, 2664–2676.

Filoteo, J. V., Friedrich, F. J., Rilling, L. M., Davis, J. D., Stricker, J. L., & Prenovitz, M. (2003). Semantic and cross-case identity priming in patients with Parkinson's disease. *J Clin Exp Neuropsyc, 25*(4), 441–456.

Frank, M. J. (2005). Dynamic dopamine modulation in the basal ganglia: A neurocomputational account of cognitive deficits in medicated and nonmedicated Parkinsonism. *J Cognitive Neurosci, 17*(1), 51–72.

Frank, M. J., Seeberger, L. C., & O'Reilly, R. C. (2004). By carrot or by stick: Cognitive reinforcement learning in Parkinsonism. *Science, 306*, 1940–1943.

Gerfen, C. R. (1992). The neostriatal mosaic: multiple levels of compart- mental organization. *Trends Neurosci, 15*, 133–139.

Gerlach, M., Double, K., Arzberger, T., Leblhuber, F., Tatschner, T., & Riederer, P. (2003). Dopamine receptor agonists in current clinical use: Comparative dopamine receptor binding profiles defined in the human striatum. *J Neural Transm, 110*, 119–1127.

Gil Robles, S., Gatignol, P., Capelle, L., Mitchell, M. C., & Duffau, H. (2005). The role of dominant striatum in language: a study using intraoperative electrical stimulations. *J Neurol Neurosurg Psychiatry, 76*, 940–946.

Grossman, M., Cooke, A., DeVita, C., Lee, C., Alsop, D., Detre, J., et al. (2003). Grammatical and resource components of sentence processing in Parkinson's disease: An fMRI study. *Neurology, 60*(5), 775–781.

Grossman, M., Glosser, G., Kalmanson, J., Morris, J., Stern, M. B., & Hurtig, H. I. (2001). Dopamine supports sentence comprehension in Parkinson's disease. *J Neurol Sci, 184*(2), 123–130.

Grossman, M., Kalmanson, J., Bernhardt, N., Morris, J., Stern, M. B., & Hurtig, H. I. (2000). Cognitive resource limitations during sentence comprehension in Parkinson's disease. *Brain Lang, 73*(1), 1–16.

Grossman, M., Zurif, E., Lee, C., Prather, P., Kalmanson, J., Stern, M. B., et al. (2002). Information processing speed and sentence comprehension in Parkinson's disease. *Neuropsychology, 16*(2), 174–181.

Henry, J. D., & Crawford, J. R. (2004). Verbal fluency deficits in Parkinson's disease: A meta-analysis. *J Int Neuropsych Soc, 10*(4), 608–622.

Herrera, E., & Cuetos, F. (2012). Action naming in Parkinson's disease patients on/off dopamine. *Neurosci Lett, 513*, 219–222.

Herrera, E., Cuetos, F., & Ribacoba, R. (2012). Verbal fluency in Parkinson's disease patients on/off dopamine medication. *Neuropsychologia, 50*, 3636–3640.

Hindle, J. V., Petrelli, A., Clare, L., & Kalbe, E. (2013). Nonpharmacological enhancement of cognitive function in Parkinson's disease: A systematic review. *Mov Disord, 28*, 1034–1049.

Huang, C., Tang, C., Feigin, A., Lesser, M., Ma, Y., Pourfar, M., Dhawan, V., & Eidelberg, D. 2007. Changes in network activity with the progression of Parkinson's disease. *Brain, 130*, 1834–1846.

Jokinen, P., Karrasch, M., Brück, A., Johansson, J., Bergman, J., & Rinne, J. O. (2013). Cognitive slowing in Parkinson's disease is related to frontostriatal dopaminergic dysfunction. *J Neurol Sci, 329*, 23–28.

Kehagia, A. A., Barker, R. A., & Robbins, T. W. (2010). Neuropsychological and clinical heterogeneity of cognitive impairment and dementia in patients with Parkinson's disease. *Lancet Neurol, 9*, 1200–1213.

Kemmerer, D. (1999). Impaired comprehension of raising-to-subject constructions in Parkinson's disease. *Brain Lang, 66*(3), 311–328.

Kischka, U., Kammer, Th., Maier, S., Weisbrod, M., Thimm, M., & Spitzer, M. (1996). Dopaminergic modulation of semantic network activation. *Neuropsychologia, 34*(11), 1107–1113.

Kish, S. J., Shannak, K., & Hornykiewicz, O. (1988). Uneven pattern of dopamine loss in the striatum of patients with idiopathic Parkinson's disease. *New Engl J Med, 318*, 876–880.

Lee, C., Grossman, M., Morris, J., Stern, M. B., & Hurtig, H.I. (2003). Attentional resource and processing speed limitations during sentence processing in Parkinson's disease. *Brain and Language, 85*(3), 347–356.

MacDonald, P. A., MacDonald, A. A., Seergobin, K. N., Tamjeedi, R., Ganjavi, H., Provost, J., & Monchi, O. (2011). The effect of dopamine therapy on ventral and dorsal striatum-mediated cognition in Parkinson's disease: Support from functional MRI. *Brain, 134*, 1447–1463.

MacDonald, A. A., Monchi, O., Seergobin, K. N., Ganjavi, H., Tamjeedi, R., & MacDonald, P. A. (2013). Parkinson's disease duration determines effect of dopaminergic therapy on ventral striatum function. *Movement Disord, 28*, 153–160.

Maril, S., Hassin-Baer, S., Cohen, O. S., & Tomer, R. (2013). Effects of asymmetric dopamine depletion on sensitivity to rewarding and aversive stimuli in Parkinson's disease. *Neuropsychologia, 51*, 818–824.

McIntyre C., Mori S., Sherman D. L., Thakor N. V., & Vitek J. L. (2004). Electric field and stimulating influence generated by deep brain stimulation of the subthalamic nucleus. *Clin Neurophysiol, 115*, 589–595.

Middleton, F. A., & Strick, P. L. (2002). Basal-ganglia 'projections' to the prefrontal cortex of the primate. *Cereb Cortex, 12*, 926–935.

Moustafa, A. A., Bell, P., Eissa, A. M., & Hewedi, D. H. (2013). The effects of clinical motor variables and medication dosage on working memory in Parkinson's disease. *Brain Cognition, 82*, 137–145.

Mueller, K., Jech, R., & Schroeter, M. L. (2013). Deep-brain stimulation for Parkinson's disease (letter). *N Engl J Med, 368*(5), 482–483.

Murray, A. M., Ryoo, H. L., Gurevich, E., & Joyce, J. N. (1994). Localization of dopamine D3 receptors to mesolimbic and D2 receptors to mesostriatal regions of human forebrain. *P Natl Acad Sci USA, 91*, 11271–11275.

Naismith, S. L., Mowszowski, L., Diamond, K., & Lewis, S. J. (2013). Improving memory in Parkinson's disease: a healthy brain ageing cognitive training program. *Mov Disord, 28*, 1097–1103.

Narayana, S., Fox, P. T., & Zhang, W. (2010). Neural correlates of efficacy of voice therapy in Parkinson's disease identified by performance-correlation analysis. *Human Brain Mapping, 31*, 222–236.

Neely, J. H. (1977). Semantic priming and retrieval from lexical memory: Roles of inhibitionless spreading activation and limited-capacity attention. *J Exp Psychol Gen, 106*(3), 226–254.

Neely, J. H. (1991). Semantic priming effects in visual word recognition: A selective review of current findings and theories. In D. Besner & G. W. Humphreys (Eds.), *Basic processes in reading: Visual word recognition* (pp. 264–336). Hillsdale, NJ: Lawrence Erlbaum.

Okun, M. (2012). Deep-brain stimulation for Parkinson's disease. *N Engl J Med, 367*, 1529–1538.

Okun, M. S., Fernandez, H. H., Wu, S. S., Kirsch-Darrow, L., Bowers, D., Bova, F., et al. (2009). Cognition and mood in Parkinson's disease in subthalamic nucleus versus globus pallidus interna deep brain stimulation: the COMPARE trial. *Ann Neurol, 65*, 586–595.

Paris, A. P., Saleta, H. G., de la Cruz Crespo Maraver, M., et al. (2011). Blind randomized controlled study of the efficacy of cognitive training in Parkinson's disease. *Mov Disord, 26*, 1251–1258.

Parsons, T. D., Rogers, S. A., Braaten, A. J., Woods, S. P., & Troster, A. I. (2006). Cognitive sequelae of subthalamic nucleus deep brain stimulation in Parkinson's disease: A meta-analysis. *Lancet Neurol, 5*, 578–588.

Péran, P., Nemmi, F., Méligne, D., Cardebat, D., Peppe, A., Rascol, O., Caltagirone, C., Demonet, J., & Sabatini, U. (2013). Effect of levodopa on both verbal and motor representations of action in Parkinson's disease: A fMRI study. *Brain Lang, 125*, 324–329.

Péran, P., Rascol, O., Démonet, J., Celsis, P., Nespoulous, J., Dubois, B., & Cardebat, D. (2003). Deficit of verb generation in nondemented patients with Parkinson's disease. *Movement Disord, 18*(2), 150–156.

Poletti, M., Frosini, D., Pagni, C., Baldacci, F., Giuntini, M., Mazzucchi, S., Tognoni, G., Lucetti, C., Dotto, P. D., Ceravolo, R., & Bonuccelli, U. (2013). The relationship between motor symptom lateralization and cognitive performance in newly diagnosed drug-naïve patients with Parkinson's disease. *J Clin Exp Neuropsychol, 35*(2), 124–131.

Portin, R., Laatu, S., Revonsuo, A., & Rinne, U. (2000). Impairment of semantic knowledge in Parkinson's disease. *Arch Neurol, 57*(9), 1338–1343.

Righi, S., Viggiano, M. P., Paganini, M., Ramat, S., & Marini, P. (2007). Recognition of category-related visual stimuli in Parkinson's disease: Before and after pharmacological treatment. *Neuropsychologia, 45*, 2931–2941.

Rodríguez-Ferreiro, J., Menéndez, M., Ribacoba, R., & Cuetos, F. (2009). Action naming is impaired in Parkinson's disease patients. *Neuropsychologia, 47*, 3271–3274.

Roesch-Ely, D., Weiland, S., Scheffel, H., Schwaninger, M., Hundemer, H., Kolter, T., & Weisbrod, M. (2006). Dopaminergic modulation of semantic priming in healthy volunteers. *Biol Psychiat, 60*, 604–611.

Ruff, R. M., Light, R. H., Parker, S. B., & Levin, H. S. (1997). The psychological construct of word fluency. *Brain & Lang, 57*, 394–405.

Sammer, G., Reuter, I., Hullmann, K., Kaps, M., & Vaitl, D. (2006). Training of executive functions in Parkinson's disease. *J Neurol Sci, 248*, 115–119.

Schroeder, U., Kuehler, A., Haslinger, B., Erhard, P., Fogel, W., Tronnier, V. M., et al. (2002). Subthalamic nucleus stimulation affects striato-anterior cingulate cortex circuit in a response conflict task: A PET study. *Brain, 125*(9), 1995–2004.

Schroeder, U., Kuehler, A., Lange, K. W., Haslinger, B., Tronnier, V., Krause, M., Pfister, R., Boecker, H., Ceballos-Baumann, A. O. (2003). Subthalamic nucleus stimulation affects a frontotemporal network: A PET study. *Ann Neurol, 54*, 445–50.

Sehm, B., Taubert, M., Conde, V., Weise, D., Classen, J., Dukart, J., et al. (2014). Structural brain plasticity in Parkinson's disease induced by balance training. *Neurobiol Aging, 35*, 232–239.

Servan-Schreiber, D., Printz, H., & Cohen, J. D. (1990). A network model of catecholamine effects: Gain, signal-to-noise ratio, and behavior. *Science, 249*, 892–896.

Shiner, T., Seymour, B., Wunderlich, K., Hill, C., Bhatia, K. P., Dayan, P., & Dolan, R. J. (2012). Dopamine and performance in a reinforcement learning task: Evidence from Parkinson's disease. *Brain, 135*, 1871–1883.

Skeel, R. L., Crosson, B., Nadeau, S. E., Algina, J., Bauer, R. M., & Fennell, E. B. (2001). Basal ganglia dysfunction, working memory, and sentence comprehension in patients with Parkinson's disease. *Neuropsychologia, 39*(9), 962–971.

Smittenaar, P., Chase, H. W., Aarts, E., Nusselein, B., Bloem, B. R., & Cools, R. (2012). Decomposing effects of dopaminergic medication in Parkinson's disease on probabilistic action selection: Learning or performance? *Eur J Neurosci, 35*, 1144–1151.

Swainson, R., Rogers, R. D., Sahakian, B. J., Summers, B. A., Polkey, C. E., & Robbins, T. W. (2000). Probabilistic learning and reversal deficits in patients with Parkinson's disease or frontal or temporal lobe lesions: Possible adverse effects of dopaminergic medication. *Neuropsychologia, 38*, 596–612.

Thomas, C., & Baker, C. I. (2013). Teaching an adult brain new tricks: A critical review of evidence for training-dependent structural plasticity in humans. *Neuroimage 73*, 225–236.

Uc, E. Y., Doerschug, K., Mehta, S., et al. (2008). Cardiovascular fitness and cognition in mild-moderate Parkinson's disease. *Neurology, 70*, A290.

Verreyt, N., Nys, G. M. S., Santens, P., & Vingerhoets, G. (2011). Cognitive differences between patients with left-sided and right-sided Parkinson's disease: A review. *Neuropsychol Rev, 21*, 405–424.

Williams-Gray, C. H., Foltynie, T., Brayne, C. E. G., Robbins, T. W., & Barker, R. A. (2007). Evolution of cognitive dysfunction in an incident Parkinson's disease cohort. *Brain, 130*, 1787–1798.

Winter, B., Breitenstein, C., Mooren, F. C., Voelker, K., Fobker, M., Lechtermann, A., . . . Knecht, S. (2007). High impact running improves learning. *Neurobiol Learn Mem, 87,* 597–609.

Ye, Z., Milenkova, M., Mohammadi, B., Kollewe, K., Schrader, C., Dengler, R., Samii, A., & Münte, T. F. (2012). Impaired comprehension of temporal connectives in Parkinson's disease: A neuroimaging study. *Neuropsychologia, 50,* 1794–1800.

Zhuang, X., Mazzoni, P., & Kang, U. J. (2013). The role of neuroplasticity in dopaminergic therapy for Parkinson's disease. *Nature Rev Neurol, 9,* 248–256.

5

Neuroplasticity in Multiple Sclerosis

Jelena Stojanovic-Radic and John DeLuca

Introduction

Multiple sclerosis (MS) is a chronic neurological disease, characterized by multiple inflammatory demyelinating processes in the brain, resulting in axonal damage (Trapp et al., 1998), brain atrophy (Bermel & Bakshi, 2006; Chard & Miller, 2009; Fisher et al., 2008) and sclerotic plaques, predominantly, but not exclusively, in the white matter of the brain (Comi, 2010). The resulting impairments, among other things, have been found to be both motor and cognitive in nature (Chiaravalloti & DeLuca, 2008). In an effort to "adjust" for these impairments, the brain has an adaptive mechanism of reorganizing its structural and functional connections in order to optimize its functional capacity. The ability to conduct such reorganization is called neuroplasticity. Neuroplasticity relies on cellular and molecular mechanisms to induce systems-level functional changes. The purpose of this chapter is to provide an overview of such neuroplasticity in MS. To do so, we will focus primarily on plasticity in the motor and cognitive domains. Due to the extensive use of neuroimaging techniques in MS, both clinically and in research, this chapter will focus primarily on studies examining neuroplasticity using magnetic resonance imaging (MRI). The first section of the chapter provides a brief overview of key terms and concepts associated with neuroplasticity, which will provide the framework from which the remainder of the chapter is presented. The second section provides reviews of neuroplasticity first within the motor system, followed by cognitive functions. The final section provides an overview of the interaction between the environment and neuroplasticity in MS and ends with a discussion of the challenges of the interpretation of such plasticity in the nervous system and future directions.

Neural Plasticity and Related Concepts

It is now well established that the central nervous system (CNS) is capable of reorganizing in response to insult or damage. This neuroplasticity has been broadly defined as "the ability of the nervous system to respond to intrinsic and extrinsic stimuli by reorganizing its structure, function and connections" (Cramer et al., 2011, p. 1591). While there are several mechanisms responsible for such reorganization, the primary mechanism is "vicariance," in which different areas of the brain "take over" functions of the damaged area (Stein et al., 1995). This can be accomplished in a variety of ways. First, reorganization can occur at the site of the lesion (e.g., expansion of cortical maps controlling the digits following deaffirnation; Merzenich et al., 1984), referred to as "local expansion." It has been shown that recovery of function is correlated with increased functional reorganization around the rim of a lesion in both animals (Dijkhuizen et al., 2003) and humans (Levy et al., 2001). A second mechanism of neuroplasticity is "homologous area adaptation" (Grafman and Litvan, 1999), which occurs when homologous regions of the contralateral hemisphere "take over" functions of the damaged brain regions. This process may come with some cost to the regular, full capacity of the functions of the contralateral area that has taken over the functions of the damaged one. In the third mechanism, other areas of the brain (e.g., distant sites) take over functional activity, referred to as "extra-region recruitment." While other mechanisms of neuroplasticity have been identified (e.g., unmasking of latent pathways), vicariance is by far the most established mechanism of reorganization and will be the primary focus of this chapter.

Unfortunately, to date, the terminology used to describe reorganized functional architecture in the brain is inconsistent. For example, brain "reorganization" and "compensation" are often used interchangeably to describe a broad spectrum of neuroplastic changes from cellular (synaptic) to systems (brain) network levels. Both refer to the fact that individuals with MS exhibit functional activations that differ from those observed in healthy individuals when performing the same task. However, some have argued that they represent different neuroplastic mechanisms (e.g., Hillary, 2008), with "compensation" referring to transient or temporary alterations in neural activity, while "reorganization" is indicative of permanent "rewiring" of brain networks. Further, both compensation and brain reorganization can result in either increased or decreased functional brain activity. However, compensatory changes are typically referred to as changes that facilitate or maintain motor or cognitive performance in neurological populations at the same level as that of healthy individuals. For the purposes of this chapter, the terms will be defined as the following: "compensation" indicates functional activation changes that facilitate performance, both transient and permanent, and "reorganization" implies fundamental changes in the networks (usually interpreted as permanent); however, both terms will be used to refer to neuroplasticity. As will be seen, while plasticity is often associated with a positive or "adaptive" outcome, this may be misleading, as such plasticity may also be "maladaptive." That is, maladaptive plasticity may also refer to cerebral inefficiency or "insufficient adaptive plasticity" (Tomassini et al., 2012b).

Motor System Plasticity in Multiple Sclerosis

The most robust findings of cortical reorganization in MS come from the observations of the motor system functional activation, derived from functional MRI (fMRI) studies. In fact, functional changes in the brain occur very early in the disease course, with several studies showing such changes in patients with clinically isolated syndrome (CIS), in which patients present with a sub-acute event involving only one functional neurological system, which marks the clinical onset of the disease in 80%–85 % of subjects but is not diagnostic of MS (DeLuca & Nocentini, 2011). Pantano et al. (2002a) examined fMRI activation in CIS patients after their first clinical attack of hemiparesis, during the performance of a sequential finger-to-thumb opposition task performed with both the previously paretic and the unaffected hand. Relative to healthy controls (HC), a significantly larger area of activation was observed in the CIS group in ipsilateral and contralateral cortical motor areas, mostly in areas not activated in HC. Further, increased activation in MS was observed primarily in ipsilateral (contralateral to the unaffected limb) brain regions relative to controls. Increased activation in CIS was also observed in regions outside the traditional motor areas (e.g., inferior parietal lobule and insula). Similar functional brain changes were observed for both the affected and unaffected hands. As such, reorganization in MS was observed as primarily pronounced by the ipsilateral activation of the motor regions (i.e., local expansion), as well as the activation of additional, non-traditional motor regions (i.e., extra-region recruitment). Harirchian et al. (2010) compared functional activation in CIS patients with clinically intact motor systems and HC while performing motor tasks across all four limbs. While performing ankle movements, relative to HC, CIS patients showed greater activation in the ipsilateral secondary somatosensory cortex, cingulate gyrus, and precuneus (i.e., local expansion). While performing the finger-tapping task, increased activity in CIS was observed in the contralateral thalamus, ipsilateral premotor cortex, and superior temporal gyrus. This study suggests that brain reorganization precedes any clinical manifestation of motor dysfunction. In addition, both Pantano et al. (2002a) and Harirchian et al. (2010) found that a greater extent of tissue damage (i.e., T2 and T1 lesion load) was associated with more extensive activation in the motor areas in MS, especially in the ipsilateral sensory-motor regions relative to controls.

Pantano et al. (2002b) examined how functional motor reorganization differs following a single attack of either specific motor damage (i.e., hemiparesis) or non-motor damage (i.e., optic neuritis) in CIS. The authors reported that MS patients with hemiparesis, and no other motor impairment prior to MS diagnosis, had marked ipsilateral motor area activation during a finger-opposition task, while patients with optic neuritis had higher contralateral motor area activation. Thus, it appears that the *nature of clinical manifestation* of MS may affect plastic changes in the motor cortex differently, such that motor impairment prior to MS diagnosis leads to the ipsilateral map expansion (i.e., increased homologous region activation), while absence of the motor impairment leads to increased contralateral motor cortex activation.

Approximately 85% of individuals with MS suffer from the relapsing-remitting type of the disease (RRMS), characterized by acute attacks, which are followed by a virtually complete recovery (Comi, 2010). A great majority (approximately 90%) of individuals with RRMS progress to a secondary progressive disease course or secondary-progressive MS (SPMS), which is marked by a continuous neurological deterioration (Comi, 2010).

Functional reorganization in the motor system is also observed in both RRMS and SPMS. Reddy et al. (2000) examined RRMS and SPMS patients with unimpaired hand function on a finger flexion-extension task. fMRI activation of the ipsilateral (the side of the moving hand) sensory motor cortex (SMC) during finger movements was increased fivefold relative to controls, and these increases were significantly correlated with decreases in neuronal integrity (i.e., decreased N-acetylaspartate [NAA] on magnetic resonance spectroscopy [MRS]). In another study, during simple extension-flexion finger movements, Lee et al. (2000) reported that RRMS and SPMS subjects showed increased ipsilateral SMC activation with increased T2 lesion load. These data are consistent with ipsilateral (unaffected hemisphere) or homologous region adaptation (see Figure 5.1). Further, there was an increasingly posterior shift in the center of SMC activation with increased T2 lesion load in the contralateral hemisphere, suggesting that the activation shifts toward the latent motor pathways. Therefore, in order to maintain motor function, latent motor pathways are being unmasked and compensate for the structural damage indicated by the T2 lesion load.

In addition to the lesion load, the age of the subjects may also affect expression of brain plasticity in MS. In a longitudinal study of MS subjects who initially showed increased bilateral sensorimotor area activation (i.e., significantly increased ipsilateral activation) during the simple finger-moving task, Pantano et al. (2005) found differences in

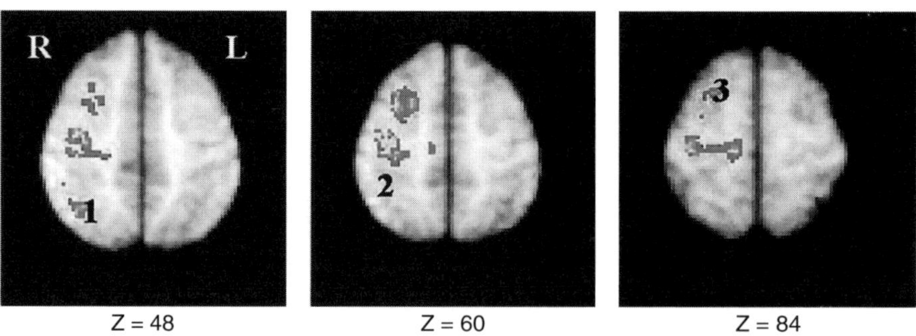

FIGURE 5.1 Ipsilateral activation in (A) inferior parietal cortex, (B) precentral gyrus (primary motor cortex), and (C) superior/middle frontal gyrus, during the right (dominant) hand movement in individuals with relapsing remitting MS. Right (R) and left (L) hemispheres are marked. From Reddy et al. (2002). *Brain*, *125*, 2646–2657, with permission.

activation at follow-up, approximately 2 years after the first scan, which correlated with the age and the structural damage observed in subjects. At time 2, the younger MS subjects showed a decrease in the ipsilateral sensorimotor area activation and less structural damage compared to the older subjects, who maintained the ipsilateral activation and showed more structural damage. The authors suggest that normalization of brain function (i.e., maintenance of contralateral activation) may be compromised in older MS patients and MS patients with more structural damage. Thus, neuroplasticity in MS appears to also be influenced by age and disease characteristics such as lesion load, relapse rate, and the extent of structural damage.

Interventions in the form of training on a visuomotor task have been shown to influence cortical plasticity and can improve MS individuals' performance of the task (e.g., Tomassini et al., 2012a). However, functional cortical reorganization following motor training appears to differ in MS patients relative to HC. RRMS patients and healthy controls were scanned prior, during, and after a 30-minute simple directional thumb-movement training (Morgen et al., 2004). Prior to training, MS subjects showed increased activation of the contralateral dorsal premotor cortex compared to controls. After training, MS subjects, unlike the HC group, did not show task-specific reductions in activation in the primary somatosensory (S1) or motor (M1) cortex, or in the adjacent parietal association cortex. Lowe et al. (2002) showed that RRMS subjects had lower functional connectivity between primary motor cortices across the two hemispheres in response to a bilateral finger-tapping exercise than the HC group. Such findings may suggest a reduced capacity to optimize compensatory recruitment of cortical motor network resources in response to the motor tasks and ultimately motor rehabilitation.

As shown by Lee et al. (2000), cortical plasticity also occurs in SPMS during the performance of the motor task. For example, Rocca et al. (2003) examined simple right flexion-extension movements of the fingers and foot during fMRI in 13 SPMS subjects. Relative to HC, during the finger movements of the affected limb, SPMS subjects showed more activation in ipsilateral inferior frontal region, bilateral middle frontal gyrus, and contralateral intraparietal sulcus. During foot flexion, SPMS subjects showed significantly more activation in contralateral SMC and thalamus, and ipsilateral upper bank of the sylvian fissure. Activation in cortical motor regions was strongly correlated with the severity of structural changes in normal-appearing white and gray matter. Thus, it is evident that functional activations correlated with the motor task in individuals with RRMS and SPMS are more widely distributed and observed in regions not found to be significantly activated in HCs.

Primary progressive MS (PPMS) is the course of the disease characterized by the continuous progression and worsening of neurological symptoms without the relapses characteristic of RRMS. Cortical reorganization during the performance of a simple motor task has been observed in PPMS. Specifically, it was found that during a motor task, functional activation in PPMS extends beyond the classical motor network (i.e., primary and supplementary motor regions, as well as sensorimotor area and cerebella; Heuninckx et al., 2008), commonly found to be activated in HC. For example, in studies by Filippi et al. (2002) and Rocca et al. (2002), patients with PPMS exhibited activations of the brain areas not commonly a part of the primary motor network (i.e., superior temporal gyrus and middle frontal gyrus), supporting the functions in response to a motor task. Activations observed were part of the multimodal sensorimotor integration network, including areas involved in motor planning and execution (i.e., SMA and cingulate region; Rocca et al., 2002) and areas extending beyond the classical motor network, including bilateral superior temporal gyrus, ipsilateral middle frontal gyrus, and contralateral insula/claustrum (Filippi et al., 2002). This "non-classical" motor network activation thus compensates for the areas of the motor network normally found to subserve the motor task in question. Even so, the authors postulated that cortical plasticity is somewhat exhausted, likely due to the irreversible tissue loss in PPMS, and may contribute to the irreversible neurological deficits. Therefore, although plastic changes do take place in PPMS, with the general accumulation of disability, adaptive properties of functional reorganization may be reduced (Filippi & Rocca, 2003).

In addition to the differences in functional activations of the motor system between individuals with MS and healthy controls, studies utilizing functional and effective connectivity have shown differences in the inter- and intrahemispheric connectivity between MS individuals with varying MS etiologies and healthy controls. Functional connectivity implies the statistical dependencies or correlations among remote neurophysiological events, while effective connectivity refers to the influence that one neural system has on another (Friston, 2003). Connectivity studies (Rocca et al., 2010a, 2011) revealed that individuals with MS, including CIS, were found to have enhanced effective and functional connectivity (Rocca et al., 2010a) between various areas of the motor network during the performance of a simple motor task, relative to healthy controls. For example, activations in one area of the motor network (e.g., supplementary motor area) correlate with activations in another area of the network (e.g., precentral gyrus) in individuals with MS. In addition, individuals with MS showed increased both inter- and intrahemispheric effective connectivity of the homologous motor regions of the two brain hemispheres. Similar to the arguments made by other authors, Rocca et al. (2010a) argue that their finding of increased effective connectivity of the motor networks contributes to the maintenance of function. Thus, arguably, homologous area adaptation of the motor network in MS is reflected both by the increased functional activations and the increased neural network connectivity relative to the healthy persons.

In summary, the type and extent of motor reorganization vary across different MS phenotypes. The magnitude of the functional reorganization is dependent on the severity of lesions in the brain (Harirchian et al., 2010; Pantano et al., 2002a, 2002b, 2005). In CIS, patients with motor impairment show preferential recruitment of the ipsilateral (contralateral to the unaffected limb) motor network. For RRMS, activations take the form of increased bilateral reorganization of sensorimotor related regions, as well as increased activations elsewhere in the brain (extra-region recruitment). It has been proposed that such bilateral recruitment may represent an adaptive mechanism limiting functional expression or reduced inter-hemispheric inhibition of the unaffected hemisphere recovery (Tomassini et al., 2012b). In the more progressive forms of the disease, specifically in SPMS, there is a notable activation of the latent motor pathways, or regions normally activated in healthy individuals during the performance of complex motor tasks. Finally, activation of the so-called multimodal sensorimotor integration network, which extends beyond the classical motor network, subserves simple motor functions in PPMS.

Cognitive Function Plasticity in MS

A number of studies have shown altered patterns of brain activation in individuals with MS relative to healthy controls during the performance of various cognitive tasks taxing working memory (e.g., Amann et al., 2011; Chiaravalloti et al., 2005; Li et al., 2004), processing speed (e.g., Audoin et al., 2008; Genova et al., 2009; Leavitt et al., 2012), and executive functions (e.g., Bonnet et al., 2010; Loitfelder et al., 2011; Smith et al., 2012). These altered activation patterns have been observed in all MS phenotypes, including CIS, RRMS, SPMS, and PPMS (Buckle, 2005; Tomassini et al., 2012b). In this section, we review these studies and discuss their implications.

Evidence of compensatory plasticity in individuals with CIS compared with healthy controls has been recorded in the absence of functional impairment. Forn et al. (2012) examined subjects within 2 months of CIS diagnosis on a processing speed and working memory task (Paced Auditory Serial Addition test; PASAT) during fMRI scanning. They found that increased cortical recruitment occurs during task performance, even in CIS subjects without cognitive impairment. Increased recruitment, reflecting the local expansion of activation, was observed in the inferior parietal lobe, precuneus, and middle frontal gyrus bilaterally, as well as the left anterior cingulate cortex, left claustrum, right thalamus, and right caudate nucleus. This suggests that such early cortical alterations may serve to limit the clinical expression of disease-related tissue damage. When cognitively impaired CIS subjects were compared to cognitively preserved CIS subjects, effective connectivity analysis showed stronger correlations in the cognitively impaired group, primarily within several regions of the right hemisphere. This finding suggests the increased need of right hemisphere activation with increased task demands. Importantly, this increased homologous hemisphere activation was associated with worse cognitive performance, and is an illustration of "maladaptive plasticity." Audoin et al. (2003) also examined functional activations in CIS patients without cognitive impairment during performance of the Paced Auditory Serial Addition Task (PASAT), with similar results. Compared with healthy controls, individuals with CIS exhibited significantly greater activation in the regions normally involved in executive functioning: orbitofrontal regions, right cerebellum, and bilateral lateral prefrontal cortex (PFC) region. Thus, in the majority of studies, patterns of activation in CIS demonstrate early plasticity of cognitive processes, including those with subclinical impairment. In addition, when task performance in individuals with CIS is unimpaired, recruitment of homologous regions of the two hemispheres, as well as the local expansion of activation, is an active compensatory mechanism, even early in the disease.

It has been shown in a healthy sample that frontal regions of the left hemisphere are the regions that are primarily active during PASAT performance (Chiaravalloti et al., 2005; Forn et al., 2011). Audoin et al. (2008) found that CIS subjects who showed improvement on the PASAT over a 12-month period showed increased right lateral PFC activation (i.e., regions involved in cognitive control) relative to CIS patients who did not show improvement over time. This right lateral PFC activation over time may suggest homologous region adaptation.

Regarding RRMS, Chiaravalloti et al. (2005) examined MS groups with and without working memory impairment, as well as healthy controls, during fMRI acquisition, using a modified PASAT. The healthy control group showed primarily left hemisphere activation during working memory performance, and the MS group without working memory impairment showed a similar pattern of left hemisphere activation. In contrast, the working memory–impaired MS group showed significantly more activation bilaterally in the parietal and frontal regions (indicative of both local expansion and homologous area adaptation). Further, the degree of extension of activation into the homologous right frontal region was correlated with worse cognitive performance, again indicative of maladaptive plasticity. This same pattern of overall results was also observed by Hillary et al. (2003) on another working memory task, which Hillary et al. (2006) interpret as neural inefficiency.

Amann et al. (2011) examined working memory (i.e., n-back), during fMRI recording in the RRMS subjects with mild cognitive impairment and healthy controls. Although the overall pattern of brain activation was similar between the HC and MS groups, the MS group showed task-related local expansion of fMRI activation around regions typically associated with working memory (i.e., anterior frontal and inferior parietal cortex). Similar findings were observed by Forn et al. (2007), who showed, in RRMS with preserved n-back performance, recruitment of brain areas adjacent to those primarily involved in working memory. Amann et al. (2011) and Forn et al. (2007) both illustrate local expansion of activation in RRMS with no to minimal cognitive impairment. Also examining working memory (i.e., PASAT), Mainero et al. (2004) studied cognitively impaired RRMS subjects and found significantly greater regional activation in areas typically associated with working memory (illustrating local expansion). The authors also found recruitment of additional areas throughout the brain not observed in HC (illustrating extra region activation). Taken together, these studies suggest that local expansion may occur when there is no or minimal cognitive decline, but that with increased cognitive impairment, there is a need for recruitment of additional areas throughout the brain in an attempt to perform cognitive tasks.

In addition to alterations in functional activation patterns, several studies have shown altered functional connectivity in individuals with RRMS during cognitive performance (Bonnet et al., 2010; Colorado et al., 2012; Leavitt et al., 2012), indicating connectivity-based neuroplasticity in MS. On a "Go/No-Go" task, Bonnet et al. (2010) showed that the RRMS group revealed a pattern of functional connectivity between the right dorsolateral PFC and medial frontal regions, whereas connectivity in healthy controls was found between the right dorsolateral PFC and cerebellar regions. This differential connectivity between the RRMS and HC groups suggests extra-region recruitment in RRMS. Leavitt et al. (2012) used effective connectivity to examine neural connections associated with processing speed in primarily RRMS. They found that in order to maintain the same level of behavioral performance (accuracy, despite being slower), the MS group required increased connections between multiple frontal regions, bilaterally. However, increased need to recruit right (but not left) frontal cortex connectivity was associated with slower reaction times within the MS group, again illustrating maladaptive plasticity.

Neuroplasticity in RRMS reflected by the recruitment of regions other than those in healthy controls is also illustrated by the work of Genova et al. (2009), who examined processing speed during fMRI recordings. In this study, the MS (primarily RRMS) and healthy control groups did not differ in accuracy; however, the MS group was significantly slower. The authors found that in the healthy control group, processing speed was mediated by the frontal, parietal, cerebellar, and thalamic regions, whereas in the MS group, processing speed was mediated by the insula, thalamus, and AC region (see Figure 5.2). Effective connectivity analyses in these subjects showed similar results (Leavitt et al.,

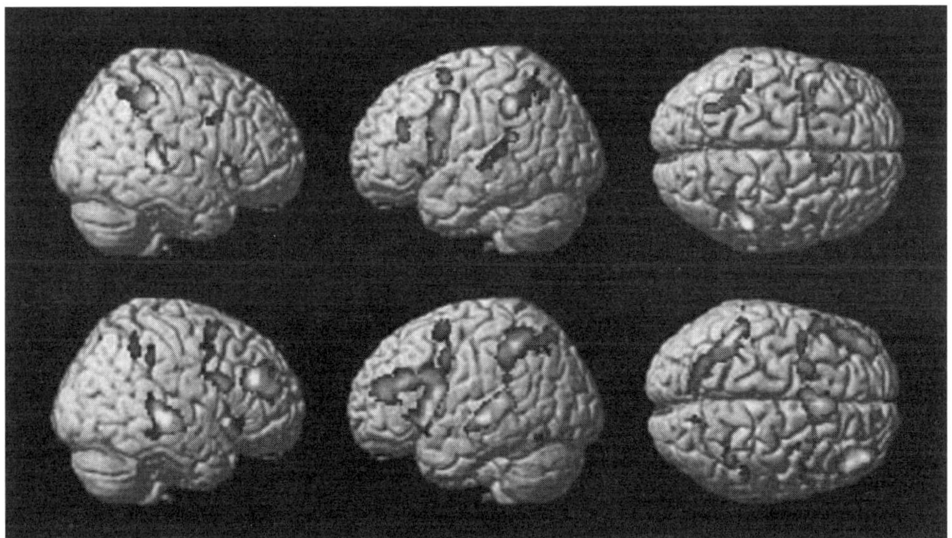

FIGURE 5.2 Cortical activation during the Paced Auditory Serial Addition Task. The top row represents HCs with activation in inferior and middle frontal gyrus, inferior parietal lobule, supplementary motor area, lateral premotor area, superior and middle temporal gyrus, insula, bilateral basal ganglia and thalamus, vermis and brainstem; the bottom row represents the MS group where, apart from the left lateral premotor area, right thalamus, and bilateral basal ganglia, there is an additional activation in the right anterior cingulate and right superior parietal lobule, illustrating extra-region activation. From Mainero et al. (2004). *NeuroImage, 21*, 858–867, with permission.

2012). Thus, activation and connectivity with other regions in the MS group were compensatory for the task accuracy, but appear to have come at the expense of the response time (i.e., maladaptive plasticity).

Neuroplasticity studies in SPMS are somewhat scarce, despite significant cognitive problems in this group (DeLuca et al., 2004; Huijbregts et al., 2004). Loitfelder et al. (2011) compared HC with CIS, RRMS, and SPMS subjects on a "Go/No-Go" task during fMRI scanning. Despite significantly more cognitive impairment in the SPMS versus CIS and RRMS, no behavioral differences were observed on the "Go/No-Go" task among groups. The HC group showed a widely distributed bilateral network activation during task performance, and the CIS group showed no difference in activation pattern from the HC group. While the RRMS group showed a relative increase in this activation pattern relative to HC and CIS groups, the SPMS group showed the most striking abnormal activation pattern. That is, SPMS subjects showed activation in regions other than the task-related network observed in the HCs (i.e., extra-region recruitment). The authors found this pattern of extensive activation to reflect neural inefficiency, accompanied by reduced ability of mediation between the fronto-parietal functional activations and the so-called default-mode network (DMN; Loitfelder et al., 2011). In addition, the degree of structural damage, measured by T2 lesion load, was not associated with functional activation patterns. This suggests that the relationship between structural and functional activation is not as straightforward as that observed in the motor system.

As with SPMS, studies on functional reorganization of cognitive functions in PPMS are scarce, likely due to the lower prevalence of this MS phenotype (Miller & Leary, 2007). Rocca et al. (2010b) examined functional activations in PPMS individuals with and without cognitive impairment and healthy controls during a working memory task (i.e., 2-back level of the n-back task). While there were no differences in performance between PPMS and healthy subjects on the task, there were several differences in activation patterns. Overall, all PPMS subjects exhibited increased activation in several regions typically observed during working memory when compared with healthy controls. These regions included bilateral cerebellum, right secondary somatosensory region, right precentral gyrus, right insula, and left cingulate region. Cognitively preserved PPMS subjects also had more significant left PFC activations when compared with healthy controls. PPMS subjects who were cognitively impaired (based on more comprehensive neuropsychological tests) exhibited more significant activations of the working memory regions outlined earlier, as well as reduced activations of the left PFC compared to both HC and the cognitively preserved PPMS group. Activation increases in both the cognitively preserved and cognitively impaired PPMS group illustrate local expansion of activation. Like the other MS phenotypes discussed earlier, local expansion of activation may reflect compensatory neuroplasticity for preserving a particular function (working memory in this case). Given that in-scanner task performance did not differ between the PPMS and healthy control groups in this study, the authors explain function maintenance by the recruitment of posterior regions. Thus, in addition to the regional expansion of activation in individuals with

PPMS, extra-region recruitment (i.e., posterior regions taking over the function of PFC) was also required to maintain task performance.

Neuroplasticity has also been observed in the hippocampus in MS. The hippocampus plays a crucial role in learning and memory and has been shown to be compromised in persons with MS. For instance, widespread hippocampal demyelination has been shown pathologically in chronic MS (Geurts et al., 2007; Vercellino et al., 2005) and is associated with neuronal loss and atrophy (Papadopoulos et al., 2009), synaptic loss, altered gene expression, and altered glutamate/GABA neurotransmission (Dutta et al., 2011). Sicotte et al. (2008) showed that hippocampal atrophy was associated with impaired verbal learning in MS patients. It is also now known that altered functional activation of the hippocampus in MS may pre-date the expression of learning and memory decline. In MS subjects without impaired memory and no hippocampal atrophy, there is less functional connectivity between the hippocampus and other areas of the brain (e.g., caudate, thalamus, anterior cingulate; Roosendall et al., 2010a). In addition, during memory encoding, memory-intact MS subjects show increased hippocampal functional activity (memory-impaired MS patients show decreased hippocampal activity), again in the absence of structural damage (Hulst et al., 2012). To address these findings, Hulst et al. (2012) proposed a functional adaptive hypothesis, which suggests that early in the disease, the hippocampus displays hyperactivation to preserve learning and memory integrity (i.e., compensation). As the disease progresses, structural damage and functional alterations ensue, leading to impairments in learning and memory.

Functional alterations in MS are also evident in the DMN both during rest (Liu et al., 2011; Roosendaal et al., 2010a) and during task performance (Sumowski et al., 2013). DMN is said to maintain a "background" level of attention, by monitoring both the internal and external environment to detect relevant events (Raichle et al., 2001). Furthermore, DMN is more active during rest than during task performance in healthy individuals than in individuals with MS (Greicius et al., 2009; Sumowski et al., 2013). In individuals with MS, it has been found that during the performance of a sustained attention task, greater deactivation of DMN was associated with worse memory performance (Sumowski et al., 2013). The need to deactivate the DMN also results in increased activation of other brain regions to perform the task (Sumowski et al., 2010a). Thus, failure to maintain DMN may represent "cerebral inefficiency," requiring the activation of other brain regions not normally responsible for task performance. Greater lifetime intellectual enrichment has been linked to greater DMN maintenance and better memory performance (Sumowski et al., 2010a, 2010b). As such, greater DMN deactivation during task performance is indicative of neural inefficiency and is correlated with worse memory performance.

Changes in functional activation during rest have been observed in individuals with MS when compared with healthy controls (Liu et al., 2011; Roosendaal et al., 2010b), as well. For example, during rest, significantly increased spontaneous (i.e., in the absence of task performance) brain activity has been noted in several brain regions in individuals with RRMS as compared with healthy controls (e.g., bilateral thalami, insula, and superior temporal gyrus; Liu et al., 2011). The authors posit that these increases in spontaneous brain activity in MS during rest may be an indication of ongoing plasticity and cortical remapping. Due to the negative association between the degree of disability (as measured by the Expanded Disability Status Scale [EDSS]) and increased spontaneous activity, the authors consider this to be adaptive plasticity in MS and to be beneficial in limiting disability. In terms of functional connectivity during rest, Roosendaal et al. (2010b) found that there is an increased synchronization (i.e., "strong temporal coherence between brain regions"; Roosendaal et al., 2010b) in six of eight resting state brain networks (i.e., DMN, executive function network, attention system, sensorimotor function network, and left and right frontoparietal network), in the earliest stages of MS, namely CIS, when compared with both RRMS subjects and healthy controls. Interestingly, the increased synchronization observed in CIS was not found in RRMS, although the RRMS group was cognitively impaired, while the CIS group was not. This increased synchronization observed in CIS suggests cortical reorganization of resting state networks, which is compensatory, as no cognitive impairment is evident in these subjects. The authors argue that the absence of increased synchronization in RRMS in these same resting state networks may indicate finite functional reorganization, which may be associated with cognitive impairment.

In summary, there is significant neuroplasticity of cognitive functions in individuals with MS. Homologous region adaptation, local activation expansion, and extra-region recruitment all occur in support of the cognitive functioning. However, this neuroplasticity can be maladaptive, especially in individuals with cognitive impairment, and it may come at the cost of other cognitive functions, such as processing speed. Nevertheless, in MS, the brain "mobilizes" compensatory properties from the earliest stages of the disease through the progression to other phenotypes, which precede overt cognitive decline. In contrast to the motor system, where structural lesions can have a direct impact on neuroplasticity, this process appears to be more complex regarding cognition, and it is an area of need of additional inquiry.

Cognitive Rehabilitation and Cognitive Reserve

Behavioral intervention for cognitive impairment can result in both changes in behavior and in brain parameters. For example, Chiaravalloti, Wylie, Leavitt, & DeLuca (2012) conducted a double-blind placebo-controlled randomized clinical trial providing a cognitive intervention to improve new learning and memory in persons with MS. Learning-impaired individuals with MS were administered a battery of neuropsychological tests and underwent an fMRI scan, and then were randomized into either the placebo and treatment group (i.e., the group receiving memory training). Following completion of the intervention, the neuropsychological battery and fMRI scan were repeated. Significant improvement in memory performance was observed only in the treatment group. At baseline,

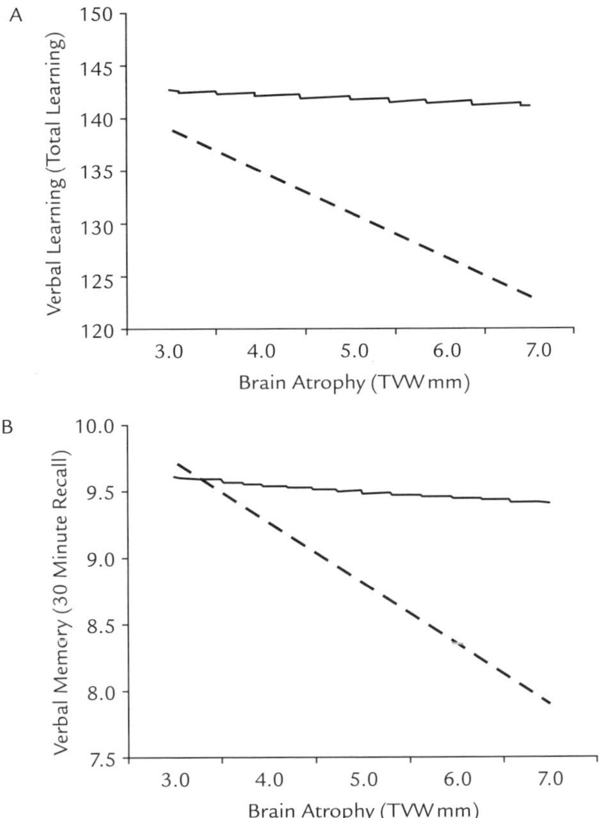

FIGURE 5.3 The figures represent the moderating effect of intellectual enrichment on brain atrophy in (A) verbal learning and (B) verbal memory. The dashed line represents subjects at the 25th percentile of intellectual enrichment and the solid line represents subjects at the 75th percentile of intellectual enrichment. From Sumowski et al. (2010). *Neurology, 74*, 1942–1945, with permission.

no functional brain activation differences were observed between the groups. However, at follow-up, when compared with the placebo group, the treatment group exhibited an increase in activation relative to baseline, within a widespread cortical network involving frontal, parietal, precuneus, and parahippocampal regions. In contrast, no significant change in brain activation was observed in the placebo group from baseline to follow-up. When examining resting state functional connectivity between the treatment and placebo groups, increased connectivity was observed only in the treatment group. That is, relative to pre-treatment baseline, increased connectivity was observed between the hippocampus and the insula bilaterally, left post central gyrus, precentral gyrus, middle frontal gyrus, and the cingulate gyrus only in the treatment group (Leavitt et al., 2012). Similar results were observed in a second randomized clinical trial by Filippi et al. (2012).

Neuropsychological expression of MS has been shown to be attenuated in individuals with MS with higher lifetime intellectual enrichment (e.g., educational attainment or high premorbid IQ; Sumowski et al., 2009, 2010), referred to as "cognitive reserve." Cognitive reserve posits that lifetime intellectual enrichment endows the brain with more fibers and connections, resulting in the brain's ability to withstand more disease before cognitive decline is clinically expressed. Sumowski et al. (2010a) showed that MS individuals with higher intellectual enrichment had better verbal learning and verbal memory scores than MS individuals with lower intellectual enrichment, in spite of having the same amount of brain atrophy (see Figure 5.3). In the functional domain, MS subjects with higher intellectual enrichment were able to perform a complex working memory task while maintaining DMN activity, and hence did not require additional cerebral resources, while the lower enrichment group needed to reduce DMN activity in order to recruit additional brain regions to perform the task (Sumowski et al., 2010b). Taken together, environmental experience can affect the brain by reducing the impact of MS neuropathology on cognitive expression. This, in turn, results in increased plasticity during one's lifetime, perhaps due to increased redundancy in cerebral architecture (Stein et al., 1995).

Conclusions

Cortical reorganization is a general response to cerebral dysfunction in MS. Neuroplasticity may be expressed through a variety of mechanisms by which the brain "reorganizes" in order to strengthen or recruit brain networks to "compensate" for neural loss or reduced efficiency. Such compensation occurs both in the motor and cognitive systems and has been noted in the earliest stages of MS, namely CIS, reflected by the homologous area adaptation (e.g., Audoin et al., 2008; Forn et al., 2012), local activation expansion (e.g., Filippi et al., 2004; Forn et al., 2012), as well as the activation of additional regions (e.g., Audoin et al., 2003). There is considerable evidence that functional brain reorganization even precedes any clinical manifestation of the disease both in motor (Harirchian et al., 2010; Reddy et al., 2000) and cognitive (e.g., Amann et al., 2011; Hulst et al., 2011) systems, and contributes to the maintenance of function (Rocca et al., 2010a, 2010b). A "functional adaptive hypothesis" suggests that early in the disease there is functional hyperactivation (using fMRI) acting as compensation to preserve cognitive or motor function. With disease progression, structural damage and functional alterations ensue, leading to cognitive and motor impairments (Hulst et al., 2011).

Despite the fact that the term "compensatory" has been generally assumed to be viewed as adaptive, there is a significant amount of evidence that brain reorganization can be maladaptive (maladaptive plasticity). Once again, this has been observed in both motor and cognitive networks. For example, homologous region recruitment has been associated with worse cognitive performance (e.g., Chiaravalloti et al., 2005; Forn et al., 2012; Hillary et al., 2003; Leavitt et al., 2012). However, some have shown that improvement over time is associated with increased homologous region adaptation (e.g., Audoin et al., 2008). Thus, assessing what is adaptive and what is maladaptive is difficult to determine, as the literature is fraught with inconsistencies (Tomassini et al., 2012a). Future studies are needed to address the issue of insufficient versus inefficient maladaptive neuroplasticity.

The term "brain reorganization" is frequently used in the literature to refer to neuroplasticity and is viewed as adaptive compensation. However, the implication that brain reorganization in neurological disorders can be measured with single time-point designs and fMRI methods has been criticized (Hillary, 2008; Medaglia et al., 2012). Rather than functional reorganizing of the brain, adaptive mechanisms may, for example, reflect unmasking of existing latent resources in the brain, during the engagement of novel or complex tasks (e.g., prolonged use of cognitive control resources; Hillary, 2008, 2011). For example, in the traumatic brain injury literature it has been demonstrated that right PFC recruitment is highly transient, even within a scanning session, and appears to be linked to task exposure (see Medaglia et al., 2012). Given the variability in this recruitment and its inconsistent relationship to task performance, the role of neural recruitment in neurological disorders, such as MS, remains unclear. In many cases, it appears necessary for task completion, but it may also be indicative of slowed information processing (neural inefficiency). Care in the use of terms such as "compensation" and "brain reorganization" needs to be considered to avoid confusion and misunderstanding regarding neuroplasticity.

Overall, neuroplasticity plays a behaviorally relevant role in the response to cerebral pathology in MS. Several factors may alter the ability of the brain to respond to such challenge (e.g., age, inflammation, lesion load, cognitive reserve; Tomassini et al., 2012). Although not well understood, such compensatory mechanisms may serve a key role in the response to interventions to improve function in MS. It is likely that functional imaging will play a critically important role in our understanding of both functional improvement and neuroplasticity.

Acknowledgments

The authors thank Dr. Frank Hillary for his review and comments on an earlier version of this manuscript. This manuscript was supported in part by grant MB 0024 from the National Multiple Sclerosis Society to J. D.

References

Amann, M., Doessegger, L. S., Penner I. K., Hirsch, J. G., Raselli, C., Calabrese, P., et al. (2011). Altered functional adaptation to attention and working memory tasks with increasing complexity in relapsing-remitting multiple sclerosis patients. *Human Brain Mapping, 32,* 1704–1719.

Audoin, B., Ibarrola, D., Ranjeva, J.-P., Confort-Gouny, S., Malikova, I., Cherif, A. A., et al. (2003). Compensatory cortical activation observed by fMRI during a cognitive task at the earliest stage of MS. *Hum Brain Mapp, 20,* 51–58.

Audoin, B., Reuter, F., Duong M. V. A., Malikova, I., Confort-Gouny, S., Cherif, A. A., et al. (2008). Efficiency of cognitive control recruitment in the very early stage of multiple sclerosis: A one-year fMRI follow-up study. *Mult Scler, 14,* 786–792.

Bermel, R. A. & Bakshi, A. (2006). The measurement and clinical relevance of brain atrophy in multiple sclerosis. *Lancet Neurol, 5,* 158–170.

Bonnet, M. C., Allard, M., Dilharreguy, B., Deloire, M., Petry, K. G., & Brochet, B. (2010). Cognitive compensation failure in multiple sclerosis. *Neurology, 75,* 1241–1248.

Buckle, G. J. (2005). Functional magnetic resonance imaging and multiple sclerosis: the evidence for neuronal plasticity. *J Neuroimaging, 15*, 82S–93S.

Chard, D., & Miller, D. (2009). Grey matter pathology in clinically early multiple sclerosis: Evidence from magnetic resonance imaging. *J Neurol Sci, 282*, 5–11.

Chiaravalloti, N. D., Hillary, F. G., Ricker, J. H., Christodoulou, C., Kalnin, A. J., Liu, W. C., et al. (2005). Cerebral activation patterns during working memory performance in multiple sclerosis using fMRI. *J Clin Exp Neuropsyc, 27*, 1–23.

Chiaravalloti, N. D., & DeLuca, J. (2008). Cognitive impairment in multiple sclerosis. *Lancet Neurol, 7*, 1139–1151.

Chiaravalloti, N. D., Wylie, G., Leavitt, V., & DeLuca, J. (2012). Increased cerebral activation after behavioral treatment for memory deficits in MS. *J Neurol, 259*, 1337–1346.

Colorado, R. A., Shukla, K., Zhou, Y., Wolinsky, J. S., & Narayana, P. A. (2012). Multi-task functional MRI in multiple sclerosis patients without clinical disability. *NeuroImage, 59*, 573–581.

Comi, G. (2010). The physiopathology of multiple sclerosis. In J. Kesselring, G. Comi, & A. Thompson (Eds.), *Multiple sclerosis recovery of function and neurorehabilitation* (pp. 8–21). New York: Cambridge University Press.

Cramer, S. C., Sur, M., Dobkin, B. H., O'Brien, C., Sanger, T. D., Trojanowski, J. Q., et al. (2011). Harnessing neuroplasticity for clinical applications. *Brain, 134*, 1591–1609.

DeLuca, J., Chelune, G. J., Tulsky, D. S., Lengenfelder, J., & Chiaravalloti, N. (2004). Is speed of processing or working memory the primary information processing deficit in multiple sclerosis? *J Clin Exp Neuropsyc, 26*, 550–562.

DeLuca, J., & Nocentini, U. (2011). Neuropsychological, medical and rehabilitative management of persons with multiple sclerosis. *NeuroRehabilitation, 29*, 197–219.

Dijkhuizen, R. M., Singhal, A. B., Mandeville, J. B., Wu, O., Halpern, E. F., Finkelstein, S. P., et al. (2003). Correlation between brain reorganization, ischemic damage, and neurologic status after transient focal cerebral ischemia in rats: A functional magnetic resonance imaging study. *J Neurosci, 23*, 510–517.

Dutta, R., Chang, A., Doud, M. K., Kidd, G. J., Ribaudo, M. V., Young, E. A., et al. (2011). Demyelination causes synaptic alterations in hippocampi from multiple sclerosis patients. *Ann Neurol, 69*, 445–454.

Filippi, M., Rocca, M. A., Falini, A., Caputo, D., Ghezzi, A., Colombo, B., et al. (2002). Correlations between structural CNS damage and functional MRI changes in primary progressive MS. *NeuroImage, 15*, 537–546.

Filippi, M., & Rocca, M. A. (2003). Disturbed function and plasticity in multiple sclerosis as gleaned from functional magnetic resonance imaging. *Curr Opin Neurol, 16*, 275–282.

Filippi, M., Rocca, M. A., Mezzapesa, D. M., Ghezzi, A., Falini, A., Martinelli, V., et al. (2004). Simple and complex movement-associated functional MRI changes in patients at presentation with clinically isolated syndromes suggestive of multiple sclerosis. *Hum Brain Mapp, 21*, 108–117.

Filippi, M., Riccitelli, G., Mattioli, F., Capra, R., Stampatori, C., Pagani, E., et al. (2012). Multiple sclerosis: effects of cognitive rehabilitation on structural and functional MR imaging measures—an explorative study. *Radiology, 262*, 932–940.

Fisher, E., Lee, J. C., Nakamura, K., & Rudick, R. A. (2008). Gray matter atrophy in multiple sclerosis: A longitudinal study. *Ann Neurol, 64*, 255–265.

Forn, C., Barros-Loscertales, A., Escudero, J., Benlloch, V., Campos, S., Parcet, M. A., et al. (2007). Compensatory activations in patients with multiple sclerosis during preserved performance of the auditory n-back task. *Hum Brain Mapp, 28*, 424–430.

Forn, C., Belenguer, A., Belloch, V., Sanjuan, A., Parcet, M. A., & Avila, C. (2011). Anatomical and functional differences between the paced auditory serial addition test and the symbol digit modalities test. *J Clin Exp Neuropsyc, 33*, 42–50.

Forn, C., Rocca, Valsasina, P., Bosca, I., Casanova, B., Sanjuan, A., et al. (2012). Functional magnetic resonance imaging correlates of cognitive performance in patients with the clinically isolated syndrome suggestive of multiple sclerosis at presentation: An activation and connectivity study. *Mult Scler J, 18*, 153–163.

Friston, K. (2003). Functional and effective connectivity: A review. *Brain Connectiv, 1*, 13–36.

Genova, H. M., Hillary, F. G., Wylie, G., Rypma, B., & DeLuca, J. (2009). Examination of processing speed deficits in multiple sclerosis using functional magnetic resonance imaging. *J Int Neuropsych Soc, 15*, 383–393.

Geurts, J. J., Bo, L., Roosendaal, S. D., Hazes, T., Daniels, R., Barkhof, F., Witter, M. P., et al. (2007). Extensive hippocampal demyelination in multiple sclerosis. *J Neuropath Exp Neur, 66*, 819–827.

Grafman, J., & Litvan, I. (1999). Evidence for four forms of neuroplasticity. In J. Grafman & Y. Christen, (Eds.), *Neuronal plasticity: Building a bridge from the laboratory to the clinic* (pp. 131–141). Heidelberg, Germany: Springer-Verlag.

Greicius, M. D., Supekar, K., Menon, V., & Dougherty, R. F. (2009). Resting-state functional connectivity reflects structural connectivity in the default mode network. *Cereb Cortex, 19,* 72–78.

Harirchian, M. H., Rezvanizadeh, A., Fakhri, M., Oghabian, M. A., Ghoreishi, A., Zarei, M., et al. (2010). Non-invasive brain mapping of motor-related areas of four limbs in patients with clinically isolated syndrome compared to healthy normal controls. *J Clin Neurosci, 17,* 736–741.

Heuninckx, S., Wenderoth, N., & Swinnen, S. P. (2008). Systems neuroplasticity in the aging brain: Recruiting additional neural resources for successful motor performance in elderly persons. *J Neurosci, 28,* 91–99.

Hillary, F. G., Chiaravalloti, N. D., Ricker, J. H., Steffener, J., Bly, B. M., Lange, G., et al. (2003). An investigation of working memory rehearsal in multiple sclerosis using fMRI. *J Clin Exp Neuropsyc, 25,* 965–978.

Hillary, F. G., Genova, H. M., Chiaravalloti, N. D., Rypma, B., & DeLuca, J. (2006). Prefrontal modulation of working memory performance in brain injury and disease. *Hum Brain Mapp, 27,* 837–847.

Hillary, F. G. (2008). Neuroimaging of working memory dysfunction and the dilemma with brain reorganization hypothesis. *J Int Neuropsych Soc, 14,* 526–534.

Hillary, F. G. (2011). Determining the nature of prefrontal cortex recruitment after traumatic brain injury: A response to Turner. *Front Syst Neurosci, 5.* doi: 10.3389/fnsys.2011.00024

Huijbregts, S. C. J., Kalkers, N. F., de Sonneville, M. J., de Groot, V., Reuling, I. E. W., & Polman, C. H. (2004). Differences in cognitive impairment of relapsing remitting, secondary, and primary progressive MS. *Neurology, 63,* 335–339.

Hulst, H. E., Schoonheim, M. M., Roosendaal, S. D., Popescu, V., Schweren, L. J. S., van der Werf, Y. D., et al. (2012). Functional adaptive changes within the hippocampal memory system of patients with multiple sclerosis. *Hum Brain Mapp, 33,* 2268–2280.

Leavitt, V. M., Wylie, G., Genova, H. M., Chiaravalloti, N. D., & DeLuca, J. (2012). Altered effective connectivity during performance of an information processing speed task in multiple sclerosis. *Mult Scler J, 18,* 409–417.

Lee, M., Reddy, H., Johansen-Berg, H., Pendlebury, S., Jenkinson, M., Smith, S., et al. (2000). The motor cortex shows adaptive functional changes to brain injury from multiple sclerosis. *Ann Neurol, 47,* 606–613.

Levy, C. E., Nichols, D. S., Schmalbrock, P. M., Keller, P., & Chakeres, D. W. (2001). Functional MRI evidence of cortical reorganization in upper-limb stroke hemiplegia treated with constraint-induced movement therapy. *Am J Phys Med Rehab, 80,* 4–12.

Li, Y., Chiaravalloti, N. D., Hillary, F. G., DeLuca, J., Liu, W. C., Kalnin, A. J., et al. (2004). Differential cerebellar activation on functional magnetic resonance imaging during working memory performance in persons with multiple sclerosis. *Arch Phys Med Rehab, 85,* 635–639.

Liu, Y., Liang, P., Duan, Y., Jia, X., Yu, C., Zhang, M., et al. (2011). Brain plasticity in relapsing-remitting multiple sclerosis: Evidence from resting-state fMRI. *J Neurol Sci, 304,* 127–131.

Loitfelder, M., Fazekas, F., Petrovic, K., Fuchs, S., Ropele, S., Wallner-Blazek, M., et al. (2011). Reorganization in cognitive networks with progression of multiple sclerosis: Insights from fMRI. *Neurology, 76,* 526–533.

Lowe, M. J., Phillips, M. D., Lurito, J. T., Mattson, D., Dzemidzic, M., & Mathews, V. P. (2002). Multiple sclerosis: Low-frequency temporal blood oxygen level-dependent fluctuations indicate reduced functional connectivity—Initial results. *Radiology, 224,* 184–192.

Mainero, C., Caramia, F., Pozzilli, C., Pisani, A., Pestalozza, I., Borriello, G., et al. (2004). fMRI evidence of brain reorganization during attention and memory tasks in multiple sclerosis. *NeuroImage, 21,* 858–867.

Medaglia, J. D., Chiou, K. S., Slocomb, J., Fitzpatrick, N. M., Wardecker, B. M., et al. (2012). The less BOLD, the wiser: Support for the latent resource hypothesis after traumatic brain injury. *Hum Brain Mapp, 33,* 979–993.

Merzenich, M. M., Nelson, R. J., Stryker, M. P., Cynader, M. S., Schoppmann, A., & Zook, J. M. (1984). Somatosensory cortical map changes following digit amputation in adult monkeys. *J Comp Neurol, 224,* 591–605.

Miller, D. H. & Leary, S. M. (2007). Primary-progressive multiple sclerosis. *Lancet Neurol, 10,* 903–912.

Morgen, K., Kadom, N., Sawaki, L., Tessitore, A., Ohayon, J., McFarland, H., et al. (2004). Training-dependent plasticity in patients with multiple sclerosis. *Brain, 127,* 2506–2517.

Pantano, P., Iannetti, G. D., Caramia, F., Mainero, C., Di Legge, S., Bozzao, L., et al. (2002a). Cortical motor reorganization after a single clinical attack of multiple sclerosis. *Brain, 125,* 1607–1615.

Pantano, P., Mainero, C., Iannetti, G. D., Caramia, F., Di Legge, S., Piattella, M. C., et al. (2002b). Contribution of corticospinal tract damage to cortical motor reorganization after a single clinical attack of multiple sclerosis. *NeuroImage, 17,* 1837–1843.

Pantano, P., Mainero, C., Lenzi, D., Caramia, F., Iannetti, G. D., Piattella, M. C., et al. (2005). A longitudinal fMRI study on motor activity in patients with multiple sclerosis. *Brain, 128,* 2146–2153.

Papadopoulos, D., Dukes, S., Patel, R., Nicholas, R., Vora, A., & Reynolds, R. (2009). Substantial archaeocortical atrophy and neuronal loss in multiple sclerosis. *Brain Pathol, 19,* 238–253.

Raichle, M. E., MacLeod, A. M., Snyder, A. Z., Powers, W. J., Gusnard, D. A., & Shulman, G. L. (2001). A default mode of brain function. *P Natl Acad Sci USA, 98,* 676–682.

Reddy, H., Narayanan, S., Woolrich, M., Mitsumori, T., Lapierre, Y., Arnold, D. L., et al. (2002). Functional brain reorganization for hand movement in patients with multiple sclerosis: Defining distinct effects of injury and disability. *Brain, 125,* 2646–2657.

Reddy, H., Narayanan, S., Arnoutelis, R., Jenkinson, M., Antel. J., Matthews, P. M., et al. (2000). Evidence for adaptive functional changes in the cerebral cortex with axonal injury from multiple sclerosis. *Brain, 123,* 2314–2320.

Rocca, M. A., Matthews, P. M., Caputo, D., Ghezzi, A., Falini, A., Scotti, G., et al. (2002). Evidence for widespread movement-associated functional MRI changes in patients with PPMS. *Neurology, 58,* 866–872.

Rocca, M. A., Gavazzi, C., Mezzapesa, D. M., Falini, A., Colombo, B., Mascalchi, M., et al. (2003). A functional magnetic resonance imaging study of patients with secondary progressive multiple sclerosis. *NeuroImage, 19,* 1770–1777.

Rocca, M. A., Absinta, M., Moiola, L., Ghezzi, A., Colombo, B., Martinelli, V., et al. (2010a). Functional and structural connectivity of the motor network in pediatric and adult-onset relapsing-remitting multiple sclerosis. *Radiology, 254,* 541–550.

Rocca, M. A., Valsasina, P., Absinta, M., Riccitelli, G., Rodegher, M. E., Misci, P., et al. (2010b). Default-mode network dysfunction and cognitive impairment in progressive MS. *Neurology, 74,* 1252–1259.

Roosendaal, S. D., Hulst, H. E., Vrenken, H., Feenstra, H. E. M., Castelijns, J. A., Pouwels, P. J. W., et al. (2010a). Structural and functional hippocampal changes in multiple sclerosis patients with intact memory function. *Radiology, 255,* 595–604.

Roosendaal, S. D., Schoonheim, M. M., Hulst, H. E., Sanz-Arigita, E. J., Smith, S. M., Geurts, J. J. G., et al. (2010b). Resting state networks change in clinically isolated syndrome. *Brain, 133,* 1612–1621.

Sicotte, N. L., Kern, K. C., Giesser, B. S., Arshanapalli, A., Schultz, A., Montag, M., et al. (2008). Regional hippocampal atrophy in multiple sclerosis. *Brain, 131,* 1134–1141.

Smith, A. M., Walker, L. A. S., Freedman, M. S., Berrigan, L. I., Pierre, J. St., Hogan, M. J., et al. (2012). Activation patterns in multiple sclerosis on the computerized tests of information processing. *J Neurol Sci, 312,* 131–137.

Stein, D. G., Brailowsky, S., & Will, B. (1995). *Brain repair.* New York: Oxford University Press.

Sumowski, J. F., Chiaravalloti, N. D., & DeLuca, J. (2009). Cognitive reserve protects against cognitive dysfunction in multiple sclerosis. *J Clin Exp Neurops, 31,* 913–923.

Sumowski, J. F., Wylie, G. R., Chiaravalloti, N., & DeLuca, J. (2010a). Intellectual enrichment lessens the effect of brain atrophy on learning and memory in multiple sclerosis. *Neurology, 74,* 1942–1945.

Sumowski, J. F., Wylie, G. R., DeLuca, J., & Chiaravalloti, N. D. (2010b). Intellectual enrichment is linked to cerebral efficiency in multiple sclerosis: functional magnetic resonance imaging evidence for cognitive reserve. *Brain, 133,* 362–374.

Sumowski, J. F., Wylie, G. R., Leavitt, V. M., Chiaravalloti, N. D., & DeLuca, J. (2013). Default network activity is a sensitive and specific biomarker of memory in multiple sclerosis. *Mult Scler J, 19,* 199–208.

Tomassini, V., Johansen-Berg, H., Jbabdi, S., Wise, R. G., Pozzilli, C., Palace, J., et al. (2012a). Relating brain damage to brain plasticity in patients with multiple sclerosis. *Neurorehab Neural Re, 26,* 581–593.

Tomassini, V., Matthews, P. M., Thompson, A. J., Fuglo, D., Geurts, J. J., Johansen-Berg, H., et al. (2012b). Neuroplasticity and functional recovery in multiple sclerosis. *Nature Rev Neurol, 8,* 635–646.

Trapp, B. D., Peterson, J., Ranshoff, R. M., Rudick, R., Mork, S., & Bo, L. (1998). Axonal transection in the lesions of multiple sclerosis. *New Engl J Med, 338,* 278–285.

Vercellino, M., Plano, F., Votta, B., Mutani, R., Giordana, M. T., & Cavalla, P. (2005). Grey matter pathology in multiple sclerosis. *J Neuropath Exp Neur, 64,* 1101–1107.

6

Plasticity of Cognition in Brain Gliomas

Hugues Duffau

Introduction

The classical concept in neuro-oncology is to see first the tumor, with very few considerations regarding the host, namely, the brain. Yet, it is crucial to take into account the "onco-functional balance" when selecting the best therapeutic strategy for each patient harboring a glioma (primary tumor of the central nervous system; Louis, Ohgaki, Wiestler, & Cavenee, 2007). To this end, although understanding the natural history of the disease is mandatory, this is, however, insufficient. One should also study the reaction of the central nervous system generated by the growth and migration of the glioma. Due to strong interactions between the tumor and the brain, cerebral adaptive phenomena often occur in order to maintain neurological and cognitive functions to compensate the spreading of the diffuse tumor (Duffau, 2005)—until limitations have been reached, with occurrence of non-adaptative responses to tumors, especially seizures.

In this chapter, the aim is to study the mechanisms underlying this plastic potential, based on lessons provided by cerebral mapping and functional outcomes in patients who underwent awake surgery for gliomas. The purpose is to switch from a localizationist view to a dynamic hodotopical framework of brain functioning. Regarding clinical implications, this fundamental knowledge will allow for tailoring the optimal therapeutic management according to the dynamic relationships between glioma's course and impact on cerebral functional reorganization at the individual level.

The Concept of Brain Plasticity

History

As early as the beginning of the ninteenth century, two opposite conceptions of the functioning of the central nervous system were suggested. First, the theory of "equipotentiality" hypothesized that the whole brain, or at least one complete hemisphere, was involved in the implementation of a functional task. By contrast, the theory of "localizationism," in which each part of the brain was supposed to correspond to a specific function, was built following the seminal description of the "phrenology." Progressively, the frequent reports of lesional studies led to an intermediate view, namely, a brain organized (1) in highly specialized functional areas, called "eloquent" regions (such as the Rolandic, Broca's, and Wernicke's areas, which were identified early on), for which any lesion gives rise to major permanent neurological deficits, and (2) in areas with no functional consequences when damaged, called "non-eloquent" regions. Based on these first anatomo-functional correlations, and despite the description by some pioneers of several observations of post-lesional recovery, the dogma of a static functional organization of the brain was settled for a long time, with the presumed inability to compensate for an injury involving the so-called eloquent areas. However, through regular reports of improved functional status following damages of cortical and/or subcortical structures considered as "critical," this view of a "fixed" central nervous system has been called into question over the past few decades. Consequently, many investigations have been conducted, initially in vitro and in animals, and more recently in humans, in order to study the mechanisms underlying these compensatory phenomena. From this, the concept of cerebral plasticity was born (for a review, see Desmurget, Bonnetblanc, & Duffau, 2007). Indeed, current developments in functional mapping and neuroimaging techniques have radically changed the classical modular model to a new dynamic and distributed perspective of brain organization, specifically, its capability to reorganize itself both during everyday life (learning) and after a pathological event (e.g., stroke or glioma; Duffau, 2008).

Definition and Mechanisms

Cerebral plasticity can be defined as the continuous processing allowing short-, middle-, and long-term remodeling of the neurono-synaptic organization, in order to optimize the functioning of the networks of the brain. It occurs during phylogenesis, ontogeny, and physiological learning, as well as following lesions involving the peripheral and the central nervous system. Several hypotheses about the pathophysiological mechanisms underlying plasticity have been considered. At a microscopic scale, these mechanisms seem to be essentially represented by synaptic efficacy modulations, unmasking of latent connections, phenotypic modifications, synchrony changes, and neurogenesis. At a macroscopic level, diaschisis, functional redundancies, cross-modal plasticity with sensory substitution, and morphological changes are suggested to be involved. Moreover, the behavioral consequences of such cerebral phenomena have been analyzed in humans in the past decade, both in physiology (ontogeny and learning) and in pathology. In particular, the ability to recover after a nervous system injury (post-lesional plasticity) and the patterns of functional reorganization within eloquent area and/or within distributed networks, allowing such compensation, have been extensively studied (Duffau, 2006).

In other words, cerebral plasticity is conceivable only in a dynamic, rather than a rigid, view of the brain. Indeed, according to new theories, the brain is an ensemble of complex networks that form, reshape, and flush information dynamically (Varela, Lachaux, Rodriguez, & Martinerie, 2001; Werner, 2007). Thus, based on the existence of multiple and overlapping redundancies hierarchically organized, reorganization could occur (Bavelier & Neville, 2002; Duffau, 2001; Duffau, Sichez, & Lehéricy, 2000; Rossini, Calautti, Pauri, & Baron, 2003; Sanes, Donoghue, Thangaraj, Edelman, & Warach, 1995). These findings have testified that neuronal aggregates around a lesion can increasingly adopt the function of the damaged area and can switch their own function to substitute for the lesioned area, while facilitating functional recovery following brain damage (Duffau, 2006).

In this setting, the concept of the brain "connectome" has recently emerged. Its aim is to capture the characteristics of spatially distributed dynamical neural processes at multiple spatial and temporal scales (Sporns, Tononi, & Kötter, 2005). The new science of brain "connectomics" is contributing both to theoretical and computational models of the brain as a complex system (Honey, Kötter, Breakspear, & Sporns, 2007). Additionally, it is contributing experimentally to new indices and metrics (e.g., nodes, hubs, efficiency, modularity) in order to characterize and scale the functional organization of the healthy and diseased nervous system (Basset & Bullmore, 2009). In pathology, brain plasticity is nonetheless possible only on the condition that the subcortical connectivity is preserved to allow spatial communication and temporal synchronization among large interconnected networks—according to the principle of hodotopy (Ius, Angelini, Thiebaut de Schotten, Mandonnet, & Duffau, 2011). Although different patterns of subcortical plasticity have recently been identified (i.e., unmasking of perilesional latent networks, recruitment of accessory pathways, introduction of additional relays within neuron-synaptic circuits, and involvement of parallel long-distance association pathways), the real capacity to build a new structural connectivity ("rewiring") leading to functional recovery has not yet been demonstrated in humans (see discussion later in this chapter; Duffau, 2009).

The Time Course of Gliomas and Brain Reorganization

In contrast with a glioblastoma (grade IV glioma according to the WHO classification, that is, a very aggressive tumor with median survival around 1 year), a diffuse low-grade glioma (DLGG, WHO grade II glioma) is a slow-growing tumor that progressively invades the brain over a period of years (Louis, Ohgaki, Wiestler, & Cavenee, 2007). This slow time course of the disease explains why numerous patients with DLGG usually have only mild or even no functional deficit, despite the frequent involvement of the so-called eloquent structures (Duffau & Capelle, 2004; Parisot, Duffau, Chemouny, & Paragios, 2011). This means that these lesions have induced progressive functional brain reshaping, as suggested by preoperative functional neuroimaging—as, for instance, language reorganization around the Broca's area (Benzagmout, Gatignol, & Duffau, 2007). Recently, it was shown that brain plasticity cannot be fully understood and fruitfully studied without considering the temporal pattern of the injury inflicted to the brain (Desmurget, Bonnetblanc, & Duffau, 2007). For instance, in acute lesion such as a stroke, only around 25% of patients fully recovered within the months following the damage (Varona, Bermejo, Guerra, & Molina, 2004). In contrast, more than 90% of patients with a DLGG (same location as the stroke) fully recovered, using the same criteria of recovery as for stoke.

Interestingly, using a neurocomputational model based on training a series of parallel distributed processing neural network models, recent work simulated acute versus slow-growing injuries (Keidel, Welbourne, & Lambon Ralph, 2010). The results showed a very different pattern emerging in the simulation of DLGG in comparison with the simulation of stroke, with slow decay of the links within the same subnetwork leading to minimal performance decline. Moreover, at the end of the decay regime, the entire affected hidden layer could be "removed" on the simulation with no effect on performance, closely matching the lack of major impairment from DLGG resection. Due to the fact that abrupt stroke occasions rapid neuronal death and DLGG initially spares neuronal tissue, only the latter allows time for cerebral remapping. Thus, functional status at the time of diagnosis may be a good reflection of the natural course of the disease.

The Patterns of Preoperative Functional Reshaping in Low-Grade Gliomas

The patterns of reorganization may differ among DLGG patients (Duffau et al., 2003; Duffau, 2006a). Indeed, preoperative functional neuroimaging has shown that four kinds of preoperative functional redistribution are possible in patients without any deficit (Desmurget, Bonnetblanc, & Duffau, 2007; Duffau, 2005). In the first type, function still persists within the tumor due to the infiltrative nature of gliomas, thus limiting the likelihood of performing a fair resection. In the second, eloquent areas are redistributed around the tumor, providing a reasonable chance of performing a near-total resection. While there are generally immediate transient deficits, secondary recovery occurs within a few weeks to months. In the third type, there is already a preoperative compensation by remote areas within the lesional hemisphere. In the fourth, a network of areas is recuited in the contralateral hemisphere; consequently, the chances of performing a total resection are very high, with only slight and very transient deficits. Finally, these different patterns of reshaping can co-occur. Therefore, in cases of brain lesions involving eloquent areas, plasticity mechanisms seem to be based on a hierarchically organized model. First, intrinsic reorganization occurs within injured areas (indice of favorable outcome). Second, when this reshaping is insufficient, other regions implicated in the functional network are recruited in the ipsilateral hemisphere (close and even remote to the damaged area) and then in the contralateral hemisphere, if necessary (Duffau, 2008). This is the reason that a contralateral compensation can be associated with an incomplete recovery, for example, some difficulties in complex movements following a supplementary motor area syndrome with recruitment of the contralateral homologous area (Krainik et al., 2001, 2004).

In summary, as recently supported by magnetoencephalography study, a focal DLGG disturbs the functional and effective connectivity within the whole brain, and not only in a restricted area around the tumor (Bartolomei et al., 2006). These network dysfunctions are related to cognitive processing in DLGG patients, with a decline in psychomotor function, information processing, and working memory (Bosma et al., 2008). Indeed, when objective neuropsychological and health-related quality of life assessments have been performed, visuo-spatial, memory, attention, planning, learning, emotional, motivational, and behavioral deficits have regularly been observed in glioma patients (Klein, Duffau, & De Witt Hamer, 2012). These results show that the potential for brain plasticity may be limited, and this potential should be studied at the individual level. In other words, because surgical treatment itself may induce changes in large-scale functional connectivity (Douw et al., 2008), such knowledge of individual pattern of remapping should be taken into account in order to elaborate personalized therapeutic management in patients bearing DLGG.

Intraoperative Plasticity

Intrasurgical Electrical Mapping

During surgery for a glioma invading both cortical and subcortical structures, especially in "eloquent areas," it has become common clinical practice to awaken patients in order to assess the functional role of restricted cerebral regions. Thanks to individual mapping, the surgeon can maximize the extent of resection, thereby improving the overall survival, preserving eloquent structures (particularly language). That is, the resection is performed according to functional boundaries (Duffau, 2012; Duffau, Gatignol, Mandonnet, Capelle & Taillandier, 2008). During the procedure, patients perform several sensory-motor, language, and cognitive tasks, while the surgeon temporarily interacts with discrete areas within the gray and white matter around the tumor, using direct electrical stimulation (DES). If the patients stops performing the task or incorrectly responds, the surgeon avoids removing the stimulated site (Duffau, 2012a). DES transiently interacts both locally with a small cortical or axonal site, and non-locally, as the focal perturbation disrupts the whole (sub)network sustaining a given function (Mandonnet, Winkler, & Duffau, 2010). Intraoperative mapping also has a prognostic value concerning the postoperative recovery for movement (Duffau, 2001a). Thus, DES represents a unique opportunity to identify with great accuracy and reproducibility the structures that are crucial for cognitive functions (particularly language), both at cortical and subcortical (white matter and deep gray nuclei) levels (Duffau, 2008a; Duffau et al., 2002).

Intrasurgical Cognitive Monitoring and Test Selection

The selection of the tasks administrated to the patient intrasurgically is crucial to the preservation of a normal life (Duffau, 2003a, 2006b, 2007, 2008a, 2010, 2013). For instance, language mapping can be performed to detect possible language epicenters in the right "non-dominant" hemisphere in left-handers or ambidextrous individuals (and even in some cases in right-handers), according to the results of the presurgical cognitive assessment (e.g., if language disturbances have been identified even in cases of left-lateralization on functional MRI) (Duffau, Leroy, & Gatignol, 2008; Vassal, Le Bars, Moritz-Gasser, Menjot, & Duffau, 2010). The goal is to map the networks underlying the different but interactive subfunctions that have to be preserved intraoperatively—and which will serve as boundaries of the resection.

Indeed, DES allows the mapping of numerous brain functions, including movement (Lafargue & Duffau, 2008; Sallard, Barral, Duffau, & Bonnetblanc, 2012; Sallard, Duffau, & Bonnetblanc, 2012; Schucht, Moritz-Gasser, Herbet, Raabe, & Duffau, 2013), somatosensory function (Duffau et al., 2003b; Schucht, Moritz-Gasser, Herbet, Raabe, & Duffau, 2013), visual function (Coello, Duvaux, de Benedictis, Matsuda, & Duffau, 2013; Duffau, Velut, Mitchell, Gatignol, & Capelle, 2004; Gras-Combe, Moritz-Gasser, Herbet, & Duffau, 2012; Mandonnet, Gatignol, & Duffau, 2009), auditory-vestibular function (Spena, Gatignol, Capelle, & Duffau, 2006), spatial awareness (Thiebaut et al., 2005), and higher-order functions (e.g., calculation, memory, attention, cognitive control, and cross-modal judgement; Duffau et al., 2002; Gil Robles, Gatignol, Capelle, Mitchell, & Duffau, 2005; Milea et al., 2002; Plaza, Gatignol, Cohen, Berger, & Duffau, 2008). As previously noted, language, including object naming, comprehension, writing, reading, syntax, bilingualism, and switching from one language to another, can also be mapped using intrasurgical DES (Duffau, Gatignol, Mandonnet, Capelle, & Taillandier, 2008; Duffau, Gatignol, Mandonnet, Peruzzi, Tzourio-Mazoyer, & Capelle, 2005; Duffau et al., 2003a; Gatignol, Capelle, Le Bihan, & Duffau, 2004; Moritz-Gasser, & Duffau, 2009; Sanai, Mirzadeh, & Berger, 2008; Vidorreta, Garcia, Moritz-Gasser, & Duffau, 2011). All these functions are equally well mapped by DES, and can show reorganization in the setting of a tumor.

Acute Functional Remapping During Glioma Surgery

Brain DES in awake patients allows a re-examination of the neural foundations of cerebral functions. In fact, intraoperative stimulation mapping before any resection has enabled the confirmation of the existence of a functional reshaping induced by brain lesions, as demonstrated using functional neuroimaging. Moreover, acute reorganization of functional maps was equally observed during the resection, likely due to the surgical act itself, which can generate a loco-regional hyperexcitability. Although stimulation of the precentral gyrus in several patients harboring a frontal lesion induced motor responses only at the level of a limited number of cortical sites before resection, an acute unmasking of redundant motor sites located within the same precentral gyrus, and eliciting the same movements than the previous adjacent sites when stimulated, was observed immediately following lesion removal (Duffau, 2001). Acute unmasking of redundant somatosensory sites was also regularly observed within the retrocentral gyrus in patients operated on for a parietal glioma. Furthermore, it was equally possible to detect a redistribution within a larger network involving the whole rolandic region, that is, with unmasking of functional homologous located in the precentral gyrus for the first cortical representation and in the retrocentral gyrus for its redundancy (or vice versa) (Duffau, Sichez, & Lehéricy, 2000).

Subcortical Connectivity as a Limitation for Cerebral Remapping: Toward Brain Hodotopy

Axonal Connectivity and the Minimal Common Brain

Although plastic potential is high at the cortical level, subcortical plasticity is low, implying that axonal connectivity should be preserved to allow post-lesional compensation. Indeed, lessons from stroke studies have taught that damage to white matter pathways generates a more severe neurological picture, worse than cortical lesions. By combining cortical function and axonal connectivity, an updated model of cerebral processing has recently been proposed, moving from a traditional "localizationist" view to a "hodotopical" framework (Catani, 2007). In pathology, according to this new concept, a topological mechanism (from the Greek *topos* = place) refers to a dysfunction of the cortex (deficit, hyperfunction, or a combination of the two), whereas a hodological mechanism (from the Greek *hodos* = road or path) refers to dysfunction related to connecting pathways (disconnection, hyperconnection, or a combination of the two; de Benedictis & Duffau, 2011). Thus, one should take into account the complex functioning of a large-scale distributed cortico-subcortical network to understand both its physiology, as well as the functional consequences of a lesion in this circuit, which depending on the location and extent of the damage (e.g., purely cortical, or purely subcortical, or both) result in different potential deficits.

Recently, development of a probabilistic postsurgical residue atlas was undertaken, and was computed on a series of patients who underwent incomplete resection for a DLGG on the basis of intraoperative electrical brain mapping (Ius, Angelini, Thiebaut de Schotten, Mandonnet, & Duffau, 2011; Mandonnet et al., 2007). The anatomo-functional correlations obtained by combining the intrasurgical functional data with postoperative anatomical MRI findings provided a greater understanding of the functional limitations of surgical removal and new insights into the potential of brain plasticity, as well as its limitations. This probabilistic atlas highlighted the crucial role of the axonal pathways in the reorganization of the brain after a lesion. Additionally, it provided a general framework to establish anatomo-functional correlations by computing the probability of each brain voxel to be preserved—due to its functional role—on the postoperative MRI. Its overlap with the cortical Montreal Neurological Institute (MNI) template and a diffusion tensor imaging tractography atlas offered a unique tool to analyze the potentialities and the limitations of inter-individual variability and plasticity, both for cortical areas and axonal pathways. As a rule, a low probability of residual tumors on the cortical surface were observed, whereas most of the regions with high probability of residual tumor were located in the deep white matter. Thus, projection and association axonal pathways seem to play a critical role in the proper functioning of the brain. The functions subserved by long-range axonal pathways seem to be less subject to inter-individual variability and reorganization than cortical sites (Ius, Angelini, Thiebaut de Schotten, Mandonnet, & Duffau, 2011). Consequently, these pathways define the surgical deep limits (Duffau, Gatignol, Mandonnet, Capelle, & Taillandier, 2008), and, since DLGGs infiltrate these tracts (Mandonnet, Capelle, & Duffau, 2006), they constitute the main obstacle to radical surgical resection. Two questions arise regarding why there is no inter-individual variability for these areas and why their resection cannot be efficiently compensated by plasticity phenomena. For some of these areas, the explanation could be that they act as input or output areas: input sites convey or are the first relay of information entering the brain, whereas output sites are the last relay for sending information outside the brain. This is a limitation of plastic potential in comparison with more distributed functions. These areas are mainly unimodal and likely serially organized, and they include the primary motor and somatosensory areas, the cortico-spinal and thalamo-cortical tracts, and the optic radiations (i.e., projection fibers). The absence of a parallel alternative pathway explains the impossibility to restore their function after any damage (Duffau, 2009).

For all other areas, their non-resectability should be analyzed within a network perspective. Higher-order cognitive processes are mediated by short- and long-range networks, with cortical epicenters connected by U-shaped fibers, associative and commissural pathways. A particular network topology (like the "small world" one) is required to allow proper synchronization between several distant areas (Stam, 2010). The link between the function and the anatomy is not as simple as for input–output areas; in fact, a local lesion can disturb a whole network topology, which in turn, could ultimately hamper the function sustained by this network. It has been hypothesized that, beyond the posterior part of the posterior temporal gyrus in the left dominant hemisphere, subcortical structures like the inferior fronto-occipital fascicle and the arcuate fascicle are non-resectable because their lesion would cause such significant changes in the network topology that any dynamical plasticity potential would be overwhelmed. Interestingly, these areas are considered "hubs" in revisited models of cognition (e.g., the posterior part of the left dominant superior temporal gyrus and its junction with the inferior parietal lobule; Hickok

& Poeppel, 2007). Indeed, these functional epicenters allow a plurimodal integration of multiple data coming from unimodal areas. In the future, this integration may lead to a new conceptualization of brain processing, performed at the level of a wide network including the hubs. As a consequence, these hubs are interconnected by subcortical pathways, themselves crucial for brain function, such as the arcuate fascicle or the inferior fronto-occipital fascicle, which enables a direct communication between the posterior temporal and frontal plurimodal regions. The reproducibility of these results, despite the inter-individual anatomo-functional variability and plastic mechanisms, may lead to the notion of a "minimal common brain" necessary for the basic cognitive functions—even if likely not sufficient for more complex functions such as multi-processing. This hypothesis is in agreement with recent biomathematical models, which have analyzed the effect of a simulated focal lesion on the whole brain network topology (Alstott, Breakspear, Hagmann, Cammoun, & Sporns, 2009). Of note, for these areas, even biological plasticity, which has been shown to offer an axonal rewiring in animal models (Dancause et al., 2005; Guleria et al., 2008), would fail in the long term to repair the connectivity required to rebuild an effective network topology, hence a functional network (Duffau, 2009).

Consequently, neurosurgeons should improve their knowledge concerning white matter circuitry. Therefore, beyond the well-known cortico-spinal (pyramidal), thalamo-cortical (somatosensory), and visual (optic radiations) pathways, subcortical connectivity subserving language and cognitive functions must be more extensively studied for each patient. Because DLGG is a tumor that migrates along the main projection of commissural and long-distance association bundles (Mandonnet, Capelle, & Duffau, 2006), it is impossible to define the optimal therapeutic strategy against invasive glioma without understanding the organization of the neural networks. Thus, cognitive neurosciences are closely related with neuro-oncology, since the use of brain mapping during DLGG surgery also provides new insights into the circuits underlying cognitive functions.

Anatomo-Functional Connectivity of Language: Naming Process Studied by DES

One of the best examples of a large-scale circuit that should be better understood is the network subserving picture naming—a task that is considered a cornerstone in intraoperative mapping of language for several decades (Ojemann, Ojemann, Lettich, & Berger, 1989; see Figure 6.1). In the naming process, the first step is visual perception and recognition. Electrical stimulation of the optic pathway may elicit phosphenes (flashes) and/or reversible visual loss in the contralateral visual field reported by the awake patients, demonstrating an inhibition of visual perception (Gras-Combe, Moritz-Gasser, Herbet, Duffau, 2012). Visual formal paraphasia has been generated by electrical interference with a second stage of visual processing, that is, visual recognition (Mandonnet, Gatignol, & Duffau, 2009). These disturbances were induced by axonal stimulation of a subpart of the posterior inferior longitudinal fascicle, which links the visual cortex to the "visual

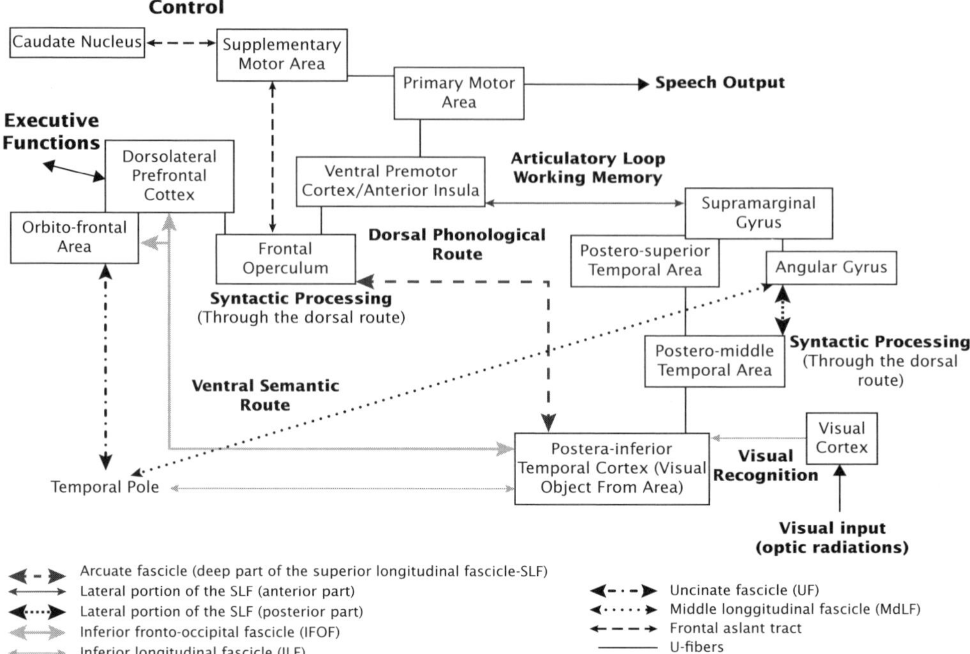

FIGURE 6.1 Proposal of a hodotopical model of language, with incorporation of anatomic constraints, elaborated on the basis of structural-functional correlations provided by intraoperative direct cortico-subcortical electrostimulation. Modified from Duffau, Moritz-Gasser, & Mandonnet, 2014.

object form area" (Mandonnet, Gatignol, & Duffau, 2009). This visual object form area, involved in object recognition, is near the visual word form area, which receives another subpart of the inferior longitudinal fascicle, a subpathway involved in reading and generating alexia when damaged (Gaillard et al., 2006).

Recently, based on functional disturbances induced by electrostimulation during picture naming, an original dual model for visual language processing in humans (after the first step of visual recognition) was suggested: a ventral stream maps visual information to meaning (the "what" pathway), and a dorsal stream maps visual information to articulation through visuo-phonological conversion. This model suggests that both processes are performed in parallel, and not serially, because double dissociation between phonemic and semantic processing has been elicited by stimulation (Maldonado, Moritz-Gasser, & Duffau, 2011). Regarding the ventral semantic stream, cortically, semantic paraphasias have been observed during intraoperative stimulation of the posterior part of superior temporal sulcus, as well as in the frontal lobe, specifically, the dorsolateral prefrontal cortex and the pars orbitaris of the inferior frontal gyrus (Bello et al., 2007; Duffau, Gatignol, Mandonnet, Peruzzi, Tzourio-Mazoyer, & Capelle, 2005). Axonally, such errors were elicited by stimulation of the left inferior fronto-occipital fascicle (Benzagmout, Gatignol, & Duffau, 2007; Duffau, Gatignol, Mandonnet, Peruzzi, Tzourio-Mazoyer, & Capelle, 2005), a pathway that connects the posterior occipital lobe and visual object form area to anterior cortical areas comprising the inferior frontal gyrus and the dorso-lateral prefrontal cortex (Martino, Brogna, Gil Robles, Vergani, & Duffau, 2010; Sarubbo, De Benedictis, Maldonado, Basso, & Duffau H, 2013). These regions are known to be involved in language semantics, as demonstrated in functional MRI studies (for a meta-analysis, see Vigneau et al., 2006) and cortical stimulation (Duffau, Gatignol, Mandonnet, Peruzzi, Tzourio-Mazoyer, & Capelle, 2005). These sites are able to make the link with higher cognitive function such as plurimodal integration and judgment (Plaza, Gatignol, Cohen, Berger, & Duffau, 2008). Thus, pretreated information by the visual recognition system is subsequently processed by the semantic system (parallel to the dorsal phonological stream, see discussion later in this chapter) before being processed by the executive system. In addition to this direct ventral route subserved by the inferior fronto-occipital fascicle, an indirect ventral semantic pathway seems to exist, with a relay at the level of the temporal pole. Indeed, the temporal pole is a "hub," that is, a functional epicenter allowing a plurimodal integration of the multiple data coming from the unimodal systems—explaining its role in semantics (Holland & Lambon-Ralph, 2010). This indirect ventral stream is constituted by the anterior part of the inferior longitudinal fascicle, connecting the visual object form area with the temporal pole (Mandonnet, Nouet, Gatignol, Capelle, & Duffau, 2007), and then is relayed by the uncinate fascicle, which links the temporal pole with the pars orbitalis of the inferior frontal gyrus (Duffau, Gatignol, Moritz-Gasser, & Mandonnet, 2009). It is nonetheless worth noting that this indirect pathway can be functionally compensated when (unilaterally) damaged, as extensively demonstrated following anterior temporal lobectomy in epilepsy surgery (Duffau, Thiebaut de Schotten, & Mandonnet, 2008). Even if a very mild and selective deficit may persist in proper name retrieval (Papagno et al., 2011), this is a good illustration of "subcortical plasticity," in which a subnetwork (direct pathway) is able to bypass and functionally compensate for another subnetwork (indirect pathway) (Duffau, Gatignol, Moritz-Gasser, & Mandonnet, 2009).

Regarding the dorsal phonological stream, cortically, phonemic paraphasias can be elicited by stimulating the inferior parietal lobule and the inferior frontal gyrus (De Witt Hamer, Moritz-Gasser, Gatignol, & Duffau, 2011; Maldonado, Moritz-Gasser, de Champfleur, Bertram, Moulinié, & Duffau, 2011). Axonally speaking, phonemic paraphasias were elicited when stimulating the arcuate fascicle, which is a fiber tract stemming from the caudal part of the temporal lobe (mainly the inferior and middle temporal gyri). It arches around the insula and advances forward to end within the frontal lobe, essentially within the ventral premotor cortex and the pars opercularis of the inferior frontal gyrus (Benzagmout, Gatignol, & Duffau, 2007; De Witt Hamer, Moritz-Gasser, Gatignol, & Duffau, 2011; Duffau et al., 2002; Maldonado, Moritz-Gasser, & Duffau 2011; Martino et al., 2013). On the basis of lesion studies, Geschwind postulated that lesions of this tract would produce conduction aphasia, including phonemic paraphasias (Geschwind, 1970), supporting the role of the subpart of the dorsal stream mediated by the arcuate fascicle in phonological processing. Interestingly, the posterior cortical origin of this tract within the posterior part of the inferior temporal gyrus (Martino et al., 2013) seems to correspond to the visual object form area. Indeed, this region represents a functional hub, involved in both semantic (see previous discussion in this chapter) and phonological processing, dedicated to visual material (Vigneau et al., 2006). Therefore, phonological processes subserved by the arcuate fascicle seem to be performed in parallel to the semantic processes underlain by the ventral route (Mandonnet, Gatignol, & Duffau, 2009). Of note, in addition to this direct dorsal route, recent tractography studies evidenced the existence of an indirect dorsal stream, running more superficially and underlying the lateral superior longitudinal fascicle (Catani, Jones, & ffytche, 2005). This pathway is implied in articulation and phonological working memory, as demonstrated by electrostimulation. Cortical areas eliciting articulatory disorders are located in the rolandic operculum, especially the ventral premotor cortex in the ventral part of the supramarginal gyrus, as well as in the posterior part of the superior temporal gyrus (Benzagmout, Gatignol, & Duffau, 2007; De Witt Hamer, Moritz-Gasser, Gatignol, & Duffau, 2011; Duffau, Gatignol, Denvil, Lopes, & Capelle, 2003). Axonally, stimulation of the white matter in the fronto-parietal operculum, as well as under the supramarginal gyrus laterally and ventrally to the arcuate fascicle, induces anarthria as well (Duffau, Gatignol, Denvil, Lopes, & Capelle, 2003; Maldonado, Moritz-Gasser, & Duffau, 2011). Interestingly, the existence of an operculo-opercular component of the superior longitudinal fascicle, named "SLF III" by some authors (Makris et al., 2005) and "anterior segment" by others (Catani, Jones, & ffytche, 2005), was recently demonstrated. This subpathway connects the supramarginal gyrus, as well as the posterior portion of the superior temporal gyrus, with the frontal operculum (Martino et al., 2013), and articulatory codes are stored in this fronto-parietal loop. Posteriorly, the ventral supramarginal gyrus receives feedback information from somatosensory and auditory areas (in the parietal lobe and superior temporal gyrus, respectively), which would explain why stimulation induces dysarthria/anarthria when applied over these posterior regions (Maldonado, Moritz-Gasser, de Champfleur, Bertram, Moulinié, & Duffau, 2011; Duffau, Gatignol, Denvil, Lopes, & Capelle, 2003). Anteriorly, the ventral premotor cortex receives afferences, bringing the phonological and/or phonetic information to be translated into articulatory motor programs, and efferences toward the primary motor area (Duffau et al., 2003a). Because these different functional pathways are part of the minimal common brain, they represent a limitation to brain plasticity.

In summary, the vision of the neural basis of cognition has begun to shift. For a long time, cognitive functions such as language were conceived in associationist terms of centers and pathways, the general assumption being that visual and auditory linguistic information was processed in localized cortical regions with the serial passage of information between regions through white matter tracts. Currently, an alternative hodotopical account is proposed, in which language is conceptualized as resulting from parallel distributed processing performed by distributed groups of connected neurons rather than individual centers (Duffau, 2008a, 2012b). In contrast with the serial model of language in which processing must be finished before the information proceeds to another level of processing, these new models of "independent networks" propose that different processing can be performed simultaneously with interactive feedbacks (Duffau et al., 2014; Figure 6.1). The next step to progress in the understanding of brain connectivity might be a more accurate analysis of the interactions between the language circuit and the networks underlying other cognitive functions, in particular, the visuo-spatial component in which the role of the superior longitudinal fasciculus has been emphasized (Thiebaut de Schotten et al., 2005), as well as the emotional and behavioral aspects. Such a multimodality approach seems to represent a unique opportunity to move toward an integrative model of the various functions. A better knowledge of these interactions is important in understanding the mechanisms underlying cross-modal plasticity.

Cerebral Reshaping: Its Implications for (Surgical) Treatment of DLGG

Maximal surgical resection is the first option in DLGG (Duffau, 2009b). Consequently, the preoperative estimation of the extent of resection should be reliable. Such prediction will directly depend on the involvement (or not) of subcortical pathways that cannot be functionally compensated, and this will lead to the selection of surgery as a first treatment or the selection of neoajuvant chemotherapy (Blonski et al., 2012). Results of the neuropsychological assessment, which should be conducted before the initiation of any treatment, will also contribute to the investigation of the individual's plasticity potential. If the patient already has experienced significant cognitive disorders and a fortiori neurological deficit, it may mean that the limits of brain plasticity have been reached—precluding functional compensation. Such parameters, in addition to the data provided by presurgical functional neuroimaging previously detailed regarding the pattern of reorganization elicited by DLGG, should be incorporated into the surgical strategy in DLGG with the goal of (1) extending the indications of the resection to eloquent structures so far considered as "inoperable," (2) maximizing the extent of glioma removal by performing the resection according to (not fixed) functional boundaries with no margin, and (3) minimizing the risk of postoperative permanent neurological worsening, and improving the quality of life (de Benedictis & Duffau, 2010; Duffau, 2006a; Duffau et al., 2005; Gil Robles & Duffau, 2010).

As mentioned, intraoperative stimulation mapping before and throughout tumor resection has allowed the confirmation of the existence of a functional reshaping induced by DLGG (Duffau, 2005). Thanks to these phenomena of preoperative and intraoperative plasticity, it was possible to remove DLGG invading the following "eloquent" brain structures with a minimal morbidity (Figure 6.2; Duffau, 2012):

• *Broca's area resection in the left dominant hemisphere*: The possibility of surgical resection of DLGG within the pars opercularis and triangularis of the left inferior frontal gyrus without generating permanent language deficits has been previously reported (Benzagmout, Gatignol, & Duffau, 2007; Lubrano, Draper, & Roux, 2010). Language compensation may be achieved by the recruitment of adjacent regions, in particular, the ventral premotor cortex, the pars orbitaris of the inferior frontal gyrus, the dorsolateral prefrontal cortex, and the insula (Benzagmout, Gatignol, & Duffau, 2007; 2012b; Lubrano, Draper, & Roux, 2010). Given the fact that Broca's area is located just in front of the non-resectable ventral premotor cortex (Ius, Angelini, Thiebaut de Schotten, Mandonnet, & Duffau, 2011), one can hypothesize that the real motor area for speech output is the ventral premotor cortex rather than Broca's area, the latter probably being involved in other components of language (such as syntactic and phonological processes) that can be compensated for (Benzagmout, Gatignol, & Duffau, 2007; Sahin, Pinker, Cash, Schomer, Halgren, 2009). A recent study with an extensive neuropsychological examination following resection of Broca's area confirmed complete functional recovery (Plaza, Gatignol, Leroy, & Duffau, 2009). Surgical approach through Broca's area, even though not invaded by the tumor, was recently reported in insular DLGG to decrease the risk of vascular injuries at the level of the Sylvian fissure (Duffau, 2012).

• *Wernicke's area resection*: Language compensation (particularly comprehension) following left dominant temporal resection could be explained by the fact that this complex function is organized in multiple parallel networks. Consequently, beyond the recruitment of areas adjacent to the surgical cavity, the long-term reshaping could be related to progressive involvement of remote regions within the left dominant hemisphere—such as the supramarginal gyrus, the pars triangularis of inferior frontal gyrus, or other left fronto-lateral regions—as well as the controlateral right non-dominant hemisphere due to a trans-callosal disinhibition phenomenon (Sarubbo, Le Bars, Moritz-Gasser, & Duffau, 2012).

• *Insular resection*: Despite a hemiparesis after right insula removal (likely because this region is a non-primary motor area) and transient speech disturbances following left dominant insula resection, all patients recovered in a personal surgical experience—except in rare cases (2%) of deep stroke due to a damage of the lenticulo-striate arteries (Duffau, 2009a; Duffau, Bauchet, Lehéricy, & Capelle, 2001; Duffau, Moritz-Gasser, & Gatignol, 2009; Duffau, Taillandier, Gatignol, & Capelle, 2006). Moreover, in right non-dominant fronto-temporo-insular DLGG involving the deep gray nuclei, the claustrum can be removed without any cognitive disorders (despite its role suggested in consciousness; Duffau; Mandonnet, Gatignol, & Capelle, 2007). Additionally, the invaded striatum can also be removed without inducing either motor deficit or movement disorder. This compensation can be explained by a recruitment of parallel subcortical circuits such as pallido-luyso-pallidal, strio-nigro-striate, cortico-strio-nigro-thalamo-cortical and cortico-luysal networks (Duffau, Denvil, & Capelle, 2002), and utilization of these alternative pathways.

• *Resection of primary sensory-motor area of the face*: The recovery of the usual transient central facial palsy, with a potential transitory Foix-Chavany-Marie syndrome when the insula is also involved (Duffau, Karachi, Gatignol, & Capelle, 2003), is likely explained by the disinhibition of the contralateral homologous sites via transcallosal pathways (LeRoux, Berger, Haglund, Pilcher, & Ojemann, 1991).

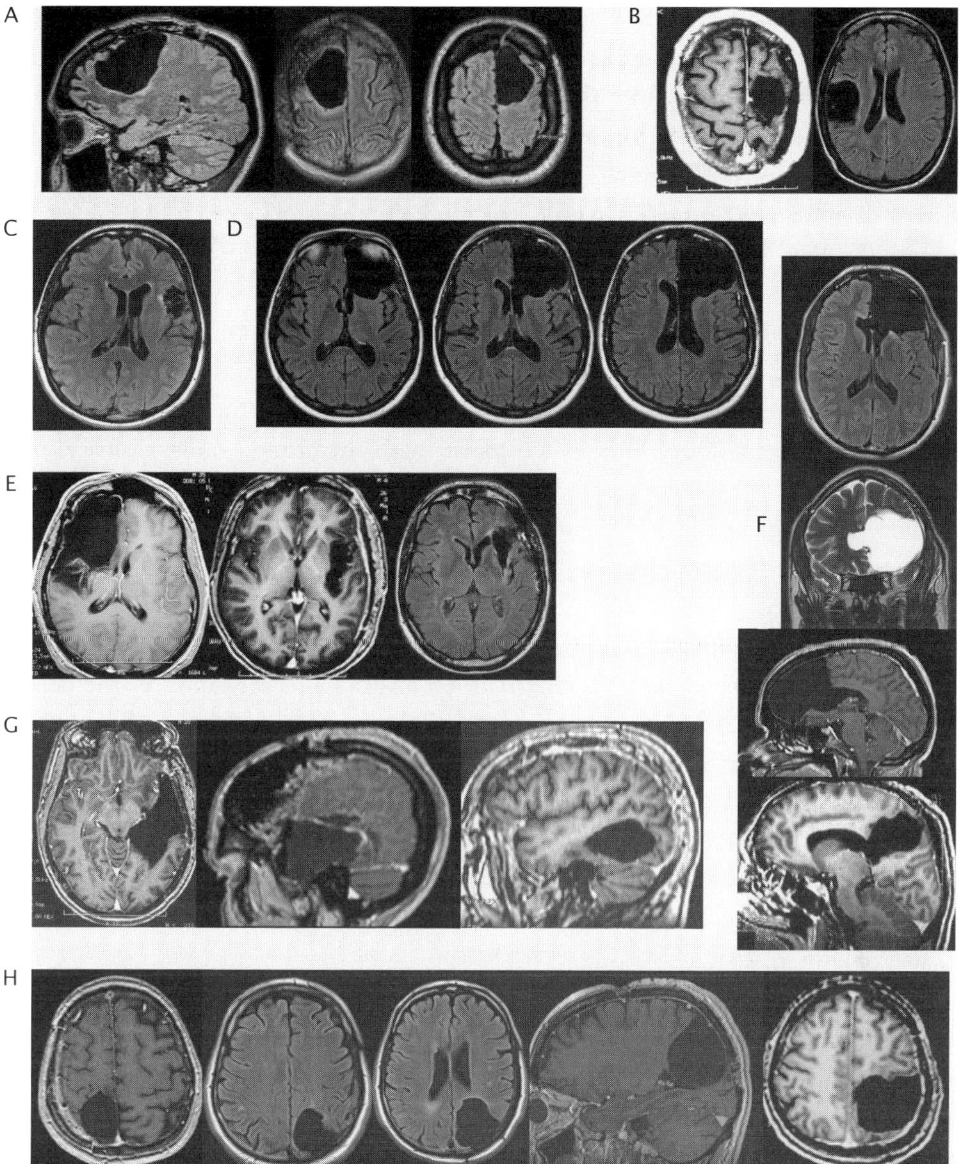

FIGURE 6.2 Examples of extensive glioma resections performed within the so-called "eloquent" areas using intraoperative electrical mapping, with preservation of the quality of life thanks to brain plasticity: (A) left and right supplementary motor area; (B) left primary motor area of the hand ("knob of the hand") and right primary sensory-motor area of the face; (C) "Broca's area" in the left dominant hemisphere; (D) entire left frontal lobe including "Broca's area"; (E) right paralimbic system and left insula; (F) corpus callosum, anterior or posterior part (splenium); (G) anterior/mid- and posterior left dominant temporal lobe, including "Wernicke's area"; and (H) parietal lobe in right and left hemispheres, including the primary somatosensory area. Modified from Duffau (2008).

- *Resection of primary motor area of the upper limb*: On the basis of the existence of multiple cortical motor representations evidenced in humans using functional neuroimaging and intraoperative stimulation mapping, the compensation of the motor function could be explained by the recruitment of parallel networks within the primary motor cortex. This would thereby allow the removal of the upper limb area, eventually using two consecutive surgeries in order to induce durable remapping following the first surgery (Duffau, 2001; Duffau, Denvil, & Capelle, 2002; see discussion later in this chapter).

- *Resection of the primary somatosensory area*: The first results using pre- and postoperative functional neuroimaging have suggested the possible recruitment of "redundant" eloquent sites around the cavity in the postcentral gyrus (Meunier, Duffau, Garnero, Capelle, & Ducorps, 2000). It is in accordance with the intraoperative electrical mapping data that show unmasking of redundant somatosensory sites during resection, which are likely explained by the decrease of the cortico-cortical inhibition. The recruitment of the second somatosensory area (i.e., posterior parietal cortex), primary motor area, and contralateral primary somatosensory area are also potential explanations of the recovery (Duffau & Capelle, 2001).

- *Supplementary motor area resection*: Removal of this area induces the delayed onset of a syndrome associated with transient akinesia and (potentially) transient mutism in the dominant hemisphere (Duffau, Lopes, Denvil, & Capelle, 2001; Krainik et al., 2001). However, all patients recovered, likely due to recuitment of the contralateral hemisphere (Krainik et al., 2003, 2004). Of note, deficits in bimanual coordination may nonetheless persist (Krainik et al., 2001), raising the question of the preservation of networks subserving motor control (Schucht, Moritz-Gasser, Herbet, Raabe, & Duffau, 2012).

- *Resection of the (dominant) parietal posterior lobe*: Such resection can be performed without inducing any sequelae, and may even result in an improvement in comparison to the preoperative status, especially using a manual pointing task with no visual feedback, in which subjects aimed at 48 targets spaced regularly around two starting positions (Desmurget, Bonnetblanc, & Duffau, 2007; Sallard, Duffau, & Bonnetblanc, 2012).

- Interestingly, some white matter pathways can be resected with no permanent functional deficit. For instance, the anterior part of the left inferior longitudinal fascicle and the left uncinate fascicle are such areas because they can be compensated for by the "direct ventral semantic pathways" subserved by the inferior fronto-occipital fascicle (as noted earlier; Duffau, Thiebaut de Schotten, & Mandonnet, 2008). The corpus callosum may also be removed with no morbidity (Duffau, Khalil, Gatignol, Denvil, & Capelle, 2004). However, as previously mentioned, in spite of these rare exceptions, the subcortical connectivity should be preserved in the vast majority of cases.

Postoperative Plasticity Evidenced by Serial Mapping: Toward a Multistage Surgical Approach

Beyond preoperative and intraoperative reshaping of brain networks, postoperative plasticity also accounts for the resectability of areas that, for a long time, were deemed "inoperable." Again, these areas should be considered as nodes within a wide network. After their removal, the whole functional network will self-reorganize by dynamical and biological plasticity, and the function will ultimately be preserved. Indeed, the positive clinical status 3 months after surgery, as evidenced by extensive neuropsychological testing, as well as the return to a normal life (including the return to work), argue for efficient plasticity mechanisms for these areas (Moritz-Gasser, Herbet, Maldonado, & Duffau, 2012; Teixidor, Gatignol, Leroy, Masuet-Aumatell, Capelle, & Duffau, 2007). Of note, early and intensive postoperative functional rehabilitation plays a major role in optimizing the neurological and cognitive recovery (Gehring et al., 2009). Such mechanisms induced by surgical resection within eloquent areas were also studied by performing postoperative functional neuroimaging once the patient had recovered preoperative functional status. In particular, several patients were examined following the resection of gliomas involving the supplementary motor area, which elicited a transient postsurgical syndrome with akinesia eventually associated with mutism in the left dominant hemisphere. In comparison to the preoperative imaging, functional MRI showed activations of the supplementary motor area and premotor cortex contralateral to the lesion, demonstrating that the contrahemispheric homologous areas participated in the postsurgical functional compensation (Krainik et al., 2004).

Sometimes, in order to achieve such favorable functional results, an incomplete resection of the glioma is required (e.g., when the tumor-invaded areas are still crucial for function). A new concept recently proposed is to more systematically use postoperative functional neuroimaging when the patient has totally recovered, since neuroimaging can be easily repeated due to its non-invasive feature. This allows for comparison between the pre-surgery and new maps. Although this method has some methodological limitations, subtraction between a pre- and postoperative acquisition may nonetheless show possible additional functional reshaping, due to (1) the resection itself, (2) the postsurgical rehabilitation, and/or (3) the regrowth of the residual DLGG (as before surgery). Such findings have led to the proposition of a new strategy based on a multistage surgical approach (Gil Robles, Gatignol, Lehéricy, & Duffau, 2008). Of note, a better understanding of mechanisms underlying this postsurgical plasticity was made possible thanks to experimentations in animals.

Experimental Observations in Animals

First, the possibility that functional recovery is modulated by kinetic factors has been addressed in a series of animal studies. The main idea behind these studies was to mimic the development of slow-growing lesions by performing successive partial surgical ablations within a cerebral structure. These partial excisions were then compared to acute resections. In most experiments a control group was included in which several surgeries were performed, but no cerebral tissue was removed ("sham" operation). Beyond some marginal disparities, the take-home message of all these studies is quite clear: the negative functional impact of large cerebral lesions is much smaller in progressive than acute lesions. For instance, in rats, it was shown that major deficits were still present 36 days after an acute ablation of the entire somatosensory cortex. These deficits were absent when the same area was removed in two stages. In this case, the experimental rats could not be differentiated from a non-operated control group (Finger, Marshak, Cohen, Scheff, Trace, & Niemand, 1971). Another similar, even more spectacular, report was provided by Adametz in cats (1959). The animals were submitted to progressive (up to 8 surgeries) or acute resection of the midbrain reticular formation. In the latter case, the cats fell into deep coma and died within a few days after the surgery. In the former case, by contrast, complete recovery occurred. Moreover, the same type of dissociation was observed in monkeys. Acute ablations of the prefrontal cortex were found to induce functional deficits that were much more severe than those produced by serial lesions (Rosen, Stein, & Butters, 1971).

Probably the most convincing demonstration that functional recovery is directly influenced by the time course of the lesion (acute versus slow-growing) inflicted to the brain has been provided by Patrissi and Stein (1975). These authors trained a group of rats to retrieve water alternatively located in the right or the left branch of a conventional T-maze. Following a period of training, the rats were divided in several subgroups: (1) one-stage bilateral resection of the frontal cortex; (2) two-stage bilateral resection of the frontal cortex (one hemisphere per operation); (3) one- or two-stage sham operations (control group). For the two-stage groups, three interlesion intervals were considered: 10, 20, or 30 days. The rats given sequential (two-stage) frontal lesions with either a 20- or 30-day interoperative interval could not be differentiated from the sham-operated controls. Animals with two-stage lesions produced 10 days apart exhibited substantial deficits when contrasted with the sham-operated, the 20-day, or the 30-day two-stage groups. However, the two-stage 10-day animals performed significantly better than the one-stage rats. Similar results were found in other studies involving resections of the frontal cortex (Glick & Zimmerberg, 1972) and the superior temporal gyri (Stewart & Ades, 1951). In all of these studies, the animals were reported to exhibit complete recovery when the different surgeries were spaced by a sufficient interval. This interval varied from study to study but it was never less than 6 days. Whatever the interlesion interval, the level of recovery was always better for the multistage surgeries than for the one-stage operations.

Of course, the positive effect of sequential lesions on functional recovery depends strongly on the amount of tissue resected at each surgical stage. This was clearly shown by Stein and colleagues in a monkey study involving the resection of the sulcus principalis. In this study, the total amount of tissue resected was kept constant. It was reported that four partial lesions

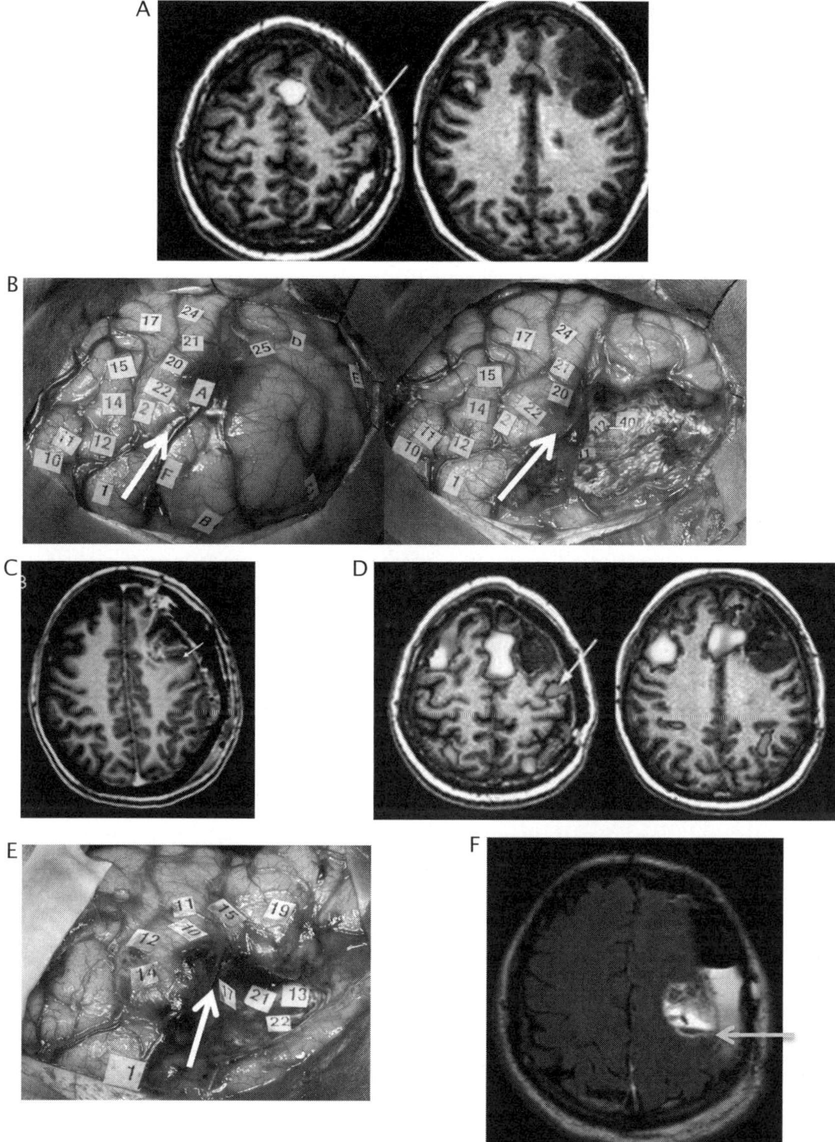

FIGURE 6.3 Illustration of the multiple-stages surgical approach: (A) Preoperative language fMRI in a patient without deficit, haboring a DLGG involving the left premotor area; language activation was very close to the posterior part of the tumor, within the precentral sulcus (white arrow). (B) Intraoperative views before (left) and after (right) resection of the glioma, delineated by letter tags. Direct electrical stimulation shows a reshaping of the eloquent maps, with a recruitment of perilesional language sites, allowing a subtotal resection with nevertheless a posterior residue due to invasion of crucial areas (number tags). The green arrow shows the precentral sulcus, demonstrating that it was not possible to remove the part of the glioma involving the precentral gyrus. (C) Immediate postoperative enhanced T1-weighted MRI showing the residue (arrow), in front of the precentral gyrus. (D) Postoperative language fMRI 4 years after the first fMRI, demonstrating a recruitment of the controlateral hemisphere, and the posterior displacement of activation previously located at the posterior border of the tumor, now within the central sulcus (white arrow). (E) Intraoperative view during the second surgery, confirming the remapping, and allowing a more extensive tumor resection posteriorly, with no permanent deficit. Again, the green arrow shows the precentral sulcus, demonstrating that, this time, it was possible to remove a part of the glioma involving the precentral gyrus. (F) Immediate postoperative axial FLAIR-weighted MRI (3 hours after surgery) showing the improvement of the extent of resection within the left precentral gyrus, thanks to functional reshaping (the blue arrow shows the central sulcus). The follow-up is now 11 years since the first surgery, with no recurrence since the second operation, in a patient enjoying a normal social and professional life. Modified from Gil Robles, Gatignol, Lehéricy, & Duffau (2008).

performed 3 weeks apart produced a greater level of recovery than two partial lesions performed 10 weeks apart (Stein, Butters, & Rosen, 1977). This result pleads directly for the idea that the progressiveness of neural destruction is a key predictor of functional recuperation.

Application to Patients With DLGG

Interestingly, recent studies demonstrated that such remapping was not a theoretical concept, but a concrete reality in humans (Duffau, 2005). Postoperative functional neuroimaging performed some months or years following the surgery for DLGG in patients with a complete recovery clearly showed a new recruitment of perilesional areas and/or remote regions within the ipsilesional hemisphere and/or a recruitment of controlateral structures (Krainik et al., 2004; Sarubbo, Le Bars, Moritz-Gasser, & Duffau, 2012). On the basis of these data, a second surgery was proposed before the occurrence of new symptoms (except possible seizures) in patients who continued to enjoy a normal life, due to a tumor relapse (Gil Robles, Gatignol, Lehéricy, & Duffau, 2008). The second surgery was also conducted using intraoperative cortical and subcortical mapping, in order to validate the mechanisms of brain reshaping, supported by preoperative functional neuroimaging (de Benectis, Moritz-Gasser, & Duffau, 2010; Martino, Taillandier, Moritz-Gasser, Gatignol, & Duffau, 2009; see Figure 6.3). Preliminary results support the efficacy and safety of such multistage resections for DLGG when located in eloquent areas. Indeed, in a recent series, 74% of resections were complete or subtotal (less than 10 ml of residue) following the second operation, despite no additional serious neurological deficit—on the contrary, with an improvement of the neurological status in 16% of cases. Furthermore, seizures were reduced or eliminated in 82% of patients with epilepsy before the second operation. The median time between the two operations was 4.1 years, and all patients were still alive with a median follow-up of 6.6 years, despite an initial incomplete resection. Therefore, these original data demonstrated that, thanks to mechanisms of cerebral plasticity, it is possible to re-operate patients with DLGG involving eloquent areas with minimal morbidity and increase in the extent of resection (Martino, Taillandier, Moritz-Gasser, Gatignol, & Duffau, 2009). This concept of multistage surgical approach was particularly useful for optimizing the extent of resection in traditional "critical" areas (Duffau, 2012) such as the left premotor region (Gil Robles, Gatignol, Lehéricy, & Duffau, 2008), rolandic area (Duffau, 2001), insula (Duffau, Taillandier, Gatignol, & Capelle, 2006), or Wernicke's area (Sarubbo, Le Bars, Moritz-Gasser, & Duffau, 2012; see Figure 6.2). Reoperations with repeated mapping in the patients over time represent a unique opportunity to demonstrate brain plasticity in humans.

In addition, one should consider performing postoperative functional neuroimaging after rehabilitation, particularly when there is significant improvement in cognition and functioning (Duffau, 2008, 2012a), as well as after recovery following a second surgery, in order to open the door to a possible third or even fourth resection several years after the previous operations. Indeed, the likelihood of subsequent surgeries will be increased in cases of good recovery. The goal is both to allow the patient to enjoy a normal life and to increase overall survival. It is also possible to integrate surgeries within a dynamic therapeutic strategy including chemotherapy and radiotherapy, especially when a wide removal is not possible for functional reasons (Duffau, 2009b). To this end, neoadjuvant (before surgery) chemotherapy was recently advocated in DLGG, with the goal of inducing a shrinkage of the tumor before an operation or a re-operation (Duffau, Taillandier, & Capelle, 2006)—but also possibly to facilitate functional brain reshaping (Blonski et al., 2012).

Conclusions and Perspectives

The combination of online intraoperative anatomo-functional correlations (transient virtual lesion) with data provided by tractography (subcortical anatomical information), magnetoencephalography (temporal data), and serial fMRI (perioperative functional data) could enable one to elaborate individual and predictive models of functioning of neurono-synaptic circuits. Such models may lead to a better knowledge of the dynamic potential of spatio-temporal reorganization of the parallel and interacting networks, namely the mechanisms of brain plasticity thought to play a major role in functional compensation following slow-growing lesions such as DLGG and in their surgical resection. In order to evolve toward a multistage surgical approach in practice (i.e., second or third surgery more extensive than the first one in cases of initial incomplete resection within eloquent areas), a dynamic strategy must be envisaged for functional neuroimaging. The goal is to switch from a "static" use of a unique preoperative functional neuroimaging assessment (limited technique with lack of reliability) to longitudinal studies based on the repetition of neuroimaging before and after surgical resection(s), with the goal of analyzing a possible brain reshaping at the individual scale and selecting the candidates for re-operation(s). The next step is to use bio-mathematical models to examine brain functional interaction through effective connectivity in order to attempt to predict the patterns of postsurgical remapping at the individual scale *before surgery* on the basis of the data provided by the preoperative functional neuroimaging. The new graph theory approach may help to move us toward this type of individual prediction (Marrelec et al., 2006, 2008). Nonetheless, it is worth noting that individualized prediction of whether a brain area could be resected or not based on non-invasive preoperative imaging and mathematical model remains a neuroscientific challenge. Once again, this underlines the inescapable importance of the individual intraoperative study with direct electrostimulation mapping in awake patients.

It could be suggested to guide brain plasticity, using notably pharmacologic drugs, functional rehabilitation, or even transcranial magnetic stimulation, to promote functional recovery not only following surgery, but also before surgery (Duffau, 2006; Gehring et al., 2012). One could hypothesize that such preoperative remapping might enable the surgeon to increase the extent of the resection (and possibly to take a margin around the lesion) while avoiding postsurgical worsening, even in the classically so-called "eloquent" areas according to anatomic criteria (Yordanova, Moritz-Gasser, & Duffau, 2011). Furthermore, the use of plasticity could lead to proposed surgery in asymptomatic patients. Indeed, thanks to the current development of neuroimaging, incidental discovery of tumors will progressively increase in the near future. Interestingly, concerning DLGG, it was recently demonstrated that their natural history was the same in the presymptomatic period as in the first symptomatic period (usually seizures; Pallud et al., 2010). Therefore, on the basis of the new neuroscientific concept of a "hodotopic and plastic brain," the next surgical goal could be to evolve toward a "prophylactic functional neurooncology" (Duffau, 2012c).

In conclusion, cognitive neurosciences represent a special means of helping neuro-oncology by opening new avenues to elaborate therapeutic strategies, thus improving both quality of life and median survival (Duffau, 2011). In other words, it is time to switch from a modular to a hodotopical (delocalized) and dynamic view of cerebral processing. Within this framework, brain functioning is implemented by large-scale subnetworks that interact together and possess the ability to compensate for each other after brain lesion (at least to some degree). This in turn allows for surgical resection of tumors in areas classically considered as "inoperable," while preserving neurological and cognitive functions. The next step is to map the neural basis subserving emotional and behavioral processing, and to develop a hodotopic approach to these functions.

References

Adametz, J. (1959). Rate of recovery of functioning in cats with rostral reticular lesions: An experimental study. *J Neurosurg, 16*, 85–97.

Alstott, J., Breakspear, M., Hagmann, P., Cammoun, L., & Sporns, O. (2009). Modeling the impact of lesions in the human brain. *PLoS Comput Biol, 5*, e1000408.

Bartolomei, F., Bosma, I., Klein, M., Baayen, J. C., Reijneveld, J. C., Postma, T. J., et al. (2006). How do brain tumors alter functional connectivity? A magnetoencephalography study. *Ann Neurol, 59*, 128–138.

Basset, D. S., & Bullmore, E. T. (2009). Human brain networks in health and disease. *Curr Opin Neurol, 22*, 340–347.

Bavelier, D., & Neville, H. J. (2002). Cross-modal plasticity: Where and how? *Nat Rev Neurosci, 3*, 443–452.

Bello, L., Gallucci, M., Fava, M., Carrabba, G., Giussani, C., Acerbi, F., et al. (2007). Intraoperative subcortical language tract mapping guides surgical removal of gliomas involving speech areas. *Neurosurgery, 60*, 67–80.

Benzagmout, M., Gatignol, P., & Duffau, H. (2007). Resection of WHO Health Organization Grade II gliomas involving Broca's area: Methodological and functional considerations. *Neurosurgery, 61*, 741–752.

Blonski, M., Taillandier, L., Herbet, G., Maldonado, I. L., Beauchesne, P., Fabbro, M., et al. (2012). Combination of neoadjuvant chemotherapy followed by surgical resection as new strategy for WHO grade II gliomas: A study of cognitive status and quality of life. *J Neuro-oncol, 106*, 353–366.

Bosma, I., Douw, L., Bartolomei, F., Heimans, J. J., van Dijk, B. W., Postma, T. J., et al. (2008). Synchronized brain activity and neurocognitive function in patients with low-grade glioma: A magnetoencephalography study. *Neuro-oncology, 10*, 734–744.

Catani, M. (2007). From hodology to function. *Brain, 130*, 602–605.

Catani, M., Jones, D. K., & ffytche, D. H. (2005). Perisylvian language networks of the human brain. *Ann Neurol, 57*, 8–16.

Coello, A. F., Duvaux, S., de Benedictis, A., Matsuda, A., & Duffau, H. (2013). Involvement of the right inferior longitudinal fascicle in visual hemiagnosia: A brain stimulation mapping study. *J Neurosurg, 118*, 202–205.

Dancause, N., Barbay, S., Frost, S. B., Plautz, E. J., Chen, D., Zoubina, E. V., et al. (2005). Extensive cortical rewiring after brain injury. *J Neurosci, 25*, 10167–10179.

de Benedictis, A., & Duffau, H. (2011). Brain hodotopy: From esoteric concept to practical surgical applications. *Neurosurgery, 68*, 1709–1723.

de Benedictis, A., Moritz-Gasser, S., & Duffau, H. (2010). Awake mapping optimizes the extent of resection for low-grade gliomas in eloquent areas. *Neurosurgery, 66*, 1074–1084.

Desmurget, M., Bonnetblanc, F., & Duffau, H. (2007). Contrasting acute and slow growing lesions: A new door to brain plasticity. *Brain, 130*, 898–914.

De Witt Hamer, P., Moritz-Gasser, S., Gatignol, P., & Duffau, H. (2011). Is the human left middle longitudinal fascicle essential for language? A brain electrostimulation study. *Hum Brain Mapp, 32*, 962–973.

Douw, L., Baayen, J. C., Bosma, I., Klein, M., Vandertop, W. P., Heimans, J. J., et al. (2008). Treatment-related changes in functional connectivity in brain tumor patients: A magnetoencephalography study. *Exp Neurol, 212*, 285–290.

Duffau, H. (2001). Acute functional reorganisation of the human motor cortex during resection of central lesions: A study using intraoperative brain mapping. *J Neurol Neurosur Ps, 70*, 506–513.

Duffau, H. (2001a). Recovery from complete hemiplegia following resection of a retrocentral metastasis: The prognostic value of intraoperative cortical stimulation. *J Neurosurg, 95*, 1050–1052.

Duffau, H. (2005). Lessons from brain mapping in surgery for low-grade glioma: Insights into associations between tumour and brain plasticity. *Lancet Neurol, 4*, 476–486.

Duffau, H. (2006). Brain plasticity: From pathophysiological mechanisms to therapeutic applications. *J Clin Neurosci, 13*, 885–897.

Duffau, H. (2006a). New concepts in surgery of WHO grade II gliomas: Functional brain mapping, connectionism and plasticity. *J Neuro-oncol, 79*, 77–115.

Duffau, H. (2006b). Intraoperative cortico-subcortical stimulations in surgery of low-grade gliomas. *Expert Rev Neurother, 5*, 473–485.

Duffau, H. (2007). Contribution of cortical and subcortical electrostimulation in brain glioma surgery: Methodological and functional considerations. *Neurophysiol Clin, 37*, 373–382.

Duffau, H. (2008). Brain plasticity and tumors. *Adv Tech Stand Neurosurg, 3*, 3–33.

Duffau, H. (2008a). The anatomo-functional connectivity of language revisited: New insights provided by electrostimulation and tractography. *Neuropsychologia, 4*, 927–934.

Duffau, H. (2009). Does post-lesional subcortical plasticity exist in the human brain? *Neurosci Res, 65*, 131–135.

Duffau, H. (2009a). A personal consecutive series of surgically treated 51 cases of insular WHO Grade II glioma: Advances and limitations. *J Neurosurg, 110*, 696–708.

Duffau, H. (2009b). Surgery of low-grade gliomas: Towards a "functional neurooncology." *Current Opinion in Oncology, 21*, 543–549.

Duffau, H. (2010). Awake surgery for nonlanguage mapping. *Neurosurgery, 66*, 523–528.

Duffau, H. (Ed.) (2011). *Brain mapping: From neural basis of cognition to surgical applications.* New York: Springer.

Duffau, H. (2012). A new concept of diffuse (low-grade) glioma surgery. *Adv Tech Stand Neurosurg, 38*, 3–27.

Duffau, H. (2012a). The challenge to remove diffuse low-grade gliomas while preserving brain functions. *Acta Neurochir (Wien), 154*, 569–574.

Duffau, H. (2012b). The "frontal syndrome" revisited: Lessons from electrostimulation mapping studies. *Cortex, 48*, 120–131.

Duffau, H. (2012c). Awake surgery for incidental WHO grade II gliomas involving eloquent areas. *Acta Neurochir (Wien), 154*, 575–584.

Duffau, H. (2013). Cognitive assessment in glioma patients. *J Neurosurg, 119*, 1348–1349.

Duffau, H., Bauchet, L., Lehéricy, S., & Capelle, L. (2001). Functional compensation of the left dominant insula for language. *Neuroreport, 12*, 2159–2163.

Duffau, H., & Capelle, L. (2001). Functional recovery following lesions of the primary somatosensory fields: Study of the compensatory mechanisms. *Neurochir, 47*, 557–563.

Duffau, H., & Capelle, L. (2004). Preferential brain locations of low-grade gliomas. *Cancer, 100*, 2622–2626.

Duffau, H., Capelle, L., Denvil, D., Sichez, N., Gatignol, P., Lopes, M., et al. (2003). Functional recovery after surgical resection of low grade gliomas in eloquent brain: Hypothesis of brain compensation. *J Neurol Neurosur Ps, 74*, 901–907.

Duffau, H., Capelle, L., Denvil, D., Gatignol, P., Sichez, N., Lopes, M., et al. (2003a). The role of dominant premotor cortex in language: A study using intraoperative functional mapping in awake patients. *NeuroImage, 20*, 1903–1914.

Duffau, H., Capelle, L., Denvil, D., Sichez, N., Gatignol, P., Taillandier, L., et al. (2003b). Usefulness of intraoperative electrical subcortical mapping during surgery for low-grade gliomas located within eloquent brain regions: Functional results in a consecutive series of 103 patients. *J Neurosurg, 98*, 764–778.

Duffau, H., Capelle, L., Sichez, N., Denvil, D., Bitar, A., Sichez, J. P., et al. (2002). Intraoperative mapping of the subcortical language pathways using direct stimulations: An anatomo-functional study. *Brain, 125,* 199–214.

Duffau, H., Denvil, D., & Capelle, L. (2002). Absence of movement disorders after surgical resection of glioma invading the right striatum. *J Neurosurg, 97,* 363–369.

Duffau, H., Denvil, D., & Capelle, L. (2002). Long term reshaping of language, sensory and motor maps following glioma resection: A new parameter to integrate in the surgical strategy. *J Neurol Neurosur Ps, 72,* 511–516.

Duffau, H., Denvil, D., Lopes, M., Gasparini, F., Cohen, L., Capelle, L., et al. (2002). Intraoperative mapping of the cortical areas involved in multiplication and subtraction: An electrostimulation study in a patient with a left parietal glioma. *J Neurol Neurosur Ps, 73,* 733–738.

Duffau, H., Gatignol, P., Denvil, D., Lopes, M., & Capelle, L. (2003). The articulatory loop: Study of the subcortical connectivity by electrostimulation. *Neuroreport, 14,* 2005–2008.

Duffau, H., Gatignol, P., Mandonnet, E., Capelle, L., & Taillandier, L. (2008). Intraoperative subcortical stimulation mapping of language pathways in a consecutive series of 115 patients with Grade II glioma in the left dominant hemisphere. *J Neurosurg, 109,* 461–471.

Duffau, H., Gatignol, P., Mandonnet, E., Peruzzi, P., Tzourio-Mazoyer, N., & Capelle, L. (2005). New insights into the anatomo-functional connectivity of the semantic system: A study using cortico-subcortical stimulations. *Brain, 128,* 797–810.

Duffau, H., Gatignol, P., Moritz-Gasser, S., & Mandonnet, E. (2009). Is the left uncinate fasciculus essential for language? A cerebral stimulation study. *J Neurol, 256,* 382–389.

Duffau, H., Karachi, C., Gatignol, P., & Capelle, L. (2003). Transient Foix-Chavany-Marie syndrome after surgical resection of a right insulo-opercular low-grade glioma. *Neurosurgery, 53,* 426–431.

Duffau, H., Khalil, I., Gatignol, P., Denvil, D., & Capelle, L. (2004). Surgical removal of corpus callosum infiltrated by low-grade glioma: Functional outcome and oncological considerations. *J Neurosurg, 100,* 431–437.

Duffau, H., Lopes, M., Arthuis, F., Bitar, A., Sichez, J. P., van Effenterre, R., et al. (2005). Contribution of intraoperative electrical stimulations in surgery of low grade gliomas: A comparative study between two series without (1985–96) and with (1996–2003) functional mapping in the same institution. *J Neurol Neurosur Ps, 76,* 845–851.

Duffau, H., Lopes, M., Denvil, D., & Capelle, L. (2001). Delayed onset of the supplementary motor area syndrome after surgical resection of the mesial frontal lobe: A time course study using intraoperative mapping in an awake patient. *Stereot Funct Neuros, 76,* 74–82.

Duffau, H., Leroy, M., & Gatignol, P. (2008). Cortico-subcortical organization of language networks in the right hemisphere: an electrostimulation study in left-handers. *Neuropsychologia, 46,* 3197–3209.

Duffau, H., Mandonnet, E., Gatignol, P., & Capelle, L. (2007). Functional compensation of the claustrum: lessons from low-grade glioma surgery. *J Neuro-oncol, 81,* 327–329.

Duffau, H., Moritz-Gasser, S., & Gatignol, P. (2009). Functional outcome after language mapping for insular World Health Organization Grade II gliomas in the dominant hemisphere: Experience with 24 patients. *Neurosurg Focus, 27,* E7.

Duffau, H., Moritz-Gasser, S., & Mandonnet, E. (2014). A re-examination of neural basis of language processing: Proposal of a dynamic hodotopical model from data provided by brain stimulation mapping during picture naming. *Brain Lang, 131,* 1–10.

Duffau, H., Sichez, J. P., & Lehéricy, S. (2000). Intraoperative unmasking of brain redundant motor sites during resection of a precentral angioma: Evidence using direct cortical stimulations. *Ann Neurol, 47,* 132–135.

Duffau, H., Taillandier, L., & Capelle, L. (2006). Radical surgery after chemotherapy: A new therapeutic strategy to envision in grade II glioma. *J Neuro-oncol, 80,* 171–176.

Duffau, H., Taillandier, L., Gatignol, P., & Capelle, L. (2006). The insular lobe and brain plasticity: lessons from tumor surgery. *Clin Neurol Neurosurg, 108,* 543–548.

Duffau, H., Thiebaut de Schotten, M., & Mandonnet, E. (2008). White matter functional connectivity as an additional landmark for dominant temporal lobectomy. *J Neurol Neurosur Ps, 79,* 492–495.

Duffau, H., Velut, S., Mitchell, M. C., Gatignol, P., & Capelle, L. (2004). Intra-operative mapping of the subcortical visual pathways using direct electrical stimulations. *Acta Neurochir (Wien), 146,* 265–269.

Finger, S., Marshak, R. A., Cohen, M., Scheff, S., Trace, R., & Niemand, D. (1971). Effects of successive and simultaneous lesions of somatosensory cortex on tactile discrimination in the rat. *J Comp Physiol Psychol*, *77*, 221–227.

Gaillard, R., Naccache, L., Pinel, P., Clémenceau, S., Volle, E., Hasboun, D., et al. (2006). Direct intracranial, fMRI, and lesion evidence for the causal role of left inferotemporal cortex in reading. *Neuron*, *50*, 191–204.

Gatignol, P., Capelle, L., Le Bihan, R., & Duffau, H. (2004). Double dissociation between picture naming and comprehension: An electrostimulation study. *Neuroreport*, *15*, 191–195.

Gehring, K., Patwardhan, S. Y., Collins, R., Groves, M. D., Etzel, C. J., Meyers, C. A., et al. (2012). A randomized trial on the efficacy of methylphenidate and modafinil for improving cognitive functioning and symptoms in patients with a primary brain tumor. *J Neuro-oncol*, *107*, 165–174.

Gehring, K., Sitskoorn, M. M., Gundy, C. M., Sikkes, S. A., Klein, M., Postma, T. J., et al. (2009). Cognitive rehabilitation in patients with gliomas: A randomized, controlled trial. *J Clin Oncol*, *27*, 3712–3722.

Geschwind, N. (1970). The organization of language and the brain. *Science*, *170*, 940–944.

Gil Robles, S., & Duffau, H. (2010). Surgical management of World Health Organization Grade II gliomas in eloquent areas: The necessity of preserving a margin around functional structures. *Neurosurg Focus*, *28*, E8.

Gil Robles, S., Gatignol, P., Capelle, L., Mitchell, M. C., & Duffau H. (2005). The role of dominant striatum in language: A study using intraoperative electrical stimulations. *J Neurol Neurosur Ps*, *76*, 940–946.

Gil Robles, S., Gatignol, P., Lehéricy, S., & Duffau, H. (2008). Long-term brain plasticity allowing multiple-stages surgical approach for WHO grade II gliomas in eloquent areas: a combined study using longitudinal functional MRI and intraoperative electrical stimulation. *J Neurosurg*, *109*, 615–624.

Glick, S. D., & Zimmerberg, B. (1972). Comparative recovery following simultaneous- and successive-stage frontal brain damage in mice. *J Comp Physiol Psychol*, *79*, 481–487.

Gras-Combes, G., Moritz-Gasser, S., Herbet, G., & Duffau, H. (2012). Intraoperative subcortical electrical mapping of optic radiations in awake surgery for glioma involving visual pathways. *J Neurosurg*, *117*, 466–473.

Guleria, S., Gupta, R. K., Saksena, S., Chandra, A., Srivastava, R. N., Husain, M., et al. (2008). Retrograde Wallerian degeneration of cranial corticospinal tracts in cervical spinal cord injury patients using diffusion tensor imaging. *J Neurosci Res*, *86*, 2271–2280.

Hickok, G., & Poeppel, D. (2007). The cortical organization of speech processing. *Nat Rev Neurosci*, *8*, 393–402.

Holland, R., & Lambon-Ralph, M. A. (2010). The anterior temporal lobe semantic hub is a part of the language neural network: Selective disruption of irregular past tense verb by rTMS. *Cereb Cortex*, *20*, 2771–2775.

Honey, C. J., Kötter, R., Breakspear, M., & Sporns, O. (2007). Network structure of cerebral cortex shapes functional connectivity on multiple time scales. *P Natl Acad Sci USA*, *104*, 10240–10245.

Ius, T., Angelini, E., Thiebaut de Schotten, M., Mandonnet, E., & Duffau, H. (2011). Evidence for potentials and limitations of brain plasticity using an atlas of functional resectability of WHO grade II gliomas: Towards a "minimal common brain." *NeuroImage*, *56*, 992–1000.

Keidel, J. L., Welbourne, S. R., & Lambon Ralph, M. A. (2010). Solving the paradox of the equipotential and modular brain: A neurocomputational model of stroke vs. slow-growing glioma. *Neuropsychologia*, *48*, 1716–1724.

Klein, M., Duffau, H., & De Witt Hamer, P. C. (2012). Cognition and resective surgery for diffuse infiltrative glioma: An overview. *J Neuro-oncol*, *108*, 309–318.

Krainik, A., Duffau, H., Capelle, L., Cornu, P., Boch, A. L., Mangin, J. F., et al. (2004). Role of the healthy hemisphere in recovery after resection of the supplementary motor area. *Neurology*, *62*, 1323–1332.

Krainik, A., Lehéricy, S., Duffau, H., Capelle, L., Chainay, H., Cornu, P., et al. (2003). Postoperative speech disorder after medial frontal surgery: Role of the supplementary motor area. *Neurology*, *60*, 587–594.

Krainik, A., Lehéricy, S., Duffau, H., Vlaicu, M., Poupon, F., Capelle, L., et al. (2001). Role of the supplementary motor area in motor deficit following medial frontal lobe surgery. *Neurology*, *57*, 871–878.

Lafargue, G., & Duffau, H. (2008). Awareness of intending to act following parietal cortex resection. *Neuropsychologia*, *46*, 2662–2667.

LeRoux, P. D., Berger, M. S., Haglund, M. M., Pilcher, W. H., & Ojemann, G. A. (1991). Resection of intrinsic tumors from nondominant face motor cortex using stimulation mapping: Report of two cases. *Surgical Neurology*, *36*, 44–48.

Louis, D. N., Ohgaki, H., Wiestler, O. D., & Cavenee, W. K. (Eds.) (2007). *WHO classification of tumours of the central nervous system*. Lyon: IARC.

Lubrano, V., Draper, L., & Roux, F. E. (2010). What makes surgical tumor resection feasible in Broca's area? Insights into intraoperative brain mapping. *Neurosurgery*, *66*, 868–875.

Makris, N., Kennedy, D. N., McInerney, S., Sorensen, A. G., Wang, R., Caviness, V. S., Jr., et al. (2005). Segmentation of subcomponents within the superior longitudinal fascicle in humans: A quantitative, in vivo, DT-MRI study. *Cereb Cortex, 15,* 854–869.

Maldonado, I. L., Moritz-Gasser, S., de Champfleur, N. M., Bertram, L., Moulinié, G., & Duffau, H. (2011). Surgery for gliomas involving the left inferior parietal lobule: New insights into the functional anatomy provided by stimulation mapping in awake patients. *J Neurosurg, 115,* 770–779.

Maldonado, I. L., Moritz-Gasser, S., & Duffau, H. (2011). Does the left superior longitudinal fascicle subserve language semantics? A brain electrostimulation study. *Brain Struct Funct, 216,* 263–264.

Mandonnet, E., Capelle, L., & Duffau, H. (2006). Extension of paralimbic low grade gliomas: Toward an anatomical classification based on white matter invasion patterns. *J Neuro-oncol, 78,* 179–185.

Mandonnet, E., Gatignol, P., & Duffau, H. (2009). Evidence for an occipito-temporal tract underlying visual recognition in picture naming. *Clin Neurol Neurosurg, 111,* 601–605.

Mandonnet, E., Jbabdi, S., Taillandier, L., Galanaud, D., Benali, H., Capelle, L., et al. (2007). Preoperative estimation of residual volume for WHO grade II glioma resected with intraoperative functional mapping. *Neuro Oncology, 9,* 63–69.

Mandonnet, E., Nouet, A., Gatignol, P., Capelle, L., & Duffau, H. (2007). Does the left inferior longitudinal fasciculus play a role in language? A brain stimulation study. *Brain, 130,* 623–629.

Mandonnet, E., Winkler, P., & Duffau, H. (2010). Direct electrical stimulation as an input gate into brain functional networks: Principles, adavantages and limitations. *Acta Neurochir (Wien), 152,* 185–193.

Marrelec, G., Bellec, P., Krainik, A., Duffau, H., Pélégrini-Issac, M., Lehéricy, S., et al. (2008). Regions, systems and the brain: Hierarchical measures of functional integration in fMRI. *Med Image Anal, 12,* 484–496.

Marrelec, G., Krainik, A., Duffau, H., Pélégrini-Issac, M., Lehéricy, S., Doyon, J., et al. (2006). Partial correlation for functional brain interactivity investigation in functional MRI. *NeuroImage, 32,* 228–237.

Martino, J., Brogna, C., Gil Robles, S., Vergani, F., & Duffau, H. (2010). Anatomic dissection of the inferior fronto-occipital fasciculus revisited in the lights of brain stimulation data. *Cortex, 46,* 691–699.

Martino, J., De Witt Hamer, P. C., Berger, M. S., Lawton, M. T., Arnold, C. M., de Lucas, E. M., et al. (2013). Analysis of the subcomponents and cortical terminations of the perisylvian superior longitudinal fasciculus: A fiber dissection and DTI tractography study. *Brain Struct Funct, 218,* 105–121.

Martino, J., Taillandier, L., Moritz-Gasser, S., Gatignol, P., & Duffau, H. (2009). Re-operation is a safe and effective therapeutic strategy in recurrent WHO grade II gliomas within eloquent areas. *Acta Neurochir (Wien), 151,* 427–436.

Meunier, S., Duffau, H., Garnero, L., Capelle, L., & Ducorps, A. (2000). Comparison of the somatosensory cortical mapping of the fingers using a whole head magnetoencephalography (MEG) and direct electrical stimulations during surgery in awake patients. *NeuroImage, 11,* 5(S868).

Milea, D., Lobel, E., Lehéricy, S., Duffau, H., Rivaud-Péchoux, S., Berthoz, A., et al. (2002). Intraoperative frontal eye field stimulation elicits ocular deviation and saccade suppression. *Neuroreport, 13,* 1359–1364.

Moritz-Gasser, S., & Duffau, H. (2009). Evidence of a large-scale network underlying language switching: A brain stimulation study. *J Neurosurg, 111,* 729–732.

Moritz-Gasser, S., Herbet, G., Maldonado, I. L., & Duffau, H. (2012). Lexical access speed is significantly correlated with the return to professional activities after awake surgery for low-grade gliomas. *J Neuro-oncol, 107,* 633–641.

Ojemann, G., Ojemann, J., Lettich, E., & Berger, M. (1989). Cortical language localization in left, dominant hemisphere: An electrical stimulation mapping investigation in 117 patients. *J Neurosurg, 71,* 316–326.

Pallud, J., Fontaine, D., Duffau, H., Mandonnet, E., Sanai, N., Taillandier, L., et al. (2010). Natural history of incidental WHO grade II gliomas. *Ann Neurol, 68,* 727–733.

Papagno, C., Miracapillo, C., Casarotti, A., Romero Lauro, L. J., Castellano, A., Falini, A., et al. (2011). What is the role of the uncinate fasciculus? Surgical removal and proper name retrieval. *Brain, 134,* 405–414.

Parisot, S., Duffau, H., Chemouny, S., Paragios, N. (2011). Graph based spatial position mapping of low-grade gliomas. *MICCAI, 14,* 508–515.

Patrissi, G., & Stein, D.G. (1975). Temporal factors in recovery of function after brain damage. *Exp Neurol, 47,* 470–480.

Plaza, M., Gatignol, P., Cohen, H., Berger, B., & Duffau, H. (2008). A discrete area within the left dorsolateral prefrontal cortex involved in visual-verbal incongruence judgment. *Cereb Cortex, 18,* 1253–1259.

Plaza, M., Gatignol, P., Leroy, M., & Duffau, H. (2009). Speaking without Broca's area after tumor resection. *Neurocase, 9*, 1–17.

Rosen, J., Stein, D., & Butters, N. (1971). Recovery of function after serial ablation of prefrontal cortex in the rhesus monkey. *Science, 173*, 353–356.

Rossini, P. M., Calautti, C., Pauri, F., & Baron, J. C. (2003). Post-stroke plastic reorganisation in the adult brain. *Lancet Neurol, 2*, 493–502.

Sahin, N. T., Pinker, S., Cash, S. S., Schomer, D., & Halgren, E. (2009). Sequential processing of lexical, grammatical, and phonological information within Broca's area. *Science, 326*, 445–449.

Sallard, E., Barral, J., Duffau, H., & Bonnetblanc, F. (2012). Manual reaction times and brain dynamics after "awake surgery" of slow-growing tumours invading the parietal area. *Brain Injury, 26*, 1750–1755.

Sallard, E., Duffau, H., & Bonnetblanc, F. (2012). Ultra-fast recovery from right neglect after "awake surgery" for slow-growing tumor invading the left parietal area. *Neurocase, 18*, 80–90.

Sanai, N., Mirzadeh, Z., & Berger, M. S. (2008). Functional outcome after language mapping for glioma resection. *New Engl J Med, 358*, 18–27.

Sanes, J. N., Donoghue, J. P., Thangaraj, V., Edelman, R. R., & Warach, S. (1995). Shared neural substrates controlling hand movements in human motor cortex. *Science, 268*, 1775–1777.

Sarubbo, S., De Benedictis, A., Maldonado, I. L., Basso, G., & Duffau, H. (2013). Frontal terminations for the inferior fronto-occipital fascicle: anatomical dissection, DTI study and functional considerations on a multi-component bundle. *Brain Struct Funct, 218*, 21–37.

Sarubbo, S., Le Bars, E., Moritz-Gasser, S., & Duffau, H. (2012). Complete recovery after surgical resection of left Wernicke's area in awake patient: A brain stimulation and functional MRI study. *Neurosurg Rev, 35*, 287–292.

Schucht, P., Moritz-Gasser, S., Herbet, G., Raabe, A., & Duffau, H. (2013). Subcortical electrostimulation to identify network subserving motor control. *Hum Brain Mapp, 34*, 3023–3030.

Spena, G., Gatignol, P., Capelle, L., & Duffau, H. (2006). Superior longitudinal fasciculus subserves vestibular network in humans. *Neuroreport, 17*, 1403–1406.

Sporns, O., Tononi, G., & Kötter, R. (2005). The human connectome: a structural description of the human brain. *PLoS Comput Biol, 1*, e42.

Stam, C. J. (2010). Characterization of anatomical and functional connectivity in the brain: a complex networks perspective. *Int J Psychophysiol, 77*, 186–194.

Stein, D. G., Butters, N., & Rosen, J. (1977). A comparison of two- and four-stage ablations of sulcus principals on recovery of spatial performance in the rhesus monkey. *Neuropsychologia, 15*, 179–182.

Stewart, J. W., & Ades, H. (1951). The time factor in reintegration of a learned habit lost after temporal lobe lesions in the monkey (Macaca mulatta). *J Comp Physiol Psychol, 44*, 479–486.

Teixidor, P., Gatignol, P., Leroy, M., Masuet-Aumatell, C., Capelle, L., & Duffau, H. (2007). Assessment of verbal working memory before and after surgery for low-grade glioma. *J Neuro-oncology, 81*, 305–313.

Thiebaut de Schotten, M., Urbanski, M., Duffau, H., Volle, E., Levy, R., Dubois, B., et al. (2005). Direct evidence for a parietal-frontal pathway subserving spatial awareness in humans. *Science, 309*, 2226–2228.

Varela, F., Lachaux, J. P., Rodriguez, E., & Martinerie, J. (2001). The brainweb: Phase synchronization and large-scale integration. *Nat Rev Neurosci, 2*, 229–239.

Varona, J. F., Bermejo, F., Guerra, J. M., & Molina, J. A. (2004). Long-term prognosis of ischemic stroke in young adults: Study of 272 cases. *J Neurol, 251*, 1507–1514.

Vassal, M., Le Bars, E., Moritz-Gasser, S., Menjot, N., & Duffau, H. (2010). Crossed aphasia elicited by intraoperative cortical and subcortical stimulation in awake patients. *J Neurosurg, 113*, 1251–1258.

Vidorreta, J. G., Garcia, R., Moritz-Gasser, S., & Duffau, H. (2011). Double dissociation between syntactic gender and picture naming processing: A brain stimulation mapping study. *Hum Brain Mapp, 32*, 331–340.

Vigneau, M., Beaucousin, V., Herve, P. Y., Duffau, H., Crivello, F., Houdé, O., et al. (2006). Meta-analyzing left hemisphere language areas: Phonology, semantics, and sentence processing. *NeuroImage, 30*, 1414–1432.

Werner, G. (2007). Brain dynamics across levels of organization. *J Physiol Paris, 101*, 273–279.

Yordanova, Y., Moritz-Gasser, S., & Duffau, H. (2011). Awake surgery for WHO grade II gliomas within "noneloquent" areas in the left dominant hemisphere: Toward a "supratotal" resection. *J Neurosurg, 115*, 232–239.

7

Connectivity Modeling and Neuroplasticity After Traumatic Brain Injury

Umesh M. Venkatesan, Sarah M. Rajtmajer, and Frank G. Hillary

Introduction

In the United States, traumatic brain injury (TBI) is one of the most common neurological disorders in young adults, occurring at a rate of approximately 1.7 million people annually, and severe TBI contributes to roughly one-third of the injury-related deaths in the United States (Faul, Xu, Wald, & Coronado, 2010). While there has been incredible progress in understanding the acute metabolic consequences after TBI (for review, see Hillered, Vespa, & Hovda, 2005), there has been far less work examining the whole-brain or "system-level" plastic changes associated with moderate and severe TBI. The terms "plasticity" or "neuroplasticity" often refer to the dynamic nature of neural processes on both micro- and macro-scales. For the purposes of this chapter, "neuroplasticity" will refer to system-level changes (large-scale, or whole brain network changes), including transient changes during new learning as well as more adaptive and permanent alterations secondary to injury.

Functional imaging methods provide unparalleled opportunity to examine the expression of neuroplasticity at the macro level through non-invasive methods and may eventually provide a means for tracking the success of rehabilitation interventions. There has been a dramatic increase in the use of functional neuroimaging techniques such as blood oxygen level dependent functional magnetic resonance imaging (BOLD fMRI) to examine cognitive, sensory, and motor dysfunction in neurologically impaired populations. To date, however, the integration of functional imaging into the assessment and treatment of neurotrauma has been slow, and we anticipate that the integration of novel methods focusing on connectivity modeling may help to bridge the gap between cognitive neurosciences and neurorehabilitation. Accordingly, the goal of this chapter is to examine the current understanding of brain changes associated with brain injury recovery from a systems neuroscience perspective.

For our purposes, "systems neuroscience" refers to the examination of macro-scale neural responses after injury, measured via functional brain imaging methods such as BOLD fMRI, magnetoencephalography (MEG), electroencephalography (EEG), positron emission tomography (PET) and others. This literature differs from comparative work focusing on cellular/synaptic mechanisms of brain change after injury by focusing instead on large-scale groups of neurons and their distributed communication. We aim to focus our summary on how entire neural systems are adapting to brain injury and how these changes may inform clinical interventions. To do so, in the first section, this chapter discusses the results of traditional functional imaging studies examining the mean signal change during task perturbation. We review current interpretations of the literature and barriers to progress in understanding plasticity in recovery after TBI. We anticipate that integrating connectivity modeling into these approaches with specific emphasis on within-subject change will provide new avenues in the study of TBI recovery. In the second section of this chapter, we offer a non-technical summary of several of the most prominent connectivity approaches in the neurosciences, including (1) effective connectivity modeling, (2) "resting-state" connectivity, and (3) graph theoretical approaches. In the final section, we offer a review of the research to date using these methods to examine whole-brain and region-of-interest changes in brain connectivity after TBI.

Understanding the Meaning of Brain Plasticity in Functional Imaging

One critical discussion point in this chapter has to do with how we interpret functional imaging data that reveal basic brain changes after TBI. We make the argument that in order to understand plasticity in dynamic neural systems, our methods should include connectivity analyses (broadly defined). Again, we use the term "plasticity" here to refer to any observable change in network connectivity, and these changes can take many forms, including transient alterations that operate to facilitate performance (e.g., neural compensation) and those that are deemed to be more long-standing and less responsive to moment-to-moment demands (e.g., brain reorganization) (for a review, see Hillary, Genova, Chiaravalloti, Rypma, & DeLuca, 2006; Hillary, 2008).

To illustrate this point, we will focus for the moment on the functional MRI literature examining working memory (WM) dysfunction after TBI. In early fMRI work examining neurological disorders, the most frequently studied cognitive domains have been attention, speed of information processing, and WM, which is the ability to maintain information in the mind for brief windows of time (i.e., seconds) for their manipulation and use (see Baddeley, 1996). From this literature examining mean signal change (i.e., aggregating "task" vs. "rest" periods), it was a primary finding that neural systems often recruit additional brain regions after injury, as opposed to using fewer resources after TBI. For example, influential work examining WM deficits in TBI patients demonstrated that injury resulted in increased involvement of neural resources in prefrontal cortex (PFC) and parietal areas (McAllister et al., 1999, 2001). Since that time, studies of cognitive deficit after injury have almost universally demonstrated (i.e., across a variety of tasks and paradigms) increased involvement of neural networks, most often involving PFC, and commonly right PFC (Perlstein et al., 2004; Sanchez-Carrion et al., 2008a). One clinically oriented goal in this literature has been to identify a primary signature or "biomarker" for deficit that might be the target of intervention. For example, with a number of studies in TBI demonstrating the recruitment of right PFC, this would appear to be a viable signature of neural disruption and compromise. However, the meaning of PFC recruitment has yet to be clarified; some investigators maintain that it represents brain reorganization (Sanchez-Carrion et al., 2008a; 2008b) or operates to facilitate performance (McAllister et al., 1999, 2001; Newsome et al., 2007; Scheibel et al., 2007), while we have maintained that the effect is a transient indicator of slowed and/or inefficient processing speed (Christodoulou et al., 2001; Hillary et al., 2010). More important, there is some evidence that this neural recruitment is a nonspecific response evident in other neurological disorders and may occur under some conditions in healthy adults (Hillary, 2008). Thus, even with a common finding appearing in most studies of TBI, the traditional approach of documenting regions of distinct "activation" in the TBI sample led to little new information for clinical intervention. To date, there remain important challenges to understanding the brain activation changes repeatedly observed in studies of deficit after neurological compromise.

There appear to be three important contributors to difficulty in interpreting the results in this literature. First, unlike behavioral studies where performance differences are often of primary interest, it is a consistent challenge in functional imaging work to guarantee identical performance between clinical and healthy adult samples; comparable between-group performance is required in order to reliably interpret altered "activation" in the clinical sample (Friston et al., 1996; Price, Crinion, & Friston, 2006). Second, it is not uncommon for there to be some variability in the functional brain activation elicited during even very well-defined tasks. That is, the degree of neural involvement in any neural network varies even between healthy adults and may be greatly influenced by demographic factors and task performance (Bergerbest, Ghahremani, & Gabrieli, 2004; Braver et al., 1997; Rypma et al., 2006). This consideration precedes the influence of clinical pathophysiology, which itself is often expressed differently between people. Third, cross-sectional studies that focus on establishing between-group differences are not able to discern why the differences exist or how they contribute to either behavioral deficits or residual skills. Thus, the focus on documenting between-group differences is accompanied by significant methodological challenges. Its most important shortcoming is conceptual; such an approach does not recognize the inherent flexibility in dynamic neural systems in both normal and damaged networks. Thus, after a decade of research examining cognitive deficits associated with TBI using advanced functional imaging methods, the question remains: What is the nature of neural recruitment after neurological disruption?

We have argued elsewhere that findings of increased prefrontal activity, occurring across a wide spectrum of neurological disorders (e.g., MS, TBI, HIV), have been misinterpreted as brain reorganization (Hillary, 2008; Hillary et al., 2006). In one study, we replicated the finding that individuals with TBI demonstrate increased PFC involvement during a rapid decision-making task (Hillary et al., 2010). However, we also demonstrated, using an independent, whole-brain analysis, that this neural recruitment could be predicted by using reaction time as a regressor of the fMRI signal and by examining within-subject, between-trial learning. We observed that these neural systems (healthy and disrupted) are more similar than different when adapting to this task, and that because it attenuates with task practice in both samples, PFC recruitment is quite transient and at least partially accounted for by time-on-task. In other words, neural recruitment emerged as a sort of transient "support mechanism," necessary for accurate performance but at the same time a marker of slow, inefficient processing. Similar findings were also observed in a different task and in a different TBI sample (Medaglia et al., 2012). Taken together, these data suggest that subtle shifts in resource use are more likely representative of temporary buttresses rather than formal brain reorganization.

The question then remains: If the neural recruitment occurring after injury is transient, mirrors what is observable in healthy adults, and can be reliably predicted by reaction time, how might it inform us about the potential for recovery? Until recently, our ability to answer this question was limited to analyses from which we could infer brain activity as being dissociable by the location and amplitude of the signal alone. While very informative in orienting scientists to key brain regions, such between-group comparisons have done little beyond helping to characterize gross differences in local signal evident in TBI. Complementary methods are needed to determine the nature of these differences and how components within complex networks interact. For functional imaging to make a significant contribution to our understanding of brain disorders and, eventually, to our clinical interventions, it must help us take critical steps to understand how *entire neural networks* accommodate insult.

The Meaning of Plasticity After TBI

If the primary goal is to use functional imaging methods evaluatively in neurorehabilitation, then there are several additional methodological caveats worth considering that will be integrated as part of this discussion. In order to ideally identify the basic brain changes associated with neurological disruption, we emphasize here two critical approaches to be integrated with connectivity modeling approaches. The first is to directly examine the relationship between altered neural networks and task performance, and the second is to focus on the capacity for network change during serial observations of the individual.

Direct Examination of Performance-Activation Relationships

An indispensable element for determining the meaning of neural recruitment in PFC (and associated network change) is the relationship between performance and activation. Work to date has attempted to equate between-group performance in order to aid in interpreting network changes in clinical samples. By maintaining a constant level of task performance, examiners have reduced between-group behavioral differences. In doing so, however, they have also reduced behavioral variance and have failed to assess network change as a function of task performance. In order to directly investigate changing task performance against neural network plasticity, examiners can (1) manipulate task load to observe attendant changes in neural activity (McAllister et al., 1999, 2001; Perlstein et al., 2004), and (2) use behavior (e.g., accuracy, RT) as a regressor to predict the brain response (Hillary et al., 2010). These methods permit examination of the relationships between discrete components of a neural network and behavior change over the course of recovery. This approach also provides the opportunity to separate the primary neural networks required for engaging in the task (e.g., visual cortex) from components in the neural network that directly modulate task performance (e.g., PFC). It may ultimately be the case that transient support mechanisms play an important role for how more permanent brain changes are expressed (i.e., the recruited support network in the short term becomes a permanent mechanism to subserve that function), but this relationship remains unclear because the existing literature has not differentiated these effects. To understand the meaning of network change in recovery, it is important to directly examine the relationship between network dynamics and task performance.

Examining Within-Subject Change

The second methodological manipulation that is essential for advancing connectivity science and its integration with rehabilitation is the need to examine within-subject change. There are two approaches that have been used in the literature to date. The first method for understanding how neural systems adapt to injury and disease is to observe how a disrupted neural system accommodates novel tasks, thereby changing during "learning" over the course of repeated trials. Even after significant neurological disruption, most individuals with TBI retain the ability to acquire new information, albeit at a reduced capacity and/or pace. Unfortunately, there is little information in humans demonstrating how damaged neural networks permit new learning after insult. If the basic parameters of change in a "learning" neural network can be determined, functional imaging methods may be paired with behavioral change as a complementary dependent variable for determining the timeline and efficacy of treatment interventions. Fortified with this information, clinical interventions may begin to use imaging results as an additional dependent variable to make determinations about treatment efficacy, including the timeline, direction, and magnitude of network change, on a case-by-case basis.

A second approach for examining within-subject change is to directly examine patient change during early critical windows of recovery. While painstaking, this approach is incredibly powerful, as it permits one to directly examine network plasticity during time periods when change is certain to occur and can be directly linked to recovery. Examples from human neurorehabilitation indicate that an important window of recovery from moderate and severe forms of TBI is during the first year following injury, with the greatest behavioral change occurring during the first 6 months following injury (Millis et al., 2001; Pagulayan, Temkin, Machamer, & Dikmen, 2006). There is some work to date examining network plasticity during this window (elaborated upon in the final section of this chapter). This approach also eliminates many of the methodological challenges facing researchers attempting to make between-group comparisons of task activation (e.g., performance, control tasks; see Price & Friston, 1999, 2002; Price et al., 2006) and circumvents the significant problems in understanding heterogeneous responses.

Overall, serial observation methods, such as those described here, may help to clarify inconsistent or nuanced findings in the literature. For example, dorsolateral PFC and ventrolateral PFC likely have distinct roles in WM and may have dissociable roles in recovery. Separately, while this chapter has focused on the increased activation typically observed in WM functioning, some work has shown decreased activation in central parts of the neural network when comparing clinical samples and healthy adults (Chen et al., 2004). In the case of very severe pathology (e.g., "catastrophic" TBI) and/or atrophy, neural recruitment may be impossible due to significant gray matter loss and the eradication of viable neural networks. Therefore, in cross-sectional work, imaging results may be highly dependent upon the time period post-injury in which data are collected. Through serial observation initiated early after injury, the evolution of neural change/recovery can be assessed, including the role of distinct substrates in recovery and potentially competing effects such as neural disconnection and neural recruitment. If functional imaging is to begin making measurable contributions to the treatment of individuals with TBI, it is imperative that fMRI methods be used to characterize the timeline, magnitude, and permanence of the system-level changes occurring in the individual. Examples of studies using the approaches outlined above are integrated in the final section of this chapter.

Connectivity Approaches: Examining an Integrated Network

The goal of this section is to provide a non-technical overview of the prominent connectivity approaches being applied in the clinical neurosciences. In turn, the final section of the chapter offers a critical summary of the work utilizing these methods as they apply to understanding TBI deficit and recovery.

Examining the Brain at "Rest"

There is growing enthusiasm in the cognitive neurosciences for examining "resting" or "intrinsic" brain activity to understand separable brain networks. While the approaches examining the intrinsic signal vary, for our discussion here, we refer to this broad category of analysis as resting-state functional connectivity (RSFC) methods. The emphasis on RSFC is relatively new, but the first study documenting RSFC effects was over 15 years ago. Biswal and colleagues demonstrated that in the absence of stimulation, voxels spatially representative of the motor cortex could be reliably observed in the baseline, or resting, data (Biswal, Yetkin, Haughton, & Hyde, 1995); these findings were extended by others (Xiong, Parson, Py, Gao, & Fox, 1998; Xiong et al., 1999). Several years later, investigators demonstrated task anticorrelations, or a "default mode" network (DMN) operating in reciprocal fashion to networks associated with volitional task processing (Fox et al., 2005; Raichle et al., 2001; Raichle & Snyder, 2007). There now exists a rapidly growing literature using RSFC methods to document the interplay between on-task and off-task networks (Fransson, 2005; Greicius, Krasnow, Reiss, & Menon, 2003; Greicius, Srivastava, Reiss, & Menon, 2004; Kelly, Uddin, Biswal, Castellanos, & Milham, 2008; Weissman, Roberts, Visscher, & Woldorff, 2006).

As an example of the "reciprocity" between these networks, Figure 7.1 demonstrates data for a group of individuals with moderate and severe TBI before and after practicing a demanding working memory task (the n-back). These data reveal tight reciprocity between the dorsal anterior cingulate, purportedly an attentional control region, and the posterior cingulate, a region with likely multiple contributions, but critical to intrinsic, or

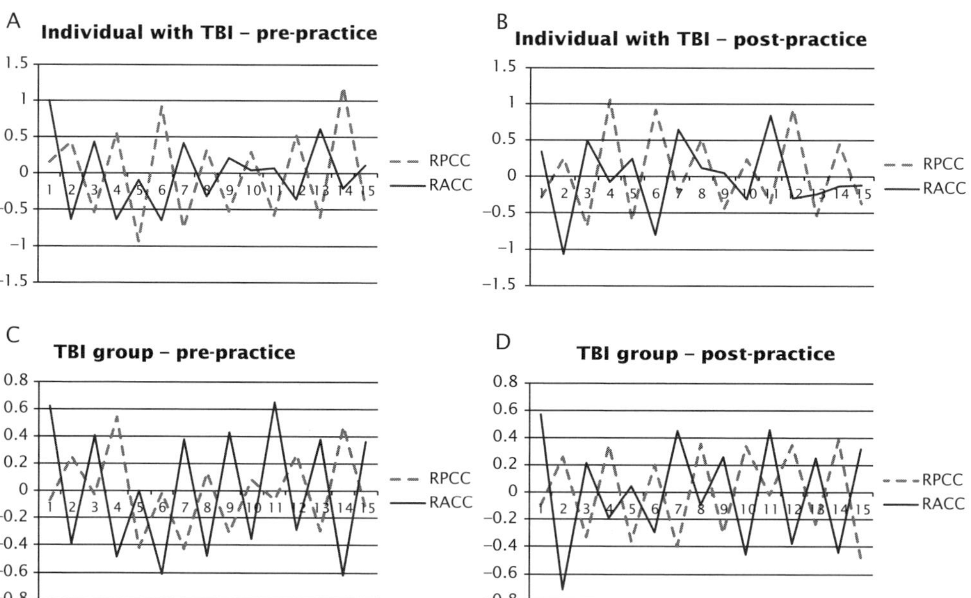

FIGURE 7.1 Reciprocity between right anterior cingulate cortex (ACC) ROI and right posterior cingulate cortex (PCC) ROI during the 1-back in (A) an individual with moderate-severe TBI before practice, (B) the same individual after practice, (C) group time series for a sample of 12 individuals with TBI before practice, and (D) the same group after practice. *Data points (one per block) represent an average of all BOLD signal time series values in that block. Vertical axes represent Pearson correlation coefficients (r). Horizontal axes represent blocks (odd = task, even = rest). Unpublished data from laboratory of Frank G. Hillary. From Venkatesan et al., in preparation.

resting-state networks. What we demonstrate here is that these networks are shifting in TBI with practice, and that (a) this reciprocity is not completely disrupted after TBI, and (b) the relationship between these networks are malleable with new learning (these data are discussed in greater detail in the final section of this chapter).

There are important advantages to using RSFC methods to understand plasticity after TBI. Methodologically, RSFC analyses circumvent dilemmas that arise when using fMRI in clinical samples: for example, it is difficult to guarantee task compliance, and assumptions surrounding cognitive subtraction or pure insertion may not be justified when comparing healthy and clinical samples (Hillary, 2008; Price & Friston, 2002). Furthermore, task-induced brain activation maps underestimate the size and number of involved regions, and the extent of functional networks are more fully revealed by RSFC analysis (Biswal et al., 1995; Xiong et al., 1998, 1999). Conceptually, resting-state network activity has been shown to be related to task-induced activation and efficient performance (Hampson, Driesen, Skudlarski, Gore, & Constable, 2006; Kelly et al., 2008; Mennes et al., 2010; for theoretical discussion, see Raichle, 2010), and altered resting-state patterns have been documented consistently in other clinical disorders (e.g., Alzheimer's disease), signifying the potential contribution of intrinsic connectivity changes to functional disturbances. Identification and characterization of resting-state networks thus offers important insights into brain functioning across cognitive states.

There are a number of methodological approaches for documenting the resting signal in functional brain data, but the most essential feature to this type of network analysis is to examine the covariance in time series between distinct regions in the brain. This can be performed by selecting specific brain regions, determined a priori, or sampling from "whole-brain" data, including or excluding task (for general review of the history of the DMN, see Raichle & Snyder, 2007). The goal is to document how brain regions (or systems) are oscillating together over time, including changes in these dynamics with perturbation/intervention. One of the most interesting findings from this growing literature is that there are a number of "subnetworks" whose constituents covary, irrespective of overt task demands (van den Heuvel & Pol, 2010). Some investigators have cautioned against interpretation of these putative covariations between regions, citing methodological issues that may induce spurious interregional relationships (e.g., Murphy, Birn, Handwerker, Jones, & Bandettini, 2009; Weissenbacher et al., 2009). However, subsequent functional connectivity work has endeavored to address these concerns (Carbonell, Bellec, & Shmuel, 2011; Chai, Castanon, Ongur, & Whitfield-Gabrieli, 2012; Fox, Zhang, Snyder, & Raichle, 2009; Keller et al., 2013), and has revealed that there are indeed brain regions that seem to reliably "hang together" across brain environments. For example, the dorsolateral prefrontal cortex and parietal regions often covary at rest or during task (i.e., an attentional control network), as do the posterior cingulate and medial prefrontal cortices (i.e., default mode network). These networks are highly interactive, and their interrelationships are a critical focus of investigation in the cognitive neurosciences (see van den Heuvel & Pol, 2010, for review).

The RSFC and related methods described here are relatively new to the clinical neurosciences and very novel in TBI research. As is discussed in the final section of this chapter, these methods provide alternative means to examine major shifts in network dynamics after TBI, which may to prove to be invaluable in our understanding of network level plasticity after neurological compromise.

Effective Connectivity

In functional imaging, the term "effective connectivity" is attributed to Friston (1994) and describes the causal nature of connections between neural nodes. In essence, the goal of effective connectivity is to isolate nodes within the network that are deemed to play the largest role in processing and to examine the directed relationships between them. This is often, but not necessarily, achieved through task perturbation, and the number of regions of interest (ROIs) can vary dramatically from two to greater than 20. One critical assumption in many methods is that causality can be inferred by temporal sequence. That is, later events should not cause earlier events. With this assumption as the basis for causal modeling, most effective connectivity modeling approaches infer causality or "influence" between any two nodes by examining the temporal sequence of covariation in the time series.

Early applications of effective connectivity used structural equation modeling in fMRI time series (McIntosh & Gonzalez-Lima, 1994) and in PET studies to identify distinct pathways in the visual perceptual systems (McIntosh et al., 1994). Over the past 20 years, there has been continued progress in the area of effective connectivity, with the goal of refining approaches to handle time series neuroimaging data (broadly defined, including fMRI, MEG, and EEG data). In time series data, methods have typically measured either simultaneous covariance between brain regions (e.g., structural equation modeling [SEM]) or time-lagged influences between nodes, or the influence that prior moments in the time series have on later moments (e.g., Granger causal modeling, vector autoregression). Dynamic causal modeling (DCM) was designed specifically for handling functional imaging time series data (and in particular fMRI) by modeling the BOLD signal. DCM also considers nonlinear relationships between network nodes and permits direct measurement of the influence of task perturbation on the network (Friston, Harrison, & Penny, 2003; Sarty, 2007).

The development of causal modeling has not been without significant criticism (see Smith et al., 2011, for a vital analysis), with specific concern given to the meaningfulness of "directed" connections in time series data where the temporal resolution is measured in the second as opposed to millisecond timescale, where much of information transfer in neural systems is happening. Moreover, methods such as SEM and DCM operate largely in a confirmatory manner, requiring some notion a priori of how network nodes should interact. Moreover, many models of the modeling techniques are deterministic, a feature that permits little flexibility for a system that is inherently fluctuating, even in the absence of perturbation (i.e., "intrinsic connectivity," described earlier). Even given these concerns, in very recent work initiated by Kim et al. (2007) and later in a series of papers by Gates and Molenaar (see Gates & Molenaar, 2012; Gates, Molenaar, Hillary, Ram, & Rovine,

2010; Gates, Molenaar, Hillary, & Slobounov, 2011), effective connectivity modeling has been refined in an attempt to address several critical methodological drawbacks, including poor reliability in determining the directness of nodal influence and poor temporal resolution afforded by imaging methods such as fMRI. While the timescale of measurement using methods like fMRI has unresolvable physiological limitations, the methods for examining covariance between multiple ROIs and examining within-subject change and small-group effects have been refined in recent developments (see Gates & Molenaar, 2012), and are essential for examining recovery in TBI. Figure 7.2 provides an example of

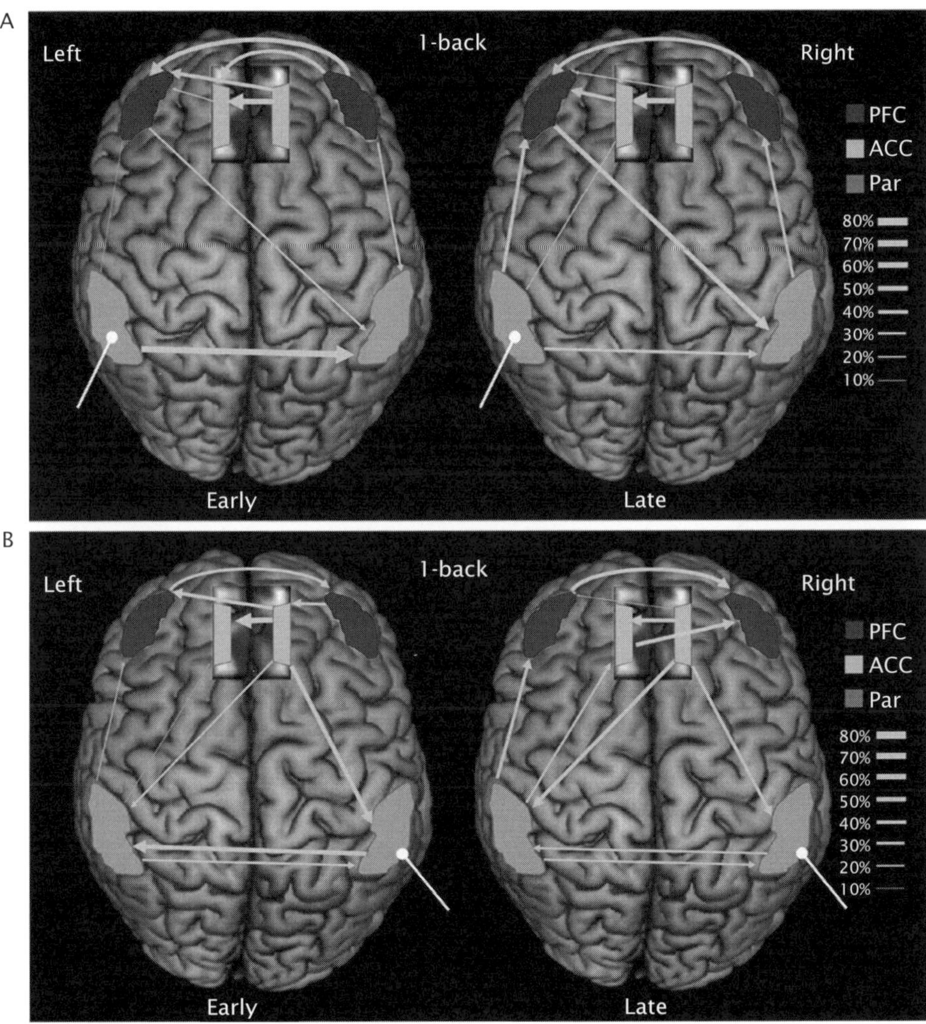

FIGURE 7.2 Group frequency data for effective connectivity in the (A) healthy control, and (B) TBI samples, for effects during earlier and later trials of the 1-back task. Line thickness indicates frequency of connections. The primary influence of "task input" is represented as a white bar. Colored Brodmann areas are a schematic representation illustrating the approximate spatial constraints for the regions of interest (i.e., peak + 5 mm sphere). ACC = anterior cingulate cortex; Par = parietal; PFC = prefrontal cortex. Reprinted with permission from Hillary et al. (2011).

this type of analysis in a group of healthy adults comparing "early" to "late" performance on a task. Overall, with continued refinement, effective connectivity methods hold the promise of adding important information about nodal interactions within neural models, with the most important added information being the direction of influence between network constituents.

Graph Theoretical Approaches

Graphs as models for complex systems have a long history, which is considered to have begun with Leonhard Euler's search for a walk through the Prussian city of Königsberg that traversed each of the city's seven bridges exactly once. He provided a formal proof that no such walk was possible by abstracting the problem to represent the bridges and land masses without consideration of distance or shape, thus establishing the foundations of *graph theory*, a branch of combinatorics and, more generally, discrete mathematics. In today's language, a *graph* is a collection of objects, called *vertices* or *nodes*, and the pairwise relationships among them, *edges, links, lines*, or *arcs*.

Early on, graph theory enjoyed primary applications in chemistry for the enumeration of isomers and description of molecular structure (Cayley, 1875; Sylvester, 1878). Modern graphical methods started to appear in the social and behavioral sciences in the 1930s (see Scott, 2000), gaining momentum and popularity following Stanley Milgram's 1967 "small-world experiment" (Milgram, 1967). Since then, graph theoretical approaches have come to the forefront in social psychology and sociology for the study of relationships within and among individuals, organizations, communities, and societies.

Modern *network science* is quite young (Barabási, 2002; Watts, 2003;), having taken on its current form at the turn of this century. Networks, as abstract structures, are simply graphs. The distinction in terms arises from the additional meaning that network graphs carry representations of real-world complex systems, typically endowed with nontrivial topological structure and often dynamic in nature. More recent advances in computing capabilities have enabled data collection and analyses on a much larger scale than ever before, and what has emerged is a series of findings revealing a few surprisingly robust, consistent self-organizing principles in networks across diverse domains.

Small-World Networks

In a landmark paper by Duncan Watts and Steven Strogatz (1998), it was demonstrated that many real-world networks have a *small-world* structure, defined primarily by two graph theoretic features. First, compared to purely random graphs, they have a high *clustering coefficient*. The clustering coefficient measures the extent to which a network is composed of smaller, tightly knit subsets of nodes that are densely linked among themselves but more sparsely linked to the rest of the graph. In a network where clustering coefficient is high and this structure is pronounced, these pockets of denser connectivity are called *communities*. Second, the average *shortest path length* tends to be low in small-world networks, so that any node in the graph can reach any other through a relatively short sequence of steps, a classic measure of information efficiency.

Critical work by Albert-László Barabási and Réka Albert (1999) arrived a year later, demonstrating that the topology of (a portion of) the World Wide Web and that of several other social and biological networks share another prominent feature, a power-law degree distribution, coining the term "scale-free" to describe this behavior. The *degree* of a node is defined as the number of links incident to it. In scale-free networks, the probability of a node having a given degree is inversely proportional to that degree, raised to a constant power. This unique structure is a consequence of network growth: over time, new nodes are added to the system; as these nodes enter the graph, they obey *preferential attachment*, being proportionally more likely to link with nodes of higher degree. Scale-free networks share the properties of small-world networks, and actually can be considered a special class of small-world networks, *ultra small-worlds*, in the sense that their average shortest path lengths are even shorter than in other small-world systems (Cohen & Havlin, 2003). In addition, they are characterized by the presence of *hubs*, a few very influential, highly connected nodes. It has been shown that while scale-free networks are quite resilient to random error, they are very vulnerable to targeted attacks on network hubs (Albert, Jeong, & Barabási, 2000).

Neural Networks

Anatomical and functional neural networks have been well-described as small-world networks (see Bassett & Bullmore, 2006, for a review), starting with the neuronal network of *Caenorhabditis elegans*, described in terms of the 2,462 synaptic connections among 282 constituent neurons (Watts & Strogatz, 1998) and followed soon after by an analysis of anatomical connectivity matrices derived from tract-tracing studies in the macaque and the cat (Hilgetag, Burns, O'Neill, & Scannell, 2000). In 2004, Cornelius Stam proposed that the functional connectivity patterns of human magnetoencephalographic recordings obeyed small-world structure. His study involved resting-state data from 126 MEG sensors whose pairwise associations were determined through synchronization likelihood analysis of the sensor signals, filtered into classical EEG frequency bands (Stam, 2004). Similar studies of MEG/EEG data soon followed in various contexts (Micheloyannis et al., 2006; Stam, Jones, Nolte, Breakspear, & Scheltens, 2007; see Sporns, 2010, for a review). Small-world properties were first demonstrated in fMRI data in 2005 (Salvador et al., 2005). Since that time, a rich body of work has emerged in *connectivity* modeling using fMRI, beyond resting-state data, toward understanding learning, memory, aging, injury, and disease (for a review, see Sporns, 2010).

A precursor to the analysis of functional brain networks is the definition of the nodes and links that determine the system, which is less straightforward than for anatomical neural networks. A number of methods for this have been proposed (see Smith et al., 2011, for a review), and certain methods are more appropriate depending on the size and nature of the dataset or the goals of the analysis, but all of these methods typically have the same general framework. Brain regions of interest (ROIs) are determined, either hand-selected or using a standard brain atlas, and these ROIs become the nodes in the functional network. Signals within each ROI are averaged to obtain a representative time series for that region, and the pairwise relationships between these regional series are determined using correlation, partial correlation, synchronization, coherence, and similar statistical methods, either on the raw signal or on a signal decomposed using the wavelet transform. Correlations are either subjected to a threshold in order to determine presence or absence of a link between respective nodes in the graph, or a *weighted* graph can be drawn preserving information about the extent of regional interactions.

That anatomical and functional brain network architectures have evolved with small-world properties is unsurprising for several reasons, the foremost being that the small-world topology allows maximal functionality with minimal wiring costs. The simultaneous presence of tightly connected clusters and short paths between distant network nodes is both locally and globally efficient, supporting segregated and distributed information processing in parallel. At the individual voxel scale, there is evidence that functional brain networks also have scale-free properties (Eguíluz, Chialvo, Cecchi, Baliki, & Apkarian, 2005; van den Heuvel, Stam, Boersma, & Pol, 2008). However, on a regional scale, the degree distribution seems to better fit an exponentially truncated power law (Achard, Salvador, Whitcher, Suckling, & Bullmore, 2006; Bassett, Meyer-Lindenberg, Achard, Duke, & Bullmore, 2006), so there are slightly fewer hubs than would be expected in a strictly scale-free network. This structure may serve as an important mediator of scale-free networks' core vulnerability, allowing brain networks to be more resilient to attack than scale-free networks, while still equally resilient to random error (Achard et al., 2006). As is seen in the following section, graph theory can be applied to understand how entire systems are changing with neurological insult.

Connectivity Dynamics After Neurotrauma: Applying the Methods

The investigation of functional connectivity in TBI is a relatively recent endeavor. Nonetheless, functional connectivity techniques, such as those discussed earlier in this chapter, have offered an initial glimpse into network dynamics following neurological compromise. Importantly, studies employing these approaches have begun to clarify the component processes of functional neural recruitment seen in traditional fMRI activation studies. Some work has also used serial observations to track these processes through acute injury recovery, providing an expanded context for interpreting neurorecovery and behavioral change. Given their potential relevance to clinical intervention, we review here the literature making use of the techniques described in the previous section to examine brain dynamics at rest, during task, and over the course of recovery.

As in the resting-state literature in healthy individuals and other clinical populations, most studies of TBI using resting paradigms have focused on the default mode network (DMN). The DMN is thought to be associated with semantic processing (Binder & Desai, 2011; Binder, Desai, Graves, & Conant, 2009) and internally focused tasks such as autobiographical memory retrieval and self-referential thought (Buckner, Andrews-Hanna, & Schacter, 2008). Kim and colleagues (2010) were the first to report on resting-state perturbations in DMN regions of those with moderate or severe TBI, and a modest number of subsequent investigations have interrogated DMN connectivity after brain injury. Through the use of independent component analysis (ICA) and dual regression techniques to identify nodes within the network, these studies have commonly observed increased functional connectivity within the DMN, featuring prominently the posterior cingulate cortex (PCC) and precuneus (Bonnelle et al., 2011; Sharp et al., 2011; review of method in Zuo et al., 2010). Importantly, they have also interrogated the relationship between resting connectivity and task performance, concluding that greater connectivity within the DMN supports quicker and more stable performance. For example, Sharp et al. (2011) noted greater connectivity of the PCC to the rest of the DMN in TBI relative to controls. PCC-DMN connectivity was positively associated with faster information processing speed in both groups (see Figure 7.3; Sharp et al., 2011). Similarly, in the same patient sample, functional connectivity of the precuneus to remaining DMN structures at the beginning of a choice reaction time task was negatively associated with change in reaction time during that task (Bonnelle et al., 2011). These authors also found that the magnitude of precuneus-DMN functional connectivity correctly classified a subgroup of individuals with TBI demonstrating deficits in sustained attention compared to both controls and brain-injured individuals with intact sustained attention.

Not all RSFC studies have shown that TBI results in DMN hyperconnectivity. Other work in severe forms of TBI has found decreases in RSFC involving the DMN (Arenivas et al., 2012), hippocampus, and frontal attentional network (Marquez de la Plata et al., 2011). Arenivas et al. (2012) investigated DMN function with three approaches to RSFC—correlations between network nodes and the entire brain, within-network interregion correlations, and direct node-node correlations—and noted that all three methods detected weaker connectivity patterns in the TBI sample. However, this apparent deficiency was not associated with functional or cognitive status. In contrast, this group previously found that diminished interhemispheric hippocampal connectivity at rest was significantly associated with delayed verbal recall ability on neuropsychological testing (Marquez de la Plata et al., 2011), concordant with the widely accepted view of hippocampal function as integral to episodic memory.

Indeed, findings from functional connectivity studies in TBI remain mixed in some regards, and they serve as a reminder of the importance of investigating functional connectivity on multiple levels, from single-region to distributed networks, in relation to recovery. In this respect, such work remains largely exploratory, and continues to benefit from innovative study designs and analytic tools. Research incorporating serial

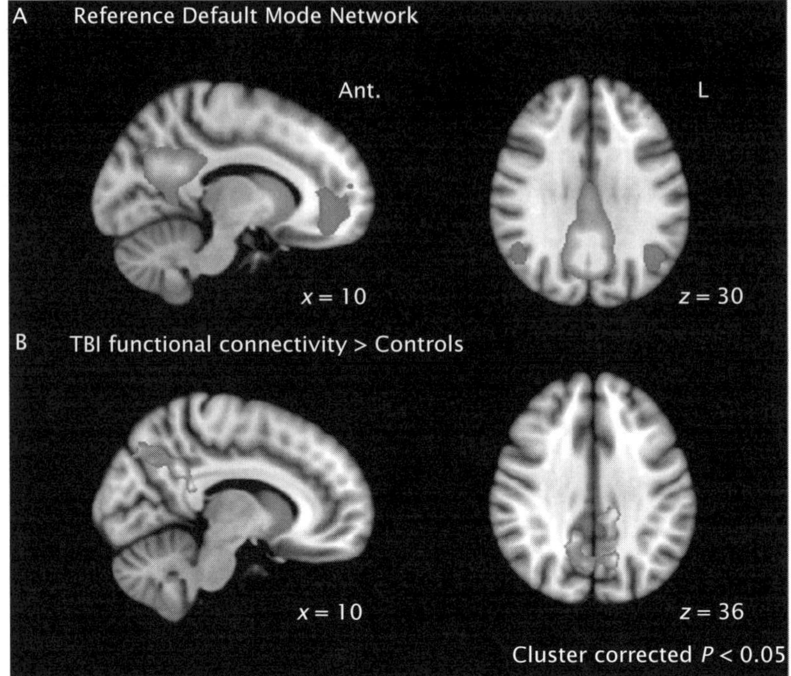

C Default mode functional connectivity and behavior

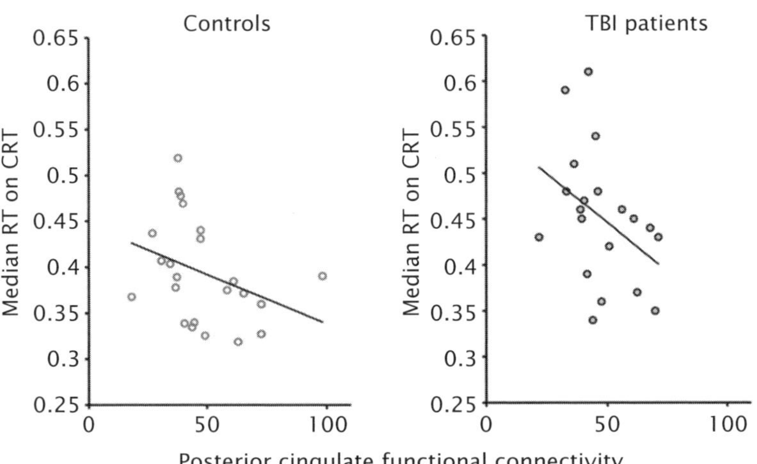

FIGURE 7.3 Functional connectivity within the DMN correlates with information processing speed
following traumatic brain injury. (A) The resting state default mode network as identified in control subjects. Voxels showing significant functional connectivity are shown in red–yellow. (B) Voxels
showing greater correlation with the time course of the DMN for patients with traumatic brain injury
than age-matched control patients are shown in red–yellow (P <0.05 threshold). Anterior (Ant.) MNI
coordinates for brain slices are shown. (C) Posterior cingulate cortex functional connectivity is plot-
ted against median reaction time (RT) on the choice-reaction time (CRT) task. L = left. Reprinted with
permission from Sharp et al. (2011).

observation as well as advanced connectivity techniques modeling both default mode and control networks has offered novel insights into the movement of large-scale networks during recovery and has provided new avenues of inquiry regarding heterogeneous brain responses.

Given the highly dynamic nature of neural networks, their relevance to recovery is most appropriately determined through longitudinal characterization of widespread resting-state connectivity patterns. Accordingly, two resting-state studies of TBI adopted graph theoretical approaches in either fMRI (Nakamura, Hillary, & Biswal, 2009) or MEG (Castellanos et al., 2011) to study global disruptions in network function at 3 months after injury and following a period of recovery, revealing remarkable consistency. Both of these investigations yielded graph theory metrics that were indicative of network inefficiency (compared to controls) at the first time point for the TBI samples. However, 3 months to 1 year later, network characteristics of those with TBI more closely approximated those seen in controls (see Figure 7.4). Furthermore, Castellanos et al. (2011) found that measures of functional network integrity were positively associated with performance on tests of intelligence. These studies, therefore, provided the first data suggesting that recovery after TBI might be observable on the network level.

In the hopes of identifying the roles of specific brain regions in recovery, another study used resting methods to examine interregional connectivity in periods of "off-task" fMRI signal at 3 and 6 months post-injury (Hillary et al., 2011b). Regions of interest were selected based on their distinct roles in integrating internal milieu with external demands ("internal-state" network; medial prefrontal cortex [MPFC] and PCC) and in "goal-directed" or on-task behavior (dorsolateral prefrontal cortex [DLPFC] and anterior cingulate cortex [ACC]). Findings revealed significant increases in connectivity in "internal-state" networks from 3 to 6 months post-injury, consistent with work in post-acute TBI populations discussed (Bonnelle et al., 2011; Sharp et al., 2011). The authors also noted that the most consistent network changes for both goal-directed and internal-state networks appeared as increased connections to insular and medial temporal regions over time, suggesting that increased insular involvement permits more fluid negotiation and shifting between internally directed and attentional control processes over time (Hillary et al., 2011b; see Figure 7.4).

While RSFC techniques have provided a basic view of how regions coactivate and cluster intrinsically, effective connectivity techniques have allowed researchers to make inferences about causality in network relationships. While still in its infancy, research into the directionality of functional relationships in TBI has begun to shed light on the mechanisms modulating complex neural systems. Some of the initial work in this area was presented by Maguire and colleagues, who examined hippocampal connectivity in an amnestic patient (Maguire, Vargha-Khadem, & Mishkin, 2001). Using structural equation modeling, their data demonstrated important connectivity shifts in the patient during episodic memory retrieval not evident in control subjects. In TBI, Hillary

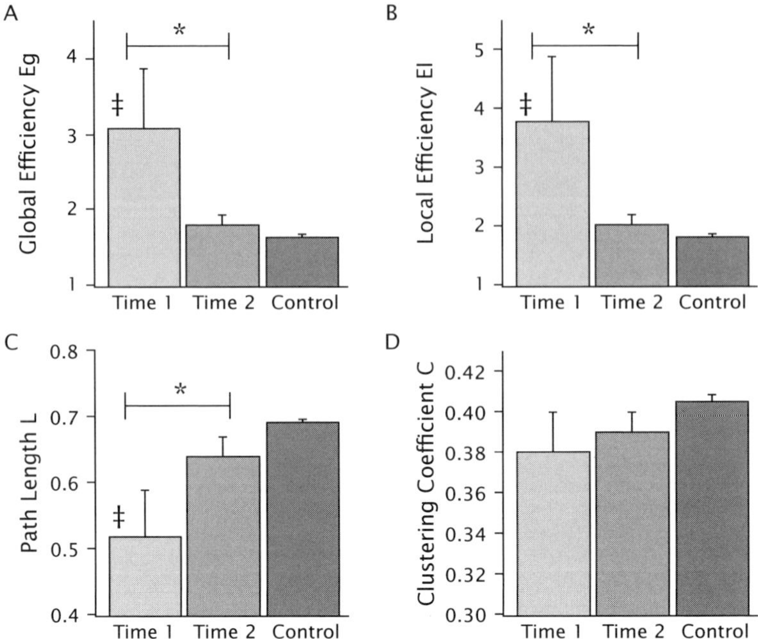

FIGURE 7.4 Functional network properties of networks with connections (edges) weighted by correlation strength (1). Results obtained from the graph theory metrics of (A) Global efficiency Eg, (B) Local efficiency El, (C) Characteristic path length L, and (D) Clustering coefficient C, for TBI and control groups. * indicates significant difference between Time 1 and Time 2. ‡ indicates significant change from control group. Reprinted via open access from Nakamura, Hillary, & Biswal (2009).

et al. (2011a) initiated this work by employing extended unified structural equation modeling (euSEM; method in Gates et al., 2011) to investigate the sequential contributions of regions activated during working memory task performance. Through this approach, their goal was to identify communication patterns between components of distributed networks, especially those underlying task-induced neural recruitment. Their results showed that the TBI group had greater right hemisphere connectivity and greater right prefrontal influence on the left hemisphere compared to controls (see Figure 7.2 in Hillary et al., 2011a), consistent with literature documenting the specificity of right prefrontal recruitment (see the first section of this chapter). Additionally, there was a greater parietal influence on anterior networks in controls, and an anterior-posterior "shift" with practice of the working memory task in the TBI sample, such that parietal versus anterior regions gradually exercised greater influence over task performance. The authors interpreted these findings as further indication that the right prefrontal cortex offers essential support, in the form of cognitive control, to tasks typically associated with the left prefrontal cortex, and that this requirement is relaxed with brief task exposure. Furthermore, the very need for additional cognitive resources denotes increased cognitive challenge (see the first section of this chapter), which is minimized gradually with task practice.

The notion that neural recruitment in TBI represents a cognitive control mechanism has been proposed by several authors, but it remains unclear whether it represents a mechanism that directly facilitates performance (e.g., Turner & Levine, 2008) or if it is an indication of a slowed and inefficient network, much like what is observed in healthy adults at lower task loads (Hillary et al., 2010; Medaglia et al., 2012; Scheibel et al., 2003; for a review, see Hillary, 2008). However, longitudinal RSFC and effective connectivity models have begun to extend this argument to include a more nuanced and integrated view of brain function after TBI, capturing the dynamic nature of networks throughout recovery and the relative influence of distinct nodes within networks during this time. Reports have documented the similarity between TBI networks and healthy control networks achieved during critical windows of recovery (Castellanos et al., 2010, 2011; Nakamura et al., 2009;) as well as during task exposure (Hillary et al., 2011a; Hillary, Medaglia, Gates, Molenaar, & Good, 2012), offering some evidence for the claim that recovery from TBI entails incremental disengagement of supportive resources as network efficiency increases over time. This has been partially corroborated by Turner and colleagues (2011), who also used effective connectivity techniques to arrive at the conclusion that those with TBI leverage support processes afforded by the right prefrontal cortex. While their interpretation differs in important ways—they interpret increased PFC involvement as "altered engagement" and "poor regulation" of neural resources—their findings are similar, and future work can help to clarify the role of these connectivity changes. Despite differences in phenomenological attributions, overall, RSFC studies and advanced connectivity approaches interrogating the DMN and attentional control networks provide unique and complementary information in order to understand the basis of neural recruitment observed in traditional imaging studies and to document network change after TBI.

Functional connectivity studies of TBI also bear clinical relevance, and the current state of the field evinces the pathophysiological and neurocognitive heterogeneity in TBI that has long been an issue in clinical intervention efforts (Doppenberg, Choi, & Bullock, 2004; Jordan, 2000; Narayan et al., 2002). For example, to examine more closely the relationship between effective connectivity characteristics and behavior, Hillary and colleagues (2012) recently extended their previous study using the euSEM technique to probe effective connectivity in TBI subgroups. They identified sustained learners, individuals who continued to show improvements in reaction time after working memory task practice, and those who demonstrated progressively slower reaction times after practice. A comparison of these two subgroups revealed distinct effective connectivity models, with the former showing diminished connectivity within frontal regions and increased connectivity between frontal and parietal regions, akin to the control sample in Hillary et al. (2011a). Individuals who were impaired in learning, however, demonstrated a pattern of frontal hyperconnectivity. Hence, these data suggested that decreasing reliance on frontal networks—notably, those involving prefrontal cortex—and increasing posterior involvement together may denote a restoration of typical network behavior and thus may be a marker of neural and cognitive recovery.

As evidenced by the preceding discussion, studies of functional connectivity after neurotrauma provide valuable and more fine-grained information about neural aberrances than that obtained by older methods. The reader is oriented here to four general findings from the contemporary literature. The first is that moderate or severe TBI results in immediate large-scale disorganization of neural networks, notably involving frontal hyperconnectivity. Such patterns are thought to reflect the compromised integrity of axonal tracts (Bonnelle et al., 2012; Palacios et al., 2013) and a resultant cerebral inefficiency, that is, higher neural costs for the same level of cognitive functioning. Moreover, inefficient network organization may be able to resolve at least partially, to what is observed in healthy individuals, with brief task exposure and during protracted recovery periods. Third, and perhaps the least understood finding to date, involves the nature of dynamic interplay between specific functional subnetworks after TBI, and the apparent necessity of DMN suppression and connectivity increases between regions negotiating network exchange (e.g., goal-directed and default mode network communication). Finally, threaded through each of the preceding conclusions is the idea that connectivity profiles are seldom universal across individuals, and may result in spurious findings if examined only on the aggregate level, without regard for individual or subgroup characteristics.

The potential clinical implications of connectivity work in TBI have been discussed by Ham and Sharp (2012), who argue that identification of individual-associated connectivity patterns may be a critical missing piece in developing effective interventions that are necessarily tailored to individual needs. Furthermore, the severity of injury and the time points at which individuals are observed are paramount to understanding network and behavioral change. For example, Ham and Sharp (2012) note that while Sharp et al. (2011) found DMN-associated connectivity increases at rest in a sample of chronic TBI, Hillary et al. (2011b) found increases in this network only after a 6-month recovery period. Thus, limited, "snapshot" views of group network function are likely insufficient for drawing meaningful conclusions about complex neurological disruption, but longitudinal tracking of individual patients' network dynamics may hold some promise for predicting clinical outcomes. This comprehensive person-specific approach has long been advocated by scientists who contend that group-level data often possess little information about any given individual, and that developmental processes—of which neurorecovery could be classified as a special case—must be studied principally on the level of dynamic intraindividual systems (Ford & Lerner, 1992; Molenaar, 2004, 2006, 2008; Molenaar, Sinclair, Rovine, Ram, & Corneal, 2009; Wohlwill, 1973; for overview of argument, see Medaglia, Ramanathan, Venkatesan, & Hillary, 2011). Coincidentally, this mirrors the fundamental clinical dilemma in the neurorehabilitation of TBI: one intervention does not (always) fit all. Indeed, connectivity modeling of individual-specific brain changes after injury presents exciting possibilities for the future study and treatment of TBI.

References

Achard, S., Salvador, R., Whitcher, B., Suckling, J., & Bullmore, E. T. (2006). A resilient, low-frequency, small-world human brain functional network with highly connected association cortical hubs. *J Neurosci, 26*, 63–72.

Albert, R., Jeong, H., & Barabási, A. L. (2000). Error and attack tolerance of complex networks. *Nature, 406*(6794), 14.

Arenivas, A., Diaz-Arrastia, R., Spence, J., Cullum, C. M., Krishnan, K., Bosworth, C., . . . Marquez de la Plata, C. (2012). Three approaches to investigating functional compromise to the default mode network after traumatic axonal injury. *Brain Imag Behav.* doi: 10.1007/s11682-012-9191-2

Baddeley, A. (1996). The fractionation of working memory. *P Natl Acad Sci USA, 93*(24), 13468–13472.

Barabási, A. L. (2002). *Linked: The new science of networks.* Cambridge, MA: Perseus Publishing.

Barabási, A. L., & Albert, R. (1999). Emergence of scaling in random networks. *Science, 286*(5439), 509–512.

Bassett, D. S., & Bullmore, R. (2006). Small-world brain networks. *Neuroscientist, 12*(6), 512–523.

Bassett, D. S., Meyer-Lindenberg, A., Achard, S., Duke, T., & Bullmore, E. T. (2006). Adaptive reconfiguration of fractal small-world human brain functional networks. *P Natl Acad Sci USA, 103*, 19518–19523.

Bergerbest, D., Ghahremani, D. G., & Gabrieli, J. D. E. (2004). Neural correlates of auditory repetition priming: Reduced fMRI activation in the auditory cortex. *J Cogn Neurosci, 16*(6), 966–977. doi: doi:10.1162/08 98929041502760

Binder, J. R., & Desai, R. H. (2011). The neurobiology of semantic memory. *Trends Cogn Sci, 15*(11), 527–536. doi: 10.1016/j.tics.2011.10.001

Binder, J. R., Desai, R. H., Graves, W. W., & Conant, L. L. (2009). Where is the semantic system? A critical review and meta-analysis of 120 functional neuroimaging studies. *Cereb Cortex, 19*(12), 2767–2796. doi: 10.1093/cercor/bhp055

Biswal, B., Yetkin, F. Z., Haughton, V. M., & Hyde, J. S. (1995). Functional connectivity in the motor cortex of resting human brain using echo-planar MRI. *Magnet Reson Med, 34*(4), 537–541.

Bonnelle, V., Ham, T. E., Leech, R., Kinnunen, K. M., Mehta, M. A., Greenwood, R. J., & Sharp, D. J. (2012). Salience network integrity predicts default mode network function after traumatic brain injury. *P Natl Acad Sci USA, 109*(12), 4690–4695. doi: 10.1073/pnas.1113455109

Bonnelle, V., Leech, R., Kinnunen, K. M., Ham, T. E., Beckmann, C. F., De Boissezon, X., . . . Sharp, D. J. (2011). Default mode network connectivity predicts sustained attention deficits after traumatic brain injury. *J Neurosci, 31*(38), 13442–13451. doi: 10.1523/jneurosci.1163-11.2011

Braver, T. S., Cohen, J. D., Nystrom, L. E., Jonides, J., Smith, E. E., & Noll, D. C. (1997). A parametric study of prefrontal cortex involvement in human working memory. *NeuroImage, 5*(1), 49–62.

Buckner, R. L., Andrews-Hanna, J. R., & Schacter, D. L. (2008). The brain's default network: anatomy, function, and relevance to disease. *Ann NY Acad Sci, 1124*, 1–38. doi: 10.1196/annals.1440.011

Carbonell, F., Bellec, P., & Shmuel, A. (2011). Global and system-specific resting-state fMRI fluctuations are uncorrelated: principal component analysis reveals anti-correlated networks. *Brain Connect, 1*(6), 496–510. doi: 10.1089/brain.2011.0065

Castellanos, N. P., Leyva, I., Buldu, J. M., Bajo, R., Paul, N., Cuesta, P., . . . del-Pozo, F. (2011). Principles of recovery from traumatic brain injury: Reorganization of functional networks. *NeuroImage, 55*(3), 1189–1199. doi: 10.1016/j.neuroimage.2010.12.046

Castellanos, N. P., Paul, N., Ordonez, V. E., Demuynck, O., Bajo, R., Campo, P., . . . Maestu, F. (2010). Reorganization of functional connectivity as a correlate of cognitive recovery in acquired brain injury. *Brain, 133*(Pt 8), 2365–2381. doi: 10.1093/brain/awq174

Cayley, A. (1875). Ueber die Analytischen Figuren, welche in der Mathematik Bäume genannt werden und ihre Anwendung auf die Theorie chemischer Verbindungen. *Ber Dtsch Chem Ges, 8*(2), 1056–1059.

Chai, X. J., Castanon, A. N., Ongur, D., & Whitfield-Gabrieli, S. (2012). Anticorrelations in resting state networks without global signal regression. *NeuroImage, 59*(2), 1420–1428. doi: 10.1016/j.neuroimage.2011.08.048

Chen, J. K., Johnston, K. M., Frey, S., Petrides, M., Worsley, K., & Ptito, A. (2004). Functional abnormalities in symptomatic concussed athletes: An fMRI study. *NeuroImage, 22*(1), 68–82.

Christodoulou, C., DeLuca, J., Ricker, J. H., Madigan, N. K., Bly, B. M., Lange, G., . . . Ni, A. C. (2001). Functional magnetic resonance imaging of working memory impairment after traumatic brain injury. *J Neurol Neurosur Ps, 71*(2), 161–168.

Cohen, R., & Havlin, S. (2003). Scale-free networks are ultrasmall. *Phys Rev Lett, 90*(5), 058701.

Doppenberg, E. M., Choi, S. C., & Bullock, R. (2004). Clinical trials in traumatic brain injury: Lessons for the future. *J Neurosurg Anesth, 16*(1), 87–94.

Eguíluz, V. M., Chialvo, D. R., Cecchi, G. A., Baliki, M., & Apkarian, A. V. (2005). Scale-free brain functional networks. *Phys Rev Lett, 94*, 018102.

Faul, M., Xu, L., Wald, M. M., & Coronado, V. G. (2010). *Traumatic brain injury in the United States: Emergency department visits, hospitalizations, and deaths.* Atlanta, GA: Centers for Disease Control and Prevention, National Center for Injury Prevention and Control.

Ford, D. H., & Lerner, R. M. (1992). *Developmental systems theory.* Newbury Park, CA: Sage Publications.

Fox, M. D., Snyder, A. Z., Vincent, J. L., Corbetta, M., Van Essen, D. C., & Raichle, M. E. (2005). The human brain is intrinsically organized into dynamic, anticorrelated functional networks. *Proc Natl Acad Sci USA, 102*, 9673–9678.

Fox, M. D., Zhang, D., Snyder, A. Z., & Raichle, M. E. (2009). The global signal and observed anticorrelated resting state brain networks. *J Neurophysiol, 101*(6), 3270–3283. doi: 10.1152/jn.90777.2008

Fransson, P. (2005). Spontaneous low-frequency BOLD signal fluctuations: An fMRI investigation of the resting-state default mode of brain function hypothesis. *Hum Brain Mapp, 26*, 15–29.

Friston, K. J. (1994). Functional and effective connectivity in neuroimaging: A synthesis. *Hum Brain Mapp, 2*, 56–78.

Friston, K. J., Harrison, L., & Penny, W. (2003). Dynamic causal modeling. *NeuroImage, 19*, 1273–1302.

Friston, K. J., Price, C. J., Fletcher, P., Moore, C., Frackowiak, R. S. J., & Dolan, R. J. (1996). The trouble with cognitive subtraction. *NeuroImage, 4*(2), 97–104.

Gates, K. M., & Molenaar, P. C. (2012). Group search algorithm recovers effective connectivity maps for individuals in homogeneous and heterogeneous samples. *NeuroImage, 63*(1), 310–319. doi: 10.1016/j.neuroimage.2012.06.026

Gates, K. M., Molenaar, P. C., Hillary, F. G., Ram, N., & Rovine, M. J. (2010). Automatic search for fMRI connectivity mapping: An alternative to Granger causality testing using formal equivalences among SEM path modeling, VAR, and unified SEM. *NeuroImage, 50*(3), 1118–1125. doi: 10.1016/j.neuroimage.2009.12.117

Gates, K. M., Molenaar, P. C., Hillary, F. G., & Slobounov, S. (2011). Extended unified SEM approach for modeling event-related fMRI data. *NeuroImage, 54*(2), 1151–1158. doi: 10.1016/j.neuroimage.2010.08.051

Greicius, M. D., Krasnow, B., Reiss, A. L., & Menon, V. (2003). Functional connectivity in the resting brain: A network analysis of the default mode hypothesis. *Proc Natl Acad Sci USA, 100*, 253–258.

Greicius, M. D., Srivastava, G., Reiss, A. L., & Menon, V. (2004). Default-mode network activity distinguishes Alzheimer's disease from healthy aging: Evidence from functional MRI. *Proc Natl Acad Sci USA, 101*, 4637–4642.

Ham, T. E., & Sharp, D. J. (2012). How can investigation of network function inform rehabilitation after traumatic brain injury? *Curr Opin Neurol, 25*(6), 662–669. doi: 10.1097/WCO.0b013e328359488f

Hampson, M., Driesen, N. R., Skudlarski, P., Gore, J. C., & Constable, R. T. (2006). Brain connectivity related to working memory performance. *J Neurosci, 26*(51), 13338–13343. doi: 10.1523/jneurosci.3408-06.2006

Hilgetag, C. C., Burns, G. A. P. C., O'Neill, M. A., & Scannell, J. W. (2000). Anatomical connectivity defines the organization of clusters of cortical areas in the macaque and the cat. *Philos Trans R Soc Lond B Biol Sci, 355*, 7–20.

Hillary, F. G. (2008). Neuroimaging of working memory dysfunction and the dilemma with brain reorganization hypotheses. *J Int Neuropsych Soc, 14*(4), 526–534. doi: 10.1017/s1355617708080788

Hillary, F. G., Genova, H. M., Chiaravalloti, N. D., Rypma, B., & DeLuca, J. (2006). Prefrontal modulation of working memory performance in brain injury and disease. *Hum Brain Mapp, 27*(11), 837–847.

Hillary, F. G., Genova, H. M., Medaglia, J. D., Fitzpatrick, N. M., Chiou, K. S., Wardecker, B. M., . . . DeLuca, J. (2010). The nature of processing speed deficits in traumatic brain injury: Is less brain more? *Brain Imaging Behav, 4*(2), 141–154. doi: 10.1007/s11682-010-9094-z

Hillary, F. G., Medaglia, J. D., Gates, K., Molenaar, P. C., Slocomb, J., Peechatka, A., & Good, D. C. (2011a). Examining working memory task acquisition in a disrupted neural network. *Brain, 134*(Pt 5), 1555–1570. doi: 10.1093/brain/awr043

Hillary, F. G., Medaglia, J. D., Gates, K. M., Molenaar, P. C., & Good, D. C. (2012). Examining network dynamics after traumatic brain injury using the extended unified SEM approach. *Brain Imaging Behav.* doi: 10.1007/s11682-012-9205-0

Hillary, F. G., Slocomb, J., Hills, E. C., Fitzpatrick, N. M., Medaglia, J. D., Wang, J., . . . Wylie, G. R. (2011b). Changes in resting connectivity during recovery from severe traumatic brain injury. *Int J Psychophysiol, 82*(1), 115–123. doi: 10.1016/j.ijpsycho.2011.03.011

Hillered, L., Vespa, P. M., & Hovda, D. A. (2005). Translational neurochemical research in acute human brain injury: The current status and potential future for cerebral microdialysis. *J Neurotrauma, 22*(1), 3–41. doi: 10.1089/neu.2005.22.3

Jordan, B. D. (2000). Cognitive rehabilitation following traumatic brain injury. *JAMA, 283*(23), 3123–3124.

Keller, C. J., Bickel, S., Honey, C. J., Groppe, D. M., Entz, L., Craddock, R. C., . . . Mehta, A. D. (2013). Neurophysiological investigation of spontaneous correlated and anticorrelated fluctuations of the BOLD signal. *J Neurosci, 33*(15), 6333–6342. doi: 10.1523/jneurosci.4837-12.2013

Kelly, A. M., Uddin, L. Q., Biswal, B. B., Castellanos, F. X., & Milham, M. P. (2008). Competition between functional brain networks mediates behavioral variability. *NeuroImage, 39*(1), 527–537.

Kim, J., Whyte, J., Patel, S., Avants, B., Europa, E., Wang, J., . . . Detre, J. A. (2010). Resting cerebral blood flow alterations in chronic traumatic brain injury: An arterial spin labeling perfusion fMRI study. *J Neurotrauma, 27*(8), 1399–1411. doi: 10.1089/neu.2009.1215

Kim, J., Zhu, W., Chang, L., Bentler, P. M., & Ernst, T. (2007). Unified structural equation modeling approach for the analysis of multisubject, multivariate functional MRI data. *Hum Brain Mapp, 28*(2), 85–93. doi: 10.1002/hbm.20259

Maguire, E. A., Vargha-Khadem, F., & Mishkin, M. (2001). The effects of bilateral hippocampal damage on fMRI regional activations and interactions during memory retrieval. *Brain, 124*(Pt 6), 1156–1170.

Marquez de la Plata, C. D., Garces, J., Shokri Kojori, E., Grinnan, J., Krishnan, K., Pidikiti, R., . . . Diaz-Arrastia, R. (2011). Deficits in functional connectivity of hippocampal and frontal lobe circuits after traumatic axonal injury. *Arch Neurol, 68*(1), 74–84. doi: 10.1001/archneurol.2010.342

McAllister, T. W., Saykin, A. J., Flashman, L. A., Sparling, M. B., Johnson, S. C., Guerin, S. J., . . . Yanofsky, N. (1999). Brain activation during working memory 1 month after mild traumatic brain injury: A functional MRI study. *Neurology, 53*(6), 1300–1308.

McAllister, T. W., Sparling, M. B., Flashman, L. A., Guerin, S. J., Mamourian, A. C., & Saykin, A. J. (2001). Differential working memory load effects after mild traumatic brain injury. *NeuroImage, 14*(5), 1004–1012.

McIntosh, A. R., & Gonzalez-Lima, F. (1994). Structural equation modeling and its application to network analysis in functional brain imaging. *Hum Brain Mapp, 2*, 2–22.

McIntosh, A. R., Grady, C. L., Ungerleider, L. G., Haxby, J. V., Rapoport, S. I., & Horwitz, B. (1994). Network analysis of cortical visual pathways mapped with PET. *J Neurosci, 14*(2), 655–666.

Medaglia, J. D., Chiou, K. S., Slocomb, J., Fitzpatrick, N. M., Wardecker, B. M., Ramanathan, D., . . . Hillary, F. G. (2012). The less BOLD, the wiser: Support for the latent resource hypothesis after traumatic brain injury. *Hum Brain Mapp, 33*(4), 979–993. doi: 10.1002/hbm.21264

Medaglia, J. D., Ramanathan, D. M., Venkatesan, U. M., & Hillary, F. G. (2011). The challenge of non-ergodicity in network neuroscience. *Network (Bristol, England), 22*(1–4), 148–153. doi: 10.3109/09638237.2011.639604

Mennes, M., Kelly, C., Zuo, X. N., Di Martino, A., Biswal, B. B., Castellanos, F. X., & Milham, M. P. (2010). Inter-individual differences in resting-state functional connectivity predict task-induced BOLD activity. *NeuroImage, 50*(4), 1690–1701. doi: 10.1016/j.neuroimage.2010.01.002

Micheloyannis, S., Pachou, E., Stam, C. J., Vourkas, M., Erimaki, S., & Tsirka, V. (2006). Using graph theoretical analysis of multi channel EEG to evaluate the neural efficiency hypothesis. *Neurosci Lett, 402*(3), 273–277.

Milgram, S. (1967). The small world problem. *Psychology Today, 1*(1), 60–67.

Millis, S. R., Rosenthal, M., Novack, T. A., Sherer, M., Nick, T. G., Kreutzer, J. S., . . . Ricker, J. H. (2001). Long-term neuropsychological outcome after traumatic brain injury. *J Head Trauma Rehab, 16*(4), 343–355.

Molenaar, P. C. (2004). A manifesto on psychology as idiographic science: Bringing the person back into scientific psychology, this time forever. *Measurement, 2*(4), 201–218.

Molenaar, P. C. (2006). The future of dynamic factor analysis in psychology and biomedicine. *B Soc Sci Med Lux*, (2), 201–213.

Molenaar, P. C. (2008). On the implications of the classical ergodic theorems: Analysis of developmental processes has to focus on intra-individual variation. *Dev Psychobiol, 50*(1), 60–69. doi: 10.1002/dev.20262

Molenaar, P. C., Sinclair, K. O., Rovine, M. J., Ram, N., & Corneal, S. E. (2009). Analyzing developmental processes on an individual level using nonstationary time series modeling. *Dev Psychol, 45*(1), 260–271. doi: 10.1037/a0014170

Murphy, K., Birn, R. M., Handwerker, D. A., Jones, T. B., & Bandettini, P. A. (2009). The impact of global signal regression on resting state correlations: Are anti-correlated networks introduced? *NeuroImage, 44*(3), 893–905. doi: 10.1016/j.neuroimage.2008.09.036

Nakamura, T., Hillary, F. G., & Biswal, B. B. (2009). Resting network plasticity following brain injury. *PloS One, 4*(12), e8220. doi: 10.1371/journal.pone.0008220

Narayan, R. K., Michel, M. E., Ansell, B., Baethmann, A., Biegon, A., Bracken, M. B., . . . Yurkewicz, L. (2002). Clinical trials in head injury. *J Neurotrauma, 19*(5), 503–557. doi: 10.1089/089771502753754037

Newsome, M. R., Scheibel, R. S., Steinberg, J. L., Troyanskaya, M., Sharma, R. G., Rauch, R. A., . . . Levin, H. S. (2007). Working memory brain activation following severe traumatic brain injury. *Cortex, 43*(1), 95–111.

Pagulayan, K. F., Temkin, N. R., Machamer, J., & Dikmen, S. S. (2006). A longitudinal study of health-related quality of life after traumatic brain injury. *Arch Phys Med Rehab, 87*(5), 611–618.

Palacios, E. M., Sala-Llonch, R., Junque, C., Roig, T., Tormos, J. M., Bargallo, N., & Vendrell, P. (2013). Resting-state functional magnetic resonance imaging activity and connectivity and cognitive outcome in traumatic brain injury. *JAMA Neurol, 70*(7), 845–851. doi: 10.1001/jamaneurol.2013.38

Perlstein, W. M., Cole, M. A., Demery, J. A., Seignourel, P. J., Dixit, N. K., Larson, M. J., & Briggs, R. W. (2004). Parametric manipulation of working memory load in traumatic brain injury: Behavioral and neural correlates. *J Int Neuropsychol Soc, 10*(5), 724–741. doi: 10.1017/s1355617704105110

Price, C. J., Crinion, J., & Friston, K. J. (2006). Design and analysis of fMRI studies with neurologically impaired patients. *J Magn Reson Imaging, 23*(6), 816–826.

Price, C. J., & Friston, K. J. (1999). Scanning patients with tasks they can perform. *Hum Brain Mapp, 8*(2–3), 102–108. doi: 10.1002/(SICI)1097-0193(1999)8:2/3<102::AID-HBM6>3.0.CO;2-J [pii]

Price, C. J., & Friston, K. J. (2002). Functional imaging studies of neuropsychological patients: Applications and limitations. *Neurocase, 8*(5), 345–354.

Raichle, M. E. (2010). Two views of brain function. *Trends Cogn Sci, 14*(4), 180–190. doi: 10.1016/j.tics.2010.01.008

Raichle, M. E., MacLeod, A. M., Snyder, A. Z., Powers, W. J., Gusnard, D. A., & Shulman, G. L. (2001). A default mode of brain function. *P Natl Acad Sci USA, 98*(2), 676–682. doi: 10.1073/pnas.98.2.676

Raichle, M. E., & Snyder, A. Z. (2007). A default mode of brain function: A brief history of an evolving idea. *NeuroImage, 37*(4), 1083–1090; discussion 1097-1089. doi: 10.1016/j.neuroimage.2007.02.041

Rypma, B., Berger, J. S., Prabhakaran, V., Bly, B. M., Kimberg, D. Y., Biswal, B. B., & D'Esposito, M. (2006). Neural correlates of cognitive efficiency. *NeuroImage, 33*(3), 969–979. doi: 10.1016/j.neuroimage.2006.05.065

Salvador, R., Suckling, J., Coleman, M. R., Pickard, J. D., Menon, D., & Bullmore, E. (2005). Neurophysiological architecture of functional magnetic resonance images of human brain. *Cereb Cortex, 15*(9), 1332–1342. doi: 10.1093/cercor/bhi016

Sanchez-Carrion, R., Fernandez-Espejo, D., Junque, C., Falcon, C., Bargallo, N., Roig, T., . . . Vendrell, P. (2008a). A longitudinal fMRI study of working memory in severe TBI patients with diffuse axonal injury. *NeuroImage, 43*(3), 421–429.

Sanchez-Carrion, R., Vendrell Gomez, P., Junque, C., Fernandez-Espejo, D., Falcon, C., Bargallo, N., . . . Bernabeu, M. (2008b). Frontal hypoactivation on functional magnetic resonance imaging in working memory after severe diffuse traumatic brain injury. *J Neurotrauma, 25*(5), 15.

Sarty, G. E. (2007). *Computing brain activity maps from fMRI time-series images.* New York: Cambridge University Press.

Scheibel, R. S., Newsome, M. R., Steinberg, J. L., Pearson, D. A., Rauch, R. A., Mao, H., . . . Levin, H. S. (2007). Altered brain activation during cognitive control in patients with moderate to severe traumatic brain injury. *Neurorehabil Neural Repair, 21*(1), 36–45. doi: 10.1177/1545968306294730

Scheibel, R. S., Pearson, D. A., Faria, L. P., Kotrla, K. J., Aylward, E., Bachevalier, J., & Levin, H. S. (2003). An fMRI study of executive functioning after severe diffuse TBI. *Brain Injury, 17*(11), 919–930.

Scott, J. P. (2000). *Social network analysis: A handbook* (2nd ed.). Thousand Oaks, CA: Sage Publications.

Sharp, D. J., Beckmann, C. F., Greenwood, R., Kinnunen, K. M., Bonnelle, V., De Boissezon, X., . . . Leech, R. (2011). Default mode network functional and structural connectivity after traumatic brain injury. *Brain, 134*(Pt 8), 2233–2247. doi: 10.1093/brain/awr175

Smith, S. M., Miller, K. L., Salimi-Khorshidi, G., Webster, M., Beckmann, C. F., Nichols, T. E., . . . Woolrich, M. W. (2011). Network modelling methods for fMRI. *NeuroImage, 54*, 875–891.

Sporns, O. (2010). *Networks of the brain.* Cambridge, MA: MIT Press.

Stam, C. J. (2004). Functional connectivity patterns of human magnetoencephalographic recordings: a "small-world" network? *Neurosci Lett, 355,* 25–28.

Stam, C. J., Jones, B. F., Nolte, G., Breakspear, M., & Scheltens, P. (2007). Small-world networks and functional connectivity in Alzheimer's disease. *Cereb Cortex, 17*(1), 92–99.

Sylvester, J. J. (1878). Chemistry and algebra. *Nature, 17,* 284.

Turner, G. R., & Levine, B. (2008). Augmented neural activity during executive control processing following diffuse axonal injury. *Neurology, 71*(11), 812–818. doi: 10.1212/01.wnl.0000325640.18235.1c

Turner, G. R., McIntosh, A. R., & Levine, B. (2011). Prefrontal compensatory engagement in TBI is due to altered functional engagement of existing networks and not functional reorganization. *Front Sys Neurosci, 5,* 9. doi: 10.3389/fnsys.2011.00009

van den Heuvel, M. P., & Pol, H. E. H. (2010). Exploring the brain network: A review on resting-state fMRI functional connectivity. *Eur Neuropsychopharmaco, 20,* 519–534.

van den Heuvel, M. P., Stam, C. J., Boersma, M., & Pol, H. E. H. (2008). Small-world and scale-free organization of voxel-based resting-state functional connectivity in the human brain. *NeuroImage, 43,* 528–539.

Watts, D. J. (2003). *Six degrees: The science of a connected age* (Vol. 1). New York: W. W. Norton.

Watts, D. J., & Strogatz, S. H. (1998). Collective dynamics of "small-world" networks. *Nature, 393*(6684), 440–442.

Weissenbacher, A., Kasess, C., Gerstl, F., Lanzenberger, R., Moser, E., & Windischberger, C. (2009). Correlations and anticorrelations in resting-state functional connectivity MRI: A quantitative comparison of preprocessing strategies. *NeuroImage, 47*(4), 1408–1416. doi: 10.1016/j.neuroimage.2009.05.005

Weissman, D. H., Roberts, K. C., Visscher, K. M., & Woldorff, M. G. (2006). The neural bases of momentary lapses in attention. *Nat Neurosci, 9,* 971–978.

Wohlwill, J. F. (1973). *The study of behavioral development.* New York: Academic Press.

Xiong, J., Parson, L. M., Py, Y., Gao, J. H., & Fox, P. T. (1998). Abstracts (Continue in Part V). Improved inter-regional connectivity mapping by use of covariance analysis within rest condition. *P Int Soc Magn Reson Med, 1998*(S1), 201–250.

Xiong, J., Parsons, L. M., Gao, J.-H., & Fox, P. T. (1999). Interregional connectivity to primary motor cortex revealed using MRI resting state images. *Hum Brain Mapp, 8*(2–3), 151–156.

Zuo, X. N., Kelly, C., Adelstein, J. S., Klein, D. F., Castellanos, F. X., & Milham, M. P. (2010). Reliable intrinsic connectivity networks: test-retest evaluation using ICA and dual regression approach. *NeuroImage, 49*(3), 2163–2177. doi: 10.1016/j.neuroimage.2009.10.080.

8

Aberrant Brain Plasticity in Autism Spectrum Disorders

Lindsay M. Oberman, Alexander Rotenberg,
and Alvaro Pascual-Leone

Introduction

Recently the field has begun to transition from referring to "autism," or even "autism spectrum disorder," to "autism spectrum disorders" (plural). This transition has come about as a result of the acknowledgment of the enormous heterogeneity in the clinical presentations of patients with disorders within the spectrum. Autism spectrum disorders (ASD) share core symptoms in the areas of social communication as well as restricted, repetitive, and stereotyped patterns of behavior, interests, and activities (APA, 2013). However, the severity of the symptoms, the presence of comorbid symptoms (including epilepsy, sleep disturbance, gastrointestinal conditions, and others), and the underlying cause and pathophysiology may differ drastically among individuals, and thus their clinical phenotype may also vary. ASD is diagnosed based on behaviors, but the exact brain dysfunction that leads to the behavioral phenotype remains unknown.

There are a number of genetic disorders that have comorbid ASD features, including fragile X syndrome, tuberous sclerosis, neurofibromatosis, and PTEN (phosphatase and tensin homolog) macrocephaly. Additionally, a number of environmental factors and physiological responses to environment have been implicated in ASD, including prenatal infection, hypo- or hyper-reactivity to sensory stimulation, and valproate exposure (see Chaste & Leboyer, 2012, for a review). Most cases of ASD, however, are idiopathic with no identifiable cause. This has led many researchers to begin to propose larger-scale mechanistic pathologies underlying ASD, that could be affected by a number of predisposing factors. One such mechanism that has been recently proposed is the idea of aberrant plasticity.

In this chapter, we present the claim and provide supporting evidence that a number of factors and primary insults that predispose an individual to developing ASD converge on the loss of inhibitory control of excitatory synaptic plasticity. *We propose that such loss of inhibitory control leads to a shift in the synaptic plasticity threshold toward a potentiated state, inducing developmental changes in the anatomical and functional connectivity of cortical circuitry and eventually giving rise to the behavioral ASD phenotype.*

Plasticity: A Double-Edged Sword

Brain function may be best conceptualized by the notion of distributed neural networks that might be widely dispersed anatomically but are structurally interconnected, and can be functionally integrated to serve a specific behavioral role. Such neural networks are dynamically plastic. The clinical phenotype of any neurological disorder, including ASD, is not simply the result of a genetic mutation or environmental insult, but rather is the consequence of how the brain is capable of sustaining function in the context of these precursors. If confronted with a genetic or acquired insult, neural plasticity can provide adaptive compensation and thus minimize or prevent the manifestation of disease, or on the contrary, confer perceptible change in the behavioral output of the brain, leading to changes that constitute symptoms of disease.

Brain plasticity is an intrinsic property of the nervous system that allows an individual to adapt to a rapidly changing environment through strengthening, weakening, pruning, or adding of synaptic connections, and by promoting neurogenesis (Feldman, 2009; Pascual-Leone, Amedi, Fregni, & Merabet, 2005). Plasticity might be conceptualized as the balanced interplay of mechanisms promoting change and those promoting stability (so-called homeostatic plasticity). At the synaptic level, this plays out in the balance of long-term potentiation (LTP), which strengthens the connections between pre-synaptic and post-synaptic neurons, and long-term depression (LTD), which weakens these connections(Bear & Abraham, 1996; Bliss & Gardner-Medwin, 1973). The propensity of a synapse to undergo LTP or LTD relies on the influence of a number of molecular mechanisms (Kandel, 2001) as well as the current state of the synapse (whether it has undergone a plastic change in the recent past, so called metaplastic influences; Abraham, 2008; Mockett & Hulme, 2008). Plasticity can be studied at the level of the synapse with slice preparations and animal models, at the level of networks as changes in functional and anatomical connectivity arguably stemming from changes at the level of the synapse, or through behavior, captured by measures of learning, memory, and adaptation. Modifications of plasticity at any level can have far-reaching consequences at other levels of analysis.

The molecular mechanisms responsible for plasticity are complex, involving multiple cascades eventually culminating in functional and structural changes. Many models of plasticity propose the involvement of the NMDA (*N-methyl-D-aspartate*) receptor which, depending on the timing and degree of depolarization of the post-synaptic neuron, leads to subsequent synaptic LTP or LTD. This process is kept in check by regulatory forms of plasticity to avoid a situation whereby certain neurons never fire and others fire constantly. These feedback mechanisms include homeostatic synaptic scaling, whereby uniform increases or decreases in network activity over several hours or days lead to an opposing increase or decrease in excitatory synaptic strength (Turrigiano & Nelson, 2004). Metaplasticity is another feedback mechanism, where experience-dependent alterations in inhibitory tone, dendritic excitability, and NMDA receptor function alter the ability of future stimuli to drive LTP and LTD (Abraham & Bear, 1996).

It is essential to recognize, as originally pointed out by William James (James, 1890), that in plasticity there is a critical functional trade-off between adaptability and stability. While a deficit in plasticity will render the brain unable to adjust to changing demands, if the brain is too plastic or lacks appropriate homeostatic brakes, excessive environmental influence on the developing brain may also lead to dysfunction. Therefore, what is crucial is to have "the correct amount of plasticity" at a given time (Pascual-Leone, et al., 2011).

The degree and duration of experience-dependent changes to cortical function and structure are very strictly regulated. During development, there are critical periods when a specific region of cortex has heightened capacity for plasticity. The onset of these critical periods is thought to be regulated by the maturation of specific gamma-aminobutyric acid (GABAergic) neurons (parvalbumin-positive basket cells; Hensch, 2005). How these cells control plasticity is not known, but the process may involve setting a permissive excitatory-inhibitory balance or editing pyramidal cell firing patterns to promote excitatory synaptic plasticity. The regulation of these critical periods during development and the resulting control of plasticity are integral to the healthy establishment of cortical circuits. Consequently, dysfunction of critical period timing, excitatory-inhibitory imbalance, and aberrant cortical plasticity have been put forth as potential pathophysiological mechanisms underlying developmental disorders such as ASD (LeBlanc & Fagiolini, 2011; Rubenstein & Merzenich, 2003).

It should also be noted that the timing of alterations in plasticity will have differential effects on various cortical regions and therefore will result in deficits in specific domains, as the timeline for synaptogenesis is different across the cortex (Huttenlocher, 2002). Consistent with the role of altered plasticity in ASD, a disorder whose behavioral symptoms are clinically evident in early childhood, regions related to language production and social skills in the frontal and prefrontal cortex have a spike in synapse development between years 1 and 3 (Huttenlocher, 2002), when behavioral symptoms become evident in these domains in children who go on to develop ASD. Excessive excitatory plasticity during this time may lead to a disorganization in the critical balance of the development of this circuitry. Other developmental disorders may also be related to altered plasticity with exact timing, direction of alteration (potentiation vs. depression), cortical network impacted, and type of synapse (excitatory versus inhibitory) dictating the specific neurological and behavioral phenotype of the given disorder (see Oberman and Pascual-Leone, 2013, for a review).

Altered Brain Plasticity as a Model for the Physiological and Behavioral Symptoms and Comorbidities of ASD

Most investigators agree that idiopathic ASD results from a number of initiating genetic and environmental factors. These genetic-environmental interactions may lead to aberrant excitatory plasticity in different neural systems, depending on the type and timing of the expression of the genetic abnormalities and the environmental factors involved. The mechanisms by which synaptic plasticity is altered likely vary across individuals with ASD, affecting specific brain areas and systems at different times in development, and thus contributing to the known heterogeneity in behavioral phenotypes, neurological impairments, and comorbid conditions in ASD. If so, any one patient's ASD clinical phenotype might reflect *which* specific neural systems and brain areas are affected by this altered state of potentiation and *when* in development this abnormal plasticity manifests itself. Despite this heterogeneity, published data suggest that many of the identified risk factors for ASD converge on a single pathophysiological mechanism: a reduction of intracortical inhibitory tone. This reduction in inhibitory tone may have two direct consequences: first, an increase in the excitation/inhibition ratio (consistent with the model proposed by Rubenstein & Merzenich, 2003), and second, aberrant connectivity, for which there is growing evidence in ASD. Some report that ASD is a developmental "disconnection" syndrome (Geschwind & Levitt, 2007), while others suggest a paradoxical increase in connectivity leading to an excess of diffuse "noise" in the local circuit (Casanova & Trippe, 2009). A recent meta-analysis (Muller et al., 2011) suggests that this inconsistency in the literature may be driven by methodological differences. Regardless, alterations in brain connectivity in ASD seem to be a consistent finding, and a recent in vitro study found that blocking GABA synthesis leads to an increase in axonal density and complexity and a reduction in synapse pruning and elimination (Wu et al., 2012), all signs of excessive uncontrolled excitatory plasticity at the cellular level. Therefore, we argue that conceptualizing ASD as a disorder of plasticity, with altered local cortical excitation/inhibition balance and brain network functional connectivity, provides a fruitful framework for understanding both the core and comorbid symptoms of ASD, accounts for and unifies theories that have been proposed at the molecular, systems, and behavioral levels, and potentially offers a target for future interventions.

Our proposed theory implicating dysfunction of mechanisms of plasticity as the proximal cause of ASD is consistent with a number of emerging theories in the literature that implicate processes of plasticity from different levels of analysis. For example, LeBlanc & Fagiolini (2011) argue for an alteration in the expression or timing of the critical period in primary sensory brain areas. The critical period is defined by an increase in excitatory synaptic plasticity, and its initiation and closure appear to be tightly regulated by GABAergic signaling (Fagiolini et al., 2004; Hensch et al., 1998). The authors of these studies claim that the critical period may be altered in

ASD, though the exact direction of alteration (precocious or delayed, decreased or extended) may differ, depending on the particular etiology. If, as we propose in ASD, there is a lack of inhibitory control on excitatory synaptic plasticity, perhaps due to a dysfunction in the GABAergic system, then this may lead to an alteration in the critical period, as proposed by LeBlanc & Fagiolini (2011).

Another theory related to the current hypothesis was originally proposed by Rubenstein and Merzenich (2003) and argues that ASD is caused by an increased ratio of excitation/inhibition (E/I) in sensory, mnemonic, social, and emotional systems, resulting from an increase in glutamatergic signaling or a decrease in GABAergic signaling. This increased ratio of excitation/inhibition may be a cause or consequence of altered plasticity. A decrease in GABAergic signaling (a lack of inhibition), as discussed earlier, may lead to increased excitatory synaptic plasticity, which in turn may lead to increased excitation.

A third theory, proposed by Markram and colleagues (Markram & Markram, 2010), suggests a mechanism whereby the brain could become hyperexcitable, the "intense world" hypothesis. This theory suggests that the symptoms of ASD emerge as a response to the environment, which the authors argue is perceived as aversively intense by the autistic brain, which they argue is hyper-reactive. Like an E/I imbalance, hyper-reactivity may underlie, or alternatively result from, alterations in excitatory synaptic plasticity. Differing from this theory, however, we contend that the symptoms of ASD can emerge outside the influence of the proposed "aversive environment." And rather than the environment being an "intense world," it may be the internal workings of the cortex that create this hyper-reactivity.

Recent studies have also linked ASD to inflammatory processes and a dysregulation in cytokines. The underlying cause of these immune abnormalities in ASD may be a result of genetic mutations, prenatal or neonatal hypoxia, or a response to maternal immune activation when the child was *in utero* (Onore, Careaga, & Ashwood, 2012; Rossignol & Frye, 2011). In addition to their role in the immune system, many cytokines play important roles in neurodevelopment and synaptic plasticity: for example, tumor necrosis factor-α (TNF-α) and interleukin-1β (IL-1β) are thought to regulate pruning and plasticity of synapses (Deverman & Patterson, 2009). Thus, exposure to a maternal infection or an early hypoxic event may trigger developmental abnormalities in synaptic plasticity and connectivity.

Our plasticity theory does not contradict or supersede prior pioneering theories, but rather provides a developmental model explaining how pathology at the level of well-characterized synaptic processes relates to the specific clinical phenotype of ASD. We will begin by providing evidence that individuals with ASD display abnormalities in plasticity and then later describe how these specific abnormalities manifest in the behavioral symptoms displayed by individuals with ASD. The heterogeneity in the population may result from the degree and exact timing of the plasticity alteration in any given individual.

Evidence for Altered Brain Plasticity in ASD

Four lines of evidence supporting our proposal of altered plasticity in ASD come from (1) genetics and molecular neuroscience, (2) animal neurophysiology, (3) human neuroimaging and neuropathology, and (4) human noninvasive brain stimulation studies.

Genetics and Molecular Neuroscience

Most candidate genes linked to ASD code for proteins that play a role in developmental and experience-dependent plasticity. For example, BDNF (brain-derived neurotrophic factor) plays a critical role in maintenance of synaptic potentiation (Akaneya, Tsumoto, Kinoshita, & Hatanaka, 1997; Huber, Sawtell, & Bear, 1998; Jiang et al., 2001; Korte et al., 1995; Patterson et al., 1996) and has been found to be elevated in postmortem tissue of individuals with ASD, specifically, in the basal forebrain (Perry et al., 2001). Additionally, multiple studies note a reduction in GABAergic receptors (Fatemi, Folsom, Reutiman, & Thuras, 2009; Fatemi et al., 2010; Fatemi, Reutiman, Folsom, & Thuras, 2009) as well as a 50% reduction in enzymes that synthesize GABA (glutamic acid decarboxylase [GAD] 65 and 67; Fatemi et al., 2002; Yip, Soghomonian, & Blatt, 2007). These changes in the GABA system may directly contribute to altered connectivity, especially between the cerebellum and the thalamus and ultimately the cerebral cortex. This may represent a mechanism by which motor as well as cognitive behaviors may be affected in ASD (Blatt & Fatemi, 2011).

Other genes coding for molecules such as neuroligin 3 and 4 that are implicated in synaptogenesis (Jamain et al., 2003), SH3 and multiple ankyrin repeat domains 3 (SHANK3) that encodes a protein involved in dendritic development (Durand et al., 2007), and chromosome 3 open reading frame 58 (c3orf58), sodium/hydrogen exchanger isoform 9 (NHE), and protocadherin-10 (PCDH10), thought to be critically involved in synaptic development and plasticity (Durand et al., 2007; Jamain et al., 2003; Morrow et al., 2008), have all been identified as candidate genes that confer increased risk of ASD (Cook, 2001; Lamb, Moore, Bailey, & Monaco, 2000; Persico & Bourgeron, 2006). In addition, single gene disorders associated with autism implicate genes that code for proteins that play important roles in synaptic plasticity. Among these are mutations in the FMR1 (fragile X mental retardation 1) gene, which codes for the protein FMRP (fragile X mental retardation protein). FMRP normally functions as an inhibitory regulator of translation of the metabotropic glutamate receptor 5 (mGluR5; Bear et al., 2004; Laggerbauer et al., 2001; Li et al., 2001; Zhang et al., 2001;). Thus the loss of FMRP results in excessive translation of mGluR5. mGluR5 plays an integral role in the establishment of new synaptic connections (Le Be & Markram, 2006) and thus is critical to stabilizing LTD and inducing LTP; (Simonyi et al., 2005).

Other examples include mutations in TSC1 and TSC2 genes that cause tuberous sclerosis, in the neurofibromin 1 (NF1) gene that causes neurofibromatosis, and in the PTEN gene that causes PTEN macrocephaly (Dolen & Bear, 2009). Although the contributions of these genes and proteins to synaptic plasticity are incompletely described, animal models of these human single gene syndromic causes of autism predictably demonstrate increases in synaptic protein synthesis and corresponding increases in synaptic connectivity (Kelleher & Bear, 2008). These genetic findings have inspired others to propose that autism should be thought of as a "synapsopathy" (Dolen & Bear, 2009) whereby proteins that are involved in synaptic development and plasticity are affected.

Animal Models and Neurophysiology

Animal ASD models reveal abnormal plasticity mechanisms (reviewed in Tordjman et al., 2007). For example, a recent study exploring the parvalbumin (PV)-positive basket cell (a key player for critical period plasticity) in two animal models of autism (valproic acid [VPA] and neuroligin3 knock-out models) found a reduction or complete lack of PV-cells in parietal and occipital cortices (Gogolla et al., 2009), suggesting a possible molecular mechanism underlying a proposed hyperpotentiated state. When the microcircuits of these animals were investigated, their reactivity to stimulation, as measured by the number of spikes and the number of post-synaptic potentials following stimulation, was nearly twice that of wild-type animals (Rinaldi, Silberberg, & Markram, 2008). This hyper-reactivity was found in multiple regions including the somatosensory cortex (Rinaldi, Silberberg, et al., 2008), prefrontal cortex (Rinaldi, Perrodin, & Markram, 2008), and amygdala (Markram, Rinaldi, La Mendola, Sandi, & Markram, 2008), thus indicating a widespread enhancement in reactivity of cortical and subcortical neurons. Synaptic responses have also been recorded in pyramidal neurons following a Hebbian pairing stimulation protocol in these animals, and though the presynaptic response was normal, the post-synaptic cell had a more than twofold increase in response, indicating a state of hyperpotentiation (Rinaldi, Kulangara, Antoniello, & Markram, 2007). Similarly, abnormal synaptic plasticity, specifically exaggerated LTD, has also been shown in mouse models of genetic disorders associated with autism, namely the FMR1-null mouse (model for fragile X syndrome) and MECP2-null mouse (model for Rett syndrome; Dani et al., 2005; Huber, Gallagher, Warren, & Bear, 2002).

Human Neuroimaging and Neuropathology

The most consistent neuroimaging finding in humans with idiopathic autism is increased brain volume, with an overall increase in both gray and white matter volume (Courchesne et al., 2001). Furthermore, there is a distinct developmental trajectory of brain size abnormalities in ASD whereby reduced or normal brain size is present at birth, followed by a rapid rate of brain growth during early childhood. This trajectory suggests that the underlying mechanism is a dynamic process with a timeline consistent with a shift toward increased potentiation of excitatory synapses during early childhood (Courchesne & Pierce, 2005). Recent studies reveal that the overall larger brain in individuals with ASD is primarily due to larger white matter volumes, particularly in the outer "radiate" regions, including the origins and terminations of projection and sensory fibers (Herbert et al., 2004). Even when accounting for the overall greater brain volume, the proportion of white matter still is greater than normal, suggesting that abnormal axons and neural connections, rather than the neuronal cell bodies themselves, may be responsible for the abnormalities in brain structure. There is also neuropathological data in postmortem tissue supporting brain overgrowth, specifically in the prefrontal cortex (Courchesne, Campbell, & Solso, 2011) and abnormalities at the minicolumn level indicating aberrant minicolumn structure with reduced neuronal size and increased density attributable to reductions in the inhibitory peripheral neuropil space (Casanova, Buxhoeveden, Switala, & Roy, 2002). The authors suggest that this lack of inhibition would lead to gross alterations in cortical connectivity. Another common neuropathological finding in ASD is a reduction in the number of cerebellar Purkinje cells (Bauman & Kemper, 1996). Such a reduction is thought to release the deep cerebellar nuclei from inhibition, producing abnormally strong physical connectivity and potentially abnormally weak computational connectivity along the cerebello-thalamocortical circuit and, furthermore, possibly aberrant activity-dependent plasticity along this pathway (Belmonte et al., 2004).

Abnormally high and indiscriminate physical connectivity may lead to abnormally low and ineffective functional connectivity due to excessive noise and poor temporal precision secondary to activity of superfluous connections. Consistent with this assertion, structural and functional MRI studies have confirmed anatomical and functional connectivity abnormalities in individuals with ASD (for a review, see Geschwind & Levitt, 2007). The specific disconnection, however, does not appear to be simple, but rather is a complex result of interactions between local "noisy" overconnectivity, perhaps stemming from increased density of cortical minicolumns (Casanova et al., 2002), leading to a breakdown in long-distance network functioning (Rippon, Brock, Brown, & Boucher, 2007). This breakdown in long-distance networks is supported by diffusion tensor imaging (DTI) studies indicating reduced white matter integrity in individuals with ASD (Alexander et al., 2007; Cheung et al., 2009; Fletcher et al., 2010; Shukla, Keehn, & Muller, 2011). Together, these studies provide indirect evidence for aberrant connectivity in ASD, likely secondary to pathology in plasticity at the synaptic level.

Human Noninvasive Brain Stimulation Studies

The capacity to safely and noninvasively assess the mechanisms of cortical plasticity in humans has been made possible with transcranial magnetic stimulation (TMS; Hallett, 2007; Pascual-Leone et al., 2011). TMS is a noninvasive procedure based on Faraday's principle of electromagnetic induction, featuring the application of rapidly changing magnetic field pulses to the scalp via a copper wire coil connected to a stimulator (Wagner, Valero-Cabre, & Pascual-Leone, 2007). These brief pulsed magnetic fields painlessly pass through the scalp and skull and create electric currents in discrete brain regions. Applied in single TMS pulses, the induced currents are of sufficient magnitude to depolarize a small population of neurons. Trains of repeated TMS (rTMS) pulses at various stimulation frequencies and patterns can induce a lasting modification of activity in the targeted brain region, which can outlast the effects of the stimulation itself.

One rTMS protocol, theta burst stimulation (TBS), involves applying bursts of 3 pulses of TMS at 50 Hz, repeated at intervals of 200 ms, and enables characterization of mechanisms of cortical plasticity in humans in vivo. After TBS is applied to the motor cortex in an intermittent fashion (iTBS), TMS-induced potentials show increased amplitude for a period of 20–30 minutes, whereas continuous TBS (cTBS) leads to a suppression of the TMS-induced potentials for approximately the same amount of time. This modulation, induced by TBS parallels that seen in theta burst protocols used for the induction of LTP and LTD in slice preparations and animal models. Physiologic and pharmacologic studies of TBS in humans reveal involvement of glutamatergic and GABAergic mediators consistent with LTP and LTD, respectively, and the effects and their time courses are consistent with the notion that TBS does indeed index mechanisms of cortical synaptic plasticity (Cardenas-Morales, Nowak, Kammer, Wolf, & Schonfeldt-Lecuona, 2010; Huang, Chen, Rothwell, & Wen, 2007; Huang, Edwards, Rounis, Bhatia, & Rothwell, 2005). Thus, post-TBS facilitation (iTBS) and suppression (cTBS) of the cortical activity are considered to index LTP-like (iTBS) and LTD-like (cTBS) induction of synaptic plasticity in the targeted brain area (though the specific neurobiological substrates remain elusive and in need of further study).

In a recent study (Oberman et al., 2012) we used TBS paradigms to evaluate LTP-like and LTD-like plasticity in vivo in 20 adults with Asperger's syndrome (high functioning ASD), and found them to show greater and longer-lasting modulation of cortical reactivity in the motor cortex following both cTBS and iTBS as compared to age-, gender-, and IQ-matched controls. The latency to return to baseline following TBS was on average 80–90 minutes in the ASD group, compared to 25–30 minutes in the controls. This finding was confirmed in a separate cohort of 15 individuals (Oberman et al., 2012). This is consistent with the current hypothesis, as a lack of inhibitory tone would lead to a greater propensity for LTP (as demonstrated in the longer duration of modulation following iTBS). In addition, as cTBS is thought to induce changes in cortical reactivity by increasing inhibition at excitatory synapses (Di Lazzaro et al., 2005), it is not surprising that LTD-like modulation is also greater in individuals with ASD. At first glance this may seem counterintuitive; however, the propensity of a synapse to undergo potentiation or depression is dynamic and dependent on its current state of activity. The BCM model (Bienenstock, Cooper, & Munro, 1982) predicts that if the synapse is already potentiated, the threshold for LTD will be lowered and incoming stimulation will generate a stronger LTD-like response than if the synapse is in a depressed or neutral state. Thus, the dynamics of the synapse in ASD may lead to increased potential for both LTP and LTD, a very unstable state. Interestingly, consistent with other studies, there was no significant group difference in measures of basic excitability, as assessed by resting and active motor thresholds (Enticott et al., 2013; Oberman et al., 2012; Theoret et al., 2005) or response to single-pulse TMS (Enticott et al., 2011; Oberman et al., 2012). Thus, the excessive modulation of excitability in response to stimulation (a putative measure of LTD-like and LTP-like plasticity) is not primarily attributable to differences in baseline excitability (see Figure 8.1).

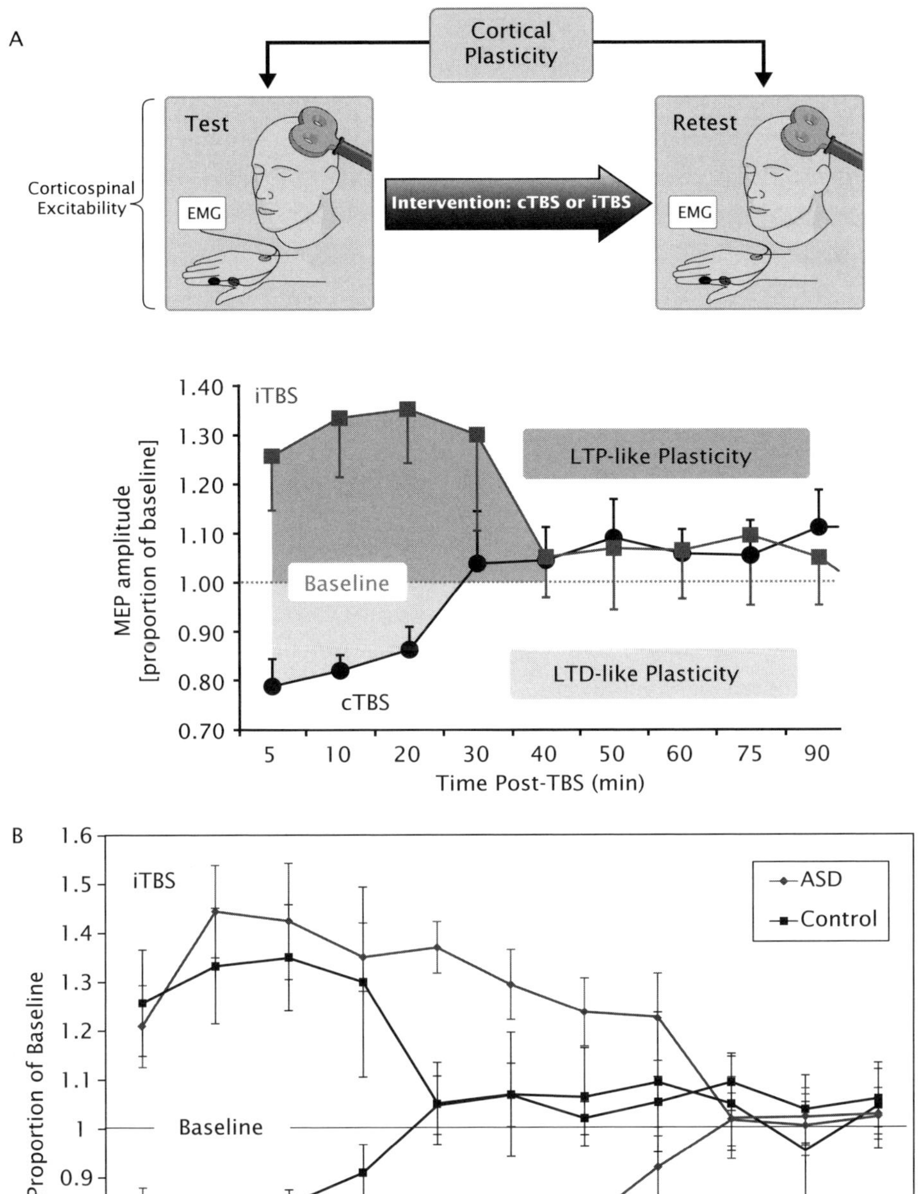

FIGURE 8.1 A. Schematic representation of TBS protocol. The amplitude of TMS-induced motor evoked potentials (MEPs) is significantly modulated by theta burst stimulation. Following TBS, there is a suppression of MEP amplitude (cTBS) and facilitation of MEP amplitude (iTBS) that in neurotypical subjects recovers back to baseline after approximately 30 min. B. Findings on measures of cortical plasticity as based on TMS-EMG method in ASD versus neurotypical controls. In adults with ASD (red) the modulation in MEP amplitude following both cTBS and iTBS lasts significantly longer than in neurotypical controls (blue).

It should be noted that the vast majority of the participants in these studies to date have been high-functioning young adults. Thus, it is unclear whether our hypothesis would be supported by experimental TMS findings in lower functioning individuals or children. These questions are currently being explored in our laboratory. Similarly, further studies are ongoing to clarify the molecular substrates of the TMS findings. Recent reports find alterations in *N*-methyl-D-aspartate (NMDA; Blundell et al., 2010; Eadie, Cushman, Kannangara, Fanselow, & Christie, 2012; Maliszewska-Cyna, Bawa, & Eubanks, 2010; Moy et al., 2008; Rinaldi et al., 2007), 2-amino-3-(3-hydroxy-5-methyl-isoxazol-4-yl) pro-panoic acid (AMPA; Purcell, Jeon, Zimmerman, Blue, & Pevsner, 2001), metabotropic glutamate (see Dolen & Bear, 2009, for a review), and GABA receptors (Fatemi, Folsom, et al., 2009; Fatemi et al., 2010; Fatemi, Reutiman, et al., 2009) in ASD: all of these receptors play critical roles in modulating reactivity at the synaptic level and all interact with one other. As the spatial resolution of TMS is at the level of millions of neurons (approximately a cubic centimeter of cortex), modulations in any combination of these neurotransmitters could be driving this effect. Translational studies with rodents and humans, combining TMS with pharmacological agents or TMS with imaging techniques such as magnetic resonance spectroscopy (MRS), may provide insight into the molecular mechanisms underlying these effects.

Accounting for Clinical Manifestation on the Basis of Altered Plasticity

The proposed theory not only aims to develop a model unifying the literature across multiple levels of analysis, but also aims to explain how alterations at the synaptic level have direct consequences on the development of cortical circuitry that in turn lead to the behavioral phenotype of ASD. Though there is an abundance of evidence of abnormalities at each of these levels, how changes at the level of the synapse generate changes at the level of functional connectivity and how those in turn lead to the specific deficits in social and communicative skills in ASD are still unanswered questions.

Despite many years of research, the exact pathology and what systems are affected in ASD remain unknown. The networks responsible for the high-level skills that are affected in the core impairments of ASD are complex and require integration of multiple, distributed brain regions. It is now well established that the pathophysiology underlying ASD is not limited to a single brain region. In this chapter we have aimed to highlight the evidence suggesting that the breakdown in functioning and integration of long-range circuits is secondary to a breakdown in the inhibitory control of excitatory synaptic plasticity on the local circuit level and a hyperpotentiated state of the synapse. This hyperpotentiated state in local microcircuits during development would be expected to lead to excessively expanded dendritic arborization, an increased number of synaptic terminals, and redundant neural connectivity. We suggest that this leads to distinct pathological consequences.

First, because of the redundant connectivity on the local level (which is supported by neuropathological evidence; Casanova et al., 2002), these local circuits may become increasingly autonomous and difficult to synchronize with other distal microcircuits, leading to reduced formation of long-range connections during development.

Despite anatomical overconnectivity, functional neuroimaging studies suggest functional underconnectivity in ASD between regions that are critical in solving a complex task, such as between inferior frontal and inferior parietal areas in sentence imagery (Kana, Keller, Cherkassky, Minshew, & Just, 2006), between dorsolateral prefrontal cortex and inferior parietal areas in problem-solving (Just, Cherkassky, Keller, Kana, & Minshew, 2007), between cingulate cortex and parietal areas in response inhibition (Kana, Keller, Minshew, & Just, 2007), and between medial/orbital prefrontal and temporoparietal areas in theory of mind tasks (Kana, Keller, Cherkassky, Minshew, & Just, 2009). Anatomical and functional underconnectivity has also been shown in the default mode network in individuals with ASD (Assaf et al., 2010; Cherkassky, Kana, Keller, & Just, 2006; Kennedy & Courchesne, 2008; Kennedy, Redcay, & Courchesne, 2006; Monk et al., 2009; Murdaugh et al., 2012). The default mode network comprises the medial prefrontal cortex, ACC, PCC, precuneus, angular gyrus, and inferior parietal lobule (Buckner, Andrews-Hanna, & Schacter, 2008). This network is said to be active during the resting state, and will deactivate for a cognitively demanding task. While resting states are task-free, such states trigger self-reflection, internally directed thought, and mentalizing, all tasks shown to be atypical in individuals with ASD (Castelli, Frith, Happe, & Frith, 2002; Frith & Happé, 1999). Dysfunction in this network has also been shown to be associated with impaired social skills and increased repetitive behaviors and restricted interests (Weng et al., 2010).

The establishment of these long-range functional networks and synchronization of signals across the cortex are particularly important for tasks that require integration of signals from multiple interconnected networks over a short temporal timescale. Thus, higher-order cognitive and social tasks may be more affected in these individuals as compared to lower-level visual-spatial tasks. Consistent with this notion, information processing in ASD appears to be intact in tasks with low cognitive demand, but it is impaired in tasks with increased cognitive demand (Luna, Doll, Hegedus, Minshew, & Sweeney, 2007). In a study involving adults with ASD, Minshew and colleagues (Minshew, Goldstein, & Siegel, 1997) found intact or even enhanced performance in certain domains, including attention, sensory perception, elementary motor ability, simple memory, formal language, rule learning, and visuospatial processing. However, they also found deficits in their participants with ASD in complex motor ability (e.g., grooved pegboard test and trail-making test), complex memory (e.g., delayed recall), complex language (e.g., metaphor and passage comprehension), and concept formation. Thus, deficits become more prominent as the complexity of the tasks increases.

In social interaction, such difficulty in rapid processing of complex stimuli can lead to unsuccessful or awkward interpersonal interactions. For example, skills such as joint attention (sharing the experience of observing an object or event using gaze or gesture) are vital in early social and cognitive development. Initiating and especially responding to joint attention requires quick processing of the object and the other people and interpreting their mental states. Skills such as interpersonal perception (Crown, 1982; Feldstein, 1982), communication of mood (Natale, 1978), empathy (Welkowitz, 1969, 1970), perceived interpersonal relatedness (Welkowitz, 1969), understanding of intentions (Baldwin, 1993; Tomasello, 1999), and theory of mind abilities (Blakemore et al., 2003) have all been shown to be particularly sensitive to very short temporal shifts and all represent fundamental cognitive deficits in ASD (APA, 2013).

Multiple studies of the temporal properties of perceptual and response systems have shown delayed and variable latencies in responses, particularly to higher level social stimuli, in individuals with ASD (McPartland, Dawson, Webb, Panagiotides, & Carver, 2004; Oberman, Winkielman, & Ramachandran, 2009; Webb, Dawson, Bernier, & Panagiotides, 2006), and the speed of such processing appears to be related to the degree of impairment in social skills (Dawson, Webb, Carver, Panagiotides, & McPartland, 2004). Processing speed can also affect problems associated with language and communication in ASD. A recent study (Oliveras-Rentas, Kenworthy, Roberson, Martin, & Wallace, 2011) found that processing speed performance on an IQ test was related to communicative symptoms and adaptive communication abilities in ASD. Speed of processing can also be critical during interpretation of figurative speech and jokes, which are commonly used in social communication. A second consequence of the hyperpotentiated state of the synapse may be related to the positive symptoms of ASD including restricted, repetitive, and stereotyped patterns of behavior, interests, and activities (APA, 2013). We suggest that hyperpotentiation of excitatory synapses underlies the formation of an excess number of synaptic terminals, which would be more sensitive to stimulation, would be more reactive, and once activated could become autonomous and difficult for top-down mechanisms to control. On a behavioral level this same autonomy of neural circuits could manifest as increased attention to a restricted domain, with difficulty breaking that attention to engage in alternative tasks (Markram & Markram, 2010). This may be mediated by the loss of inhibition that, in a healthy brain, would work against such over-reactivity. The increase in sensitivity and reactivity, paired with the loss of significant control from inhibitory innervation, may also explain the increased risk of epilepsy in this population (epilepsy affects approximately 30% of individuals with ASD as compared to less than 1% in the general population; Hirtz et al., 2007). Recent histopathological and electrophysiological data strongly suggest that the selective loss of GABAergic interneurons paired with axon sprouting and progressive formation of new recurrent excitatory circuits directly contribute to the emergence of epileptogenesis (see Dudek & Staley, 2012, for a review).

The hyperpotentiated state of the cortex and the resulting increase in synapses may also account for the anecdotal and empirical evidence for sensory hypersensitivity in individuals with ASD (Blakemore et al., 2006; Cascio et al., 2008; Grandin, 1992, 2000; Jones et al., 2003). Temple Grandin, an individual with high-functioning ASD and author of several books on her experiences of being a person with ASD, writes, "The nerve endings on my skin were supersensitive. Stimuli that were insignificant to most people were like Chinese water torture" (Grandin, 1992, page 108). Empirical studies show superior detection of high-frequency skin vibration in adults with ASD (Blakemore et al., 2006) and increased sensitivity to vibration and thermal pain in adults with ASD (Cascio et al., 2008). Relevant to the current plasticity theory, a conceptual model has been proposed suggesting an interaction between sensory thresholds (i.e., the amount of stimuli needed for the nervous system to notice or react to stimuli) and the manner in which the young child responds in relation to the thresholds (Dunn, 1997). This model suggests that when young children have low thresholds (as is suggested in ASD), neurons trigger more readily and, therefore, cause more frequent reactions to stimuli in the environment. Furthermore, under this model, children with high sensory sensitivity will engage in sensory avoidance behaviors, thus reducing unpredictable stimuli that occur during activities (making routines and rituals predictable patterns of input and responses; Dunn, 1997). Though intriguing as a theoretical model, it is not wholly consistent with the previous TMS findings suggesting typical baseline motor cortical excitability in response to single pulses of TMS. However, it is possible that lowered sensory thresholds could depend on increased sensory cortical excitability, leaving motor cortical excitability unchanged. Further research into the physiological basis of sensory sensitivity is warranted.

It is important to remember that the brain does not develop in a vacuum. The environment in which the child is placed has a great influence on developmental and learning-based plasticity. Arguably, children growing up in recent years are being exposed to an ever more diverse and stimulating environment, packed with stimuli to process from very early on. Plasticity exists to cope with a rapidly changing environment; however, for a brain in a chronic hyperpotentiated state, a very rich and over-stimulating environment may lead to excessive modification beyond what may be neurologically beneficial. In a child who has limited control over the degree of excitatory synaptic plasticity, this overly stimulating environment may lead to negative consequences. Markram and colleagues have argued along these lines in their "intense world" hypothesis (Markram & Markram, 2010). In this framework, our rich and stimulating society may be the catalyst for the increased prevalence of ASD, as it triggers the clinical relevance of otherwise relatively silent predisposing genes. If our ever more complex environment is actually triggering an increase in the prevalence of ASD, then one would expect to see a smaller increase in ASD in developing countries. In fact, a recent epidemiology network has been set up as a joint effort between Autism Speaks Foundation and the CDC to investigate this very question. No data have been published to date and there are many confounding factors that may contribute to the lower prevalence of ASD in developing countries, including, for example, access to services and cultural factors.

On the other hand, many individuals with ASD have a distinctively uneven cognitive profile, with intact and often supranormal abilities in specific domains (for example, in their understanding of physical properties and relationships; Baron-Cohen, Ashwin,

Ashwin, Tavassoli, & Chakrabarti, 2011). Altered excitatory synaptic plasticity may explain this fact also and may offer an evolutionary argument for the persistence of ASD. Though this reduction in inhibitory control of excitatory synaptic plasticity might lead to deficits in certain domains, it would also be predicted to facilitate reactivity and promote a potentially more evolutionarily adaptive cognitive style. In primary sensory cortices, for example, a hyperpotentiated state of the cortex may lead to an enhanced ability to detect changes in the environment that may have provided an evolutionary advantage in our ancestors. Another potential advantage of a hyperpotentiated state might be enhanced skill acquisition in certain domains. This may explain the fact that savantism (having an area of skill that is significantly superior relative to the other skills) is found more commonly in ASD than in any other neurological group, and the majority of people with savant skills have an ASD (Hermelin, 2002). The relationship between savantism and an evolutionary benefit of genes related to ASD is speculative at this point. Further research would be needed to empirically support such claims.

Finally, increased plasticity may also prove beneficial with increasing age, as plasticity generally shows age-related decreases that may be linked to cognitive and behavioral decline (Pascual-Leone et al., 2011). If one begins with a greater propensity for potentiation, one is less likely to become deficient in older age (Oberman & Pascual-Leone, in press). It has been suggested that increased capacity for plastic change may be related to the concept of cognitive reserve (Bartres-Faz & Arenaza-Urquijo, 2011). When age-related or neuropathological brain changes emerge in later life, this higher baseline plasticity may provide greater dynamic capacity for adjusting and remodeling cortical circuits when necessary to counteract pathological or age-related decline. Whether individuals with ASD are protected from developing age-related cognitive decline is an open question and one that is being explored in our laboratory.

Conclusions

Here we have outlined a theory for both the core symptoms and comorbidities associated with ASD. We argue that the behavioral symptoms that define ASD are a consequence of developmental abnormalities in the basic structures and functions of neural circuits as a result of a reduction in inhibitory control of excitatory synaptic plasticity. Thus, if, as we suggest, the diagnostic behavioral deficits of ASD develop as a consequence of altered plasticity, specific testable predictions can be explored. For example, if the core deficit is that of plasticity in early postnatal development, it follows that brain anatomy and physiology may be relatively free from pathology initially in life. Additionally, abnormalities in the control of plasticity of excitatory synapses would pre-date any structural or functional brain alterations or any behavioral symptom. Most important, one could design interventions aimed at modulating plasticity mechanisms that, if effective, could prevent the resulting structural and functional pathology so that the behavioral symptoms that define ASD might not have an opportunity to develop.

References

Abraham, W. C. (2008). Metaplasticity: Tuning synapses and networks for plasticity. *Nat Rev Neurosci*, *9*(5), 387.

Abraham, W. C., & Bear, M. F. (1996). Metaplasticity: The plasticity of synaptic plasticity. *Trends Neurosci*, *19*(4), 126–130.

Akaneya, Y., Tsumoto, T., Kinoshita, S., & Hatanaka, H. (1997). Brain-derived neurotrophic factor enhances long-term potentiation in rat visual cortex. *J Neurosci*, *17*(17), 6707–6716.

Alexander, A. L., Lee, J. E., Lazar, M., Boudos, R., DuBray, M. B., Oakes, T. R., et al. (2007). Diffusion tensor imaging of the corpus callosum in autism. *NeuroImage*, *34*(1), 61–73.

APA (2013). *Diagnostic and statistical manual of mental disorders* (5th ed.). Arlington, VA: American Psychiatric Publishing.

Assaf, M., Jagannathan, K., Calhoun, V. D., Miller, L., Stevens, M. C., Sahl, R., et al. (2010). Abnormal functional connectivity of default mode sub-networks in autism spectrum disorder patients. *NeuroImage*, *53*(1), 247–256.

Baldwin, D. A. (1993). Early referential understanding: Infant's ability to recognize referential acts for what they are. *Dev Psychol*, *29*, 832–843.

Baron-Cohen, S., Ashwin, E., Ashwin, C., Tavassoli, T., & Chakrabarti, B. (2011). The paradox of autism: Why does disability sometimes give rise to talent? In N. Kapur (Ed.), *The paradoxical brain* (pp. 274–288). New York: Cambridge University Press.

Bartres-Faz, D., & Arenaza-Urquijo, E. M. (2011). Structural and functional imaging correlates of cognitive and brain reserve hypotheses in healthy and pathological aging. *Brain Topogr*, *24*(3–4), 340–357.

Bauman, M., & Kemper, T. (1996). Observations of the Purkinje cells in the cerebellar vermis in autism. *Neuropath Exp Neurol*, *55*, 613.

Bear, M. F., Huber, K. M., and Warren, S.T. (2004). The mGluR theory of fragile X mental retardation. *Trends Neurosci*. 27, 370–377.

Bear, M. F., & Abraham, W. C. (1996). Long-term depression in hippocampus. *Annu Rev Neurosci*, *19*, 437–462.

Belmonte, M. K., Allen, G., Beckel-Mitchener, A., Boulanger, L. M., Carper, R. A., & Webb, S. J. (2004). Autism and abnormal development of brain connectivity. *J Neurosci*, *24*(42), 9228–9231.

Bienenstock, E. L., Cooper, L. N., & Munro, P. W. (1982). Theory for the development of neuron selectivity: Orientation specificity and binocular interaction in visual cortex. *J Neurosci*, *2*(1), 32–48.

Blakemore, S. J., Boyer, P., Pachot-Clouard, M., Meltzoff, A., Segebarth, C., & Decety, J. (2003). The detection of contingency and animacy from simple animations in the human brain. *Cereb Cortex*, *13*(8), 837–844.

Blakemore, S. J., Tavassoli, T., Calo, S., Thomas, R. M., Catmur, C., Frith, U., et al. (2006). Tactile sensitivity in Asperger syndrome. *Brain Cogn*, *61*(1), 5–13.

Blatt, G. J., & Fatemi, S. H. (2011). Alterations in GABAergic biomarkers in the autism brain: Research findings and clinical implications. *Anat Rec (Hoboken)*, *294*(10), 1646–1652.

Bliss, T. V., & Gardner-Medwin, A. R. (1973). Long-lasting potentiation of synaptic transmission in the dentate area of the unanaestetized rabbit following stimulation of the perforant path. *J Physiol*, *232*(2), 357–374.

Blundell, J., Blaiss, C. A., Etherton, M. R., Espinosa, F., Tabuchi, K., Walz, C., et al. (2010). Neuroligin-1 deletion results in impaired spatial memory and increased repetitive behavior. *J Neurosci*, *30*(6), 2115–2129.

Buckner, R. L., Andrews-Hanna, J. R., & Schacter, D. L. (2008). The brain's default network: Anatomy, function, and relevance to disease. *Ann NY Acad Sci*, *1124*, 1–38.

Cardenas-Morales, L., Nowak, D. A., Kammer, T., Wolf, R. C., & Schonfeldt-Lecuona, C. (2010). Mechanisms and applications of theta-burst rTMS on the human motor cortex. *Brain Topogr*, *22*(4), 294–306.

Casanova, M., Buxhoeveden, D. P., Switala, A. E., & Roy, E. (2002). Minicolumnar pathology in autism. *Neurology*, *58*(3), 428–432.

Casanova, M., & Trippe, J. (2009). Radial cytoarchitecture and patterns of cortical connectivity in autism. [Review]. *Philos Trans Roy Soc Lond B Biol Sci*, *364*(1522), 1433–1436.

Cascio, C., McGlone, F., Folger, S., Tannan, V., Baranek, G., Pelphrey, K. A., et al. (2008). Tactile perception in adults with autism: a multidimensional psychophysical study. *J Autism Dev Disord*, *38*(1), 127–137.

Castelli, F., Frith, C., Happe, F., & Frith, U. (2002). Autism, Asperger syndrome and brain mechanisms for the attribution of mental states to animated shapes. *Brain*, *125*(Pt 8), 1839–1849.

Chaste, P., & Leboyer, M. (2012). Autism risk factors: Genes, environment, and gene-environment interactions. *Dialogues Clin Neurosci*, *14*(3), 281–292.

Cherkassky, V. L., Kana, R. K., Keller, T. A., & Just, M. A. (2006). Functional connectivity in a baseline resting-state network in autism. *Neuroreport, 17*(16), 1687–1690.

Cheung, C., Chua, S. E., Cheung, V., Khong, P. L., Tai, K. S., Wong, T. K., et al. (2009). White matter fractional anisotrophy differences and correlates of diagnostic symptoms in autism. *J Child Psychol Psychiatry, 50*(9), 1102–1112.

Cook, E. H., Jr. (2001). Genetics of autism. *Child Adolesc Psychiatr Clin N Am, 10*(2), 333–350.

Courchesne, E., Campbell, K., & Solso, S. (2011). Brain growth across the life span in autism: Age-specific changes in anatomical pathology. *Brain Res, 1380*, 138–145.

Courchesne, E., Karns, C. M., Davis, H. R., Ziccardi, R., Carper, R. A., Tigue, Z. D., et al. (2001). Unusual brain growth patterns in early life in patients with autistic disorder: An MRI study. *Neurology, 57*(2), 245–254.

Courchesne, E., & Pierce, K. (2005). Brain overgrowth in autism during a critical time in development: Implications for frontal pyramidal neuron and interneuron development and connectivity. *Int J Dev Neurosci, 23*(2–3), 153–170.

Crown, C. L. (1982). Impression formation and the chronography of dyadic interactions. In M. Davis (Ed.), *Interaction rhythms: Periodicity in communicative behavior* (pp. 225–248). New York: Human Sciences Press.

Dani, V. S., Chang, Q., Maffei, A., Turrigiano, G. G., Jaenisch, R., & Nelson, S. B. (2005). Reduced cortical activity due to a shift in the balance between excitation and inhibition in a mouse model of Rett syndrome. *P Natl Acad Sci USA, 102*(35), 12560–12565.

Dawson, G., Webb, S. J., Carver, L., Panagiotides, H., & McPartland, J. (2004). Young children with autism show atypical brain responses to fearful versus neutral facial expressions of emotion. *Dev Sci, 7*(3), 340–359.

Deverman, B. E., & Patterson, P. H. (2009). Cytokines and CNS development. *Neuron, 64*(1), 61–78.

Di Lazzaro, V., Pilato, F., Saturno, E., Oliviero, A., Dileone, M., Mazzone, P., et al. (2005). Theta-burst repetitive transcranial magnetic stimulation suppresses specific excitatory circuits in the human motor cortex. *J Physiol, 565*(Pt 3), 945–950.

Dolen, G., & Bear, M. F. (2009). Fragile x syndrome and autism: From disease model to therapeutic targets. *J Neurodev Disord, 1*(2), 133–140.

Dudek, F. E., & Staley, K. J. (2012). The time course and circuit mechanisms of acquired epileptogenesis. In J. L. Noebels, M. Avoli, M. A. Rogawski, R. W. Olsen, and A. V. Delgado-Escuita (Eds.), *Jasper's Basic Mechanisms of Epilepsies. [Internet]. 4th edition.* Bethesda: National Center for Biotechnology Information.

Dunn, W. (1997). The impact of sensory processing abilities on the daily lieves of young children and their families: A conceptual model. *Inf Young Children, 9*, 23–35.

Durand, C. M., Betancur, C., Boeckers, T. M., Bockmann, J., Chaste, P., Fauchereau, F., et al. (2007). Mutations in the gene encoding the synaptic scaffolding protein SHANK3 are associated with autism spectrum disorders. *Nat Genet, 39*(1), 25–27.

Eadie, B. D., Cushman, J., Kannangara, T. S., Fanselow, M. S., & Christie, B. R. (2012). NMDA receptor hypofunction in the dentate gyrus and impaired context discrimination in adult Fmr1 knockout mice. *Hippocampus, 22*(2), 241–254.

Enticott, P. G., Kennedy, H. A., Rinehart, N. J., Tonge, B. J., Bradshaw, J. L., & Fitzgerald, P. B. (2013). GABAergic activity in autism spectrum disorders: An investigation of cortical inhibition via transcranial magnetic stimulation. *Neuropharmacology, 68*, 202–209.

Enticott, P. G., Kennedy, H. A., Rinehart, N. J., Tonge, B. J., Bradshaw, J. L., Taffe, J. R., et al. (2011). Mirror neuron activity associated with social impairments but not age in autism spectrum disorder. *Biol Psychiatry, 71*(5), 427–433.

Fagiolini, M., Fritschy, J. M., Low, K., Mohler, H., Rudolph, U., & Hensch, T. K. (2004). Specific GABAA circuits for visual cortical plasticity. *Science, 303*(5664), 1681–1683.

Fatemi, S. H., Folsom, T. D., Reutiman, T. J., & Thuras, P. D. (2009). Expression of GABA(B) receptors is altered in brains of subjects with autism. *Cerebellum, 8*(1), 64–69.

Fatemi, S. H., Halt, A. R., Stary, J. M., Kanodia, R., Schulz, S. C., & Realmuto, G. R. (2002). Glutamic acid decarboxylase 65 and 67 kDa proteins are reduced in autistic parietal and cerebellar cortices. *Biol Psychiatry, 52*(8), 805–810.

Fatemi, S. H., Reutiman, T. J., Folsom, T. D., Rooney, R. J., Patel, D. H., & Thuras, P. D. (2010). mRNA and protein levels for GABAAalpha4, alpha5, beta1 and GABABR1 receptors are altered in brains from subjects with autism. *J Autism Dev Disord, 40*(6), 743–750.

Fatemi, S. H., Reutiman, T. J., Folsom, T. D., & Thuras, P. D. (2009). GABA(A) receptor downregulation in brains of subjects with autism. *J Autism Dev Disord, 39*(2), 223–230.

Feldman, D. E. (2009). Synaptic mechanisms for plasticity in neocortex. *Annu Rev Neurosci, 32*, 33–55.

Feldstein, S. (1982). Impression formation in dyads: the temporal dimension. In M. Davis (Ed.), *Interaction rhythms: Periodicity in communicative behavior* (pp. 207–224). New York: Human Sciences Press.

Fletcher, P. T., Whitaker, R. T., Tao, R., DuBray, M. B., Froehlich, A., Ravichandran, C., et al. (2010). Microstructural connectivity of the arcuate fasciculus in adolescents with high-functioning autism. *NeuroImage, 51*(3), 1117–1125.

Frith, U., & Happé, F. (1999). Theory-of-mind and self-consciousness: What is it like to be autistic? *Mind Lang, 14*, 1–22.

Geschwind, D. H., & Levitt, P. (2007). Autism spectrum disorders: Developmental disconnection syndromes. *Curr Opin Neurobiol, 17*(1), 103–111.

Gogolla, N., Leblanc, J. J., Quast, K. B., Sudhof, T. C., Fagiolini, M., & Hensch, T. K. (2009). Common circuit defect of excitatory-inhibitory balance in mouse models of autism. *J Neurodev Disord, 1*(2), 172–181.

Grandin, T. (1992). An inside view of autism. In E. Schopler & G. B. Mesibov (Eds.), *High functioning individuals with autism.* New York: Plenum Press.

Grandin, T. (2000). My experiences with visual thinking, sensory problems, and communication difficulties. Available online: http://www.autism.org/temple/visual/html.

Hallett, M. (2007). Transcranial magnetic stimulation: A primer. *Neuron, 55*(2), 187–199.

Hensch, T. K. (2005). Critical period plasticity in local cortical circuits. [Review]. *Nat Rev Neurosci, 6*(11), 877–888.

Hensch, T. K., Fagiolini, M., Mataga, N., Stryker, M. P., Baekkeskov, S., & Kash, S. F. (1998). Local GABA circuit control of experience-dependent plasticity in developing visual cortex. *Science, 282*(5393), 1504–1508.

Herbert, M. R., Ziegler, D. A., Makris, N., Filipek, P. A., Kemper, T. L., Normandin, J. J., et al. (2004). Localization of white matter volume increase in autism and developmental language disorder. *Ann Neurol, 55*(4), 530–540.

Hermelin, B. (2002). *Bright splinters of the mind: A personal story of research with autistic savants.* London: Jessica Kingsley.

Hirtz, D., Thurman, D. J., Gwinn-Hardy, K., Mohamed, M., Chaudhuri, A. R., & Zalutsky, R. (2007). How common are the "common" neurologic disorders? *Neurology, 68*(5), 326–337.

Huang, Y. Z., Chen, R. S., Rothwell, J. C., & Wen, H. Y. (2007). The after-effect of human theta burst stimulation is NMDA receptor dependent. *Clin Neurophysiol, 118*(5), 1028–1032.

Huang, Y. Z., Edwards, M. J., Rounis, E., Bhatia, K. P., & Rothwell, J. C. (2005). Theta burst stimulation of the human motor cortex. *Neuron, 45*(2), 201–206.

Huber, K. M., Gallagher, S. M., Warren, S. T., & Bear, M. F. (2002). Altered synaptic plasticity in a mouse model of fragile X mental retardation. *P Natl Acad Sci USA, 99*(11), 7746–7750.

Huber, K. M., Sawtell, N. B., & Bear, M. F. (1998). Brain-derived neurotrophic factor alters the synaptic modification threshold in visual cortex. *Neuropharmacology, 37*(4–5), 571–579.

Huttenlocher, P. R. (2002). *Neural plasticity.* Cambridge, MA: Harvard University Press.

Jamain, S., Quach, H., Betancur, C., Rastam, M., Colineaux, C., Gillberg, I. C., et al. (2003). Mutations of the X-linked genes encoding neuroligins NLGN3 and NLGN4 are associated with autism. *Nat Genet, 34*(1), 27–29.

James, W. (1890). *The principles of psychology.* New York: Henry Holt.

Jiang, B., Akaneya, Y., Ohshima, M., Ichisaka, S., Hata, Y., & Tsumoto, T. (2001). Brain-derived neurotrophic factor induces long-lasting potentiation of synaptic transmission in visual cortex in vivo in young rats, but not in the adult. *Eur J Neurosci, 14*(8), 1219–1228.

Jones, R. P., Quigney, C., and Huws, J.C. (2003). First-hand accounts of sensory perceptual experiences in autism: A qualitative analysis. *J Intellect Dev Dis, 28*, 112–121.

Just, M. A., Cherkassky, V. L., Keller, T. A., Kana, R. K., & Minshew, N. J. (2007). Functional and anatomical cortical underconnectivity in autism: Evidence from an fMRI study of an executive function task and corpus callosum morphometry. *Cereb Cortex, 17*(4), 951–961.

Kana, R. K., Keller, T. A., Cherkassky, V. L., Minshew, N. J., & Just, M. A. (2006). Sentence comprehension in autism: Thinking in pictures with decreased functional connectivity. *Brain, 129*(Pt 9), 2484–2493.

Kana, R. K., Keller, T. A., Cherkassky, V. L., Minshew, N. J., & Just, M. A. (2009). Atypical frontal-posterior synchronization of Theory of Mind regions in autism during mental state attribution. *Soc Neurosci, 4*(2), 135–152.

Kana, R. K., Keller, T. A., Minshew, N. J., & Just, M. A. (2007). Inhibitory control in high-functioning autism: Decreased activation and underconnectivity in inhibition networks. *Biol Psychiatry, 62*(3), 198–206.

Kandel, E. R. (2001). The molecular biology of memory storage: A dialogue between genes and synapses. *Science, 294*(5544), 1030–1038.

Kelleher, R. J., III, & Bear, M. F. (2008). The autistic neuron: Troubled translation? *Cell, 135*(3), 401–406.

Kennedy, D. P., & Courchesne, E. (2008). The intrinsic functional organization of the brain is altered in autism. *NeuroImage, 39*(4), 1877–1885.

Kennedy, D. P., Redcay, E., & Courchesne, E. (2006). Failing to deactivate: Resting functional abnormalities in autism. *P Natl Acad Sci USA, 103*(21), 8275–8280.

Korte, M., Carroll, P., Wolf, E., Brem, G., Thoenen, H., & Bonhoeffer, T. (1995). Hippocampal long-term potentiation is impaired in mice lacking brain-derived neurotrophic factor. *P Natl Acad Sci USA, 92*(19), 8856–8860.

Laggerbauer, B., Ostareck, D., Keidel, E.M., Ostareck-Lederer, A., and Fischer, U. (2001). Evidence that fragile X mental retardation protein is a negative regulator of translation. *Hum Mol Genet, 10*, 329–338.

Lamb, J. A., Moore, J., Bailey, A., & Monaco, A. P. (2000). Autism: Recent molecular genetic advances. *Hum Mol Genet, 9*(6), 861–868.

Le Be, J. V., and Markram, H. (2006). Spontaneous and evoked synaptic rewiring in the neonatal neocortex. *P Natl Acad Sci USA, 103*, 13214–13219.

LeBlanc, J. J., & Fagiolini, M. (2011). Autism: a "critical period" disorder? *Neural Plast, 2011*, 921680.

Li, Z., Zhang, Y., Ku, L., Wilkinson, K. D., Warren, S. T., and Feng, Y. (2001). The fragile X mental retardation protein inhibits translation via interacting with mRNA. *Nucleic Acids Res, 29*, 2276–2283.

Luna, B., Doll, S. K., Hegedus, S. J., Minshew, N. J., & Sweeney, J. A. (2007). Maturation of executive function in autism. *Biol Psychiatry, 61*(4), 474–481.

Maliszewska-Cyna, E., Bawa, D., & Eubanks, J. H. (2010). Diminished prevalence but preserved synaptic distribution of N-methyl-D-aspartate receptor subunits in the methyl CpG binding protein 2(MeCP2)-null mouse brain. *Neuroscience, 168*(3), 624–632.

Markram, K., & Markram, H. (2010). The intense world theory: A unifying theory of the neurobiology of autism. *Front Hum Neurosci, 4*, 224.

Markram, K., Rinaldi, T., La Mendola, D., Sandi, C., & Markram, H. (2008). Abnormal fear conditioning and amygdala processing in an animal model of autism. *Neuropsychopharmacol, 33*(4), 901–912.

McPartland, J., Dawson, G., Webb, S. J., Panagiotides, H., & Carver, L. J. (2004). Event-related brain potentials reveal anomalies in temporal processing of faces in autism spectrum disorder. *J Child Psychol Psychiatry, 45*(7), 1235–1245.

Minshew, N. J., Goldstein, G., & Siegel, D. J. (1997). Neuropsychologic functioning in autism: Profile of a complex information processing disorder. *J Int Neuropsychol Soc, 3*(4), 303–316.

Mockett, B. G., & Hulme, S. R. (2008). Metaplasticity: New insights through electrophysiological investigations. *J Integr Neurosci, 7*(2), 315–336.

Monk, C. S., Peltier, S. J., Wiggins, J. L., Weng, S. J., Carrasco, M., Risi, S., et al. (2009). Abnormalities of intrinsic functional connectivity in autism spectrum disorders. *NeuroImage, 47*(2), 764–772.

Morrow, E. M., Yoo, S. Y., Flavell, S. W., Kim, T. K., Lin, Y., Hill, R. S., et al. (2008). Identifying autism loci and genes by tracing recent shared ancestry. *Science, 321*(5886), 218–223.

Moy, S. S., Nadler, J. J., Poe, M. D., Nonneman, R. J., Young, N. B., Koller, B. H., et al. (2008). Development of a mouse test for repetitive, restricted behaviors: relevance to autism. *Behav Brain Res, 188*(1), 178–194.

Muller, R. A., Shih, P., Keehn, B., Deyoe, J. R., Leyden, K. M., & Shukla, D. K. (2011). Underconnected, but how? A survey of functional connectivity MRI studies in autism spectrum disorders. *Cereb Cortex, 21*(10), 2233–2243.

Murdaugh, D. L., Shinkareva, S. V., Deshpande, H. R., Wang, J., Pennick, M. R., & Kana, R. K. (2012). Differential deactivation during mentalizing and classification of autism based on default mode network connectivity. *PLoS One, 7*(11), e50064.

Natale, M. (1978). Perceived empathy, warmth, and genuineness, as effected by interviewer timing of speech in a telephone interview. *Psychother, 12*, 145–152.

Oberman, L. M., Eldaief, M., Fecteau, S., Ifert-Miller, F., Tormos, J. M., & Pascual-Leone, A. (2012). Abnormal modulation of corticospinal excitability in adults with Asperger's syndrome. *Eur J Neurosci, 36*(6), 2782–2788.

Oberman, L.M., & Pascual-Leone, A. (2013). Changes in plasticity across the lifespan: Cause of disease and target for intervention. In M. Nahum, T. Vanvleet, & M. Merzenich (Eds.), *Progress in brain research: Changing brains—applying brain plasticity to advance and recover human ability.* Oxford: Elsevier Press.

Oberman, L. M., & Pascual-Leone, A. (in press). Hyperplasticity in autism spectrum disorder confers protection from Alzheimer's disease. *Medical Hypotheses.*

Oberman, L. M., Winkielman, P., & Ramachandran, V. S. (2009). Slow echo: Facial EMG evidence for the delay of spontaneous, but not voluntary, emotional mimicry in children with autism spectrum disorders. *Dev Sci, 12*(4), 510–520.

Oliveras-Rentas, R. E., Kenworthy, L., Roberson, R. B., III, Martin, A., & Wallace, G. L. (2011). WISC-IV profile in high-functioning autism spectrum disorders: Impaired processing speed is associated with increased autism communication symptoms and decreased adaptive communication abilities. *J Autism Dev Disord, 42*(5), 655–664.

Onore, C., Careaga, M., & Ashwood, P. (2012). The role of immune dysfunction in the pathophysiology of autism. *Brain Behav Immun, 26*(3), 383–392.

Pascual-Leone, A., Amedi, A., Fregni, F., & Merabet, L. B. (2005). The plastic human brain cortex. *Annu Rev Neurosci, 28,* 377–401.

Pascual-Leone, A., Freitas, C., Oberman, L., Horvath, J. C., Halko, M., Eldaief, M., et al. (2011). Characterizing brain cortical plasticity and network dynamics across the age-span in health and disease with TMS-EEG and TMS-fMRI. *Brain Topogr, 24*(3–4), 302–315.

Patterson, S. L., Abel, T., Deuel, T. A., Martin, K. C., Rose, J. C., & Kandel, E. R. (1996). Recombinant BDNF rescues deficits in basal synaptic transmission and hippocampal LTP in BDNF knockout mice. *Neuron, 16*(6), 1137–1145.

Perry, E. K., Lee, M. L., Martin-Ruiz, C. M., Court, J. A., Volsen, S. G., Merrit, J., et al. (2001). Cholinergic activity in autism: abnormalities in the cerebral cortex and basal forebrain. *Am J Psychiatry, 158*(7), 1058–1066.

Persico, A. M., & Bourgeron, T. (2006). Searching for ways out of the autism maze: Genetic, epigenetic and environmental clues. *Trends Neurosci, 29*(7), 349–358.

Purcell, A. E., Jeon, O. H., Zimmerman, A. W., Blue, M. E., & Pevsner, J. (2001). Postmortem brain abnormalities of the glutamate neurotransmitter system in autism. *Neurology, 57*(9), 1618–1628.

Rinaldi, T., Kulangara, K., Antoniello, K., & Markram, H. (2007). Elevated NMDA receptor levels and enhanced postsynaptic long-term potentiation induced by prenatal exposure to valproic acid. *P Natl Acad Sci USA, 104*(33), 13501–13506.

Rinaldi, T., Perrodin, C., & Markram, H. (2008). Hyper-connectivity and hyper-plasticity in the medial prefrontal cortex in the valproic Acid animal model of autism. *Front Neural Circuits, 2,* 4.

Rinaldi, T., Silberberg, G., & Markram, H. (2008). Hyperconnectivity of local neocortical microcircuitry induced by prenatal exposure to valproic acid. *Cereb Cortex, 18*(4), 763–770.

Rippon, G., Brock, J., Brown, C., & Boucher, J. (2007). Disordered connectivity in the autistic brain: challenges for the "new psychophysiology." *Int J Psychophysiol, 63*(2), 164–172.

Rossignol, D. A., & Frye, R. E. (2011). A review of research trends in physiological abnormalities in autism spectrum disorders: Immune dysregulation, inflammation, oxidative stress, mitochondrial dysfunction and environmental toxicant exposures. *Mol Psychiatry, 17*(4), 389–401.

Rubenstein, J. L., & Merzenich, M. M. (2003). Model of autism: Increased ratio of excitation/inhibition in key neural systems. *Genes Brain Behav, 2*(5), 255–267.

Shukla, D. K., Keehn, B., & Muller, R. A. (2011). Tract-specific analyses of diffusion tensor imaging show widespread white matter compromise in autism spectrum disorder. *J Child Psychol Psychiatry, 52*(3), 286–295.

Simonyi, A., Schachtman, T. R., and Christofferson, G. R. (2005). The role of metabotropic glutamate receptor 5 in learning and memory processes. *Drug News Perspect, 18,* 353–361.

Theoret, H., Halligan, E., Kobayashi, M., Fregni, F., Tager-Flusberg, H., & Pascual-Leone, A. (2005). Impaired motor facilitation during action observation in individuals with autism spectrum disorder. *Curr Biol, 15*(3), R84–85.

Tomasello, M. (1999). *The cultural origins of human cognition.* Cambridge, MA: Harvard University Press.

Tordjman, S., Drapier, D., Bonnot, O., Graignic, R., Fortes, S., Cohen, D., et al. (2007). Animal models relevant to schizophrenia and autism: Validity and limitations. *Behav Genet, 37*(1), 61–78.

Turrigiano, G. G., & Nelson, S. B. (2004). Homeostatic plasticity in the developing nervous system. [Review]. *Nat Rev Neurosci, 5*(2), 97–107.

Wagner, T., Valero-Cabre, A., & Pascual-Leone, A. (2007). Noninvasive human brain stimulation. *Annu Rev Biomed Eng, 9*, 527–565.

Webb, S. J., Dawson, G., Bernier, R., & Panagiotides, H. (2006). ERP evidence of atypical face processing in young children with autism. *J Autism Dev Disord, 36*(7), 881–890.

Welkowitz, J. (1969). *Dyadic interaction and induced differences in perceived similarity*. Paper presented at the 77th Annual Convention of the American Psychological Association.

Welkowitz, J. (1970). *Relation of experimentally manipulated interpersonal perception and psychological differentiation to be the temporal patterning of conversation*. Paper presented at the 78th Annual Convention of the American Psychological Association.

Weng, S. J., Wiggins, J. L., Peltier, S. J., Carrasco, M., Risi, S., Lord, C., et al. (2010). Alterations of resting state functional connectivity in the default network in adolescents with autism spectrum disorders. *Brain Res, 1313*, 202–214.

Wu, X., Fu, Y., Knott, G., Lu, J., Di Cristo, G., & Huang, Z. J. (2012). GABA signaling promotes synapse elimination and axon pruning in developing cortical inhibitory interneurons. *J Neurosci, 32*(1), 331–343.

Yip, J., Soghomonian, J. J., & Blatt, G. J. (2007). Decreased GAD67 mRNA levels in cerebellar Purkinje cells in autism: Pathophysiological implications. *Acta Neuropathol, 113*(5), 559–568.

Zhang, Y. Q., Bailey, A. M., Matthies, H.J., Renden, R. B., Smith, M. A., Speese, S. D., Rubin, G. M., and Broadie, K. (2001). Drosophila fragile X-related gene regulates the MAP1B homolog Futsch to control synaptic structure and function. *Cell 107*, 591–603.

9

Cognitive Plasticity in Healthy Older Adults, Mild Cognitive Impairment, and Alzheimer's Disease

Contributory Factors and Treatment Responses

Benjamin M. Hampstead and K. Sathian

Introduction

Aging is an unavoidable part of life that is accompanied by substantial changes in virtually all aspects of our bodies. Age-restrictive colloquialisms, such as "you can't teach an old dog new tricks," are likely founded on observations that older adults have more difficulty learning new information and on empirical evidence that "fluid" cognitive abilities (e.g., episodic learning/memory, executive functions) show substantial decline with age (see Salthouse, 2010, for a review). Such sentiments also correspond with the long-standing belief that the human brain only sheds, but does not create, neurons during one's lifetime. In reality, however, neurogenesis has been documented throughout the life span within the subventricular zone and the dentate gyrus of the hippocampus (see Braun & Jessberger, 2014, for a review). As discussed in detail later in this chapter, it is now clear that the brain remains plastic throughout the life span and even produces neuroplastic responses in the setting of degenerative diseases, such as Alzheimer's disease (AD). The critical question is whether the observed neuroplastic changes are adaptive or maladaptive in nature and whether they are amenable to external interventions.

This chapter integrates evidence from both structural and functional neuroimaging research to describe the neuroplastic changes that occur during "normal" aging, as well as the changes that occur during the pathological states of mild cognitive impairment (MCI) and AD. We will generally limit our focus to the cognitive domains of explicit learning and memory, as well as executive functioning, given the often highly interactive and even interdependent nature of these skills. As will be seen, age- and disease-related changes are evident within the brain networks mediating these particular cognitive abilities.

Defining the Populations

As noted, we discuss three primary groups of older adults throughout the chapter: cognitively intact, MCI, and AD. Cognitively intact older adults are generally defined as those whose neuropsychological functioning falls within normal limits on standardized testing. These individuals are also fully independent in everyday life. The diagnosis of AD lies at the other end of this spectrum as patients demonstrate progressive cognitive decline that affects multiple cognitive domains (McKhann et al., 2011). Learning and memory are typically the most severely affected domains, while impairments in executive functioning, language, and visuospatial abilities are also common. These patients demonstrate functional decline, with instrumental activities of daily living (i.e., more complex tasks like managing bills, appointments, cooking) typically affected before more basic activities (e.g., grooming, dressing, hygiene). While the characteristics of these two groups are quite clearly defined, conceptualization of MCI as an entity has evolved and therefore warrants closer discussion.

Identifying those at risk of converting to AD while they are still relatively early in the disease course provides a window of opportunity for treatments aimed at delaying progression or otherwise modifying the course of the disease. Petersen and colleagues coined the term "mild cognitive impairment" over a decade ago (Petersen, 2004; Petersen et al., 1999), and the National Institute on Aging and the Alzheimer's Association (Albert et al., 2011) recently accepted the diagnosis of MCI as a pre-AD state. Because multiple age-related conditions can cause cognitive impairment, the diagnostic criteria specify guidelines for establishing MCI that are consistent with underlying Alzheimer's pathology. These patients present with (1) subjective complaints of progressive cognitive decline (via self- or informant report), especially in the areas of learning and memory; (2) objective evidence of cognitive impairment (via neuropsychological testing); and (3) intact activities of daily living. Learning and memory deficits are the most common presenting problems (Albert et al., 2011; Petersen, 2004), and are associated with medial temporal lobe atrophy and hippocampal dysfunction (Jack, 2012). This combination of cognitive and atrophic changes was previously referred to as amnestic MCI (Petersen, 2004). Additional cognitive deficits may be evident (e.g., executive functioning, language, visuospatial abilities), depending on when the patient presents clinically (i.e., additional deficits are typically evident later in the disease course as patients progress toward AD). Importantly, the diagnosis of MCI specifies that the cognitive deficits cannot be accounted for by vascular, traumatic, or other medical conditions (Albert et al., 2011). Approximately 8% of individuals over age 70 likely meet criteria for MCI (Ferri et al., 2005), and nearly 80% of those diagnosed with MCI will convert to dementia within 6 years (Petersen, 2004). Such findings are consonant with evidence of high rates of cerebral beta-amyloid ($A\beta$) and neurofibrillary tau (both characteristic of AD) in patients with MCI (see Jack, 2012).

In order to appreciate the neuroplastic changes affecting cognition during "healthy" aging, MCI, and AD, it is first necessary to briefly review the neuroanatomy of "normal" learning and memory.

"Normal" Memory Processing

Thousands of empirical research papers have examined the way in which memories are encoded and retrieved, so a full review is beyond the scope of this chapter. Two general findings have emerged that are central to the thesis of this chapter. First, medial temporal lobe (MTL) structures, especially the hippocampus, are vital for forming new memories (Squire & Zola, 1996). An important caveat is that this region primarily mediates explicit (i.e., declarative) rather than implicit (i.e., procedural or habit) memory.[1] Classic examples of this distinction come from amnestic patients, including H. M., who retained the ability to learn and perform tasks dependent on implicit memory, despite the substantial bilateral MTL damage that led to severe explicit memory deficits (see Milner, Squire, & Kandel, 1998, for a review). Thus, our primary focus will be on changes in explicit memory as a function of age and disease (defined here as MCI and AD). Although information can be learned through both active (i.e., intentional) and passive (i.e., incidental) mechanisms, it has long been known that intentional encoding that enhances the depth of processing through "top-down" cognitive control mechanisms facilities learning and memory (Craik & Lockhart, 1972). Such knowledge contributes to the second general finding, which is that this core MTL memory system closely interacts with other brain regions/networks during encoding and retrieval. For instance, the lateral prefrontal cortex (PFC) is known to mediate cognitive control mechanisms like working memory (Baddeley, 2003), task coordination, and interference control (Derrfuss, Brass, & von Cramon, 2004). Such abilities are undoubtedly necessary during intentional learning and memory. It is therefore not surprising that functional neuroimaging meta-analyses have revealed activation of both the lateral PFC and hippocampus during trials in which stimuli are successfully encoded (Spaniol et al., 2009).

---

1. It is worthwhile to note that there is now a reasonable body of evidence that the hippocampus also contributes to implicit forms of memory, although this point remains controversial (see Hannula & Greene, 2012, for a review).

Age- and Disease-Related Cognitive and Structural Changes

It is now well established that cognitive abilities like processing speed, executive functioning, and explicit memory decline with age, whereas over-learned abilities (e.g., vocabulary) remain relatively stable (see Salthouse, 2010, for a review).[2] Age-related structural changes in the brain are also widely reported and are observed in areas typically associated with the above noted cognitive abilities. For example, PFC and hippocampal volumes are inversely associated with age, and appear to demonstrate decline over a 5-year follow-up (Rodriguez & Raz, 2004). Similarly, atrophic change occurs around the major cerebral sulci over a 2-year period in healthy older adults, particularly the superior frontal sulcus—presumably reflecting atrophy of the superior and dorsolateral PFC (Liu, Sachdev, et al., 2013). In addition to these "normal" age-related changes, MCI patients demonstrated an accelerated rate of sulcal widening in this study. Dickerson and colleagues (2009) have demonstrated that a specific pattern of cortical thinning is highly reproducible in AD and, therefore, can be considered one of its key characteristics. This thinning occurs bilaterally in the rostral medial temporal lobes, inferior temporal gyrus, temporal pole, angular and supramarginal gyri, superior parietal lobule, precuneus, and both the inferior and superior frontal gyri.

As would be expected with age- and disease-related changes in learning and memory, the MTL also shows substantial change. Small and colleagues (2011) posited that "normal" aging preferentially targets the dentate gyrus subregion of the hippocampus, which is the only site of hippocampal neurogenesis. Conversely, AD has long been known to preferentially target the entorhinal cortex (Brodmann's area 28) during the earliest stages—which is meaningful since this region is considered the "gateway" between the rest of the neocortex and hippocampus (see De Lacoste & White, 1993; Small et al., 2011). In fact, the entorhinal cortex receives dense inputs from multiple limbic, neocortical, and thalamic (midline nuclei) structures. In turn, it projects to hippocampal subregions via the perforant pathway, as well as to the amygdala, basal forebrain, and multiple neocortical regions, including the parahippocampal gyrus (De Lacoste & White, 1993; Kandel, Schwartz, & Jessell, 2000). Longitudinal studies have supported the importance of the entorhinal cortex in anterograde learning and memory as atrophic changes are related to memory decline over 2–5-year time frames in older adults (McDonald et al., 2012; Rodrigue & Raz, 2004). AD-related changes are also found in the parahippocampal gyrus, which projects to the hippocampus and has reciprocal connections with the entorhinal cortex and other neocortical regions (see De Lacoste & White, 1993). As discussed in the next section, these structural changes are often accompanied by functional alterations during task performance.

---

2. While this is an accepted finding, it is now clear that a sizable proportion of cognitively "healthy" older adults demonstrate pathologic levels of beta-amyloid and tau; associated changes are discussed later.

Hippocampal Activation

Given the well-documented pathological changes in the MTL described above, it would be reasonable to conclude that functional neuroimaging studies would reveal dysfunction, as measured by hypoactivation, within the MTL of MCI patients. Indeed, this appears to be the case. For instance, a recent functional magnetic resonance imaging (fMRI) meta-analysis revealed consistent hypoactivation in an MTL region that centered on Brodmann's area 28, which includes the entorhinal cortex, and appeared to extend into the hippocampus (Browndyke et al., 2013). Several studies have also reported encoding-related hypoactivation in the hippocampi of those with MCI relative to healthy controls (Hampstead et al., 2011a; Johnson et al., 2004; Machulda et al., 2003, 2009; Petrella et al., 2007). Thus, there is a sizable body of work indicating that the MTL memory system is, in fact, dysfunctional by the time individuals become cognitively symptomatic (i.e., MCI).

Interestingly, however, Browndyke and colleagues' (2013) meta-analysis also found an area of consistent hyperactivation in the MCI group that was centered in the right parahippocampal gyrus (BA 35). This raises the possibility that activity in this region is upregulated in order to compensate for dysfunction in other MTL regions; this possibility is supported by previous research findings. For example, Dickerson and Sperling (2008) proposed an inverse U model of hippocampal functioning (as measured by the fMRI-measured blood oxygen level dependent [BOLD] signal relative to cognitively healthy controls) wherein less impaired MCI patients demonstrate a hyperactive pattern that gradually declines toward hypoactivation as patients progress toward AD. Several subsequent studies have supported this model and have suggested that initial hyperactivation is a harbinger of cognitive decline over a 2-year follow-up (O'Brien et al., 2010). Putcha and colleagues (2011) found that encoding-related hippocampal hyperactivation in MCI patients was inversely related to the thickness of neocortical regions included in the characteristic AD pattern of thinning shown by Dickerson and colleagues (2009). Together, these findings suggest that the hippocampus and associated neocortical regions attempt to compensate for early structural, and presumably functional, decline in the more extended memory network.

We examined this inverse U model during a recent fMRI study in which healthy older adults and patients with MCI encoded object-location associations (OLA) (Hampstead et al., 2011a). Among the advantages of this OLA paradigm are that associative memory is dependent on the MTL memory system (Mayes et al., 2007; Postma et al., 2008) and that the task holds ecological relevance since many patients complain of misplacing objects. Importantly, brain volumes (including MTL regions) were comparable between groups, and we included only correctly encoded trials in the fMRI analyses in order to avoid confounding encoding success with unsuccessful attempts. Our primary between-group contrasts revealed hippocampal *hypo*activation in the MCI patients relative to controls. We then examined the magnitude of the BOLD signal relative to two measures of disease severity: hippocampal volumes and the total score on the Repeatable Battery for Neuropsychological Status (RBANS). As seen in Figure 9.1, only the healthy control group demonstrated significant and positive relationships between right hippocampal BOLD signal and both volume and the RBANS. While a potential inverse relationship emerged between BOLD and volume in the left hippocampus of the MCI group, it fell short of statistical significance (possibly due to our sample size). No other relationship even approached significance in the MCI group. The combination of our results and those of other groups (Johnson et al., 2004; Machulda et al., 2003, 2009; Petrella et al., 2007) indicates that the inverse U model is not universally supported.

An interesting pattern emerged, however, when we examined the relationship between BOLD signal and performance on our OLA task. Activation in the body of the left hippocampus was related to performance in the healthy control group and may reflect the associative and episodic aspects of the task, as proposed by Postma et al. (2008). The MCI group also demonstrated a positive relationship between performance and activation in the left hippocampus, but in the posterior region (i.e., tail). This finding is intriguing, given the possible anterior to posterior pattern of hippocampal atrophy in MCI (Apostolova, Mosconi, et al., 2010; Apostolova, Thompson, et al., 2010), since

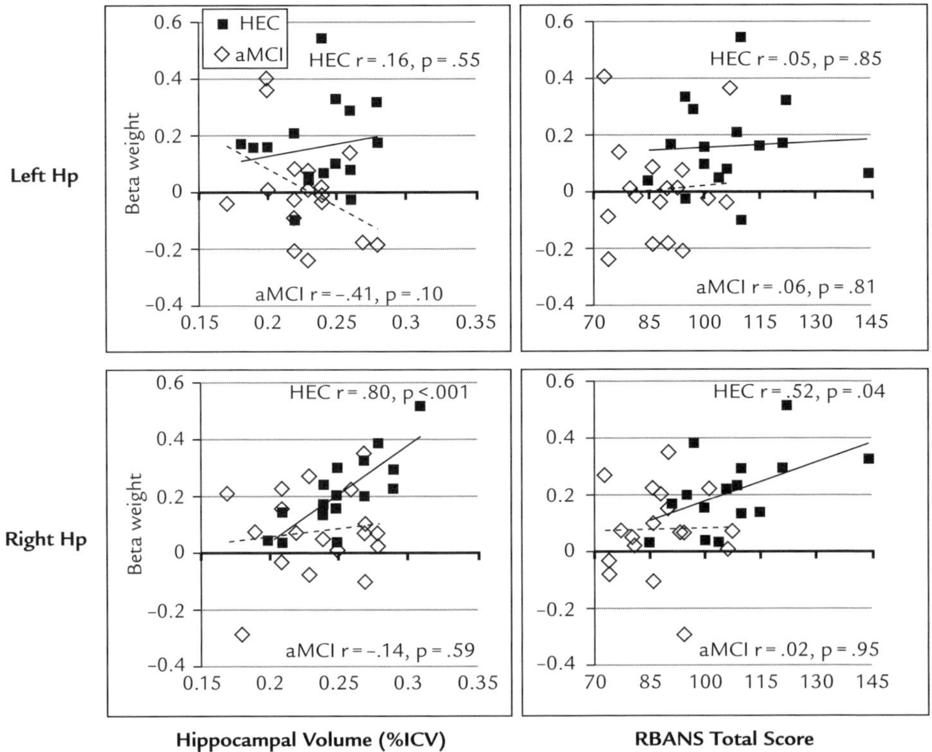

FIGURE 9.1 Relationship between average hippocampal beta-weights and hippocampal volume (left) and RBANS Total Score (right). From Hampstead et al. (2011a). *Neuropsychologia, 49,* 2349–2361.

it suggests that patients adaptively utilized relatively preserved portions of the hippocampus to maximize task performance. As discussed in the final section of this chapter, however, we demonstrated increased activation in the left hippocampal body of MCI patients who received mnemonic strategy training. This finding raises the possibility that the patients' initial approach to learning the OLAs was suboptimal and that enhancing "top-down" control re-engaged age-appropriate regions of the hippocampus, a possibility further supported by the marked increases in concomitant PFC activation (see discussion later in this chapter).

Several studies have indicated that genetic factors are also important to consider when identifying disease-related changes in activation of the hippocampus (and other parts of the MTL). To date, the apolipoprotein E ε4 allele is the single best genetic predictor of late-onset AD. In fact, compared to those with the neutral ε3 allele, ε4 heterozygotes are 4 times as likely to develop AD while ε4 homozygotes are 15 times more likely (Ashford & Mortimer, 2002). Thus, examining cognitive and neural differences between ε4 carriers versus non-carriers may provide critical information about early neuroplastic change during task performance. Unfortunately, a recent meta-analysis failed to resolve this issue as it revealed evidence of both hyper- and hypo activation in ε4 positive versus negative individuals (Trachtenberg, Filippini, & Mackay, 2012). However, Filippini and colleagues (2011) reported an ε4–by-age interaction in which the hippocampus and other regions are hyperactive in young carriers but hypoactive in older carriers relative to age-matched non-carriers. Similarly, genetic studies of early onset familial AD have revealed that individuals with the presenilin-1 (PS1) mutation become symptomatic in their mid-forties. As a result, studying a group with this mutation avoids age-related confounds that could affect neuropsychological and neuroimaging findings. Consistent with the ε4 data, PS1 positive individuals in their thirties showed greater hippocampal activation during encoding than did the PS1 negative group, who were also in their thirties (Quiroz et al., 2010). Importantly, these between-group differences were evident despite comparable neuropsychological performances and hippocampal volumes. Such findings raise the possibility of early compensatory changes in those who are genetically susceptible to developing AD.

Taken as a whole, there is evidence that individuals who are at risk of developing AD demonstrate structural and functional changes within the hippocampus and other regions of the MTL memory system; however, it appears likely that at least a subset of these individuals show some degree of adaptive reliance on relatively preserved portions of this network. As discussed below, "normal" age-related changes in the structure and function of the MTL memory system may be mitigated by increased reliance on the lateral PFC. However, this process appears to reverse in patients with MCI, raising the possibility that a loss of prefrontally mediated cognitive control interacts with MTL dysfunction and contributes to the clinically significant memory impairment that characterizes MCI.

Evidence of Neuroplasticity in Healthy Aging

By the early 2000s, functional neuroimaging research had consistently revealed significant differences in the patterns of activation in healthy young and older adults. For example, there is a well-described increase in PFC activation that appears to come at the expense of activation in posterior neocortical regions (Davis et al., 2008). Such increased PFC activation is generally independent of modality (i.e., verbal vs. visuospatial), and is evident across tasks of explicit (both episodic and semantic) learning and memory, working memory, and inhibitory control (Cabeza, 2002). Given the structural changes noted earlier, it would be reasonable to assume that older adults simply showed a pattern of reduced activation. The opposite is true, however, as older adults can demonstrate bilateral prefrontal activation during tasks on which young adults showed a unilateral pattern. This finding is described by a model termed "hemispheric asymmetry reduction in old age" (HAROLD; see Cabeza, 2002).

The functional implications of the HAROLD effect center on two primary possibilities. First, the de-differentiation view holds that the additional activation is simply a byproduct of the aging process and plays no specific role in cognition. This view was based on the notion that age-related decline in catecholamines reduces the signal-to-noise ratio in neuronal activity, thereby leading to greater "noise" in the aging brain (Li & Lindenberger, 1999). While this view may be true for some cognitive or motor processes, the evidence presented later in this chapter indicates that this explanation fails to fully account for all of the available data, especially for executive and memory related abilities.

The second interpretation of HAROLD is that the additional activation allows older adults to maximize cognitive performance. It is worthwhile to acknowledge a more recent model, termed "compensatory-related utilization of neural circuits" (CRUNCH), which holds that older adults respond to increased task demands by recruiting additional brain regions in a compensatory manner (Reuter-Lorenz & Cappell, 2008). However, CRUNCH posits that the magnitude/extent of recruitment will eventually reach a biologically defined limit that demarcates maximal cognitive performance (see Mattay et al., 2006, for an example). Because these newly recruited brain regions are associated with a given cognitive task, this compensatory response is not limited to the contralateral PFC—as implied by the HAROLD model. Rather, the individual may recruit any brain region that contributes to performance (e.g., recruiting additional language-processing areas during a verbal encoding paradigm). Cross-paradigm evidence supporting CRUNCH as opposed to HAROLD is presented elsewhere (Berlingeri, Danelli, Bottini, Sberna, & Paulesu, 2013). The critical feature of both models as they relate to the current chapter is the presence of adaptive neuroplastic change that presumably allows cognitively intact older adults to maximize their performance. Within this context, it is worthwhile to note the importance of understanding the mechanisms that govern such compensatory recruitment (e.g., redundancy, substitution), which are discussed in detail elsewhere in this volume (see Chapter 2 by Tracy, Pustina, Doucet, & Osipowicz).

This general compensatory view is supported by research showing a relationship between cognitive performance and additional prefrontal activation. For example, Reuter-Lorenz and colleagues (2000) reported faster performances during a verbal working memory task in older adults showing bilateral PFC activation relative to those who did not. Cabeza and colleagues (2002) further investigated whether bilateral PFC activation was beneficial using a source memory task. Importantly, the investigators grouped older adults based on performance (i.e., low performing vs. high performing) and compared the patterns of activation between these groups as well as with a healthy young control group. As expected, the healthy young group demonstrated a unilateral pattern of PFC activation. The low-performing older adults showed a local expansion of this unilateral pattern (i.e., the topographical extent of the PFC activation was greater than in the young group). Only the high-performing older adults demonstrated a bilateral pattern of activation, thereby supporting the adaptive function of the contralateral PFC. A relatively recent fMRI meta-analysis examined age-related differences in activation across cognitive tasks (e.g., executive functions, encoding, retrieval, perception; Spreng, Wojtowicz, & Grady, 2010). Across all domains, the results revealed significantly greater activation in the ventrolateral and dorsolateral PFC bilaterally in older relative to younger adults. However, subsequent analyses revealed left PFC hyperactivation in the older adults when task performance was equivalent, whereas right PFC hyperactivation was evident when older adults performed worse than the young. This finding suggests that older adults disproportionately recruit the right PFC when performing a cognitively demanding task and is especially interesting within the context of additional right PFC activation in other clinical populations.

Other studies have reported increased functional connectivity between the PFC and MTL memory system that may be compensatory in nature. For example, Dennis and colleagues (2008) examined the effects of age on the successful encoding of items (i.e., faces or scenes) and associative memories (i.e., particular face-scene combinations). Older adults demonstrated greater dorsolateral PFC activation during scene encoding, whereas young adults showed greater PFC activation during face and associative encoding. The authors then used a hippocampal seed region to examine differences in functional connectivity between the groups. Young adults showed greater connectivity between the hippocampus and posterior/inferior brain regions that are involved in perceptual processing, whereas the older group showed greater connectivity between the hippocampus and multiple PFC regions, especially the ventrolateral PFC. Other connectivity studies have essentially replicated these results. For example, healthy young adults demonstrated greater activation in general during scene encoding when compared with amyloid-negative healthy older adults (as measured through positron emission tomographic [PET] scanning with Pittsburgh imaging compound B, an amyloid-specific tracer; Oh & Jagust, 2013). However, the older adults demonstrated significantly greater connectivity between the parahippocampal gyrus (a region that is known to be critical for scene processing/encoding) and a number of brain regions, including the ventrolateral prefrontal cortex. Taken together, these findings indicate that older adults attempt to encode information in a different way than do the young, with seemingly increased reliance on brain regions that mediate aspects of cognitive control.

Together, the studies described above suggest that increased activation and connectivity of the PFC play an adaptive role in cognitive aging during memory and executive tasks. A potential limitation of these studies is their observational nature—meaning that neither cognition nor the underlying brain regions were directly manipulated. In this respect, studies using non-invasive brain stimulation, such as transcranial magnetic stimulation (TMS), may prove especially valuable given their ability to transiently excite (high frequency) or suppress (low frequency) a targeted brain region. A recent study used high frequency (20Hz) repetitive TMS (rTMS) to specifically investigate the hemispheric contributions of the PFC to memory encoding and retrieval (Manenti, Cotelli, & Minussi, 2011). In this study, older adults completed a verbal paired associates task in which they learned either related or unrelated word pairs—the latter of which is more cognitively demanding and of particular interest given the known importance of the MTL memory system in this process (see Mayes, Montaldi, & Migo, 2007, for a review). Stimulus presentation was time-locked with excitatory rTMS to either the left or right dorsolateral PFC. To examine the effects of stimulation, participants were grouped based on their task performance during a baseline condition (i.e., high vs. low performing). During encoding, rTMS to the right PFC improved subsequent memory for the unrelated pairs (77% correct), but only in the low-performing group (no effects were found in the high-performing group). Critically, performance after left PFC stimulation was comparable to a sham control condition in this group (64% vs. 68.5%, respectively). These findings indicate that low-performing older adults failed to spontaneously recruit the right PFC, instead relying on a unilateral (left hemisphere) approach. These TMS findings are consonant with the HAROLD/CRUNCH models presented earlier and again reinforce that recruitment of bilateral PFC can be an adaptive response to cognitive brain aging.

Further Neuroplastic Change in MCI and AD

There is now a substantial body of evidence indicating neuroplastic change in those with MCI, though it is unclear whether such change represents an adaptive and/or maladaptive response to a compromised brain. In addition to the MTL changes reported earlier, Browndyke and colleagues' (2013) recent meta-analysis revealed significantly less activation in the left ventrolateral PFC of MCI patients relative to controls. This finding is meaningful within the context of the above literature, as well as findings that the left ventrolateral PFC plays an important role in memory encoding (Köhler, 2004; Kuhl, Bainbridge, & Chun, 2012; Spaniol et al., 2009). Again, these findings raise the possibility that memory dysfunction in MCI arises following dysfunction of PFC regions that adaptively respond to aging.

In addition to the hippocampal hypoactivation discussed earlier, we found evidence of widespread neocortical dysfunction, relative to controls, as MCI patients encoded OLAs (Hampstead et al., 2011a). To appreciate the particular areas showing dysfunction, it is useful to consider Postma and colleagues' (2008) model in which each major cognitive process is preferentially mediated by a particular brain region/network. Specifically, the ventral visual stream mediates object identification, while the dorsal visual stream mediates spatial information. This information is held in mind via the lateral frontoparietal network, which mediates working memory until it is bound into a "long-term" memory by the hippocampus. Given this model, our primary question was whether MCI patients demonstrated dysfunction that was limited to the MTL memory system or if it was more widespread. Not surprisingly, controls remembered significantly more of the OLAs than did patients. Therefore, we included only correctly encoded trials in the primary analysis in order to eliminate any activation that may be associated with an unsuccessful attempt. Both groups demonstrated significant activation in each of the proposed regions; however, the magnitude and extent of activation was significantly greater in the control participants in virtually every region (see Figure 9.1). Although the MCI patients showed greater activation in the left precuneus, supramarginal gyrus, and angular gyrus, these differences were due to less negative BOLD signal in the patients relative to controls and therefore cannot be considered true hyperactivation.[3]

These results indicate that widespread dysfunction in the form of hypoactivation underlies reduced OLA memory in those with MCI. A primary limitation of standard contrast-based analyses is that they do not necessarily reflect the brain regions associated with successful task performance. Therefore, we performed whole-brain correlations between activation and behavioral performance on the OLA task. The control group again demonstrated correlated activation within each of the networks proposed by Postma et al. (2008). However, correlated activation in the MCI patients was largely restricted to the primary motor and somatosensory cortices (Figure 9.2). These results led us to conclude that patients are approaching the task in a fundamentally different way than are the controls, potentially by relying more on the physical and motor aspects of a given object. If true, then this maladaptive shift occurs at the expense of the seemingly adaptive increased top-down control mediated by the PFC that characterizes healthy aging.

To directly assess this possibility, we recently completed a series of effective connectivity analyses, using Granger causality analysis, to examine whether the co-activated areas in controls and MCI patients were, in fact, interacting differently during trials in which stimuli were successfully encoded (Hampstead et al., in preparation). In selecting the brain regions for connectivity analysis, we first performed a conjunction analysis of brain regions activated during successful encoding trials in both groups. We then selected approximately 50 areas and examined the patterns of intra- and interhemispheric

---

3. It is unclear whether the hyperactivation in MCI reported in previous studies is due to greater positive or simply less negative BOLD signal.

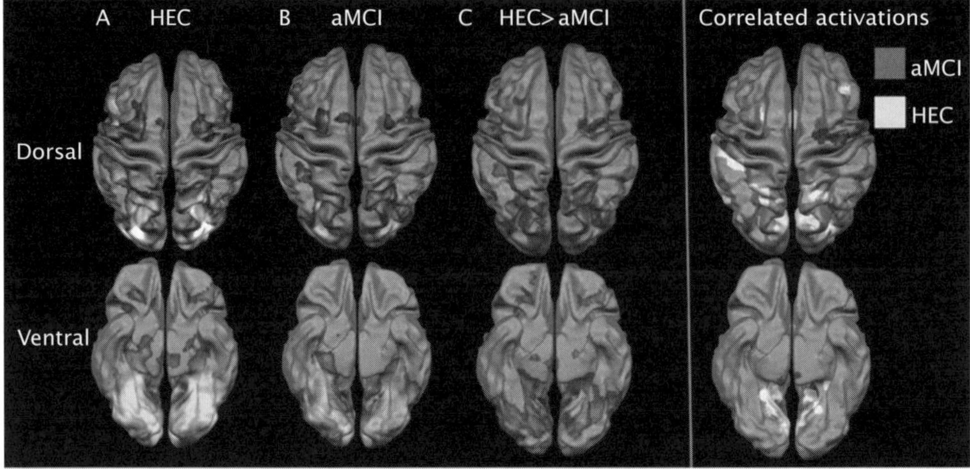

FIGURE 9.2 Patterns of activation during object-location association encoding using standard contrast analyses (columns a, b, c). The right most column shows activation that was significantly related to performance on the object-location task. HEC = healthy elderly controls; aMCI = amnestic mild cognitive impairment. Modified from Hampstead et al. (2011a). *Neuropsychologia*, *49*, 2349–2361. (see color insert)

connectivity within each group. The results were striking. Healthy controls relied on three primary brain regions in the left hemisphere that drove activity in other areas, findings that support the importance of the left hemisphere during encoding (Nyberg, Cabeza, & Tulving, 1996). Two of these areas (the inferior frontal junction and the intraparietal sulcus) are known to be involved in cognitive control and working memory, while the third (posterior cingulate cortex) is highly connected to the MTL memory system. In contrast, two regions emerged as drivers in the MCI patients, with the left posterior cingulate being the weaker of the two. The right frontal eye field (FEF) was the most robust, as it drove activation in several right hemisphere regions and virtually every left hemisphere region selected. The FEFs are known to be involved in eye movements and attentional saccades, the latter of which raises the possibility that patients were using more basic attentional processes at the expense of cognitive control mechanisms. Alternatively, these findings may suggest that patients are forced to exert additional attentional resources to optimize task performance. In either case, the combination of the correlated activations and effective connectivity results clearly indicate that MCI patients were processing information far differently than were the controls. These findings are especially important within the context of treatment-induced neuroplastic changes that are discussed later in this chapter.

Other groups have also demonstrated altered connectivity in MCI patients during encoding. For example, Protzner and colleagues (2011) found that both MCI patients and healthy controls activated a common set of brain regions during encoding, similar to those found in our study (Hampstead et al., 2011a) and in meta-analyses (Spaniol et al., 2009). While activation of this network facilitated subsequent memory in the controls, it was unrelated to memory test performance in the MCI patients. Instead, MCI patients became increasingly reliant on the left inferior temporal gyrus that appeared to be a critical "hub" within a modified encoding network that was positively related to memory test performance. This inferior temporal region is known to receive direct projections from the posterior parahippocampal gyrus (De Lacoste et al., 1993). These findings are especially interesting given Browndyke and colleagues' (2013) findings of increased parahippocampal activation in MCI patients relative to controls. Thus, the results suggest that MCI patients shifted from more global (or at least extended) toward more local network interactions. Although the cognitive implications are unclear, functional connectivity results from resting-state data have also revealed reduced connectivity between the hippocampus and multiple PFC regions (medial, superior, anterior cingulate), but increased connectivity with primary visual cortices and medial posterior regions (precuneus) in MCI patients relative to healthy controls (Wang et al., 2011). Such findings may relate to evidence of reduced connectivity between regions of the frontoparietal cognitive control network in MCI patients relative to controls, even after controlling for gray matter atrophy (Liang et al., 2011).

In sum, evidence suggests that MCI patients show decline in lateral PFC contributions to memory encoding. In response, patients begin using altered neural networks that support more basic cognitive processes. While our primary focus is on neuroplastic changes at the milder end of the AD spectrum (i.e., healthy aging and MCI), it is also useful to briefly review the additional changes that have been reported in AD.

Further Decline in AD

Two meta-analyses have examined memory encoding in patients with AD. In the first, Schwindt and Black (2009) reported that AD patients demonstrated significantly less activation than controls in a number of regions, including the hippocampus bilaterally and in the left ventrolateral and rostral PFC—findings that reinforce the patterns of change in MCI noted earlier. Other areas of activity reduction included the precuneus and superior parietal lobule, which are known sites of early Aβ deposition and cortical thinning. Additional reductions were found in the cingulate gyrus, insula, and thalamus—all of which can play a role in cognitive control. Interestingly, AD patients showed greater activation in an alternative set of PFC regions, possibly reflecting either an adaptive response to compensate for decline (e.g., local expansion) and/or an increasingly inefficient neural network (consistent with de-differentiation). A more recent and methodologically selective review found that AD patients showed less activation than controls in the right cerebellum, anterior parahippocampal gyrus, and lingual gyrus but greater activation in the precuneus, superior temporal gyrus, and superior frontal gyrus than controls (Browndyke et al., 2013). Several methodological factors likely contribute to these discrepant results, but both indicate some degree of hyperactivation in areas associated with the dorsal attention network (Spreng, Sepulcre, Turner, Stevens, & Schacter, 2012) that may suggest a shift toward more basic cognitive processing, as suggested by the MCI results described earlier. Thus, it is critical that we understand the factors contributing to this shift since this may ultimately facilitate more effective interventions that allow patients with MCI, and perhaps even AD, to re-engage or prolong use of the PFC-MTL network. Therefore, we now examine several factors that appear to be important in age- and disease-related neuroplasticity.

Factors Contributing to Neuroplastic Change: Structure-Function Relationships

Logan and colleagues (2002) provided evidence that age may play an important role in neuroplastic change, as they found bilateral PFC activation during word encoding in older adults aged 73+ whereas a unilateral pattern was evident in "young-old" (i.e., those <72 years old). A possible explanation for this finding may be related to the cumulative effects of medical conditions. Vascular health is an important factor to consider given the prevalence of vascular risk factors in older adults (e.g., hypertension, hyperlipidemia, diabetes). Liu and colleagues (2013) reported that vascular reactivity may be a critical factor to consider when examining age-related neuroplastic change. Specifically, these authors reported that older adults demonstrated reduced posterior and increased anterior (ventrolateral PFC) activation relative to their younger counterparts when standard analytic methods were employed. However, only bilateral ventrolateral PFC increases were found in older participants after accounting for cerebrovascular reactivity.

Li and colleagues (2009) provided intriguing data suggesting that white matter integrity plays a critical role in cognitive neuroplasticity. Specifically, they reported that task-related BOLD signal was upregulated in order to compensate for reduced connectivity in the lateral frontoparietal network and that the magnitude of this upregulation was inversely related to white matter integrity (measured via diffusion tensor imaging). Thus, weaker structural connectivity appears to disrupt spontaneous communication within a given network and necessitates additional neural resources to overcome this communication deficit. Similarly, Burzynska and colleagues (2013) reported that, regardless of age, BOLD signal was inversely related to white matter integrity, as measured by fractional anisotropy (FA) on diffusion tensor imaging (DTI) and that this relationship strengthened as the cognitive load increased, especially in the lateral frontoparietal network. Ansado and colleagues (2013) also demonstrated that white matter integrity facilitates the more efficient recruitment of bilateral PFC during cognitively demanding tasks.

Not surprisingly, evidence suggests that gray matter integrity also plays a role in neuroplastic change. A recent meta-analysis provided strong evidence linking age-related functional hyperactivation and gray matter atrophy (Di et al., 2014). To establish this link, the authors performed two separate meta-analyses. First, they examined age-related differences in BOLD during tasks of executive functioning (working memory, executive control, inhibition); these same abilities are important during memory encoding. This meta-analysis revealed significantly greater activation in older adults, relative to the young,

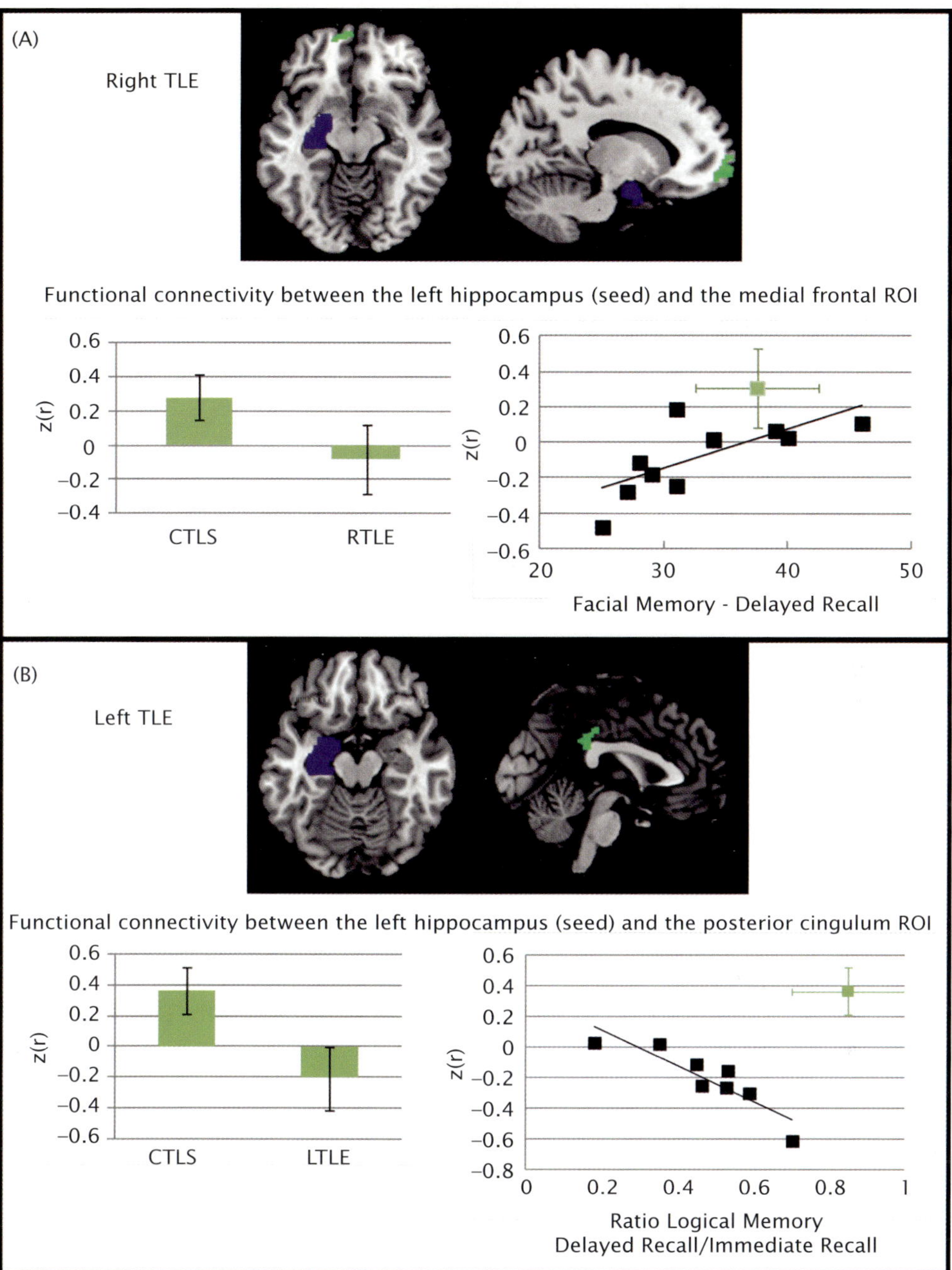

FIGURE 2.3 Correlation between FC values with the left hippocampal seed in right mesial TLE (RTLE), panel A, and in left mesial TLE (LTLE), panel B, with episodic memory scores. A: Reduced FC between the left hippocampal seed (blue) and medial frontal cortex (green, x = −14, y = 56, z = −10) in right mesial TLE patients compared with controls (*left bottom plot*); positive correlation between FC values between these two regions and the Facial Memory II Delayed Recall scores (*right bottom plot*, Spearman correlation, r = 0.78; p = 0.0045). The normative values of the controls on the right bottom plot are shown by the green data point where the *y axis* indicates the average FC value of the controls' data and the *x axis* is the normative value of age-matched healthy controls of the Facial Memory II Delayed Recall scores (Wechsler, 1997). Bars indicate standard deviation.B: Reduced FC between the left seed (blue) and posterior cingulate cortex (green, x = 2, y = −36, z = 32) in left mesial TLE patients compared with controls (*left bottom plot*); negative correlation between the FC values between these two regions and the ratio Logical Memory II Delayed Recall scores/Logical memory I Immediate Recall scores (*right bottom plot*, Spearman correlation, r = −0.93; p = 0.001). The normative values of the controls are shown through the green data point where the *y axis* indicates the average FC value of the controls' data and the *x axis* is the normative value of age-matched healthy controls of the Logical Memory ration (II/I) score (Wechsler, 1997). Bars indicate standard deviation. Modified and reprinted with permission from *Human Brain Mapping*, Doucet et al. (2013a), John Wiley and Sons.

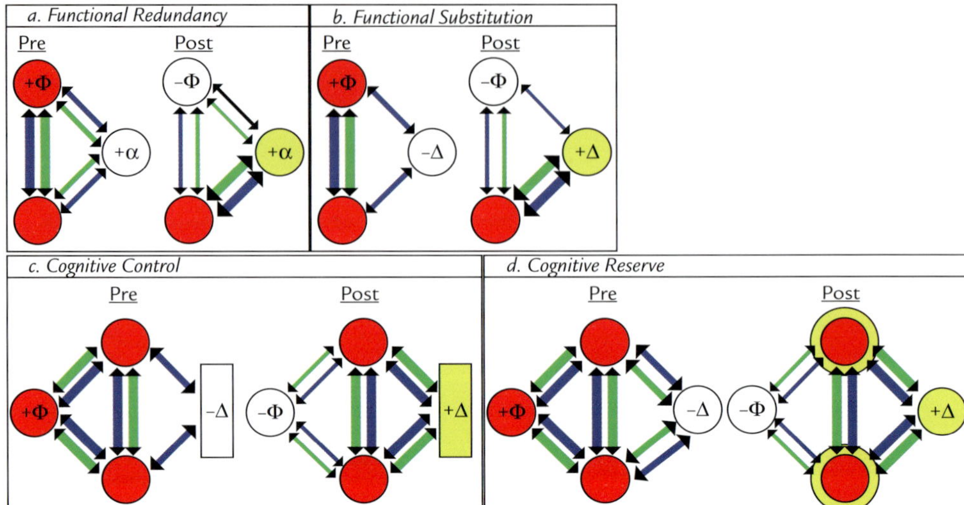

FIGURE 2.6 Graphical depiction of multimodal neuroimaging frameworks. *Panel A*: Functional redundancy. *Panel B*: Functional substitution. *Panel C*: Cognitive control. *Panel D*: Cognitive reserve. Legend: White indicates no fMRI activity in the region. Red circles indicate an area of cognitive functionality as revealed by fMRI. Yellow indicates a new region of fMRI activity, and in the case of cognitive reserve also reflects a change in the spatial extent or intensity of activation within the network (n.b., the yellow halo around the red circles of the network). Arrows indicate connectivity, with green lines depicting the rsfMRI findings and blue lines depicting the DTI findings; the arrows indicate the specific brain areas connected. The strength of connectivity is indicated by the thickness of the line, with thicker lines indicating stronger connectivity. The + and − indicate the presence or absence of fMRI activity in cases where a change in fMRI occurs across the two time points measured. The Greek letter α indicates a brain area that becomes unmasked at the second scan (e.g., after intervening event such as lesion, brain injury, or surgery); Δ marks and highlights an area that becomes newly active on the second scan; Φ indicates a brain area where fMRI activation is lost or drops out of the second scan. From Tracy & Osipowicz (2011). Copyright permission from *Journal of NeuroRehabilitation*, IOS Press.

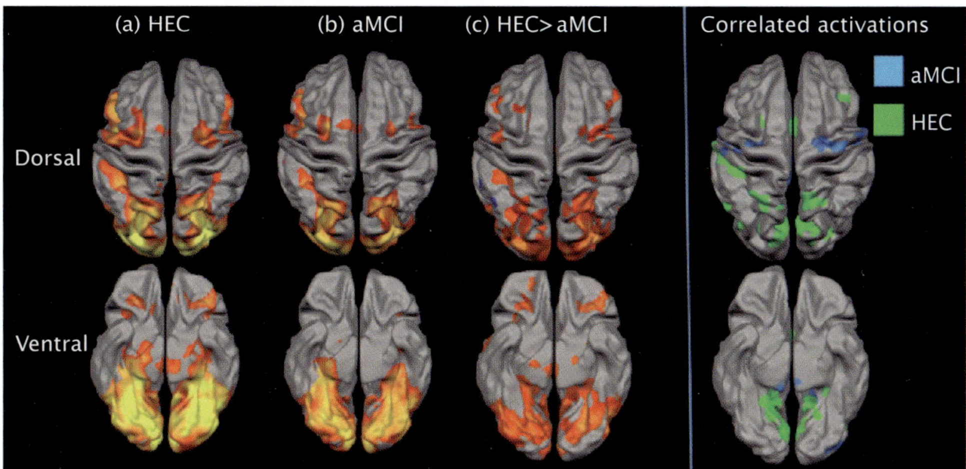

FIGURE 9.2 Patterns of activation during object-location association encoding using standard contrast analyses (columns a, b, c). The right most column shows activation that was significantly related to performance on the object-location task. HEC = healthy elderly controls; aMCI = amnestic mild cognitive impairment. Modified from Hampstead et al. (2011a). *Neuropsychologia, 49,* 2349–2361.

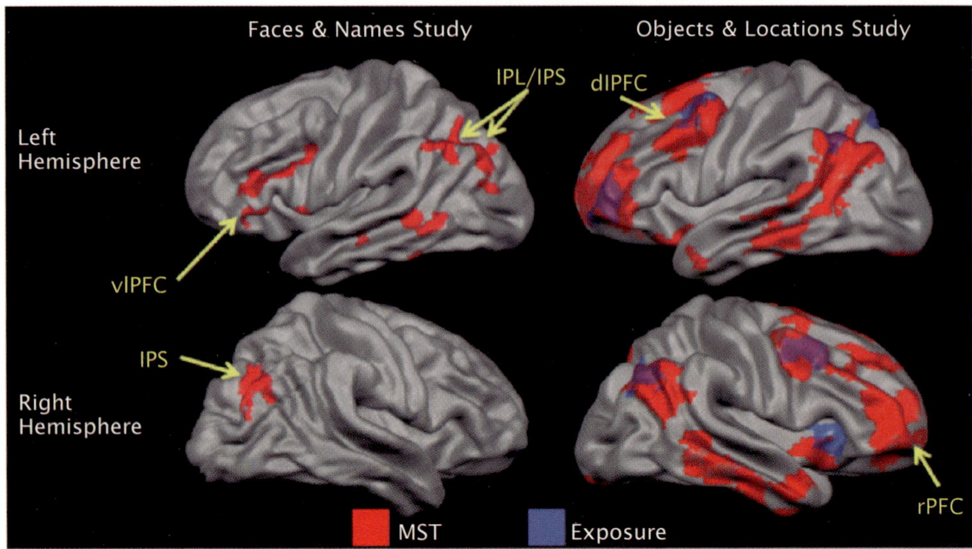

FIGURE 9.3 Areas showing increased encoding-related activity for the faces & names (left) and objects & locations (right) that were learned during the training sessions. dlPFC = dorsolateral prefrontal cortex; IPL = inferior parietal lobule; IPS = intraparietal sulcus; MFG = middle frontal gyrus; rPFC = rostral prefrontal cortex; vlPFC = anterior ventrolateral prefrontal cortex.

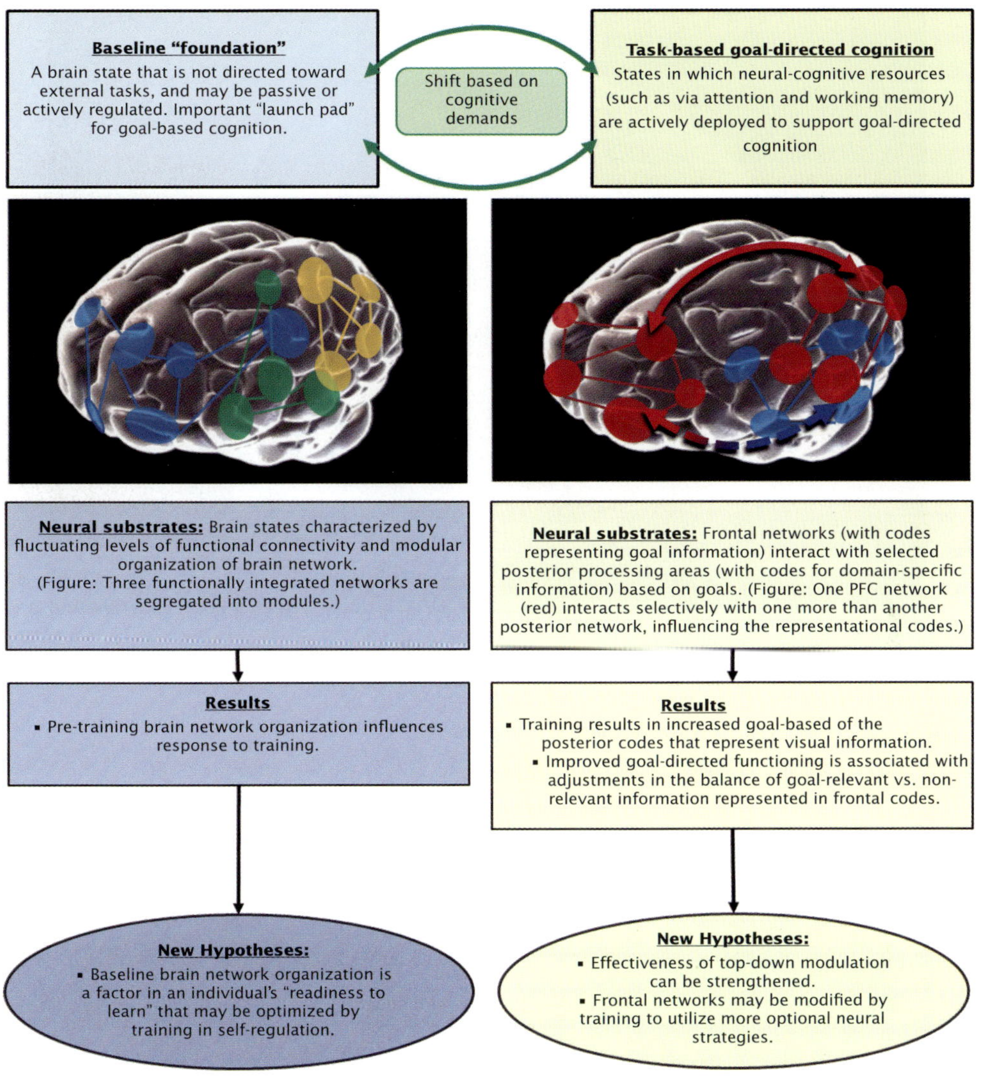

FIGURE 10.1 Lines of investigation addressing two complementary functions of plasticity in goal-directed cognition.

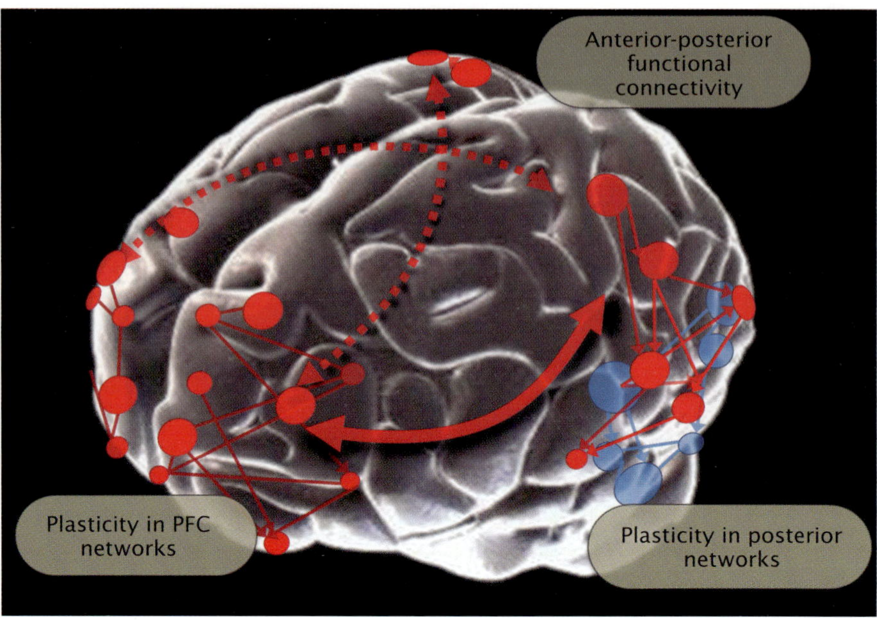

FIGURE 10.2 A summary model of network mechanisms that support plasticity in goal-directed control functioning.

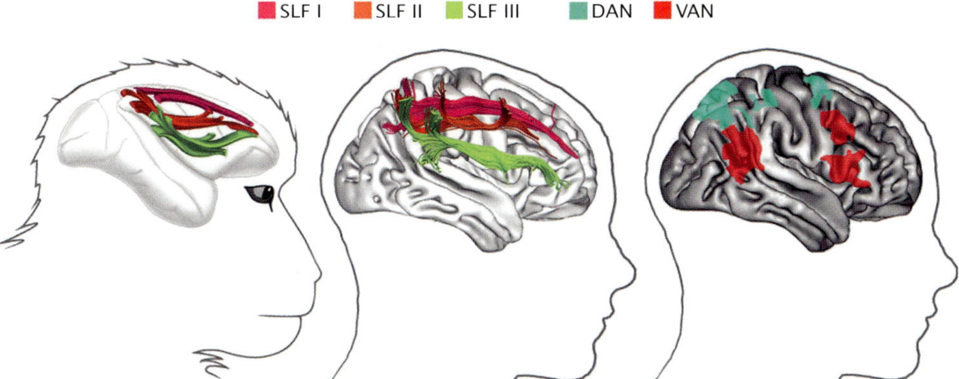

FIGURE 13.2 Frontoparietal networks in the monkey (left, from Schmahmann & Pandya, 2006) and in the human right hemisphere (middle, from Thiebaut de Schotten et al., 2011). Right: attentional networks in the right hemisphere according to Corbetta and Shulman (2002). Figure as originally published in *Frontiers in Human Neuroscience 6*, 110, 2012 "Brain networks of visuospatial attention and their disruption in visual neglect", by Paolo Bartolomeo, Michel Thiebaut de Schotten, Ana B. Chica.

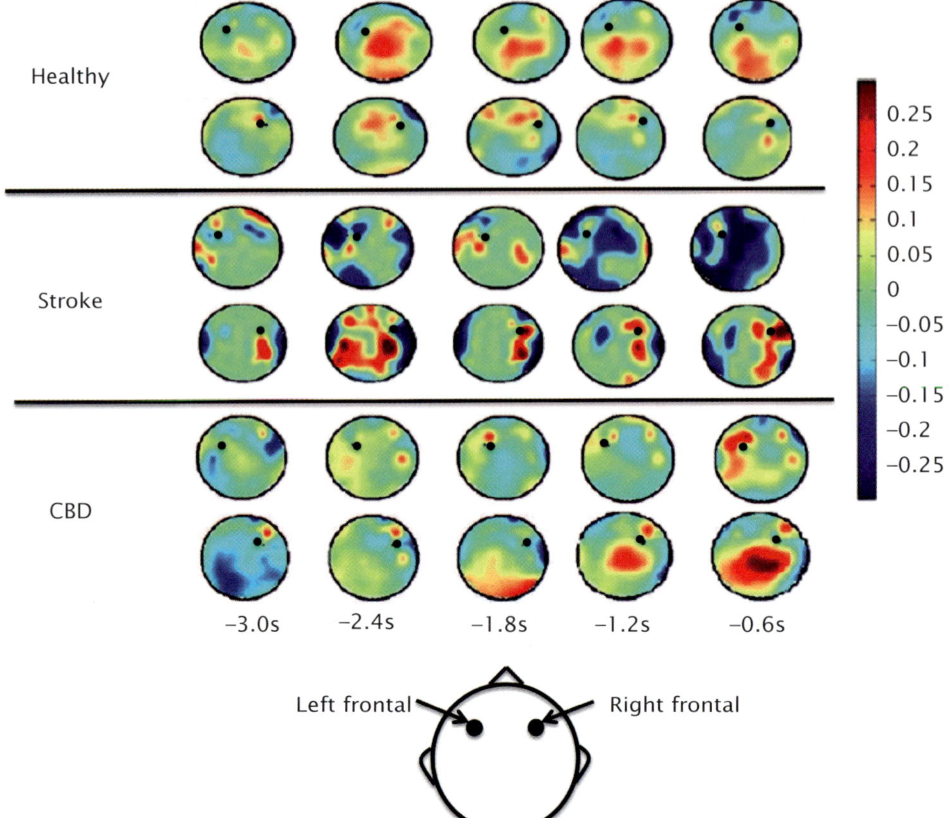

FIGURE 14.4 Head plots of a top-down view of the head (see inset for orientation) of whole brain EEG coherence relative to electrodes over left and right premotor cortex (as indicated by black dots) during motor planning (from 3 seconds before to 0.6 seconds before execution). Top shows coherence patterns in normal subjects, a stroke patient (middle), and corticobasal degeneration (CBD) patient (bottom). Coherence increases are shown in red; decreases in blue. Reprinted with permission from Wheaton et al. (2008), Elsevier.

in the ventrolateral and dorsolateral PFC bilaterally, thereby replicating most of the findings described above. Second, the authors used voxel-based morphometry to identify areas showing consistent age-related gray matter atrophy. These results revealed gray matter reduction within the PFC, insula, caudate, and thalamus of the old relative to the young, again generally replicating previous results. Di and colleagues (2014) then performed a conjunction analysis using these two meta-analyses, which revealed overlap between the hyperactive PFC regions and those with the most significant gray matter reduction. These overlapping clusters spanned aspects of both the ventrolateral and dorsolateral PFC bilaterally, supporting the notion that hyperactivity is an adaptive response to regional gray matter volume loss.

Maillet and Rajah (2013) reached a similar conclusion in their recent review that included studies examining structure-function relationships across cognitive domains. However, their findings suggested that the inverse activation-volume relationship in the PFC existed only when performance was comparable between older and younger participants. A positive relationship between activation and gray matter volume was evident when older adults performed worse than the young, especially for the right PFC. This positive structure-function relationship was evident in three of the four studies that examined memory encoding specifically, though the particular relationship was between MTL volumes and increased PFC activation. Such findings support the PFC-MTL link as well as a biologically defined limit to any potential compensatory process, as suggested by the CRUNCH model.[4] Similarly, Meunier and colleagues (2014) reported that age-related decline in the gray matter density of a left hemisphere language network mediated increased functional connectivity during a comprehension task. Although these findings suggest a degree of spontaneous reorganization/compensation, this modified network was less efficient, as measured by graph theory analyses, than that demonstrated by a group of young adults.

Together, these findings suggest that older adults undergo spontaneous reorganization of cognitive networks that interact with the MTL memory system. These neuroplastic changes appear to arise as a result of structural compromise and may allow individuals to maximize their cognitive performance, at least under some conditions. However, it is also clear that both genetic and other Alzheimer's-related risk factors can influence the neuroplastic response in the aging brain.

Genetic Factors

In addition to the MTL changes described above, there is substantial evidence that APOEε4 affects the patterns of neocortical activation. Supporting this possibility is a recent comprehensive review of the fMRI literature on the effects of APOEε4 across cognitive domains in

---

4. It should be noted that the authors discuss alternative explanations that include complex structure-function-behavior interactions. Their conclusion is that some degree of de-differentiation and compensatory neuroplastic change likely co-occur in the aging brain.

which 81% (22/27 studies) reported significant differences between ε4 positive versus negative individuals (Trachtenberg, Filippini, Mackay, 2012). Unfortunately, the pattern of results was ambiguous since 37% of the studies reported increased activation, 26% reported decreased activation, and 19% reported both increased and decreased activation. This ambiguous pattern persisted when the authors examined findings based on cognitive task/domain, family history of AD, and age. In respect to age, however, BOLD signal differences (in both directions) were evident in participants who were 20–30 years old—findings that the authors interpreted as potential evidence of an underlying fundamental difference in the neurophysiology of those with versus without ε4.[5]

A subsequent study by this group that appears to have been completed while this review was in press clarifies some of this age-related ambiguity (Filippini et al., 2011). Using an fMRI memory-encoding task, the authors discovered a significant age by ε4 status effect on the patterns of BOLD signal. Specifically, young carriers showed hyperactivation in several areas, including the hippocampi, rostral PFC, and lateral temporal cortices relative to non-carriers. Conversely, older carriers showed hypoactivation in these same regions, which was accompanied by reduced cerebral blood flow but preserved gray matter volume relative to non-carriers. Another study reported hypoactivation in a group of ε4 positive, compared to negative, cognitively intact older adults during an fMRI navigational encoding task (Borghesani et al., 2008). This hypoactivation was evident in a number of brain regions with those in the PFC, parietal, and MTL regions (including the hippocampus) being of primary interest for the current chapter. Similarly, cognitively intact ε4 positive older adults demonstrated less hippocampal activation during a spatial encoding task relative to those who were ε4 negative (Adamson, Hutchinson, Shelton, Wagner, & Taylor, 2011). Although Nichols and colleagues (2012) failed to replicate such results, the mean age of their "old" group was approximately 10 years younger than in the previously cited studies (early sixties vs. early seventies, respectively). This age difference is likely meaningful given the above noted evidence of a hyper- to hypo-active shift with age in ε4 carriers.

As with the hippocampus, young adults (mean age ~34 years) with the PS1 mutation demonstrated significantly less activation in a number of posterior brain regions bilaterally (e.g., ventral and lateral temporal lobe) but greater activation in a right-hemisphere dominant network that included the ventrolateral and dorsolateral PFC (Quiroz et al., 2010). These findings were within the context of comparable neuropsychological and experimental test performances. Thus, AD-related genetic factors appear to play an important role in neuroplastic change, though considerably more work is needed to clarify the nature of this role. In this respect, large datasets like those collected as part of the Alzheimer's Disease Neuroimaging Initiative (ADNI) are already being used to examine the relationship between genetics and structural changes in the brain (e.g., see Meda et al., 2012).

---

5. The interested reader is referred to a thorough review article by Wolf, Caselli, Reiman, & Valla (2013), *Neurobiology of Aging, 34,* 1007–1017.

Aβ deposition

It is now clear that Aβ begins to accumulate years before the onset of clinically significant cognitive deficits (e.g., see Jack, 2012), which is consistent with findings that APOE plays a role in Aβ clearance. Such findings are also significant since recent data indicate that cognitive and neuroplastic changes have already begun by the time Aβ accumulation is evident. For example, inverse relationships have consistently been reported between Aβ load and memory test performances in cognitively intact older adults (Oh et al., 2012; Sperling et al., 2013; also see meta-analysis by Hedden, Oh, Younger, & Patel, 2013). Further, stepwise discriminant function analyses revealed that the combination of visual memory, executive functioning, and working memory was optimal for predicting whether a cognitively intact older adult was Aβ negative or positive (Oh et al., 2012). Thus, there appear to be subtle cognitive changes that occur in those who are at risk of progressing through the AD spectrum; these changes are evident on tasks that depend on the lateral frontoparietal control network and MTL memory system.

From a structural standpoint, Aβ positive, cognitively intact older adults have demonstrated reduced cortical thickness in the posterior cingulate, precuneus, lateral parietal, and prefrontal cortices relative to those who were Aβ negative (Becker et al., 2011). Similarly, a study using whole-brain voxel-based morphometry found that left inferior frontal gyrus (IFG) volume was inversely related to Aβ load in cognitively healthy older adults (Oh et al., 2011). Subsequent analyses demonstrated that the volume of the IFG was associated with the structural integrity of a larger bilateral PFC network that included both ventrolateral and dorsolateral PFC regions. Further, the integrity of this larger network was associated with working memory abilities—findings that are consonant with the hyperactivity and connectivity with the MTL seen in these regions during healthy aging and seemingly lost during MCI (see discussion earlier in this chapter). In a subsequent study, Oh and colleagues (2014) used a multivariate approach to examine the relationship between relative values of Aβ, glucose metabolism (measured using fluorodeoxyglucose ([18]FDG)-PET), and gray matter volume in cognitively healthy older adults. Aβ deposition in the expected medial and lateral prefrontal, posterior cingulate, precuneus, and lateral parietal cortices was associated with relative decreases in gray matter volume but increases in glucose metabolism in these same regions. These findings are consistent with an earlier study from this same group, which reported increased encoding-related activation in prefrontal, parietal, and medial temporal cortices of amyloid positive versus amyloid negative older adults despite comparable behavioral performances (Oh & Jagust, 2013). However, the amyloid positive group showed reduced connectivity between the parahippocampal cortex and many of these task-relevant brain regions.

Additional evidence of disrupted connectivity in Aβ positive cognitively healthy older adults comes from studies using resting state connectivity. Functional neuroimaging studies have established the presence of multiple large-scale networks that are associated with different aspects of cognition (Spreng, Sepulcre, Turner, Stevens, & Schacter, 2012). The so-called default mode network (DMN) is composed of the medial PFC, posterior cingulate cortex, precuneus, and inferior parietal lobule, all of which are sites of early Aβ deposition. This network is believed to mediate internally directed cognition (e.g., self-relevance, episodic memory; Buckner, Andrews-Hanna, & Schacter, 2008) and connectivity between the DMN hubs is disrupted in both MCI (Sorg et al., 2007) and AD (Buckner, Andrews-Hanna, & Schacter, 2008; Greicius et al., 2004). Perhaps not surprisingly then, Aβ positive, cognitively intact older adults were found to have significantly reduced functional connectivity between the DMN hubs as well as between the posterior cingulate cortex and the hippocampus when compared to those who were Aβ negative (Hedden et al., 2009). Importantly, these findings persisted after controlling for age and gray matter volume.

Taken as a whole, these findings raise the possibility that the accumulation of Aβ reduces the efficiency of neural interactions, initially leading to hyperactivation (as measured through both glucose metabolism and BOLD signal magnitude) and ultimately hypoactivation of brain regions that interact with the MTL memory system. A key finding is that the loss of the increased PFC activation seen during "normal" aging appears to roughly coincide with the onset of clinically significant memory deficits that characterize MCI but may also be related to the accumulation of Aβ. Thus, treatments that enhance cognitive control and bolster cortical integrity may be especially effective at maximizing and prolonging learning and memory in those with MCI.

Treatment-Related Changes: Pharmacologic Agents

To date, the primary treatment options for AD have focused on pharmacologic agents that target the cholinergic system (e.g., donepezil, galantamine) or N-methyl-D-aspartate (NMDA) receptors (memantine). Functional neuroimaging studies have provided evidence of physiologic effects of these agents. For example, a single dose of galantamine increased retrieval-based activation in patients with MCI and AD, whereas more consistent drug use (5 days) generally resulted in decreased activation relative to baseline (Goekoop et al., 2006). While the latter results could be interpreted as increased neural efficiency, medication use failed to improve memory test performance (accuracy and latency) in either group. In a separate report, this same group showed increased encoding-related activation in the left ventrolateral and dorsolateral PFC, hippocampus, occipital cortex, and the right superior PFC and anterior cingulate of MCI patients after 5 consecutive days of galantamine treatment (Goekoop et al., 2004). Again, however, memory test performance was unchanged. Grön and colleagues (2006) administered galantamine for 7 consecutive days in a group of MCI patients and found improvements on the encoding and delayed recall of word lists, as well as increased hippocampal activation during spatial navigation.

Several studies have demonstrated similar changes following treatment with donepezil. Zaidel and colleagues (2012) recently reported increased functional connectivity between the left and right dorsolateral PFC following 8 weeks of treatment with donepezil in a small group of patients with mild AD. Another study randomized a small group of AD patients to either donepezil (n = 8) or a control condition (n = 7) (Solé-Padullés et al., 2013). After 3 months, neuropsychological functioning remained comparable between the groups, but the authors reported some evidence of increased resting state connectivity between the right parahippocampal gyrus and other DMN regions, as well as increased encoding-related activation in the right precuneus of the treated patients relative to controls. Pa and colleagues (2013) performed a double blind, placebo controlled, randomized controlled trial (RCT) in which patients with AD were treated for 3 months with either donepezil (n = 13) or placebo (n = 13). Participants encoded faces and scenes at baseline and 3 months. Compared to baseline, there were no treatment effects on accuracy for either stimulus type, but the donepezil group became significantly faster than the controls during facial recognition. This was associated with significant increased activation in the left fusiform face area as well as increased functional connectivity between this region and the right inferior frontal junction and hippocampus. Changes in this network were significantly related to the reaction time improvements in the treatment group. Thus, it appears that donepezil allowed patients to re-engage the PFC-MTL network and improve facial recognition speed but not accuracy.

As shown by these studies, existing pharmacological agents may alter neurophysiology, but this does not necessarily result in cognitive improvement. In fact, there is considerable debate about whether these medications improve cognitive functioning (Daviglus et al., 2010) and whether they delay disease progression—typically defined as conversion from MCI to AD (pro: Diniz et al., 2009; con: Daviglus et al., 2010; Raschetti et al., 2007). The most recent meta-analysis found no effect of cognitive enhancers on cognition or everyday functioning in those with MCI (Tricco et al., 2013). The authors concluded that the results do not support the use of these medications in MCI patients, especially given the significantly increased gastrointestinal side effects relative to placebos (Tricco et al., 2013).

As is clear from the literature reviewed in the first two sections of this chapter, the structural, functional, and cognitive changes in MCI and AD occur over a period of years. This gradual progression appears to result in an altered cognitive approach. However, the assumption in medication trials is that simply enhancing cholinergic (or other neurotransmitter) levels will "restore" premorbid functioning. We posit that patients may need to re-learn how to effectively learn new information since they have been relying on a progressively more ineffective network for years. As discussed in the next section, cognitive rehabilitation may be especially beneficial in this regard since it can enhance top-down control and re-engage dysfunctional brain regions.

Cognitive Rehabilitation

While cognitive rehabilitation is considered a treatment standard for some populations (e.g., traumatic brain injury; Cicerone et al., 2011), its use in older adults and patients with MCI or AD is more contentious. We recently examined several methodological factors that contribute to this controversy in those with MCI (Hampstead, Gillis, & Stringer, 2014). Here, we focus on evidence supporting the use of mnemonic strategies, which is a particular category of interventions that fall under the general umbrella of cognitive rehabilitation. Mnemonic strategies provide cognitive "tools" that facilitate a deeper level of processing by improving the organization and association of to-be-learned information. Not surprisingly, then, a meta-analysis (Verhaeghen, Marcoen, & Goossens, 1992) and several large-scale studies that included mnemonic strategies in larger programs (Craik et al., 2007; Oswald et al, 1996; Willis et al., 2006) found that older adults benefit from these techniques, as reflected by improved learning and memory performance. Other groups have demonstrated that intensive spatial navigation training was neuroprotective against age-related hippocampal volume loss (Lövdén et al., 2012). Far fewer studies have investigated the behavioral benefits of these strategies in patients with MCI, and even fewer still have examined the neuroplastic changes associated with training.

We have been systematically examining the conditions under which mnemonic strategies can be beneficial in patients with MCI using ecologically relevant paradigms that were designed to emulate the types of real-world problems that patients often encounter. We have used the same general 3-step process across studies, which we refer to as "FRI," for feature (F), reason (R), and image (I). In the first step, a salient feature is identified. Participants are encouraged to select something that is especially unique or unusual about the stimulus (e.g., the smooth skin of a face). Next, a verbally based reason for selecting that specific feature is developed. This reason should integrate the feature with the targeted information (e.g., the name). Finally, participants imagine and integrate these previous steps using mental imagery (i.e., by creating a mental "picture" or "movie"). On each subsequent trial, we require participants to recall the feature, the reason, the image, and then the targeted information (e.g., the name) in that specific order. To reinforce the use of the FRI approach, we have provided extensive practice (between 270–450 trials, depending on the study). Most of our participants have also undergone structural and fMRI before and after three training sessions.

Using this approach, we demonstrated that patients with MCI remember significantly more face-name associations both immediately after training and at a 1-month follow-up, compared to baseline (Hampstead et al., 2008). "Early" MCI patients showed greater improvement, as there was an inverse relationship between the number of training trials required and subsequent memory of the trained stimuli. Additionally, these patients showed significantly increased activation in, and effective connectivity between, a number of brain regions, including the left ventrolateral PFC and intraparietal sulcus/inferior parietal lobule (Hampstead et al., 2011b). This pattern of increased activation was evident as patients re-encoded stimuli they had learned during the training sessions and also as they encoded novel stimuli (see Figure 9.3). This latter finding raises the possibility that patients had altered the manner in which they were attempting to learn the stimuli, presumably by generalizing the strategies.

To rule out the possibility that these findings were paradigm-specific (i.e., with face-name associations) or due to practice effects, we performed a single-blind RCT wherein both healthy older adults and MCI patients underwent either mnemonic strategy training or an active exposure-matched control condition (Hampstead et al., 2012a). This study used the OLA paradigm described earlier. As before, participants randomized to the mnemonic strategy groups practiced using the FRI approach during 150 trials in each of three training sessions (450 total trials). Participants in the exposure group also received 150 trials during each of three sessions, just without any strategy training, in essence leaving them to learn and remember information as they normally would. Most participants underwent fMRI scanning before and again after these training sessions and also returned for a 1-month follow-up.

Results revealed that both treatment groups demonstrated improvement; however, there was a main effect of intervention wherein the mnemonic strategy-trained participants (both controls and MCI) demonstrated significantly more improvement than did those in the exposure group. These benefits persisted at 1 month. We also examined the neuropsychological and neuroanatomical factors (via volumetric analyses of the MTL) associated with this behavioral improvement. Mnemonic strategy training was most effective in "early" MCI (i.e., those with better executive and memory abilities and smaller inferior lateral ventricles), whereas exposure training was equally effective regardless of MCI severity. Overall, then, these results replicate our face-name study (Hampstead et al., 2008) and clearly indicate that mnemonic strategies can be effective in those with MCI, especially in the early stage.

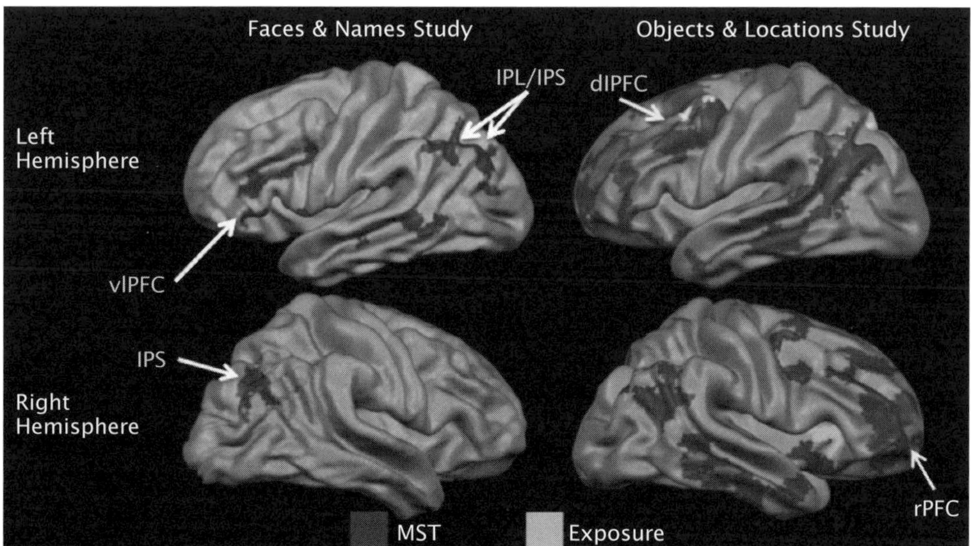

FIGURE 9.3 Areas showing increased encoding-related activity for the faces & names (left) and objects & locations (right) that were learned during the training sessions. dlPFC = dorsolateral prefrontal cortex; IPL = inferior parietal lobule; IPS = intraparietal sulcus; MFG = middle frontal gyrus; rPFC = rostral prefrontal cortex; vlPFC = anterior ventrolateral prefrontal cortex. (see color insert)

Turning to the neural mechanisms underlying this behavioral improvement, the mnemonic strategy trained groups consistently demonstrated increased activation in the lateral PFC (and other regions) during encoding (Hampstead et al., in preparation). In the healthy older adults, the mnemonic strategy group showed significantly greater activation in the right ventrolateral PFC than did the exposure group when they re-encoded stimuli learned during training, as well as when they encoded novel stimuli. These findings may be especially meaningful within the context of the HAROLD/CRUNCH models discussed earlier since the right lateral PFC is often associated with improved task performance. Other studies have also shown increased ventrolateral PFC activation in healthy older adults. For example, Logan and colleagues (2002) reported that semantic processing resulted in increased ventrolateral PFC activation during encoding. However, Belleville and colleagues (2011) reported reduced activation in the right ventrolateral and dorsolateral PFC of healthy older adults after mnemonic strategy training—possibly indicating increased processing efficiency within the context of improved performance on a verbally based encoding task.

Returning to our RCT, the MCI mnemonic strategy group (Figure 9.3) demonstrated robust increases in virtually every area of the PFC as they re-encoded stimuli learned during training. The magnitude of such activation was significantly greater than in the exposure group within the left rostral and medial PFC (including the anterior cingulate). Although there were no significant between-group differences as the MCI groups encoded novel stimuli, the exposure group demonstrated increased activation in only a subset of the PFC regions shown by the mnemonic strategy group. Consistent with the interactions between the PFC and MTL discussed earlier, we found a partial restoration in hippocampal activation only in the mnemonic strategy–trained MCI patients (Figure 9.4; Hampstead et al., 2012b). Belleville and colleagues (2011) reported increased activation in the superior PFC and inferior parietal cortex, among other regions, after MCI patients learned to use mnemonic strategies during a rehabilitation program. The magnitude of the activation increase in the inferior parietal cortex was significantly related to memory test

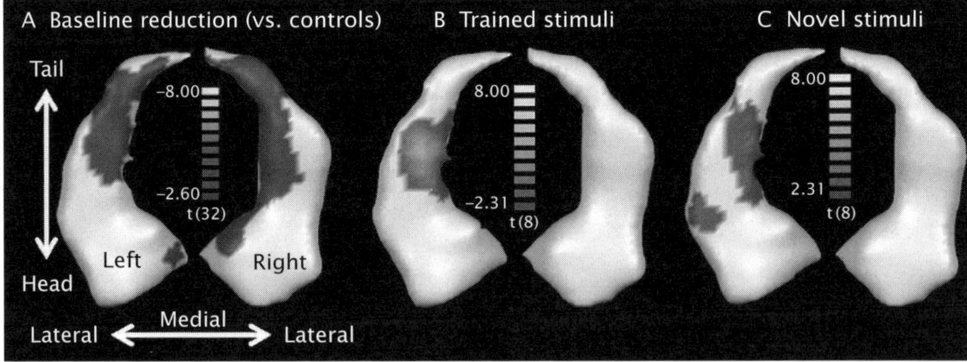

FIGURE 9.4 Encoding-related activity in the mnemonic strategy group from the object & location study. Despite showing reduced activation relative to healthy controls at baseline (A), mnemonic strategy training partially restored hippocampal activation for both trained (B) and novel (C) stimuli during the post-training fMRI session. No changes were evident in the exposure group.

performance—a finding that the authors interpreted as evidence of compensation. Such findings are consistent with our evidence of increased activation in the frontoparietal network that is known to mediate cognitive control.

Together, these studies indicate that mnemonic strategies (1) can be effective in those with MCI, (2) engage PFC regions involved in top-down cognitive control, (3) re-engage previously dysfunctional MTL regions, and (4) potentially recruit additional brain regions in a compensatory manner. Our ongoing studies are investigating whether patients are capable of independently generalizing the mnemonic strategies to other types of information and whether these seemingly adaptive neuroplastic changes persist over time.

Conclusions

The literature reviewed in this chapter highlights the cognitive, structural, and functional changes that occur across the spectrum from "normal" aging through MCI and into AD. Cognitively intact older adults often demonstrate (1) increased activation within the frontoparietal network subserving cognitive control, and (2) increased connectivity between PFC and MTL regions critical for learning and memory. These seemingly adaptive changes appear to recede with progression into MCI and ultimately AD, with changes in the role of the PFC being most striking. Several factors likely affect the functional changes, including the structural integrity of both gray and white matter, cerebrovascular functioning, genetics (e.g., APOE ε4 and PS1 status), and Aβ deposition. While existing pharmacologic agents may enhance functioning within brain regions associated with learning and memory, there is little evidence that they improve cognition in those with MCI. This apparent contradiction may arise because patients have gradually become increasingly reliant on altered or otherwise suboptimal networks as the disease has progressed. Conversely, cognitive rehabilitation techniques, especially mnemonic strategies, hold promise for re-engaging PFC and MTL regions critical for learning and memory, thereby more closely approximating "normal" aging. However, considerably more work is needed to understand the conditions under which various cognitive rehabilitation techniques are effective, especially at the individual patient level, and whether there are synergistic effects of combining pharmacologic and non-pharmacologic approaches.

References

Adamson, M. M., Hutchinson, J. B., Shelton, A. L., Wagner, A. D., & Taylor, J. L. (2011). Reduced hippocampal activity during encoding in cognitively normal adults carrying the epsilon 4 allele. *Neuropsychologia, 49*(9), 2448–2455.

Albert, M. S., et al. (2011). The diagnosis of mild cognitive impairment due to Alzheimer's disease: Recommendations from the National Institute on Aging and Alzheimer's Association workgroup. *Alzheimers Dement, 7*(3), 270–279.

Ansado, J., Collins, L., Joubert, S., Fonov, V., Monchi, O., Brambati, S. M., et al. (2013). Interhemispheric coupling improves the brain's ability to perform low cognitive demand tasks in Alzheimer's Disease and high cognitive demand tasks in normal aging. *Neuropsychology, 27*(4), 464–480.

Apostolova, L. G., Mosconi, L., Thompson, P. M., Green, A. E., Hwang, K. S., Ramirez, A., et al. (2010). Subregional hippocampal atrophy predicts Alzheimer's dementia in the cognitively normal. *Neurobiol Aging, 31*, 1077–1088.

Apostolova, L. G., Thompson, P. M., Green, A. E., Hwang, K. S., Zoumalan, C., Jack, C. R., et al. (2010). 3D comparison of low, intermediate, and adanced hippocampal atrophy in MCI. *Hum Brain Mapp, 31*, 786–797.

Ashford, J. W., & Mortimer, J. A. (2002). Non-familial Alzheimer's disease is mainly due to genetic factors. *J Alzheimers Dis, 4*, 169–177.

Baddeley, A. (2003). Working memory: Looking back and looking forward. *Nat Rev Neurosci, 4*(10), 829–839

Becker, J. A., Hedden, T., Carmasin, J., Maye, J., Rentz, D. M., Putcha, D., Fischl, B., et al. (2011). Amyloid-β associated cortical thinning in clinically normal elderly. *Anna Neurol, 69*, 1032–1042.

Belleville, S., Clement, F., Mellah, S., Gilbert, B., Fontaine, F., & Gauthier, S. (2011). Training-related brain plasticity in subjects at risk of developing Alzheimer's disease. *Brain, 134*, 1623–1634.

Berlingeri, M., Danelli, L., Bottini, G., Sberna, M., Paulesu, E. (2013). Reassessing the HAROLD model: Is the hemispheric reduction in older adults a special case of compensatory-related utilization of neural circuits? *Exp Brain Res, 224*(3), 393–410.

Borghesani, P. R., Johnson, L. C., Shelton, A. L., Peskind, E. R., Aylward, E. H., Schellenberg, G. D., & Cherrier, M. M. (2008). Altered medial temporal lobe responses during visuospatial encoding in healthy ε4 carriers. *Neurobiol Aging, 29*, 981–991.

Braun, S. M. G. & Jessberger, S. (2014). Review: Adult neurogenesis and its role in neuropsychiatric disease, brain repair and normal brain function. *Neuropath Applied Neuro, 40*, 3–12.

Browndyke, J. N., Giovanello, K., Petrella, J., Hayden, K., Chiba-Falek, O., Tucker, K. A., Burke, J. R., & Welsh-Bohmer, K. A. (2013). Phenotypic regional functional imaging patterns during memory encoding in mild cognitive impairment and Alzheimer's disease. *Alzheimers Dement, 9*, 284–294.

Buckner, R. L., Andrews-Hanna, J. R., & Schacter, D. L. (2008). The brain's default network: Anatomy, function, and relevance to disease. *Ann NY Acad Sci, 1124*, 1–38.

Burzynska, A. Z., Garrett, D. D., Preuschhof, C., Nagel, I. E., Li, S. C. Backman, L., Heekeren, H. R., Lindenberger, U. (2013). A scaffold for efficiency in the human brain. *J Neurosci, 33*(43), 17150–17159.

Cabeza, R. (2002). Hemispheric asymmetry reduction in older adults: The HAROLD model. *Psychol Aging, 17*(1), 85–100.

Cabeza, R., Anderson, N. D., Locantore, J. K., & McIntosh, A. R. (2002). Aging gracefully: Compensatory brain activity in high-performing older adults. *NeuroImage, 17*, 1394–1402.

Cicerone, K. D., Langenbahn, D. M., Braden, C., Malec, J. F., Kalmar, K., Fraas, M., et al. (2011). Evidence-based cognitive rehabilitation: Updated review of the literature from 2003 through 2008. *Arch Phys Med Rehab, 92*(4), 519–530.

Craik, F. I. M. & Lockhart, R. S. (1972). Levels of processing: A framework for memory research. *J Verb Learn Verb Be, 11*, 671–684.

Craik, F. I. M., Winocur, G., Palmer, H., Binns, M. A., Edwards, M., Bridges, K., Glazer, P., Chavannes, R., & Stuss, D. T. (2007). Cognitive rehabilitation in the elderly: Effects on memory. *J Int Neuropsychol Soc, 13*, 132–142.

Davis, S. W., Dennis, S. A., Daselaar, S. M., Fleck, M. S., Cabeza, R. (2008). Que PASA? The posterior-anterior shift in aging. *Cereb Cortex, 18*, 1201–1209.

Daviglus, M. L., Bell, C. C., Berrettini, W., Bowen, P. E., Connolly, E. S., Cox, N. J., et al. (2010). National Institutes of Health State-of-the-Science Conference Statement: Preventing Alzheimer's disease and cognitive decline. *NIH Consens State Sci Statements, 27*(4), 1–30.

De Lacoste, M. C. & White, C. L. (1993). The role of cortical connectivity in Alzheimer's disease pathogenesis: A review and model system. *Neurobiol Aging, 14*(1), 1–16.

Dennis, N. A., Hayes, S. M., Prince, S. E., Madden, D. J., Huettel, S. A., & Cabeza, R. (2008). Effects of aging on the neural correlates of successful item and source memory encoding. *J Exp Psychol, 34*(4), 791–808.

Derrfuss, J., Brass, M., & von Cramon, D. Y. (2004). Cognitive control in the posterior frontolateral cortex: Evidence from common activations in task coordination, interference control, and working memory. *NeuroImage, 23*, 604–612.

Di, X., Rypma, B., & Biswal, B. B. (2014). Correspondence of executive function related functional and anatomical alterations in aging brain. *Prog Neuro-Psychoph, 48*, 41–50.

Dickerson, B. C., Bakkour, A., Salat, D. H., Feczko, E., Pacheco, J. Greve, D. N., et al. (2009) The cortical signature of Alzheimer's disease: Regionally specific cortical thinning relates to symptom severity in very mild to mild AD dementia and is detectable in asymptomatic amyloid-positive individuals. *Cereb Cortex*, *19*, 497–510.

Dickerson, B. C., & Sperling, R. A. (2008). Functional abnormalities of the medial temporal lobe memory system in mild cognitive impairment and Alzheimer's disease: Insights from functional MRI studies. *Neuropsychologia*, *46*(6), 1624–1635.

Diniz, B. S., Pinto, J. A., Gonzaga, M. L. C., Guimaraes, F. M., Gattaz, W. F., & Forlenza, O. V. (2009). To treat or not to treat? A meta-analysis of the use of cholinesterase inhibitors in mild cognitive impairment for delaying progression to Alzheimer's disease. *Eur Arch Psychiat Clin Neurosci*, *259*(4), 248–256.

Ferri, C. P., Prince, M., Brayne, C., Brodaty, H., Fratiglioni, L., Ganguli, M., et al. (2005). Global prevalence of dementia: A Delphi consensus study. *Lancet*, *366*(9503), 2112–2117.

Filippini, N., Ebmeier, K. P., MacIntosh, B. J., Trachtenberg, A. J., Frisoni, G. B., Wilcock, G. K., Beckmann, C. F., Smith, S. M., Matthews, P. M., & Mackay, C. E. (2011). Differential effects of the genotype on brain function across the lifespan. *NeuroImage*, *54*, 602–610.

Goekoop, R., Scheltens, P., Barkhof, F., & Rombouts, S. A. R. B. (2006). Cholinergic challenge in Alzheimer patients and mild cognitive impairment differentially affects hippocampal activation: A pharmacological fMRI study. *Brain*, *129*, 141–157.

Goekoop, R., Rombouts, S. A. R. B., Jonker, C., Hibbel, A., Knol, D. L., Truyen, L., Barkhof, F., & Scheltens, P. (2004). Challenging the cholinergic system in mild cognitive impairment: A pharmacological fMRI study. *NeuroImage*, *23*, 1450–1459.

Greicius, M. D., Srivastava, G., Reiss, A. L., Menon, V. (2004). Default-mode network activity distinguishes Alzheimer's disease from healthy aging: Evidence from functional MRI. *P Natl Acad Sci USA*, *101*, 4637–442.

Grön, G., Brandenburg, I., Wunderlich, A. P., & Riepe, M. W. (2006). Inhibition of hippocampal function in mild cognitive impairment: Targeting the cholinergic hypothesis. *Neurobiol Aging*, *27*, 78–87.

Hampstead, B. M., Sathian, K., Moore, A. B., Nalisnick, C., & Stringer, A. Y. (2008). Explicit memory training leads to improved memory for face-name pairs in patients with mild cognitive impairment: Results of a pilot study. *J Int Neuropsychol Soc*, *14*, 883–889.

Hampstead, B. M., Stringer, A. Y., Stilla, R. F., Amaraneni, A., & Sathian, K. (2011a). Where did I put that? Patients with amnestic mild cognitive impairment demonstrate widespread reductions in activity during the encoding of ecologically relevant object-location associations. *Neuropsychologia*, *49*, 2349–2361.

Hampstead, B. M., Stringer, A. Y., Stilla, R. F., Deshpande, G., Hu, X., Moore, A. B., & Sathian, K. (2011b). Activation and effective connectivity changes following explicit-memory training for face-name pairs in patients with mild cognitive impairment: A pilot study. *Neurorehab Neural Re*, *25*, 210–222.

Hampstead, B. M., Sathian, K., Phillips, P. A., Amaraneni, A., Delaune, W. R., & Stringer, A. Y. (2012a). Mnemonic strategy training improves memory for object location associations in both healthy elderly and patients with amnestic mild cognitive impairment: A randomized, single-blind study. *Neuropsychology*, *26*(3), 385–399.

Hampstead, B. M., Stringer, A. Y., Stilla, R. F., Giddens, M., & Sathian, K. (2012b). Mnemonic strategy training partially restores hippocampal activity in patients with mild cognitive impairment. *Hippocampus*, *22*, 1652–1658.

Hampstead, B. M., Gillis, M. M., & Stringer, A. Y. (2014). Cognitive rehabilitation of memory for mild cognitive impairment: A methodological review and model for future research. *J Int Neuropsychol Soc*, *20*(2), 135–151.

Hampstead, B. M., Stringer, A. Y., Stilla, R. F., & Sathian, K. (in preparation). Mnemonic strategy training enhances activation during memory encoding and retrieval in patients with mild cognitive impairment relative to repeated exposure.

Hannula, D. E., & Greene, A. J. (2012). The hippocampus reevaluated in unconscious learning and memory: At a tipping point? *Front Human Neurosci*. doi: 10.3389/fnhum.2012.00080

Hedden, T., Van Dijk, K. R. A., Becker, J. A., Mehta, A., Sperling, R. A., Johnson, K. A., & Buckner, R. L. (2009). Disruption of functional connectivity in clinically normal older adults harboring amyloid burden. *J Neurosci*, *29*(40), 12686–12694.

Hedden, T., Oh, H., Younger, A. P., & Patel, T. A. (2013). Meta-analysis of amyloid-cognition relations in cognitively normal older adults. *Neurology*, *80*, 1341–1348.

Jack, C. R. (2012). Alzheimer disease: New concepts on its neurobiology and the clinical role imaging will play. *Radiology*, *263*(2), 344–361.

Johnson, S. C., Baxter, L. C., Susskind-Wilder, L., Connor, D. J., Sabbagh, M. N., & Caselli, R. J. (2004). Hippocampal adaptation to face repetition in healthy elderly and mild cognitive impairment. *Neuropsychologia, 42*(7), 980–989. doi: 10.1016/j.neuropsychologia.2003.11.015

Li, S. C., & Lindenberger, U. (1999). Cross-level unification: A computational exploration of the link between deterioration of neurotransmitter systems and dedifferentiation of cognitive abilities in old age. In L.-G. Nilsson & H. J. Markowitsch (Eds.), *Cognitive neuroscience of memory* (pp. 103–146). Seattle, WA: Hogrefe & Huber.

Li, Z., Moore, A. B., Tyner, C., & Hu, X. (2009). Asymmetric connectivity reduction and its relationship to "HAROLD" in aging brain. *Brain Res, 1295*, 149–158.

Liang, P., Wang, Z., Yang, Y., Jia, X., & Li, K. (2011). Functional disconnection and compensation in mild cognitive impairment: Evidence from DLPFC connectivity using resting-state fMRI. *PLoSOne, 6*(7): e22153. doi: 10.1371/journal.pone.0022153.

Liu, T., Sachdev, P. S., Lipnicki, D. M., Jiang, J., Cui, Y., Kochan, N. A., et al. (2013). Longitudinal changes in sulcal morphology associated with late-life aging and MCI. *NeuroImage, 74*, 337–342.

Liu, P., Hebrank, A. C., Rodrigue, K. M., Kennedy, K. M., Section, J., Park, D. C., & Lu, H. (2013). Age-related differences in memory-encoding fMRI responses after accounting for decline in vascular reactivity. *NeuroImage, 78*, 415–425.

Logan, J. M., Sanders, A. L., Snyder, A. Z., Morris, J. C., & Buckner, R. L. (2002). Under-recruitment and non-selective recruitment: Dissociable neural mechanisms associated with aging. *Neuron, 33*, 827–840.

Lövdén, M., Schaefer, S., Noack, H., Bodammer, N. C., Kühn, S., Heinze, H. J., et al. (2012). Spatial navigation training protects the hippocampus against age-related changes during early and late adulthood. *Neurobiol Aging, 33*, 620.e9–620.e22

Kandel, E. R., Schwartz, J. H., & Jessell, T. M. (2000). *Principles of neural science* (4th ed.). New York: McGraw-Hill.

Hampstead, B. M., Khoshnoodi, M., Deshpande, G., Yan, W., & Sathian, K. (in preparation). Effective connectivity differences during memory encoding and retrieval in healthy elderly and patients with mild cognitive impairment.

Köhler, S., (2004). Effects of left inferior prefrontal stimulation on episodic memory formation: A two-stage fMRI-rTMS study. *J Cogn Neurosci, 16*(2), 178–188.

Kuhl, B., Bainbridge, W., & Chun, M. (2012). Neural reactivation reveals mechanisms for updating memory. *J Neurosci, 32*(10), 3453–3461.

Machulda, M. M., Senjem, M. L., Weigand, S. D., Smith, G. E., Ivnik, R. J., Boeve, B. F., et al. (2009). Functional magnetic resonance imaging changes in amnestic and nonamnestic mild cognitive impairment during encoding and recognition tasks. *J Int Neuropsychol Soc, 15*(3), 372–382.

Machulda, M. M., Ward, H. A., Borowski, B., Gunter, J. L., Cha, R. H., O'Brien, P. C., et al. (2003). Comparison of memory fMRI response among normal, MCI, and Alzheimer's patients. *Neurology, 61*(4), 500–506.

Maillet, D., & Rajah, M. N. (2013). Association between prefrontal activity and volume change in prefrontal and medial temporal lobes in aging and dementia: A review. *Ageing Res Rev, 12*, 479–489.

Manenti, R., Cotelli, M., & Minussi, C. (2011). Successful physiological aging and episodic memory: A brain stimulation study. *Behav Brain Res, 216*, 153–158.

Mattay, V. S., Fera, F., Tessitore, A., Hariri, A. R., Berman, K. F., Das, S., Meyer-Lindenberg, A., Goldberg, T. E., Callicott, J. H., & Weinberger, D. R. (2006). Neurophysiological correlates of age-related changes in working memory capacity. *Neurosci Lett, 392*, 32–37.

Mayes, A., Montaldi, D., & Migo, E. (2007). Associative memory and the medial temporal lobes. *Trends Cogn Sci, 11*, 126–135.

McDonald, C. R., Gharapetian, L., McEvoy, L. K., Fennema-Notestine, C., Hagler, D. J., Holland, D., et al. (2012). Relationship between regional atrophy rates and cognitive decline in mild cognitive impairment. *Neurobiol Aging, 33*, 242–253.

McKhann, G. M., Knopman, D. S., Chertkow, H., Hyman, B. T., Jack, C. R., Kawas, C. H., et al. (2011). The diagnosis of dementia due to Alzheimer's disease: Recommendations from the National Institute on Aging-Alzheimer's Association workgroups on diagnostic guidelines for Alzheimer's disease. *Alzheimers Dement, 7*, 263–269.

Meda, S. A., Narayanan, B., Liu, J., Perrone-Bizzozero, N. I., Stevens, M. C., Calhoun, V. D., et al., (2012). A large scale multivariate parallel ICA method reveals novel imaging-genetic relationships for Alzheimer's disease in the ADNI cohort. *NeuroImage, 60*, 1608–1621.

Meunier, D., Stamatakis, E. A., & Tyler, L. K. (2014). Age-related functional reorganization, structural changes, and preserved cognition. *Neurobiol Aging, 35,* 42–54.

Milner, B., Squire, L. R., & Kandel, E. R. (1998). Cognitive neuroscience and the study of memory. *Neuron, 20,* 445–468.

Nichols, L. M., Masdeu, J. C., Mattay, V. S., Kohn, P., Emery, M., Sambataro, F., Kolachana, B., et al. (2012). Interactive effect of apolipoprotein E genotype and age on hippocampal activation during memory processing in healthy adults. *Arch Gen Psychiat, 69*(8), 804–813.

Nyberg, L., Cabeza, R., & Tulving, E. (1996). PET studies of encoding and retrieval: The HERA model. *Psychon B Rev, 3*(2), 135–148.

O'Brien, J. L., O'Keefe, K. M., LaViolette, P. S., DeLuca, A. N., Blacker, D., Dickerson, B. C., & Sperling, R. A. (2010). Longitudinal fMRI in elderly reveals loss of hippocampal activation with clinical decline. *Neurology, 74,* 1969–1976.

Oh, H., Habeck, C., Madison, C., & Jagust, W. (2014). Covarying alterations in Aβ deposition, glucose metabolism, and gray matter volume in cognitively normal elderly. *Hum Brain Mapp, 35,* 297–308.

Oh, H., & Jagust, W. J. (2013). Frontotemporal network connectivity during memory encoding is increased with aging and disrupted by beta-amyloid. *J Neurosci, 33*(47), 18425–18437.

Oh, H., Madison, C., Haight, T. J., Markley, C., & Jagust, W. J. (2012). Effects of age and β-amyloid on cognitive changes in normal elderly people. *Neurobiol Aging, 33,* 2746–2755.

Oh, H., Mormino, E. C., Madison, C., Hayenga, A., Smiljic, A., Jagust, W. J. (2011). β-Amyloid affects frontal and posterior brain networks in normal aging. *NeuroImage, 54,* 1887–1895.

Oswald, W. D., Rupprecht, R., Cunzelmann, T., & Tritt, K. (1996). The SIMA-project: Effects of 1-year cognitive and psychomotor training on cognitive abilities of the elderly. *Behav Brain Res, 78,* 67–72.

Pa, J., Berry, A. S., Compagnone, M., Boccanfuso, J., Greenhouse, I., Rubens, M. T., et al. (2013). Cholinergic enhancement of functional networks in older adults with mild cognitive impairment. *Ann Neurol, 73,* 762–773.

Petersen, R. C. (2004). Mild cognitive impairment as a diagnostic entity. *J Int Med, 256,* 183–194.

Petersen, R. C., Smith, G. E., Waring, S. C., Ivnik, R. J., Tangalos, E. G., & Kokmen, E. (1999). Mild cognitive impairment: Clinical characterization and outcome. *Arch Neurol, 56*(6), 303–308.

Petrella, J. R., Wang, L. H., Krishnan, S., Slavin, M. J., Prince, S. E., Tran, T. T. T., & Doraiswamy, P. M. (2007). Cortical deactivation in mild cognitive impairment: High-field strength functional MR imaging. *Radiology, 245*(1), 224–235.

Postma, A., Kessels, R. P. C., & van Asselen, M. (2008). How the brain remembers and forgets where things are: The neurocognition of object-location memory. *Neurosci Biobehav Rev, 32*(8), 1339–1345.

Protzner, A. B., Mandiza, J. L., Black, S. E., & McAndrews, M. P. (2011). Network interactions explain effective encoding in the context of medial temporal damage in MCI. *Hum Brain Mapp, 32,* 1277–1289.

Putcha, D., Brickhouse, M., O'Keefe, K., Sullivan, C., Rentz, D., Marshall, G., Dickerson, B., & Sperling, R. (2011). Hippocampal hyperactivation associated with cortical thinning in Alzheimer's disease signature regions in non-demented elderly adults. *J Neurosci, 31*(48), 17680–17688.

Quiroz, Y. T., Budson, A. E., Celone, K., Ruiz, A., Newmark, R., Castrillon, G., Lopera, F., & Stern, C. E. (2010). Hippocampal hyperactivation in presymptomatic familial Alzheimer's disease. *Ann Neurol, 68,* 865–875.

Raschetti, R., et al. (2007). *Cholinesterase inhibitors in mild cognitive impairment: A systematic review of randomised trials. Plos Med, 4*(11): 1818–1828.

Reuter-Lorenz, P., & Cappell, K. A. (2008). Neurocognitive aging and the compensation hypothesis. *Curr Dir Psychol Sci, 17*(3), 177–182.

Reuter-Lorenz, P. A., Jonides, J., Smith, E. E., Hartley, A., Miller, A., Marshuetz, C., & Koeppe, R. A. (2000). Age differences in the frontal lateralization of verbal and spatial working memory revealed by PET. *Journal of Cognitive Neuroscience, 12*(1), 174–187.

Rodriguez, K. M., & Raz, N. (2004). Shrinkage of the entorhinal cortex over five years predicts memory performance in healthy adults. *J Neurosci, 24*(4), 956–963.

Salthouse, T. A. (2010). Selective review of cognitive aging. *J Int Neuropsychol Soc, 16,* 754–760.

Schwindt, G. C., & Black, S. E. (2009). Functional imaging studies of episodic memory in Alzheimer's disease: A quantitative meta-analysis. *NeuroImage, 45,* 181–190.

Small, S. A., Schobel, S. A., Buxton, R. B., Witter, M. P., & Barnes, C. A. (2011). A pathophysiological framework of hippocampal dysfunction in ageing and disease. *Nat Rev Neurosci, 12*(10), 585–601.

Solé-Padullés, C., Bartrés-Faz, D., Lladó, A., Bosch, B., Peña-Gómez, C., Castellvi, M., et al. (2013). Donepezil treatment stabilizes functional connectivity during resting state and brain activity during memory encoding in Alzheimer's disease. *J Clin Psychopharm, 33,* 199–205.

Sorg, C., Riedi, V., Muhlau, M., Calhoun, V. D., Eichele, T., Laer, L., et al. (2007). Selective changes of resting-state networks in individuals at risk for Alzheimer's disease. *P Natl Acad Sci USA, 104*(47), 18760–18765.

Spaniol, J., Davidson, P. S. R., Kim, A. S. N., Han, H. Moscovitch, M., & Grady, C. L. (2009). Event-related fMRI studies of episodic encoding and retrieval: Meta-analyses using activation likelihood estimation. *Neuropsychologia, 47,* 1765–1779.

Spreng, R. N., Wojtowicz, M., & Grady, C. L. (2010). Reliable differences in brain activity between young and old adults: A quantitative meta-analysis across multiple cognitive domains. *Neurosci Biobehav Rev, 34,* 1178–1194.

Spreng, R. N., Sepulcre, J., Turner, G. R., Stevens, W. D., & Schacter, D. L. (2012). Intrinsic architecture underlying the relations among the default, dorsal attention, and frontoparietal control networks of the human brain. *J Cognitive Neurosci, 25*(1), 74–86.

Sperling, R. A., Johnson, K. A., Doraiswmy, P. M., Reiman, E. M., Fleisher, A. S., Sabbagh, M. N., et al. (2013). Amyloid deposition detected with florbetapir F 18 (F-18-AV-45) is related to lower episodic memory performance in clinically normal older individuals. *Neurobiol Aging, 34*(3), 822–831.

Squire, L. R. & Zola, S. M. (1996). Memory, memory impairment, and the medial temporal lobe. *Cold Spring Harb Sym Quantitative Biology, 61,* 185–195.

Trachtenberg, A. J., Filippini, N., & Mackay, C. E. (2012). The effects of APOEε4 on the BOLD response. *Neurobiol Aging, 33,* 323–334.

Tricco, A. C., Soobiah, C., Berliner, S., Ho, J. M., Ng, C.H., Ashoor, H. M., et al. (2013). Efficacy and safety of cognitive enhancers for patients with mild cognitive impairment: A systematic review and meta-analysis. *Can Med Assoc Journal, 185*(16), 1393–1401.

Verhaeghen, P., Marcoen, A., & Goossens, L. (1992). Improving memory performance in the aged through mnemonic training—a meta-analytic study. *Psychol Aging, 7*(2), 242–251.

Wang, Z., Liang, P., Jia, X., Qi, Z., Yu, L., Yang, Y., Zhou, W., Lu, J., & Li, K. (2011). Baseline and longitudinal patterns of hippocampal connectivity in mild cognitive impairment: Evidence from resting state fMRI. *J Neurolog Sci, 309,* 79–85.

Willis, S. L., Tennstedt, S. L., Marsiske, M., Ball, K., Elias, J., Koepke, K. M., et al. (2006). Long-term effects of cognitive training on everyday functional outcomes in older adults. *JAMA, 296*(23), 2805–2814.

Zaidel, L., Allen, G., Cullum, C. M., Briggs, R. W., Hynan, L. S., Weiner, M. F., et al. (2012). Donepezil effects on hippocampal and prefrontal functional connectivity in Alzheimer's disease: Preliminary Report. *J Alzheimers Dis, 31*(3), S221–S226.

PART TWO

Plasticity of Cognition in Neurologic Syndromes

10

Plasticity in Prefrontal Cortical Networks After Brain Injury

Finding the Optimal Paths

Anthony J. W. Chen and Mark D'Esposito

Introduction

Traumatic brain injuries often disrupt the ability of an individual to successfully navigate the complexity of the modern world. The abilities of paying attention, holding information in mind, organizing, and developing efficient strategies for completing activities are particularly vulnerable to TBI. These processes come together to regulate and control other, more basic neural processes based on goals. Deficits in such aspects of goal-directed cognitive processes are among the most likely to become chronic, resulting in long-lasting disruptions of a patient's capacity to accomplish life pursuits. These functions are fundamental for successful independent living, and deficits may directly contribute to poor functional outcomes. Deficits may adversely affect the pursuit of educational and occupational goals, for example, resulting in an increased rate of job turnover (Doctor et al., 2005; Drake, Gray, Yoder, Pramuka, & Llewellyn, 2000; Machamer, Temkin, Fraser, Doctor, & Dikmen, 2005; Ownsworth & McKenna, 2004).

Poor goal-directed functioning may affect the process of recovery from brain injury in even more fundamental ways. In this chapter, we explore the possible contributions of goal-directed control and the underlying brain systems in supporting plasticity and learning after injury. We argue that these systems play fundamental roles in guiding changes in brain functioning. These roles are important for learning in the healthy brain and arguably even more important for functional improvement after brain injury. What happens if these systems are injured? For centuries, it was assumed that little could be changed or improved once a brain injury becomes chronic. We explore questions regarding the potential for plasticity in goal-directed control functions, and brain mechanisms that might support plasticity and improved functioning. What mechanisms underlie improvements with cognitive training? Are there parameters of brain functioning that are most conducive to plasticity and learning? A better understanding of the nature of such mechanisms may be important for advancing treatment development (A. J. W. Chen, Abrams, & D'Esposito, 2006; D'Esposito & Chen, 2006a; D'Esposito & Gazzaley, 2006).

What Are the Contributions of Goal-Directed Control and the Underlying Brain Systems in Supporting Plasticity and Learning After Injury?

First, we highlight that goal-directed control functions, and the prefrontal cortex (PFC) systems that subserve them, play fundamental roles in modulating how the brain functions. Clinicians are sensitive to the empiric understanding that if certain cognitive functions are not intact, other attempts at rehabilitation are made much more difficult. Individuals who are unable to set learning goals, pay attention, hold relevant information in mind, and work through multistep goals are less likely to benefit from rehabilitation training. In general, patients with deficits in these and related areas of higher order cognition may have reduced benefit with training in other neurologic domains, such as motor, speech, or other basic functions (Fischer, Gauggel, & Trexler, 2004; Hyndman & Ashburn, 2003; Ozdemir, Birtane, Tabatabaei, Ekuklu, & Kokino, 2001; Prigatano & Wong, 1999; Tatemichi et al., 1994). Their broad importance in recovery further motivates the need to understand how these functions themselves might be improved after injury.

Further evidence for the importance of PFC systems stems from a common phenomenon observed with functional brain imaging after brain injuries. Functional "activation" for patients performing various cognitive tasks may involve wider areas of PFC than might otherwise be observed for non-injured individuals (Christodoulou et al., 2001; Hillary, 2008; Hillary, Genova, Chiaravalloti, Rypma, & DeLuca, 2006; T. McAllister et al., 2001). This finding has generated hypotheses regarding the importance of engaging PFC during cognitive functioning after injury. It is possible that such engagement is simply a nonspecific reflection of increased "effort." However, it may be possible to hypothesize more specific contributions. Given that PFC networks play a central role in the integration of functions in order to facilitate goal-relevant processes (Curtis & D'Esposito, 2003; Fuster, 2000; E. K. Miller & Cohen, 2001), we propose that engagement of PFC networks may play a specific role or roles in supporting functions that are impaired by injury.

What role(s) might neural mechanisms of goal-directed control play in learning and improved functioning after brain injury? We consider several possibilities.

Resources to Support Performance of Challenging Tasks After Brain Injury

There are a number of potential functions that can provide "scaffolding" to support cognitive functioning in ways that are general to the specific domain of functioning. Probably the most basic hypothesis of a supportive role for PFC engagement after injury relates to an extension of the "increased cognitive effort" logic. First, any challenging task requires increased effort. This may include tasks that were once performed easily by the individual prior to injury. Basic concepts along these lines have been discussed in some reviews, highlighting the role of PFC systems for "scaffolding" the performance of challenging tasks (A. M. Kelly & Garavan, 2005; C. Kelly, Foxe, & Garavan, 2006).

The neural correlates of "effort" have not been perfectly well defined, but it is reasonable to hypothesize that neural mechanisms involved with alertness/arousal (Aston-Jones & Cohen, 2005), motivation (Krawczyk & D'Esposito, 2011), and "energization" (D. T. Stuss & Alexander, 2007) are important for driving cognitive functioning with increased challenge. All of these functions require engagement of coordinated networks of PFC subregions (e.g., ventro-medial prefrontal, anterior cingulate, dorsal lateral, and fronto-polar). Perhaps more fundamentally, any task that requires learning or adaptation to accomplish, such as a task that requires impaired neurologic functions, will require increased "effort" to drive the engagement of mechanisms for change.

At the next, yet still basic level, we would hypothesize that there is a need for the engagement of mechanisms of "attention" when performing a task is made more difficult by neurologic damage. In particular, we would highlight that engagement of PFC networks is vital whenever tasks require increased goal-direction. The construct of attention has numerous potential definitions, but at the core we highlight the importance of mechanisms for selecting information and actions relevant to a specified goal, in preference to alternatives that may compete for limited processing resources. The effective selection of goal-relevant processes may be of particular importance when alternative tasks are easier to perform. For example, there may be a tendency to use an intact limb when the other limb is paretic. Increased effort and explicit attention may be required to engage and use the paretic limb for a task. We would suggest that similar issues arise with cognitive functions that are more difficult to accomplish after an injury.

In clinical settings, deficiencies in these general functions translate not only to difficulties with task performance, but fundamentally to reduced progress with rehabilitation. We argue next that these functions serve a fundamental role in learning and are an important initial target of treatment.

Fundamental Mechanisms to Support Learning

We propose that mechanisms of goal-direction, mediated by PFC systems, play a role in modulating and changing brain function at an even more fundamental level. PFC systems play a role in the *learning of "new" skills* (including skills that were once available to an individual prior to injury). We propose a general framework, in which there are at least three key pillars needed to support learning—goal-direction, energy to support learning efforts ("energization," motivation, effort, focus, perseverance), and domain-specific learning (e.g., learning of a specific motor skill). In this chapter, we focus mostly on the first pillar, which encompasses important mechanisms not specific to a particular domain of learning. Ultimately, however, these complementary functions need to be integrated for effective learning.

The goal-directed guidance of neural processes is arguably particularly important during the course of learning and recovery after injury, when achieving a learning goal may require effort and multiple steps, spanning an extended period of time. The sustained coordination of brain networks required for learning will be susceptible to disruption by processes less relevant to the end goal. Thus, the integrity of various aspects of goal-direction will be important for effective and efficient learning. This includes processes sometimes referred to as goal setting, providing guidance by a goal template, selectively attending to and holding in mind relevant information, monitoring and correcting approaches throughout the learning process, as well as goal maintenance through the multiple steps.

Various aspects of support for learning may be linked to different PFC network functions. For example, processes important for establishing an attentional set, selectively attending to and holding in mind relevant information appropriate to the current goal, appear to depend particularly on lateral PFC networks (D'Esposito et al., 1995; Rogers, Andrews, Grasby, Brooks, & Robbins, 2000). Determining the congruence of information or action with a goal and monitoring for a match between an intermediate outcome and a goal during the learning process likely depend on anterior cingulate cortex (Cohen, Botvinick, & Carter, 2000). There may be other domain-general functions crucial for learning, such as for the initiation, energization, and sustainment of goal-directed activities, more reliant on right PFC (D. Stuss, 2006). Right PFC seems to be increasingly engaged with increased task difficulty, across different pathological states (Hillary, 2008), though it may not be adequately engaged after injury (S. H. Chen, Kareken, Fastenau, Trexler, & Hutchins, 2003). Overall, it is likely that the coordinated involvement of multiple nodes and configurations of PFC networks contributes crucial functional scaffolding for learning.

These functions are likely to be particularly important for intentional or explicit, goal-based learning efforts, and less important for learning via such mechanisms as classical conditioning or, more generally, when learning can occur passively. This framework also highlights that there may be a need for engagement of active, explicit goal-based control for tasks that might have been "automatic" prior to injury. For example, learning with the goal of performing a previously easy occupational task may require increased attention to the rehabilitation goals and specific subordinate steps required to reach the goals, while there may be a number of action choices or other potential foci of attention that are not relevant to the learning goal during rehabilitation.

However, even when learning aims toward more automatic performance, there may be a stage of skill acquisition that involves explicit, goal-directed learning. As an example, a transient stage of "scaffolding" seems to precede the automatization of even motor or verbal skills (Peterson et al., 1998). In general, scaffolding mechanisms are beneficial but tend to be effortful. In some circumstances, the explicit control that is imposed may impede effective automatic functioning. For example, learning a golf swing requires a period of explicit, scaffolded effort, during which the desired movement needs to be held as a goal, movements need to be guided to try to match that goal, and outcomes need to be compared to adjust one's movements. However, once the skill is automatized, the engagement of scaffolding mechanisms is no longer required and may impair performance. The engagement of PFC networks during the training of some basic functions thus appears to be specific to certain phases of learning (Debaere, Wenderoth, Sunaert, Van Hecke, & Swinnen, 2004; Jueptner et al., 1997; Karni et al., 1998; Sakai et al., 1998). As another example (one that has not been explored as extensively), there is evidence that recovery of language functioning in post-stroke aphasia may be associated with the functional connectivity of a so-called "executive network," which includes PFC as well as parietal and other regions (not specifically associated with language processing; Sharp et al., 2011).

We contend that analogous processes are important for the learning of various skills after brain injury. The nature and duration of engagement of PFC networks over the course of learning will depend on the particular skills to be learned. In some cases, such as with learning organizational skills, PFC engagement needs to be sustained. In other cases, such as with learning speech production skills that are meant to become automatic, PFC engagement is beneficial during a transient phase but needs to taper off for efficient task performance.

One challenge in interpreting empiric findings with functional imaging after brain injury is in understanding the significance of the levels of activation of PFC regions. "Activation" may not be a simple, linear indication of the contribution of PFC systems to a learning process. Indeed, based on the above arguments, PFC activation may be seen when performance is either decreased or improved. Furthermore, engagement of PFC networks may be better reflected in the functional interactions of PFC regions with other relevant brain regions, rather than in activation levels per se.

As an ancillary but clinically relevant note, the need to engage more neural resources for scaffolding might help to explain increased fatigue with cognitive activity after brain injury (perhaps the most common and debilitating symptom after injury), where fatigue leads to the reduced sustainment of goal-directed activities (A. J. W. Chen & Novakovic-Agopian, 2012). Interestingly, given an understanding that limited resources are required in these contexts, one useful rehabilitation approach has been to train basic tasks to the point of automaticity. Where such tasks are consistent or even stereotyped, task performance can be trained to the point that they require little top-down control. We contend that this approach is helpful because it achieves an unloading of core PFC systems so that they may be allocated for other efforts (Doyon & Benali, 2005; Floyer-Lea & Matthews, 2004).

Finding the Best Paths for Plasticity and Learning After Injury

The functional reorganization of available brain resources is likely an important mechanism of plasticity during recovery and rehabilitation. What mechanisms guide such reorganization? Key neural systems must be available for providing such guidance after injury has occurred. Certain functions subserved by PFC systems are arguably vital for modulating brain systems to guide neural changes. Just as higher order cognitive functions are important for problem-solving and, in particular, the ability to search for new approaches or strategies to new problems, PFC systems logically play a role in finding alternative pathways or solutions at the neural level to accomplish tasks or functions. We propose that PFC networks play a central role in the processes of searching for, testing, and establishing new pathways (new connections and/or new network configurations) during the learning of neurologic skills.

One function that is required for guiding brain plasticity is the provision of a "goal-based template" that can be used to guide the organization of networks toward a goal of performing a particular neural-behavioral function. PFC networks, especially anterior and dorsolateral PFC, are likely important for establishing and maintaining such a learning template, given roles in goal-subgoal management and maintenance (Badre & D'Esposito, 2009; Badre, Hoffman, Cooney, & D'Esposito, 2009; Badre, Kayser, & D'Esposito, 2010; Braver & Bongiolatti, 2002; Burgess et al., 2006; Koechlin, Basso, Pietrini, Panzer, & Grafman, 1999; Koechlin, Ody, & Kouneiher, 2003). We would hypothesize that the establishment and maintenance of a learning template in the form of a network configuration are needed for accomplishing that "proposed" network configuration.

Another function is the search for, and perhaps "testing" of, various potential neural solutions to achieve a particular learning goal. Lateral PFC has been shown to be engaged with the application of cognitive strategies (Miotto et al., 2006). At the neural level, the successful application of new strategies would need to involve finding different pathways from the pathways available prior to injury. We hypothesize that control functions play a role in searching for, modulating, engaging, and integrating alternative neural pathways into newly configured functional networks during the process of learning to accomplish a function.

One step up is the challenge of finding the *optimal* pathway (perhaps among a number of non-optimal options after injury). In order to test and optimize any given neural solution, networks must first be temporarily integrated, or bound together in trying to accomplish a function, and this binding must be maintained to sufficiently evaluate the given solution against experienced outcomes or other alternatives. This is likely an effortful process that requires top-down control, and we suggest that this is a major contribution of engaged PFC networks after injury.

This raises the particularly important implication for what happens if PFC systems function suboptimally—important aspects of learning and recovery would be impeded. It is observable in clinical practice that the very functions that are subserved by PFC networks are those functions that are prerequisites for maximizing success in rehabilitation after brain injury. Individuals may have difficulty with various aspects of goal-directed learning, involving deficiencies in establishing clear learning goals, establishing attentional sets supportive of learning, maintaining key information during learning, redirecting resources when distracted, as well as monitoring and assessing progress relative to a learning goal. It is possible that without optimized PFC systems, alternative strategies may not be found, and problem-solving, at the level of neural networks, might not advance to the optimal solution.

In a hypothetical scenario, multifocal injury to cortex and white matter may occur after TBI, thus disrupting both nodes and interconnections in various brain networks. In order to accomplish a behavioral function that has become deficient, new network configurations may be required. This might involve engagement of nodes in new functional network configurations, in particular during an active learning and recovery phase. A number of different network configurations may need to be tried for an individual to settle on the most optimal solution. In many cases, an overall network configuration very similar to a pre-injury configuration may be the most optimal. However, there may be other circumstances in which an alternative configuration is best. This might occur when particular nodes or connections are too extensively damaged, or more generally, when a different strategy for accomplishing a particular function is applied. An example of the latter might be the use of right hemisphere networks to accomplish verbal communication when an individual learns to apply melodic intonation to accomplish speech after severe left hemisphere injury (Norton, Zipse, Marchina, & Schlaug, 2009).

We argue that the remediation of goal-directed control functions may be valuable for influencing learning and recovery in multiple neurologic domains, as these goal-directed "learning functions" relate to an individual's ability to *self-teach* skills and self-adjust to residual deficits of almost any sort. For example, improved goal-directed functioning may enhance an individual's ability to actively participate in attempts to rehabilitate motor, speech, perceptual, and other cognitive functions, allowing an individual to hold learning goals in mind, selectively focus attention to learning activities, and solve problems in the numerous intervening steps between a current state and the achievement of a learning goal.

By extension, individuals who suffer concurrent injury that affects goal-directed control, in addition to other domains, may recover more slowly or may recover with less efficient, perhaps maladaptive solutions. In extreme, though well-known examples, damage to PFC networks can lead to "static" functional outcomes. In short-term timescales, individuals are observed to perseverate on particular behaviors. In long-term timescales, recovery appears not to progress, that is, the deficits are observed to be "static." It is sometimes observed that behavior can be altered during training, but one of the biggest frustrations is that behavior tends to revert to baseline (especially in contexts beyond that of training). In other words, with PFC dysfunction, behavior tends to be "elastic," rather than plastic.

If damage to goal-directed control systems plays such a vital role in learning and recovery, then it would seem that damage to these systems would lead to very poor prognosis. It becomes important to ask the question, to what extent can the functions of goal-directed control systems be improved?

Is There Plasticity in PFC Goal-Directed Control Functions? What Neural Mechanisms Support This Plasticity?

Regulation of a Series of Neural Processes for Successful Goal-Directed Behavior

Accomplishing goals may require the regulation of multiple neural processes, including perception and cognitive processing, motor actions, and emotional functioning, as well as other aspects of behavior. Higher order cognitive functions that direct other, more basic processes are particularly important for helping individuals achieve goals in the complex settings of the real world. These functions must regulate a continuum of cognitive processes, from the selection of information for more in-depth processing (often referred to as attention and working memory) up through processes that guide the organization and execution of activities based on goals. Coordination processes need to effectively span "time and space," organizing functions across different domains (and different functional networks) across the time that is needed to achieve all the steps required to reach an end goal. Regulatory functions that span cognition, emotion, and behavior are crucial, especially in the context of distractions, disruptions, stress, and other challenges, because the goal-attainment process may be disrupted at any point in the continuum. In such contexts, regulatory functions are crucial for basic processes to be smoothly coordinated, so that individuals may function effectively and efficiently in achieving a goal.

Plasticity in Goal-Directed Selective Attention and Working Memory Processes

Selective processing of goal-relevant information is a crucial gateway that filters the information that gains access to more in-depth processing (Awh & Vogel, 2008; Baddeley, 2001; Cowan & Morey, 2006; Repovs & Baddeley, 2006; Vogel, McCollough, & Machizawa, 2005). The integrity of information processing across the continuum of processes required for goal accomplishment requires mechanisms of selection, maintenance, and protection from disruption during working memory, learning, decision-making, and/ or problem-solving. The protection of information processing from distractions anywhere along this pathway is crucial to efficient and effective goal attainment, especially when extended time or multiple steps are required.

Some recent approaches to training of "selective attention" and "working memory" processes have yielded evidence of plasticity in these processes, for individuals without brain injury. In a series of studies utilizing computer-based practice of tasks that progressively engage spatial working memory, Klingberg and colleagues have shown improvements in working memory functioning as well as transfer to higher-level cognitive functions that presumably rely on working memory (Klingberg, 2010; Olesen, Westerberg, & Klingberg, 2004; Westerberg et al., 2007). In healthy subjects, improvements were correlated with changes in activation in PFC and parietal regions, as well as changes in dopamine receptor binding (McNab et al., 2009; Olesen, Westerberg, & Klingberg, 2004). The specific explanation for changes in activation remains an area of active debate, and changes may depend on the particular domain being examined, the phase of learning, testing contexts, as well as the nature of the underlying injury. Other recent studies have generated excitement by demonstrating that improvements in specific aspects of goal-directed control and even general fluid intelligence may be possible (Dahlin, Neely, Larsson, Backman, & Nyberg, 2008; Erickson et al., 2007; Jaeggi, Buschkuehl, Jonides, & Perrig, 2008; Persson & Reuter-Lorenz, 2008). The transfer of gains to non-trained cognitive domains is an active area of inquiry, with mixed results (Anguera et al., 2013; Salminen, Strobach, & Schubert, 2012). To what extent similar task-based training approaches may alter functioning for individuals with brain injury, with improvements that generalize to real world functioning, will be worth further investigation.

There is some evidence that goal-directed cognitive functioning can be altered, even in the chronic phase of brain injury recovery. For example, training of a proposed hierarchy of attention processes after brain injury has been performed with Attention Process Training, originally formulated by Sohlberg and Mateer (Sohlberg & Mateer, 1987; Sohlberg, McLaughlin, Pavese, Heidrich, & Posner, 2000), and a number of other protocols (Cicerone et al., 2000, 2005; Kennedy et al., 2008; Levine, Turner, & Stuss, 2008; Rohling, Faust, Beverly, & Demakis, 2009). Approaches that target isolated processes, including several that use computer-based tasks, have been demonstrated to improve functioning on targeted measures. However, the transfer and generalization of gains from task practice have proved to be limited in many trials (D'Esposito & Gazzaley, 2006). This raises important questions regarding the nature of transfer beyond practiced tasks (discussed later in this chapter).

When change does occur in goal-directed control functions, in particular, for aspects of attention and working memory, what are the neural bases of these changes? Information regarding neural mechanisms of improvement in goal-directed control functions after brain injury has been sparse. Even the extent to which the neural systems that underlie control are plastic, if at all, has remained an open question. Only a handful of functional magnetic resonance imaging (fMRI) studies to date have examined cognitive rehabilitation following traumatic brain injury (Laatsch, Thulborn, Krisky, Shobat, & Sweeney, 2004; Strangman et al., 2008), and even fewer have examined the effects of training-based interventions on control functions (Kim et al., 2009).

We attempted to identify neural mechanisms that underlie improvements in goal-directed control for patients with chronic brain injury. Based on recent work from our efforts and others, we highlight several possible contributing mechanisms. These mechanisms relate to changes in the levels of top-down modulation of posterior brain regions and neural codes by PFC network, changes in the interactions between PFC and posterior regions, changes between right and left PFC, as well as changes within PFC neural codes.

Investigations of Neural Mechanisms of Improved Goal-Directed Cognition in Chronic Brain Injury

We have been investigating neural mechanisms of plasticity separable into two complementary lines, summarized in Figure 10.1, each described in detail in the next sections. These lines investigate plasticity in relation to task-based, goal-directed cognition (flow chart on the right) and baseline states that are a foundation for episodes of task-based cognition (flow chart on the left).

We have examined neural and behavioral changes with an intervention that targets goal-oriented attention regulation (Novakovic-Agopian et al., 2010). Participants with acquired brain injury and chronic executive dysfunction completed a training intervention

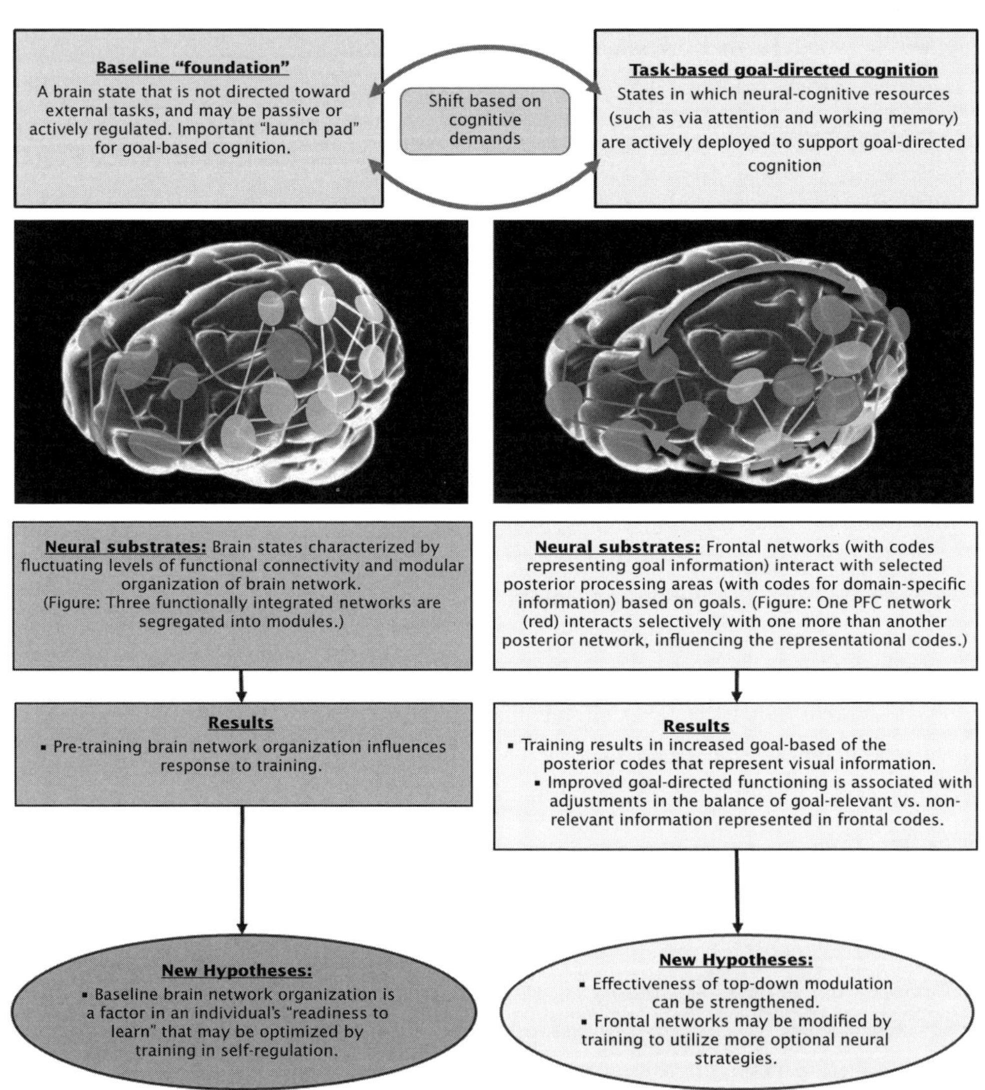

FIGURE 10.1 Lines of investigation addressing two complementary functions of plasticity in goal-directed cognition. (see color insert)

for goal-oriented attentional self-regulation that takes into account the links connecting attention, working memory, and goal-based direction of behavior in the contexts of complex, real-life goals. This intervention was developed based on the rationale that pathways from perception to action require mechanisms for the selection of information for in-depth processing, as well as the maintenance and protection of this information from disruption during working memory and subsequent learning, decision-making, and/or problem-solving. We reasoned that the selective maintenance of goal-related information is important for guiding sequences of steps (subgoals) required to accomplish the goal. Therefore, intervening on these processes may help to ameliorate symptoms of "goal neglect" (Duncan, Burgess, & Emslie, 1995; Duncan, Emslie, Williams, Johnson, & Freer, 1996). The experimental training protocol was based on training interventions that have been applied to patients with brain injury as well as other populations (D'Zurilla TJ & Goldfried, 1971; Levine et al., 2000, 2007; Nezu, Nezu, & D'Zurilla, 2007; Rath, Simon, Langenbahn, Sherr, & Diller, 2003; VonCramon, Cramon, & Mai, 1991), with special emphasis on mindfulness-based attention-regulation strategies applied to daily life situations and complex, project-based functional tasks.

It may be argued that the highest levels of goal-directed control are engaged in the low-structure environments of the real world. These environments differ from many formalized assessment contexts in that specific instructions for how to accomplish a goal are not provided, and a number of challenges may disrupt goal processes. Therefore, in order to assess the most distal effects of these interventions, we assessed changes in participant functioning during performance in "real-life" low-structure settings. Following training, participants showed improvements in accomplishing multiple errands tasks, missing fewer tasks during a limited time period for task accomplishment. This type of observed functional assessment helps to confirm generalization of training effects to complex settings. Preliminary results with a new functional assessment instrument, the Goal Processing Scale (Novakovic-Agopian et al., 2011), have been consistent with these prior findings (unpublished data).

In testing to what extent there might be plasticity in the neural-cognitive systems supporting the targeted cognitive processes, we also assessed changes in performance in specific cognitive domains utilizing neuropsychological testing tasks. Participants who completed a course of goal-oriented attentional self-regulation training improved on measures of complex attention and executive functions, including working memory, mental flexibility, inhibition, and sustained attention. Changes in performance were not observed after a comparison education intervention that did not include active skill training. These findings suggest that functional improvements may be supported by improvements in these particular domains.

Plasticity in Goal-Directed Modulation of Information Representations in the Brain

At the simplest level, cognitive control involves the top-down modulation of neural activity based on goals, as well as the coordination and monitoring of distributed neural networks in the brain. The modulation of neural processes from the "top down" is accomplished by at least two interlinked mechanisms: *selection* and *maintenance* of goal-relevant neural processes for the accomplishment of tasks.

Neural representations of information are coded in distributed networks of neurons. For example, visual objects are represented in distributed codes in the inferior temporal cortex (Haxby et al., 2001), and the representation of information in these codes can be modulated by goal-direction (A. J. W. Chen et al., 2012). This is particularly important, as information can be coded in the brain with varying levels of clarity. This may be relevant in individuals who have suffered acquired brain injury with potentially a "dis-integration" of brain networks. Whether the information represents stimuli in the external world, or representations of more abstract information, such as for the goal relevance of external stimuli, greater clarity in the neural codes that represent such information would logically support goal-directed behavior. We tested the hypothesis that training to improve goal-directed attention would increase the clarity of information representations in the brain for individuals with brain injury as a reflection of enhanced goal-based modulatory control of neural processing. Functional MRI methods adapted for testing the effects of intervention for patients with varied injury pathology were used to index modulatory control of neural processing (A. J. W. Chen et al., 2011). In order to test hypotheses at the level of distributed neural codes, we applied measurements that "read the *information*" coded in brain networks, rather than simply quantifying brain activity levels. Methods for decoding neural information representations using pattern classification of multivoxel fMRI patterns provide tools for gauging the functional integration of networks.

In order to probe the neural mechanisms supporting goal-directed selective information processing, functional MRI data were acquired during performance of a visual task that abstracts the common situation in everyday life in which multiple incoming streams of information compete for attention. For example, although multiple images (such as of faces, scenery, and other objects) may be viewed, a person may be interested in learning the faces of individuals in one moment, but identifying scenic views in another. This task was designed to require perception of all images, each resulting in representations within brain networks, but selective processing of some images in preference to others, depending on the task goals. Thus, neural codes would need to be modulated based on goal relevance to favor clearer representation of some images over others during more in-depth processing. Of note, the training interventions described in the preceding section did not involve training on the tasks used during fMRI.

We specifically measured the clarity of information representations in distributed neural codes, reasoning that increased goal-directed control would modify the clarity of goal-relevant and non-relevant information in posterior cortex. Thus, we indexed goal-based modulation of neural processing with fMRI data using a pattern classifier method by measuring the tuning of neural representations within extrastriate cortex. This measurement indexed the relative balance of representation of relevant versus non-relevant information. Our findings suggested that training led to changes in the tuning of neural representations such that the balance of representation favored goal-relevant information. In other words, the tuning of networks within the extrastriate cortex was shifted to increase the clarity of goal-relevant information relative to non-relevant. At a broad level, goal-directed control of neural processing in the posterior cortex was significantly enhanced by attention regulation training. Thus, as summarized in Figure 10.1, the modulation of posterior neural codes is plastic and can be altered by cognitive training.

Plasticity in PFC Neural Codes: Strategic Adjustments to Improve Functioning?

Changes in the extrastriate cortex are most likely a downstream effect of changes in PFC-mediated modulatory control. Lateral PFC has been strongly implicated as a source of attentional control signals that could bias neural processing in posterior cortex (Desimone, 1998; Lee & D'Esposito, 2012; B. T. Miller & D'Esposito, 2005; E. K. Miller & Cohen, 2001). For PFC to provide such guidance, representations of relevant and/or non-relevant information must be coded in PFC as well, though the specific nature of these representations may differ from the stimulus-driven representations coded in the posterior cortex. When we examined changes in lateral PFC after training using the pattern classifier methods earlier, we found that our fMRI index of the balance of representation of goal-relevant and non-relevant information shifted for each individual. The direction and degree of these depended on each individual's baseline measurement. For those with baselines tuned to represent non-relevant information more strongly than goal-relevant, the balance shifted toward the goal-relevant after training, and vice versa. This pattern of findings suggests that different strategic "adjustments" to PFC codes may be made for different individuals in order to improve personal functioning. One particularly important but challenging area for further investigation will be to understand the variability in mechanisms by which different individuals may achieve improvement in functioning after brain injury.

Plasticity in Strategic Learning: Sharpened Neural Representations of the Goal-Relevance of Perceived Information

We are all constantly faced with sources of information that either contain too much information or are ambiguous with respect to one's goals. The ability to synthesize core meaning from incoming information (i.e., "get the gist") is important for goal-directed behavior in everyday life, and relies on the integration of a number of cognitive processes. Chapman and colleagues have developed protocols to train gist-based strategic reasoning, guiding individuals through steps that engage attention (repeating and filtering the information), working memory (integration of information), and higher-level elaborative reasoning (expanding, extracting; Chapman et al., 2006; Reyna & Brainerd, 1995). Training has been shown to improve the ability to extract gist, as well as other aspects of learning and reasoning for children, as well as adults with traumatic brain injury (Vas, Chapman, Cook, Elliott, & Keebler, 2011). Vas and colleagues evaluated gist-reasoning performance and other behavioral measures in patients with chronic TBI before and after completion of 8 weeks of strategic memory and reasoning training (SMART) versus an active comparison protocol involving education regarding brain health (adapted from Binder et al., 2008) in which participants were taught general principles about brain anatomy, the effect of diet and exercise on brain activity, and cognitive changes after TBI. They found that patients who completed SMART had enhanced gist-reasoning, an effect that was sustained at 6-month follow-up. Performance on tests of attention and working memory also improved. This raises the interesting possibility that training in higher-level *integrative* abilities may either focus the direction of more basic abilities or even potentially improve more basic functions.

Critical to the process described above is the ability to distinguish goal-relevant from non-relevant information, and selectively process relevant information. Could an increase in the clarity of neural representations of goal relevance be a mechanism of plasticity with training? A subset of the patients in the strategic memory and reasoning intervention study (n = 19; Vas et al., 2011) participated in the same fMRI tasks described in the prior section (A. J. W. Chen et al., 2011), designed to engage the goal-directed selection of relevant stimuli over non-relevant stimuli during a selective, jittered, and variable n-back task. The task included alternate stimulus sets to support repeated testing, and the training interventions did not involve the fMRI tasks.

For this investigation, we applied information-decoding techniques to a hypothesis-driven novel analysis method. The analysis protocol involved gathering whole-brain voxel activations during the task, and then training a pattern classifier to distinguish between patterns of activation associated with goal-relevant stimuli, and patterns associated with non-relevant stimuli. Note that this classification is orthogonal to the classification of the presented stimulus object categories (faces and scenes), described previously (A. J. W. Chen et al., 2011), and is meant to decode a more abstract information property. We posited that the classifier's accuracy in decoding goal relevance would reflect the clarity with which representations of the goal relevance of a perceived stimulus were coded in the brain. We then determined to what extent training altered the accuracy of decoding of goal relevance. Classifier accuracy for detection of relevant and non-relevant stimuli was not different between the two groups of participants before training. After SMART, but not the education intervention, classifier accuracy was significantly greater in extrastriate cortex (p = 0.002) (M Shah et al., 2013). This study demonstrates a potential mechanism of plasticity with training in goal-based strategic memory and reasoning that is congruent with the theoretical underpinnings of the intervention.

Dynamic Plasticity in Engagement of PFC Across Hemispheres

PFC lesions do not invariably result in severe deficits in the cognitive functions thought to be subserved by these regions. Indeed, quite often with unilateral lesions, specific deficits are difficult to detect on a clinical basis or with basic cognitive testing. For example, a patient's working memory functioning may be relatively unimpaired after unilateral dorsolateral PFC damage (Badre et al., 2009; D'Esposito & Postle, 1999). This suggests that there are mechanisms of post-injury plasticity that support the recovery of cognitive function; however, the specific mechanisms for such plasticity in humans have not been clear. It has previously been proposed that when a component of PFC networks is damaged, other network components may be engaged to support the deficit functions (A. J. W. Chen et al., 2006). At the phenomenologic level, broader areas of PFC, including contralateral PFC, appear to be engaged after various forms of injury (S. H. Chen et al., 2003; Christodoulou et al., 2001; Levine et al., 2002; T. W. McAllister et al., 2001). Intact components might also include perilesional tissue, intact contralateral homologous regions (Wundt, 1902), or subcortical structures (Van Vleet et al., 2003).

Compensatory Engagement of Contralateral PFC After Unilateral Stroke

When an area of PFC is damaged, does the recovery of behavior depend on functioning of the intact contralateral PFC? Available evidence supports mechanisms in which the engagement of contralateral, intact PFC provides support for behavioral functions that might otherwise be impaired. For example, although individuals with no injury show predominantly left-lateralized PFC networks correlating with verbal working memory functioning, individuals with a history of TBI may show a positive correlation between right PFC activity and working memory functioning (Turner, McIntosh, & Levine, 2011).

Pushing beyond the general concept of intact regions of PFC engaging to "compensate" for damaged regions, the temporal dynamics of such functional compensation has been further elucidated with electrophysiologic studies involving patients with unilateral PFC damage. Evoked response potentials from patients with unilateral PFC strokes have been compared against healthy individuals with performance on lateralized attention and working memory tasks (Voytek et al., 2010). The design of the tasks allowed stimuli to be presented either to the lesioned hemisphere or non-lesioned hemisphere, even switching randomly on a trial-by-trial basis. This allowed within-subjects analyses of the interactions of stimulus location (right or left visual field) and hemisphere. This study provided evidence that intact PFC compensates for damage in the lesioned PFC on a rapid timescale, trial-by-trial in cognitive tasks. Transient increases in electrophysiologic potentials associated with attention and memory were observed in intact PFC, detectable in less than one second after stimulus presentation.

Furthermore, during a working memory task, frontal theta (4–8 Hz) oscillatory EEG activity was observed only over the intact hemisphere for patients, and this activity was increased for correctly performed task trials. Additionally, engagement of intact PFC depended on cognitive load, such that intact PFC was engaged with increasing load demands to the lesioned hemisphere. With an attention task, a late frontal positivity (450–650 ms) increased in amplitude in the intact hemisphere, for correctly performed trials. In general, evidence of engagement of intact PFC was only observed when the lesioned hemisphere was challenged. Together, these findings support the interpretation that intact PFC is engaged to provide compensatory functioning for the lesioned hemisphere. This compensatory engagement occurs flexibly and dynamically, based on cognitive demands.

Intact PFC appears to assume control of task processing on a sub-second time scale. Of note, electrophysiologic studies in nonhuman primates have shown that PFC neurons are highly adaptable, that is, physiologic properties may be altered quickly in the course of behavioral learning. For example, PFC neurons can rapidly change firing patterns in response to learning stimulus categories (Freedman, Riesenhuber, Poggio, & Miller, 2001) and learning new stimulus-response associations with a small number of trials (Asaad, Rainer, & Miller, 1998).

How might the intact PFC be engaged with posterior visual processing across hemispheres? In the setting of reduced fronto-frontal connectivity across hemispheres, and reduced fronto-parietal connectivity within the damaged hemisphere (Alstott, Breakspear, Hagmann, Cammoun, & Sporns, 2009), the most likely route through which the intact PFC can process visual information from the posterior cortex would be through the posterior corpus callosum. This pathway may provide an alternative route for interhemispheric communication, and this has implications for a prediction of worsened recovery with injury to the corpus callosum, common with traumatic multifocal axonal injury.

The importance of cross-regional connections and dynamic engagement of distant regions is highlighted in this mechanism of functional plasticity. The importance of the integrity of inter-regional connections in functional plasticity suggests a reason that axonal injury may add an impediment to recovery when such "dis-connection" injuries occur together with focal injury. This may also have implications for understanding the observation of reduced speed of processing despite intact performance in some settings, as well as increased likelihood for deficits to be observable with time limitations. Furthermore, this provides a potential basis for the value of rehabilitation techniques that emphasize utilizing increased processing time to effectively accomplish functional goals.

Evidence for Dynamic Engagement of Contralateral PFC From a Transient Disruption Model

Transcranial magnetic stimulation (TMS) provides methods for functionally disrupting anatomically localized regions to test hypotheses regarding putative mechanisms of plasticity. TMS can be used to transiently disrupt brain function in a focal region in healthy individuals, creating a "virtual lesion." In a TMS experiment, Lee disrupted functioning of lateral PFC in one hemisphere to investigate the effects on neural processing and behavior (Lee & D'Esposito, 2012).

TMS was placed over unilateral PFC to functionally disrupt this focal region prior to fMRI and performance of a task requiring selective information processing for working memory (A. J. W. Chen et al., 2011). In order to achieve a longer lasting disruption effect from TMS, continuous theta burst parameters were applied (50 Hz trains of three

TMS pulses repeated every 200 ms continuously over a period of 40 seconds; Huang, Edwards, Rounis, Bahatia, & Rothwell, 2005). Continuous theta burst has been shown to depress activity in the stimulated region for up to 60 minutes following stimulation, and this is better suited for studying the effects of TMS with fMRI given that acquisition runs last over 30 minutes. The left inferior frontal gyrus (LIFG) was chosen as the site of stimulation, because it was determined to be a likely source of top-down modulation based on functional connectivity analyses from the cognitive task applied during fMRI. In this task, images of faces and scenes were sequentially presented and participants were instructed to selectively attend to and maintain images from the relevant category while ignoring those from the irrelevant category (A. J. W. Chen et al., 2011). The task utilized in this TMS-fMRI study was designed to allow isolation of separate patterns corresponding to the perception of faces versus scenes, and thus allowed analyses of attention effects on the perceptual codes embedded in these patterns. The task was also designed with alternate stimulus sets to allow for repeated testing, vital to the repeated measurements needed for testing mechanisms of plasticity, learning, and recovery. Importantly, by examining neural data using fMRI in association with TMS disruption, hypotheses regarding the neural and behavioral effects of focal disruption, as well as neural-behavioral relationships, could be tested.

With fMRI, differential activation of the left inferior frontal gyrus (LIFG) during different attention conditions (attend vs. ignore faces) was found to correlate with behavioral performance accuracy. TMS disruption led to measurable behavioral deficits on the task. In particular, the relationship between LIFG activation and performance was disrupted by TMS over the LIFG (but not with TMS over somatosensory cortex). Importantly, after LIFG TMS, a new relationship developed between right IFG and behavioral performance. These findings suggest that the non-disrupted right IFG plays a role in compensating for disrupted left IFG function and supporting behavioral performance requiring working memory.

How might non-lesioned PFC support functioning involving posterior cortical regions? In this study, lesioning left PFC was associated with increased functional connectivity of right PFC with posterior cortical regions for some individuals. Increased connectivity of posterior brain regions (extrastriate cortex regions activated by the stimuli) with the non-disrupted PFC appeared to mitigate the disruptive effect of TMS over left PFC. This suggests that the critical factor providing compensatory functioning might be a dynamic increase in functional interactions of intact PFC regions with the domain-specific posterior regions important for task processing. Furthermore, individuals with greater PFC-posterior functional connectivity at baseline were most resistant to PFC disruption by TMS.

This same study also examined the effects of PFC disruption on properties of distributed neural codes, specifically the distinctiveness of spatially distributed neural codes in different cognitive conditions. Analyzing information represented in spatially distributed codes, rather than activation magnitudes alone, is an important conceptual as well as methodological advance. More precise information can be coded in distributed networks than in a code represented simply by magnitude increases or decreases in a single region. Measurements in the more precise distributed codes should be more sensitive to changes than more limited measurements of magnitudes in a single region. Furthermore, spatial correlation analyses are relatively insensitive to differences in the magnitude of activation (A. J. W. Chen et al., 2012) that might occur with different TMS stimulation conditions. We have previously shown that the distinctiveness of activity patterns in extrastriate cortex is modulated by attention (A. J. W. Chen et al., 2012).

The distinctiveness of brain activity patterns in selected regions can be indexed by the correlation of the spatial patterns—the stronger the correlations, the less distinctive the patterns are. TMS disruption of the left IFG was found to ablate the relationship between left IFG and the modulatory effects of attention on posterior neural codes in the extrastriate cortex. Effects of TMS disruption were not evident with simple analyses of activation levels within a selected extrastriate cortex region (the fusiform face area). Supporting the behavioral importance of these codes, the greater the left IFG TMS-induced decrease in distinctiveness between extrastriate cortex activity patterns for faces and scenes, the greater the decrement in performance accuracy on the working memory task.

In sum, by functionally disrupting PFC unilaterally, this study provides direct evidence that PFC contributes to the tuning of extrastriate cortex codes, and that measurements of this top-down influence relate to behavioral performance requiring working memory.

What Network Mechanisms Support Plasticity in Goal-Directed Control Functioning? A Summary Model

In sum, we have presented the following mechanisms of plasticity in the brain networks that subserve goal-directed cognition (see Figure 10.2).

Neural codes that represent information within posterior regional brain networks may be modified by training. There is plasticity in the representation of basic perceptual constructs, from basic visual features up through representations of objects in the visual world. It appears that modulatory control of these representations based on goals can be enhanced by training. Furthermore, codes representing more abstract information, such as the goal-relevance of any given percept or event, may also be enhanced by training.

Neural codes representing information in prefrontal cortical networks may be shaped as a mechanism of learning. Plasticity within prefrontal cortical networks may occur in different forms. The balance of information represented in PFC networks may shift with training. For example, the relative strength of representation of visual information

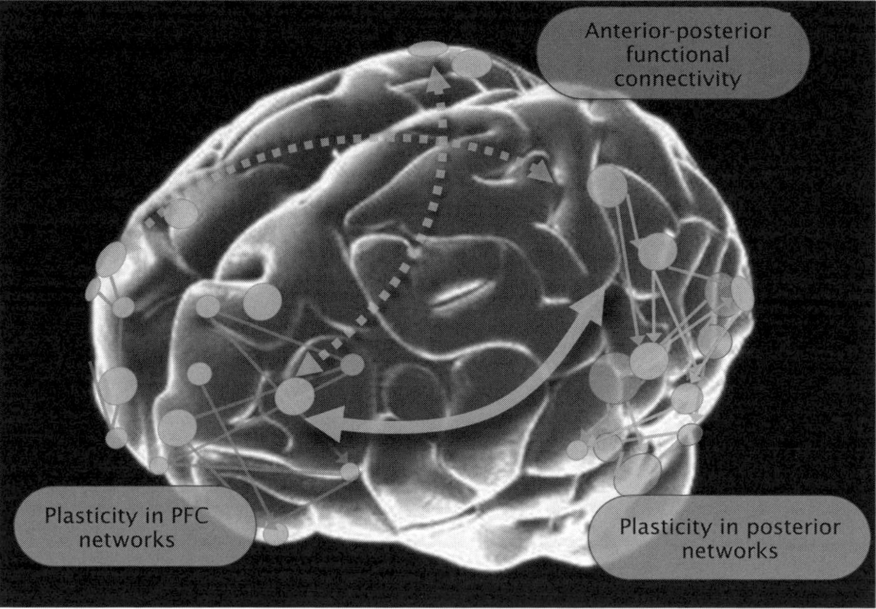

FIGURE 10.2 A summary model of network mechanisms that support plasticity in goal-directed control functioning. (see color insert)

that is goal-relevant versus non-relevant may shift. This suggests a mechanism for a "neural strategy shift," where PFC utilizes differing information to accomplish end goals. Representational codes in PFC may be plastic at a rapid time scale, changing quickly during learning trials. Furthermore, in the context of PFC injury, PFC networks may rapidly shift to engage different regions in accomplishing necessary functions. There is evidence that this occurs across hemispheres, such that functions previously subserved by injured PFC may be subsumed by engagement of intact, contralateral PFC. It is possible that the relative balance of engagement across different subregions of PFC may also be plastic, though this needs to be further examined.

Shifts in engagement of PFC subregions may be expressed not only through changes in activation and alterations in neural information representation, but importantly, *shifts in connectivity with other regions of the brain.* Indeed, one could hypothesize that it is the selective engagement of PFC networks with specific networks in other parts of the brain that is particularly important for mediating changes in goal-directed control. Furthermore, the representational codes within PFC are likely modulated by the contents of the regions that are functionally connected. Further work addressing these putative mechanisms will be valuable for determining mechanisms of plasticity in cognition and potential approaches to intervention after injury.

Having discussed mechanisms that may mediate plasticity in goal-directed cognition, we now turn to another frontier. What factors might influence the malleability of brain networks? In other words, what aspects of brain functioning might make the brain more responsive to training?

Frontiers: What Factors Encourage Plasticity and Learning in Goal-Directed Neural-Behavioral Control Functions?

The Importance of Brain State Regulation in an Individual's "Readiness to Learn"

Cognitive actions always occur in the context of a pre-existing brain state. This brain state, which could be described with particulars of ongoing activity and parameters of brain network interactions, is an important foundation from which "phasic" cognitive actions, such as in the context of externally driven tasks, are launched. The ability to regulate one's "baseline" state likely influences performance during goal-directed cognitive task action. Parameters of brain state dynamically shift between what has been called a "resting state" and a "working state," depending on cognitive demands (Kitzbichler, Henson, Smith, Nathan, & Bullmore, 2011). Fluctuations in this state influence behavioral responses and associated brain activity (Fox, Snyder, Zacks, & Raichle, 2006). The ability to regulate brain state between episodes of goal-directed cognitive task action likely influences performance during those episodes of action (Papo, 2013). Within an individual there are subtle fluctuations in modularity over time, which appear to track within-individual variability in working memory performance (Stevens, Tappon, Garg, & Fair, 2012).

Of particular importance for this discussion, opportunities for goal-directed learning (i.e., change) also must occur in the context of a pre-learning brain state. We posit that parameters of a brain state exert an important influence on an individual's ability to learn and to improve cognitive functioning. Is it possible that one could optimize parameters of a brain state to support plasticity and learning after injury?

Certain parameters of brain network organization may be particularly important in supporting the potential for learning and plasticity. Functional connectivity or functional organization between phasic deployments of cognitive resources may "tune" how the brain responds during tasks, influencing the responsiveness, efficiency, and, potentially, the plasticity of brain networks. This may be a basis for a person's ability to optimize computational capabilities, information transmission and storage, response to external information, and, ultimately, ability to learn (Haldeman & Beggs, 2005; Kinouchi & Copelli, 2006; Papo, 2013).

In particular, the modularity of brain network organization has been theorized to support learning and plasticity by enhancing the adaptivity, robustness, and evolvablity of network function (Bassett & Bullmore, 2006; Meunier, Achard, Morcom, & Bullmore, 2009). All neurologic functions are implemented through a combination of both local and distributed processes. Quantitative measures that characterize large-scale brain network organization complement the assessment of local brain properties. The organizational structure of functional brain networks may play an important role in goal-directed cognition by regulating the flow of information across the brain, constraining how efficiently goal-relevant information ("signal") is transmitted relative to irrelevant information ("noise"). Modularity is a summary of the extent to which a large-scale brain network can be characterized by subnetworks (i.e., modules) with high within-module connectivity and low between-module connectivity. Integration within modules allows for efficient local processing, while segregation between modules reduces noise propagation or intrusive crosstalk across modules (Rubinov & Sporns, 2010). Modular organization enables systems to rapidly adapt and evolve in response to the environment (Meunier, Lambiotte, & Bullmore, 2010). Cortical lesions and subcortical axonal damage may directly or indirectly disrupt the functional integration of information across distributed brain regions, leading to widespread disruptions to functional brain network organization (Crofts et al., 2011; Gratton et al., 2012; Nakamura et al., 2009; Sharp et al., 2011).

A brain state characterized by modular network configuration may serve as the optimal launching platform for engaging in goal-directed cognition, including for directed lea rning, for example through training. These arguments also suggest that network parameters of brain state may explain variability in response to training. We examined the extent to which regulation of functional organization of large-scale brain networks prior to training, indexed by network modularity, might determine an individual's response to subsequent cognitive training.

We acquired fMRI data sets from brief (5 minute) sessions prior to their participation in the cognitive training. In order to obtain an assay of functional network organization, patients were given instructions aimed at trying to achieve a relaxed but focused resting state. We indexed the modularity of brain networks by computing the proportion of within- compared to between-network connections for each individual for the 5 minute scans. A thresholded connectivity matrix of time-series correlations among 90 brain regions was used to generate a brain graph. Separate functional networks (brain modules) were determined by optimizing Newman's modularity for each individual brain graph.

We determined to what extent there was a relationship between pre-training brain network modularity and changes after training in cognitive performance relating to attention and executive functions. Pre-training measurements of brain modularity predicted the degree of improvement in attention and executive functioning with training, such that those individuals with higher baseline modularity exhibited greater improvements with cognitive training (r = −0.75, p<0.02) (publication in preparation). Baseline neuropsychological test scores did not predict treatment effects. These results support the contention that the functional organization of brain networks influences learning with attention regulation training.

These findings suggest a framework where parameters of brain networks reflect a brain *state*, and it will be worth exploring to what extent brain network states can be modified by cognitive training. Indeed, there is now accumulating evidence that regulation of baseline brain networks can be changed with training for individuals without brain injury (Brewer et al., 2011; Kilpatrick et al., 2011; Malinowski, 2013), although this has not previously been examined in patients with brain injuries. We propose that changes in modularity induced by attention regulation training may influence the ability of participants to engage in and benefit from future learning. In other words, certain forms of training may optimize an individual's "readiness to learn" by improving the regulation of brain network states. Improved regulation of brain networks might enable patients to more fully engage in broader aspects of rehabilitation, such as goal-directed learning in motor, speech, vocational, or scholastic settings.

Frontiers: On the Challenge of Enhancing Transfer and Generalization of Gains

Can training improve cognitive task performance? For many tasks, the answer is "yes." Within specific contexts, training gains have been prominent and reproducible. In addition to studies mentioned previously in this chapter, there have been numerous examples of task-based practice resulting in changes in behavioral performance. A classic example is the documented effects of practice on tasks well-designed to target specific cognitive functions, such as the famous Stroop task (Melara, 1993; Reisberg, Baron, & Kemler, 1980). Yet there still remains a large chasm between such successes and clinically relevant gains in cognitive functioning. Despite significant improvements on the practiced tasks, transfer to new tasks and/or new contexts can be quite limited. For example, practice on tasks designed to highlight the Stroop effect revealed consistent improvements in reduction of the conflict effect, suggesting improved inference resolution, and consistent lack of transfer to other task designs. Furthermore, training gains may be well retained over long periods of time, while transfer does not occur. Thus, the factors that determine transfer effectiveness are likely separate from those that determine retention of gains within the training context.

Poor transfer has been a particular challenge in training patients with acquired brain injury (S. H. Chen, Thomas, Glueckauf, & Bracy, 1997; Sohlberg & Mateer, 2001). This gap raises a number of questions regarding the nature of transfer and generalization of learning contexts outside training. What neural factors support transfer? Are these factors adversely affected by brain injury? It is worthwhile to consider the implications for defining *intervention methods* that enhance transfer of gains.

We propose two particularly important factors that support effective transfer of plasticity in goal-directed control functioning: (1) effective training of the core target functions that are required for goal-directed control in any context, and (2) effective engagement of higher-level cognition for the abstraction of learning goals, supporting the application of learning gains to contexts that were not experienced during training. There are other, less general, factors that we do not discuss in depth. For example, similarities between the training contexts and personal life contexts may influence transfer of gains. The mode of training in these contexts may also be important. For example, training of strategies that are applicable beyond the specific training context may result in greater transfer than rote practice of specific actions in a specific context.

Engagement of Core Neural Systems Supports Transfer of Gains Across Contexts

First, effective engagement and modification of PFC networks is arguably a fundamental factor for supporting successful transfer of cognitive skill gains beyond the training context. If training effectively changes core systems, then gains should be apparent across contexts that engage these systems.

This raises the question of how best to train the core systems of goal-directed control. We submit that it is the processing demands of training tasks, and not the specific stimuli, action steps, or knowledge to be learned, that engage PFC networks. For example, lateral PFC networks are engaged during working memory tasks regardless of the type of information (e.g., words or objects) that must be remembered (D'Esposito et al., 1998). More generally, we propose that the persistent integration and coordination of subordinate neural networks based on goals are the crucial factors for training. Conversely, training that leads to disengagement of PFC networks during repeated task performance is likely to result in low transfer. A basic example is training that leads to more automatic responses to the task demands, with reinforcement of task-specific networks, resulting in more efficient performance on the particular tasks but also disengagement of PFC networks (Jansma, Ramsey, Slagter, & Kahn, 2001; Peterson, 1998). This includes other examples of procedural learning, and potentially experiences that lead to repetition suppression effects (Sayres & Grill-Spector, 2006).

We have proposed some training principles to effectively target and improve goal-directed control functions (D'Esposito & Chen, 2006b). Training with a range of modalities, task content, and contexts may be necessary for effectively modifying the underlying neural systems, given their broad connectivity and multimodal nature. Furthermore, knowing that PFC networks can be rapidly, but transiently, plastic (that is, adapting to any given task quickly), one would hypothesize that challenging flexible adaptation (rather than adaptation to any specific task) is itself an important principle of training. This would require a wide range of tasks, rather than repetition of specific tasks. There is a small amount of evidence currently to support the contention that transfer effects might be enhanced if training engages higher-level executive control processes instead of focusing on basic processing or context-specific strategies (Lustig, Shah, Seidler, & Reuter-Lorenz, 2009; Noack, Lovden, Schmiedek, & Lindenberger, 2009).

In considering target neural systems, it may be valuable to look beyond task-based cognition. Training that alters the neural systems important for self-regulation, including a person's ability to regulate parameters of brain state (not specific to a particular task), may be important for supporting improvements in functioning across contexts. This is a major reason that we have emphasized the importance of training functions that regulate brain state *between*, and as well as *during*, episodes of task-based goal-directed cognition. In addition to skills explicitly taught with self-regulation or mindfulness-based training, as discussed in a prior section, it may be valuable to consider the self-regulatory functions engaged during task-based training as well. For example, aspects of self-regulation required for sustained effort and perseverance during difficult or even boring time periods of training may contribute to the transferable benefits of training.

What Brain Functions Enhance Transfer of Training Gains?

We argue that the cognitive function of *abstraction* supports the transcendence of learning beyond a specific context. Within each context that a given task is practiced, a specific set of cues and structure are available to scaffold actions. We argue that the ability to explicitly set out a generalizable learning goal at the outset of training, or later to abstract that learning goal, should facilitate transfer to other contexts. Supporting this hypothesis, more basic studies of training have found that transfer may be enhanced if the training regime taps higher-level executive control processes instead of focusing on basic processing or context-specific strategies (Karbach & Kray, 2009; Karbach & Shubert, 2013; Lustig et al., 2009; Noack et al., 2009).

Clinical observations also support this hypothesis. Indeed, it is empirically observed that patients with severe deficits in frontal cognition have difficulty learning skills and applying them across contexts, even while they may learn specific functional tasks well. A common clinical experience is successfully training such patients to perform tasks well in the treatment setting, only later to find that the patient had no improvement in functioning elsewhere. In other words, behavior has the appearance of being "plastic" in the training setting, but then is apparently "elastic," reverting to baseline automatic behaviors outside the training context. Thus, a *functional* approach has been suggested in preference to *skills-based* approaches for patients with severe acquired brain injury—these patients may successfully learn specific functional tasks in the contexts that these tasks will be needed, but will have difficulty learning more generalizable skills (Giles, 2010).

Frontiers: Understanding the Nature of Plasticity Versus Elasticity After Brain Injury

This set of hypotheses is worth further investigation, as they carry important implications for understanding individual variability in the ability to learn and transfer gains across contexts. The optimal choice of rehabilitation approach may depend on understanding the nature and severity of cognitive deficits, and the relationship of these deficits to the potential for generalizable learning.

Ultimately, in order for training-related plasticity to be of clinical relevance, it is vital that we achieve a better understanding of the neural bases that support transfer of learning gains *to personally relevant life situations*. Life situations can be much more complex contexts in which to use cognitive skills. To achieve significant generalized gains, it is likely that a combination of the above proposed factors will be needed, including engagement of higher-level cognitive functions, effective training of the core target functions that are required across contexts, and abstraction of learning goals and application across contexts. Additional factors that enhance effective functional plasticity, rather than just context-specific behavioral elasticity, will be worth further delineation.

Frontiers: Understanding Plasticity in the Functional Coordination of Goal-Directed Cognition

Deficits in goal-directed control functions are generally attributable to damage to pre-frontal systems, which include not only the prefrontal cortex per se, but extensive inter-connections with subcortical and posterior cortical structures (D'Esposito & Chen, 2006a). Although it is known that goal-directed cognitive processes are dependent on the integration of multimodal inputs distributed throughout the cortex (Mesulam, 1990), we do not yet fully understand the complex interplay of brain networks that support plasticity in cognition with training (A. J. Chen, Abrams, & D'Esposito, 2006; A. J. W. Chen, Thompson, et al., 2006; A. J. W. Chen, Thompson, Lee, Gazzaley, & D'Esposito, 2006). These networks serve a number of inter-related processes that are important for effective goal-direction. An important principle is that the component processes need to be *coordinated* or *functionally integrated* in the accomplishment of any particular goal. Goals may be conceptualized as serving to functionally organize the multiple neural processes necessary for accomplishing the goal. This includes select-ing the relevant pathways or processes (while excluding others), coordinating them at any given moment in time, and dynamically adjusting this coordination while main-taining the central goal across time to eventually accomplish the goal. Thus, plasticity in not only isolated component processes, but their functional coordination via goals, will be important targets of investigation.

Looking to the Future

Understanding the neural bases of plasticity in cognition may provide guidance for the development of treatments to enhance functioning (A. J. Chen et al., 2006; D'Esposito & Chen, 2006a; Kennedy et al., 2008; Levine et al., 2008). Intervening via rehabilitation after acquired brain injury provides further opportunities for the neuroscientific investi-gation of patient-relevant mechanisms of plasticity.

Acknowledgments

We would like to express much appreciation to Erica Pool for assistance in editing. Special thanks to Tatjana Novakovic-Agopian, Terry Nycum, Katelyn Begany, and Maulik Shah for work that has provided an important foundation for this chapter.

References

Alstott, J., Breakspear, M., Hagmann, P., Cammoun, L., & Sporns, O. (2009). Modeling the impact of lesions in the human brain. *PLoS Comput Biol, 5*(6), e1000408.

Anguera, J. A., Boccanfuso, J., Rintoul, J. L., Al-Hashimi, O., Faraji, F., Janowich, J., . . . Gazzaley, A. (2013). Video game training enhances cognitive control in older adults. *Nature, 501*(7465), 97–101.

Asaad, W. F., Rainer, G., & Miller, E. K. (1998). Neural activity in the primate prefrontal cortex during associative learning. *Neuron, 21*(6), 1399–1407.

Aston-Jones, G., & Cohen, J. D. (2005). An integrative theory of locus coeruleus-norepinephrine function: Adaptive gain and optimal performance. *Annu Rev Neurosci, 28*, 403–450.

Awh, E., & Vogel, E. K. (2008). The bouncer in the brain. *Nat Neurosci, 11*(1), 5–6.

Baddeley, A. D. (2001). Is working memory still working? *Am Psychol, 56*(11), 851–864.

Badre, D., & D'Esposito, M. (2009). Is the rostro-caudal axis of the frontal lobe hierarchical? *Nat Rev Neurosci, 10*(9), 659–669.

Badre, D., Hoffman, J., Cooney, J. W., & D'Esposito, M. (2009). Hierarchical cognitive control deficits following damage to the human frontal lobe. *Nat Neurosci, 12*(4), 515–522.

Badre, D., Kayser, A. S., & D'Esposito, M. (2010). Frontal cortex and the discovery of abstract action rules. *Neuron, 66*(2), 315–326.

Bassett, D. S., & Bullmore, E. (2006). Small-world brain networks. *Neuroscientist, 12*(6), 512–523.

Binder, D., Turner, G., Chen, A. J.-W., Novakovic-Agopian, T. (2008). Brain Health Workshop. *Instructor's manual, participant materials, knowledge tests.*

Braver, T., & Bongiolatti, S. (2002). The role of frontopolar cortex in subgoal processing during working memory. *NeuroImage, 15*(3), 523–536.

Brewer, J. A., Worhunsky, P. D., Gray, J. R., Tang, Y., Weber, J., Kober, H. (2011). Meditation experience is associated with differences in default mode network activity and connectivity. *P Natl Acad Sci, 108*(50), 20254–20259.

Burgess, P. W., Alderman, N., Forbes, C., Costello, A., Coates, L. M., Dawson, D. R., . . . Channon, S. (2006). The case for the development and use of "ecologically valid" measures of executive function in experimental and clinical neuropsychology. *J Int Neuropsychol Soc, 12*(2), 194–209.

Chapman, S. B., Gamino, J. F., Cook, L. G., Hanten, G., Li, X., & Levin, H. S. (2006). Impaired discourse gist and working memory in children after brain injury. *Brain Lang, 97*(2), 178–188.

Chen, A. J., Abrams, G. M., & D'Esposito, M. (2006). Functional reintegration of prefrontal neural networks for enhancing recovery after brain injury. *J Head Trauma Rehabil, 21*(2), 107–118.

Chen, A. J., Novakovic-Agopian, T., Nycum, T. J., Song, S., Turner, G. R., Hills, N. K., . . . D'Esposito, M. (2011). Training of goal-directed attention regulation enhances control over neural processing for individuals with brain injury. *Brain, 134*(Pt 5), 1541–1554.

Chen, A. J. W., Abrams, G. M., & D'Esposito, M. (2006). Functional re-integration of prefrontal neural networks for enhancing recovery after brain injury. *J Head Trauma Rehabil, 21*(2), 107–118.

Chen, A. J. W., Britton, M., Turner, G. R., Vytlacil, J., Thompson, T. W., & D'Esposito, M. (2012). Goal-directed attention alters the tuning of object-based representations in extrastriate cortex. *Front Hum Neurosci, 6*, 187.

Chen, A. J. W., & Novakovic-Agopian, T. (2012). Interventions to improve cognitive functioning after traumatic brain injury. In J. Tsao (Ed.), *Traumatic brain injury: A clinician's guide to diagnosis, management, and rehabilitation* (pp. 273–312). New York: Springer.

Chen, A. J. W., Thompson, T. W., La, C., Sedley, J., Sheng, T., Nir, T., . . . D'Esposito, M. (2006). *Dissociable effects of attention practice on prefrontal and visual cortex activity.* Paper presented at the Cognitive Neuroscience Society, San Francisco.

Chen, A. J. W., Thompson, T. W., Lee, J., Gazzaley, A., & D'Esposito, M. (2006). *Neural changes induced by cognitive task practice: An fMRI model for studying cognitive rehabilitation.* Paper presented at the American Academy of Neurology Annual Conference, San Diego.

Chen, A. J. W., Novakovic-Agopian, T., Nycum, T. J., Song, S., Turner, G. R., Hills, N. K., . . . D'Esposito, M. (2011). Training of goal-directed attention regulation enhances control over neural processing for individuals with brain injury. *Brain, 134*(Pt 5), 1541–1554.

Chen, S. H., Kareken, D. A., Fastenau, P. S., Trexler, L. E., & Hutchins, G. D. (2003). A study of persistent post-concussion symptoms in mild head trauma using positron emission tomography. *J Neurol Neurosurg Ps, 74*(3), 326–332.

Chen, S. H., Thomas, J. D., Glueckauf, R. L., & Bracy, O. L. (1997). The effectiveness of computer-assisted cognitive rehabilitation for persons with traumatic brain injury. *Brain Inj, 11*(3), 197–209.

Christodoulou, C., DeLuca, J., Ricker, J. H., Madigan, N. K., Bly, B. M., Lange, G., . . . Ni, A. C. (2001). Functional magnetic resonance imaging of working memory impairment after traumatic brain injury. *J Neurol Neurosurg P, 71*(2), 161–168.

Cicerone, K. D., Dahlberg, C., Kalmar, K., Langenbahn, D. M., Malec, J. F., Bergquist, T. F., . . . Morse, P. A. (2000). Evidence-based cognitive rehabilitation: Recommendations for clinical practice. *Arch Phys Med Rehabil, 81*(12), 1596–1615.

Cicerone, K. D., Dahlberg, C., Malec, J. F., Langenbahn, D. M., Felicetti, T., Kneipp, S., . . . Catanese, J. (2005). Evidence-based cognitive rehabilitation: Updated review of the literature from 1998 through 2002. *Arch Phys Med Rehabil, 86*(8), 1681–1692.

Cohen, J. D., Botvinick, M., & Carter, C. S. (2000). Anterior cingulate and prefrontal cortex: Who's in control? *Nat Neurosci, 3*(5), 421–423.

Cowan, N., & Morey, C. C. (2006). Visual working memory depends on attentional filtering. *Trends Cogn Sci, 10*(4), 139–141.

Crofts, J. J., Higham, D. J., Bosnell, R., Jbabdi, S., Matthews, P. M., Behrens, T. E., & Johansen-Berg, H. (2011). Network analysis detects changes in the contralesional hemisphere following stroke. *NeuroImage, 54*(1), 161–169.

Curtis, C. E., & D'Esposito, M. (2003). Persistent activity in the prefrontal cortex during working memory. *Trends Cogn Sci, 7*(9), 415–423.

D'Esposito, M., Aguirre, G. K., Zarahn, E., Ballard, D., Shin, R. K., & Lease, J. (1998). Functional MRI studies of spatial and nonspatial working memory. *Brain Res Cogn Brain Res, 7*(1), 1–13.

D'Esposito, M., & Chen, A. J.-W. (2006a). Neural mechanisms of prefrontal cortical function. Implications for cognitive rehabilitation. In A. Moller, S. B. Chapman, & S. G. Lomber (Eds.), *Reprogramming the Human Brain: Progress in Brain Research* (Vol. 157, pp. 123–139). Elsevier.

D'Esposito, M., & Chen, A. J.-W. (2006b). Neural mechanisms of prefrontal cortical function: Implications for cognitive rehabilitation. *Prog Brain Res, 157*, 123–139.

D'Esposito, M., Detre, J. A., Alsop, D. C., Shin, R. K., Atlas, S., & Grossman, M. (1995). The neural basis of the central executive system of working memory. *Nature, 378*, 279–281.

D'Esposito, M., & Gazzaley, A. (2006). Neurorehabilitation and executive function. In M. E. Selzer, L. Cohen, F. H. Gage, S. Clarke, & P. W. Duncan (Eds.), *Neural rehabilitation and repair* (pp. 475–487). Cambridge: Cambridge University Press.

D'Esposito, M., & Postle, B. R. (1999). The dependence of span and delayed-response performance on prefrontal cortex. *Neuropsychologia, 37*(11), 1303–1315.

D'Zurilla, T. J., & Goldfried, M. (1971). Problem solving and behavior modification. *Journal of Abnormal Psychology, 78*, 107–126.

Dahlin, E., Neely, A. S., Larsson, A., Backman, L., & Nyberg, L. (2008). Transfer of learning after updating training mediated by the striatum. *Science, 320*(5882), 1510–1512.

Debaere, F., Wenderoth, N., Sunaert, S., Van Hecke, P., & Swinnen, S. P. (2004). Changes in brain activation during the acquisition of a new bimanual coodination task. *Neuropsychologia, 42*(7), 855–867.

Desimone, R. (1998). Visual attention mediated by biased competition in extrastriate visual cortex. *Philos Trans R Soc Lond B Biol Sci, 353*(1373), 1245–1255.

Doctor, J. N., Castro, J., Temkin, N. R., Fraser, R. T., Machamer, J. E., & Dikmen, S. S. (2005). Workers' risk of unemployment after traumatic brain injury: A normed comparison. *J Int Neuropsychol Soc, 11*(6), 747–752.

Doyon, J., & Benali, H. (2005). Reorganization and plasticity in the adult brain during learning of motor skills. *Curr Opin Neurobiol, 15*(2), 161–167.

Drake, A. I., Gray, N., Yoder, S., Pramuka, M., & Llewellyn, M. (2000). Factors predicting return to work following mild traumatic brain injury: A discriminant analysis. *J Head Trauma Rehabil, 15*(5), 1103–1112.

Duncan, J., Burgess, P., & Emslie, H. (1995). Fluid intelligence after frontal lobe lesions. *Neuropsychologia, 33*(3), 261–268.

Duncan, J., Emslie, H., Williams, P., Johnson, R., & Freer, C. (1996). Intelligence and the frontal lobe: The organization of goal-directed behavior. *Cognit Psychol, 30*(3), 257–303.

Erickson, K. I., Colcombe, S. J., Wadhwa, R., Bherer, L., Peterson, M. S., Scalf, P. E., . . . Kramer, A. F. (2007). Training-induced functional activation changes in dual-task processing: An fMRI study. *Cereb Cortex, 17*(1), 192–204.

Fischer, S., Gauggel, S., & Trexler, L. E. (2004). Awareness of activity limitations, goal setting and rehabilitation outcome in patients with brain injuries. *Brain Inj, 18*(6), 547–562.

Floyer-Lea, A., & Matthews, P. M. (2004). Changing brain networks for visuomotor control with increased movement automaticity. *J Neurophysiol, 92*(4), 2405–2412.

Fox, M. D., Snyder, A. Z., Zacks, J. M., & Raichle, M. E. (2006). Coherent spontaneous activity accounts for trial-to-trial variability in human evoked brain responses. *Nat Neurosci, 9*(1), 23–25.

Freedman, D. J., Riesenhuber, M., Poggio, T., & Miller, E. K. (2001). Categorical representation of visual stimuli in the primate prefrontal cortex. *Science, 291*(5502), 312–316.

Fuster, J. M. (2000). Executive frontal functions. *Exp Brain Res, 133*(1), 66–70.

Giles, G. M. (2010). Cognitive versus functional approaches to rehabilitation after traumatic brain injury: Commentary on a randomized controlled trial. *Am J Occup Ther, 64*(1), 182–185.

Gratton, C., Nomura, E. M., Perez, F., & D'Esposito, M. (2012). Focal brain lesions to critical locations cause widespread disruption of the modular organization of the brain. *J Cognitive Neurosci, 24*(6), 1275–1285.

Haldeman, C., & Beggs, J. (2005). Critical branching captures activity in living neural networks and maximizes the number of metastable states. *Phys Rev Lett, 94*(5), 058101.

Haxby, J. V., Gobbini, M. I., Furey, M. L., Ishai, A., Schouten, J. L., & Pietrini, P. (2001). Distributed and overlapping representations of faces and objects in ventral temporal cortex. *Science, 293*(5539), 2425–2430.

Hillary, F. G. (2008). Neuroimaging of working memory dysfunction and the dilemma with brain reorganization hypotheses. *J Int Neuropsychol Soc, 14*(4), 526–534.

Hillary, F. G., Genova, H. M., Chiaravalloti, N. D., Rypma, B., & DeLuca, J. (2006). Prefrontal modulation of working memory performance in brain injury and disease. *Hum Brain Mapp, 27*(11), 837–847.

Huang, Y.-Z., Edwards, M. J., Rounis, E., Bahatia, K. P., & Rothwell, J. C. (2005). Theta burst stimulation of the human motor cortex. *Neuron, 45*, 201–206.

Hyndman, D., & Ashburn, A. (2003). People with stroke living in the community: Attention deficits, balance, ADL ability and falls. *Disabil Rehabil, 25*(15), 817–822.

Jaeggi, S. M., Buschkuehl, M., Jonides, J., & Perrig, W. J. (2008). Improving fluid intelligence with training on working memory. *P Natl Acad Sci USA, 105*(19), 6829–6833.

Jansma, J. M., Ramsey, N. F., Slagter, H. A., & Kahn, R. S. (2001). Functional anatomical correlates of controlled and automatic processing. *J Cogn Neurosci, 13*(6), 730–743.

Jueptner, M., Stephan, K. M., Frith, C. D., Brooks, D. J., Frackowiak, R. S. J., Passingham, R. E. (1997). Anatomy of motor learning: I. Frontal cortex and attention to action. *J Neurophysiol, 77*, 1313–1324.

Karbach, J., & Kray, J. (2009). How useful is executive control training? Age differences in near and far transfer of task-switching training. *Dev Sci, 12*(6), 978–990.

Karbach, J., & Shubert, T. (2013). Training-induced cognitive and neural plasticity. *Front Hum Neurosci, 7*, 1.

Karni, A., Meyer, G., Ray-Hipolito, C., Jezzard, P., Adams, M. M., Turner, R., & Ungerleider, L. G. (1998). The acquisition of skilled motor performance: Fast and slow experience-driven changes in primary motor cortex. *P Natl Acad Sci USA, 95*, 861–868.

Kelly, A. M., & Garavan, H. (2005). Human functional neuroimaging of brain changes associated with practice. *Cereb Cortex, 15*(8), 1089–1102.

Kelly, C., Foxe, J. J., & Garavan, H. (2006). Patterns of normal human brain plasticity after practice and their implications for neurorehabilitation. *Arch Phys Med Rehabil, 87*(12 Suppl 2), S20–S29.

Kennedy, M. R., Coelho, C., Turkstra, L., Ylvisaker, M., Moore Sohlberg, M., Yorkston, K., . . . Kan, P. F. (2008). Intervention for executive functions after traumatic brain injury: A systematic review, meta-analysis and clinical recommendations. *Neuropsychol Rehabil, 18*(3), 257–299.

Kilpatrick, L. A., Suyenobu, B. Y., Smith, S. R., Bueller, J. A., Goodman, T., Creswell, J. D., . . . Naliboff, B. D. (2011). Impact of mindfulness-based stress reduction training on intrinsic brain connectivity. *Neuroimage, 56*(1), 290–298.

Kim, Y. H., Yoo, W. K., Ko, M. H., Park, C. H., Kim, S. T., & Na, D. L. (2009). Plasticity of the attentional network after brain injury and cognitive rehabilitation. *Neurorehabil Neural Repair, 23*(5), 468–477.

Kinouchi, O., Copelli, M. (2006). Optimal dynamical range of excitable networks at criticality. *Nat Physics, 2*, 348–351.

Kitzbichler, M. G., Henson, R. N., Smith, M. L., Nathan, P. J., & Bullmore, E. T. (2011). Cognitive effort drives workspace configuration of human brain functional networks. *J Neurosci, 31*(22), 8259–8270.

Klingberg, T. (2010). Training and plasticity of working memory. *Trends Cogn Sci, 14*(7), 317–324.

Koechlin, E., Basso, G., Pietrini, P., Panzer, S., & Grafman, J. (1999). The role of the anterior prefrontal cortex in human cognition. *Nature, 399*(6732), 148–151.

Koechlin, E., Ody, C., & Kouneiher, F. (2003). The architecture of cognitive control in the human prefrontal cortex. *Science, 302*(5648), 1181–1185.

Krawczyk, D. C., & D'Esposito, M. (2011). Modulation of working memory function by motivation through loss-aversion. *Hum Brain Mapp, 34*(4), 762–774.

Laatsch, L. K., Thulborn, K. R., Krisky, C. M., Shobat, D. M., & Sweeney, J. A. (2004). Investigating the neurobiological basis of cognitive rehabilitation therapy with fMRI. *Brain Inj, 18*(10), 957–974.

Lee, T. G., & D'Esposito, M. (2012). The dynamic nature of top-down signals originating from prefrontal cortex: A combined fMRI-TMS study. *J Neurosci, 32*(44), 15458–15466.

Levine, B., Cabeza, R., McIntosh, A. R., Black, S. E., Grady, C. L., & Stuss, D. T. (2002). Functional reorganisation of memory after traumatic brain injury: A study with H(2)(15)0 positron emission tomography. *J Neurol Neurosurg Ps, 73*(2), 173–181.

Levine, B., Robertson, I. H., Clare, L., Carter, G., Hong, J., Wilson, B. A., . . . Stuss, D. T. (2000). Rehabilitation of executive functioning: An experimental-clinical validation of goal management training. *J Int Neuropsychol Soc, 6*(3), 299–312.

Levine, B., Stuss, D. T., Winocur, G., Binns, M. A., Fahy, L., Mandic, M., . . . Robertson, I. H. (2007). Cognitive rehabilitation in the elderly: Effects on strategic behavior in relation to goal management. *J Int Neuropsychol Soc, 13*(1), 143–152.

Levine, B., Turner, G. R., & Stuss, D. T. (2008). Rehabilitation of frontal lobe functions. In D. T. Stuss, G. Winocur, & I. H. Robertson (Eds.), *Cognitive neurorehabilitation: Evidence and applications* (pp. 464–486). Cambridge: Cambridge University Press.

Lustig, C., Shah, P., Seidler, R., & Reuter-Lorenz, P. A. (2009). Aging, training, and the brain: A review and future directions. *Neuropsychol Rev, 19*(4), 504–522.

M Shah, A. J.-W. C., Yang, F. C., Begany, K., Nycum, T., Krawczyk, D., Vas, A., D'Esposito, M., & Chapman, S. (2013). Targeted cognitive training improves the clarity of neural representation of goal-relevant stimuli in individuals with traumatic brain injury. *Abstract presented at American Academy of Neurology, March 2013, San Diego.*

Machamer, J., Temkin, N., Fraser, R., Doctor, J. N., & Dikmen, S. (2005). Stability of employment after traumatic brain injury. *J Int Neuropsychol Soc, 11*(7), 807–816.

Malinowski, P. (2013). Neural mechanisms of attentional control in mindfulness meditation. *Front Neurosci, 7*, 8.

McAllister, T., Sparling, M., Flashman, L., Guerin, S., Mamourian, A., & Saykin, A. (2001). Differential working memory load effects after mild traumatic brain injury. *Neuroimage, 14*(5), 1004–1012.

McAllister, T. W., Sparling, M. B., Flashman, L. A., Guerin, S. J., Mamourian, A. C., & Saykin, A. J. (2001). Differential working memory load effects after mild traumatic brain injury. *Neuroimage, 14*(5), 1004–1012.

McNab, F., Varrone, A., Farde, L., Jucaite, A., Bystritsky, P., Forssberg, H., & Klingberg, T. (2009). Changes in cortical dopamine D1 receptor binding associated with cognitive training. *Science, 323*(5915),

Melara, R., & Mounts, J. R. W. (1993). Selective attention to Stroop dimensions: Effects of baseline discriminability, response mode, and practice. *Mem Cognition, 21*(5), 627–645.

Mesulam, M. M. (1990). Large-scale neurocognitive networks and distributed processing for attention, language, and memory. *Ann Neurol, 28*(5), 597–613.

Meunier, D., Achard, S., Morcom, A., & Bullmore, E. (2009). Age-related changes in modular organization of human brain functional networks. *NeuroImage, 44*(3), 715–723.

Meunier, D., Lambiotte, R., & Bullmore, E. T. (2010). Modular and hierarchically modular organization of brain networks. *Front Neurosci, 4*, 200.

Miller, B. T., & D'Esposito, M. (2005). Searching for "the top" in top-down control. *Neuron, 48*(4), 535–538.

Miller, E. K., & Cohen, J. D. (2001). An integrative theory of prefrontal cortex function. *Annu Rev Neurosci, 24*, 167–202.

Miotto, E. C., Savage, C. R., Evans, J. J., Wilson, B. A., Martins, M. G., Iaki, S., & Amaro, E., Jr. (2006). Bilateral activation of the prefrontal cortex after strategic semantic cognitive training. *Hum Brain Mapp, 27*(4), 288–295.

Nakamura, T., Hillary, F. G., Biswal, B. B. (2009). Resting network plasticity following brain injury. *PLoS One, 4*(12), e8220.

Nezu, A. M., Nezu, C. M., & D'Zurilla, T. J. (2007). *Solving life's problems.* New York: Springer Publishing.

Noack, H., Lovden, M., Schmiedek, F., & Lindenberger, U. (2009). Cognitive plasticity in adulthood and old age: Gauging the generality of cognitive intervention effects. *Restor Neurol Neurosci, 27*(5), 435–453.

Norton, A., Zipse, L., Marchina, S., & Schlaug, G. (2009). Melodic intonation therapy: Shared insights on how it is done and why it might help. *Ann NY Acad Sci, 1169,* 431–436.

Novakovic-Agopian, T., Chen, A. J.-W., Rome, S., Abrams, G., Castelli, H., Rossi, A., . . . D'Esposito, M. (2011). Rehabilitation of executive functioning with training in attention regulation applied to individually defined goals: A pilot study bridging theory, assessment and treatment. *J Head Trauma Rehabil, 26*(5), 325–338.

Novakovic-Agopian, T., Chen, A. J.-W., Rome, S., Abrams, G., Castelli, H., Rossi, A., . . . D'Esposito, M. (2011). Rehabilitation of executive functioning with training in attention regulation applied to individually defined goals: A pilot study bridging theory, assessment, and treatment. *J Head Trauma Rehabil, 26*(5), 325–338.

Olesen, P. J., Westerberg, H., & Klingberg, T. (2004). Increased prefrontal and parietal activity after training of working memory. *Nat Neurosci, 7*(1), 75–79.

Ownsworth, T., & McKenna, K. (2004). Investigation of factors related to employment outcome following traumatic brain injury: A critical review and conceptual model. *Disabil Rehabil, 26*(13), 765–783.

Ozdemir, F., Birtane, M., Tabatabaei, R., Ekuklu, G., & Kokino, S. (2001). Cognitive evaluation and functional outcome after stroke. *Am J Phys Med Rehabil, 80*(6), 410–415.

Papo, D. (2013). Why should cognitive neuroscientists study the brain's resting state? *Front Hum Neurosci, 7,* 45.

Persson, J., & Reuter-Lorenz, P. A. (2008). Gaining control: Training executive function and far transfer of the ability to resolve interference. *Psychol Sci, 19*(9), 881–888.

Peterson, S., van Mier, H., Fiez, J. A., & Raichle, M. (1998). The effects of practice on the functional anatomy of task performance. *P Natl Acad Sci USA, 95,* 853–860.

Prigatano, G. P., & Wong, J. L. (1999). Cognitive and affective improvement in brain dysfunctional patients who achieve inpatient rehabilitation goals. *Arch Phys Med Rehabil, 80*(1), 77–84.

Rath, J., Simon, D., Langenbahn, D. M., Sherr, R., & Diller, L. (2003). Group treatment of problem-solving deficits in outpatients with traumatic brain injury: A randomised outcome study. *Neuropsychol Rehabil, 13*(4), 461–488.

Reisberg, D., Baron, J., & Kemler, D. (1980). Overcoming Stroop interference: The effects of practice on distractor potency. *J Exp Psychol, 6*(1), 140–150.

Repovs, G., & Baddeley, A. (2006). The multi-component model of working memory: Explorations in experimental cognitive psychology. *Neuroscience, 139*(1), 5–21.

Reyna, V., & Brainerd, C. J. (1995). Fuzzy-trace theory: An interim synthesis. *Learn Individ Differ, 7*(1), 1–75.

Rogers, R. D., Andrews, T. C., Grasby, P. M., Brooks, D. J., & Robbins, T. W. (2000). Contrasting cortical and subcortical activations produced by attentional-set shifting and reversal learning in humans. *J Cogn Neurosci, 12*(1), 142–162.

Rohling, M. L., Faust, M. E., Beverly, B., & Demakis, G. (2009). Effectiveness of cognitive rehabilitation following acquired brain injury: A meta-analytic re-examination of Cicerone et al.'s (2000, 2005) systematic reviews. *Neuropsychology, 23*(1), 20–39.

Rubinov, M., & Sporns, O. (2010). Complex network measures of brain connectivity: Uses and interpretations. *Neuroimage, 52*(3), 1059–1069.

Sakai, K., Hikosaka, O., Miyauchi, S., Takino, R., Sasaki, Y., & Putz, B. (1998). Transition of brain activation from frontal to parietal areas in visuomotor sequence learning. *J Neurosci, 18*(5), 1827–1840.

Salminen, T., Strobach, T., & Schubert, T. (2012). On the impacts of working memory training on executive functioning. *Front Hum Neurosci, 6,* 166.

Sayres, R., & Grill-Spector, K. (2006). Object-selective cortex exhibits performance-independent repetition suppression. *J Neurophysiol, 95*(2), 995–1007.

Sharp, D. J., Beckmann, C. F., Greenwood, R., Kinnunen, K. M., Bonnelle, V., De Boissezon, X., . . . Leech, R. (2011). Default mode network functional and structural connectivity after traumatic brain injury. *Brain, 134*(Pt 8), 2233–2247.

Sohlberg, M. M., & Mateer, C. A. (1987). Effectiveness of an attention-training program. *J Clin Exp Neuropsychol, 9*(2), 117–130.

Sohlberg, M. M., & Mateer, C. A. (2001). Improving attention and managing attentional problems: Adapting rehabilitation techniques to adults with ADD. *Ann NY Acad Sci, 931,* 359–375.

Sohlberg, M. M., McLaughlin, K. A., Pavese, A., Heidrich, A., & Posner, M. I. (2000). Evaluation of attention process training and brain injury education in persons with acquired brain injury. *J Clin Exp Neuropsychol, 22*(5), 656–676.

Stevens, A. A., Tappon, S. C., Garg, A., & Fair, D. A. (2012). Functional brain network modularity captures inter- and intra-individual variation in working memory capacity. *PLoS One, 7*(1), e30468.

Strangman, G. E., Goldstein, R., O'Neil-Pirozzi, T. M., Kelkar, K., Supelana, C., Burke, D., . . . Glenn, M. B. (2008). Neurophysiological alterations during strategy-based verbal learning in traumatic brain injury. *Neurorehabil Neural Repair, 23*(3), 226–236.

Stuss, D. (2006). Frontal lobes and attention: Processes and networks, fractionation and integration. *J Int Neuropsychol Soc, 12*(261–271).

Stuss, D. T., & Alexander, M. P. (2007). Is there a dysexecutive syndrome? *Philos Trans R Soc Lond B Biol Sci, 362*(1481), 901–915.

Tatemichi, T. K., Paik, M., Bagiella, E., Desmond, D. W., Pirro, M., & Hanzawa, L. K. (1994). Dementia after stroke is a predictor of long-term survival. *Stroke, 25*(10), 1915–1919.

Turner, G. R., McIntosh, A. R., & Levine, B. (2011). Prefrontal compensatory engagement in tbi is due to altered functional engagement of existing networks and not functional reorganization. *Front Syst Neurosci, 5*, 9.

Van Vleet, T., Heldt, S. A., Pyter, B., Corwin, J. V., Reep, R. L. (2003). Effects of light deprication on recovery from neglect and extinction induced by unilateral lesions of the medial agranular cortex and dorsocentral striatum. *Behav Brain Res, 138*, 165–178.

Vas, A., Chapman, S., Cook, L., Elliott, A., & Keebler, M. (2011). Higher-order reasoning training years after traumatic brain injury in adults. *J Head Trauma Rehabil, 26*(3), 224–239.

Vogel, E. K., McCollough, A. W., & Machizawa, M. G. (2005). Neural measures reveal individual differences in controlling access to working memory. *Nature, 438*(7067), 500–503.

VonCramon, D., Cramon, G. M.-v., & Mai, N. (1991). Problem-solving deficits in brain-injured patients: A therapeutic approach. *Neuropsychol Rehabil, 1*, 45–64.

Voytek, B., Davis, M., Yago, E., Barcelo, F., Vogel, E. K., & Knight, R. T. (2010). Dynamic neuroplasticity after human prefrontal cortex damage. *Neuron, 68*(3), 401–408.

Westerberg, H., Jacobaeus, H., Hirvikoski, T., Clevberger, P., Ostensson, M. L., Bartfai, A., & Klingberg, T. (2007). Computerized working memory training after stroke: A pilot study. *Brain Inj, 21*(1), 21–29.

Wundt, W. (1902). *Outlines of psychology* (2nd ed.). Leipzig: Engelmann.

11

Organic Amnesia
What Factors Determine How Much It Recovers Over Time?

Andrew Mayes

Introduction

The main aim of the chapter is to consider to what degree there is recovery over time from memory disorders that are caused by brain damage, and what factors determine the degree of this recovery. The focus will be on one kind of human memory disorder: organic amnesia. This syndrome can be caused by largely reversible pathologies (for example, transient global amnesia), stable pathologies that do not reverse and usually have a rapid onset (for example, hypoxic amnesia), and, finally, pathologies that progress usually fairly slowly (for example, Alzheimer's disease). The syndrome is often caused by damage to more than one system of structures, each of which mediates different memory-related functions. More research has been done on this syndrome than any of the other kinds of memory impairment in humans that result from brain damage. Although there is agreement about the broad kinds of memory impaired in organic amnesia and what brain lesions cause the syndrome, there is still considerable disagreement and uncertainty about the details of this story. This uncertainty particularly applies to the appropriate measurement of amnesic severity and limits our ability to measure the factors underlying recovery when it occurs. Given that there has been very little systematic research on what these factors are and, indeed, even on how much recovery amnestics of various etiologies show, it is not surprising that very little is known about recovery from amnesia. As future effective treatment of amnesia will probably need to be built on a good understanding of the factors underlying recovery, this chapter will highlight how we can most rapidly enhance this understanding.

There has been extensive work on the factors underlying recovery from *other* kinds of cognitive disorders, such as those involving motor function and language, and this work has examined how recovery may be enhanced through rehabilitation procedures (see Robertson & Murre, 1999, for a review). Among other things, this research has high-lighted what cognitive changes may drive recovery, or, more probably, partial recovery. A distinction has been drawn between restitution and compensation. Restitution is the return (to whatever degree) of the impaired processes that drove the function (a complex of interacting processes) previously mediated by whatever is left of the original structures that mediated these processes. In contrast, compensation involves the replacement of some or all of the impaired processes by other processes that are mediated by different structures: these new processes work together to support the same function that was impaired by the original trauma. Whereas restitution may only occur if some of the damaged structure remains in a potentially working state, compensation is more likely to occur when the damaged structure is completely destroyed. Both restitution and compensation must involve plastic processes that help reconnect or connect neurons that support the same or new processes, respectively.

One major apparent exception to the relative lack of systematic research on the factors underlying restitution and compensation in amnesia has been the extensive and systematic research on cognitive rehabilitation by Barbara Wilson and her colleagues (see Wilson, 2009, for a review). However, this rehabilitation research has rightly been mostly focused on easing the misery and disablement of severe amnesia. It has done this by simplifying and adapting the patient's environment, providing memory aids, such as computer diaries and SenseCam (a camera that records pictures at regular intervals throughout the day, typically from the level of the carrier's neck, in order to provide a short history of what has been done), and encouraging the use of learning procedures that enhance memory, such as mnemonics, the vanishing cues technique, and spaced learning. None of this work has produced clear evidence of an increase in the restoration of the same processes that the trauma disrupted (restitution). Although procedures such as the use of mnemonics and spaced learning can loosely be described as involving compensation in some sense, they also produce improvements in normal memory and, therefore, involve using better learning strategies, which have been taught. With a few exceptions (for example, Hampstead et al., 2012), the rehabilitation methods have not been shown to alter brain functions in structures so as to link a new set of processes together in order to mediate the same broad memory function. This does not mean that the research is not beneficial to patients and, therefore, very important, but little of this research has yet addressed the aim of this chapter.

The chapter is divided into the following sections. It begins by considering the nature, etiology, underlying brain disruption, and theories about this syndrome. This section considers some of the disagreements that remain unresolved concerning amnesia. These controversies relate to how the severity of amnesia should be measured, a topic that is considered more extensively in the next section. With these two sections providing essential background, the third section discusses the factors that influence recovery from the syndrome. In reviewing the literature, it becomes clear that we know relatively little about the factors that underlie recovery from amnesia. So the final brief section considers what needs to be done to improve knowledge in the future.

Organic Amnesia: Its Nature, etiologies, Underlying Brain Damage, and Theories

Pure organic amnesia is characterized by two kinds of memory disorder: anterograde amnesia (AA) and retrograde amnesia (RA). AA is a deficit in the ability to recall and recognize recently encountered personal experiences (episodic memory) and facts and concepts (semantic memory): this deficit may become apparent as soon as an amnesic patient is distracted after encountering any new information. RA is a similar kind of deficit, except that the recall and recognition impairment is for personal experiences and/or facts that were encountered and turned into normal episodic and/or semantic long-term memories (i.e., learned) before the amnesia-triggering brain damage occurred. AA and RA typically occur together, although measures of the severity of each are often noisy, have uncertain reliability, and blur together dissociable memory deficits. Furthermore, measurement of RA is made even harder by the long-standing, but still controversial view that RA shows a temporal gradient, with older memories being relatively more spared. Unsurprisingly, therefore, whether AA and RA can be found in isolation from each other is still an unresolved issue.

Some researchers have mistakenly claimed that organic amnesia is a selective impairment of episodic memory. There are two reasons for thinking that the claim is wrong. The first reason is that episodic and semantic memories are heterogeneous kinds of associative memory that comprise many overlapping components. For example, semantic memory may concern highly variable knowledge of oneself and one's life history, the auditory and visual spatiotemporal information of films, or conceptual information about word or sentence meanings. Episodic memories are experiences that may contain these kinds of information, but that tend to be more highly variable in their content. The only consistent difference between episodic and semantic memories is that episodic memories are always framed by the spectacles of one's conscious self as it was at the time of encoding. It is this that enables an earlier experience to be partially recreated. But it is clear that AA and RA disrupt associative memory for more than just episodic memories. Although it is sometimes argued that AA and RA are worse for episodic than semantic memory, the evidence is unconvincing (for example, see Moscovitch & Nadel, 1998; Squire & Zola, 1998).

The second reason for thinking that amnesia is not a selective disorder of episodic memory is that semantic memories are often based on more learning trials and rehearsal than are episodic memories, which, by definition, can have only one learning trial, albeit with an uncertain amount of subsequent rehearsal, some of which is believed to occur in sleep (see Inostroza & Born, 2013, for a review). The tendency for semantic memories to undergo more learning matters because over-learning protects these memories from being affected by RA. Therefore, the only relevant comparison is of episodic and semantic memories that have undergone similar, and presumably, relatively modest amounts of learning and rehearsal. Rather than a distinction based on episodic and semantic memories, it is more heuristically valuable to view AA and RA as impairments of aware memory (supporting recall and recognition) involving associations of any kind, but often between distinct items or items and their contexts (backgrounds, usually including spatiotemporal information). Item aware memory (e.g., recognition of a face) is also often impaired in organic amnesia. This is a different kind of associative aware memory, often referred to as unitized memory. For example, if the aware item memory is of faces, the components of each remembered face are bound within a "face" framework so that face components are quite hard to access individually (see Mayes et al., 2007). So, when face recognition involves recalling associations with the face from the study context, such as recalling that you felt the face was unpleasant during the study session, this is an aware item-context kind of associative memory. Only when aware memory is solely for a kind of unitized representation of face's component parts is the memory specifically for the kind of association that can appropriately be described as item memory.

In pure amnesia, AA and RA have been claimed to be accompanied by preservation of cognition and other memory functions. Thus, general intelligence is believed to be preserved. This preservation (particularly of fluid intelligence) strongly suggests that processing of new inputs should be carried out in a flexible way that relates these inputs to established knowledge normally. Not surprisingly, in people with intact brains, intelligence correlates positively with aware memory. The same relationship seems to hold in organic amnesics in whom intelligence varies because of individual differences rather than as a consequence of brain damage (unless floor effects with memory conceal this). So, AA is measured by identifying how much worse a patient's new learning and memory of events and facts are than would be expected in the average healthy person of similar intelligence. The preserved intelligence that is measured also includes crystallized intelligence, which reflects learned skills and knowledge. Thus, it is often noted that memory for pre-morbidly over-learned semantic information, such as word meanings, is unaffected in pure amnesia. In addition, it also has long been claimed that pure amnesics show preserved attention and executive functions and that their perception of incoming information is normal. According to the claim, only when amnesia is caused by more extensive brain damage—as it is, for example, in Alzheimer's disease—are these kinds of function impaired. However, recently this claim has been challenged by evidence that some authors have interpreted as meaning that hippocampal damage, which causes amnesia, also disrupts integrated, high-level visual perception of spatial scenes. In a similar way, it has been argued that perirhinal cortex lesions disrupt integrated, high-level visual perception of objects (e.g., see Lee et al., 2012, for a review of evidence about these perceptual deficit views).

The above evidence has attempted to remove the need for memory by testing discrimination immediately in the presence of the just-encountered visual stimulus. Criticism of the interpretation that high-level visual perception is impaired in amnesia has been mainly based on the argument that, although not essential, performance is still enhanced by using memory, so the impaired performance of these tasks depends on some form of memory; this might be short-term memory, or more established long-term memory, or both. The impaired perception interpretation is, however, encouraged by the consistent finding that, when memory for short sequences of spoken numbers or spatial locations is tested immediately, performance is completely preserved in amnesics, which suggests that at least some forms of short-term or working memory are completely normal in pure organic amnesia and, therefore, should be available to bolster perceptual judgments up to normal levels, provided that perception itself was preserved (see Lee et al., 2012, for this kind of argument).

However, the generality of the claim that working memory is preserved has recently been challenged because it has been found that item-location associative memory is impaired at very short delays (e.g., Pertzov et al., 2013), although the nature of this deficit has been challenged by Jeneson and Squire (2012). These researchers have used arguments similar to those made against the view that amnesics have high-level visual perception deficits. They have proposed that the almost immediate associative memory deficits reflect impaired long-term, not short-term, memory, even though the delays are short. Jeneson and Squire believe that these kinds of long-term memory deficits can be identified when tests contain materials that are hard to rehearse, involve diverting attention, and/or exceed working memory capacity (e.g., supraspan). However, characterizing the impaired forms of memory as long term in this way is in danger of being circular because the short-term/long-term memory distinction is conceptually unclear. If valid, the distinction should ultimately reflect different physiological storage mechanisms for short- and long-lasting memories, but the evidence is currently insufficient to determine whether immediately tested item/location associative memory depends on the same synaptic storage mechanisms as memories, typically regarded as long term, that are tested following a clear distraction.

Acquisition of all non-aware forms of memory that are described as long term by psychologists has generally been believed to be preserved in amnesia. These kinds of memory include skills, habits, priming, and various forms of conditioning. So, AA has usually been characterized as a selective deficit in acquiring long-term aware memories for personal experiences and facts. Even this belief has been challenged recently, at least with respect to priming, that is, stimulus-specific memory indicated by enhanced processing that does not need memory to be aware (e.g., Henke, 2010). There is also abundant evidence that the neural systems mediating aware memory and some of the kinds of unaware memory (e.g., skills) interact in both excitatory and inhibitory ways (e.g., Poldrack & Packard, 2003).

Pure organic amnesia is not caused by damage to only one brain structure, such as the hippocampus. It, or a similar amnesia-like memory disorder, can be caused by trauma to quite a few brain structures that interconnect with each other. Individual disruption of any one of these structures is sufficient to cause an amnesic-like condition. The implicated structures include distinct components of the medial temporal lobes (MTL: comprising the hippocampus, perirhinal cortex, parahippocampal cortex, entorhinal cortex, and amygdala), structures in the midline diencephalon (comprising the mammillary bodies, anterior thalamus, dorsomedial thalamus, and probably some other thalamic nuclei), structures in the basal forebrain (including the septum and diagonal band of Broca), the ventral tegmental nucleus of Guddens, the retrosplenial cortex, and possibly parts of the frontal and parietal cortices. These structures are highly interconnected. This explains why damage to the fornix, which mainly connects the hippocampus to the mammillary bodies and anterior thalamus, or damage to the mammillothalamic tract, which connects the mammillary bodies to the anterior thalamus, causes AA. This indicates that the memory functions, disrupted in amnesia, are mediated by neural circuits of connected MTL, midline diencephalic, and other structures. Indeed, there is direct evidence that damage to non-MTL structures in these circuits not only causes amnesia, but disturbs activity in the structurally intact MTL (Snaphaan et al., 2009). This strongly suggests that it is disturbed activity in these memory circuits that determines how bad the amnesia is.

The organic amnesia syndrome (i.e., AA and RA) has several distinct etiologies each of which disrupts the ability of one or more of the brain structures to mediate aware memory functions. These etiologies include side effects of neurosurgery, both infarctions and hemorrhagic stroke (particularly, ruptured aneurysms of the anterior communicating artery), tumors, temporal lobe epilepsy and related epileptic tissue removal, hypoxia, chronic alcoholism in which an associated thiamine deficiency is probably the key factor (Korsakoff syndrome), neurotoxins (e.g., domoic acid), autoimmune conditions such as voltage-gated potassium channel complex antibody-associated limbic encephalitis, viral or bacterial infection of the brain (e.g., Herpes simplex encephalitis), head injury, and some dementing conditions (e.g., the typical form of Alzheimer's disease). These etiologies differ with respect to the brain regions that they typically disrupt. For example, whereas Herpes simplex encephalitis typically disrupts the MTL, the midline diencephalon is typically disrupted in Korsakoff syndrome. Different patients with organic amnesia differ considerably with respect to how bad their amnesia is. For example, hypoxia can cause dramatic amnesia, or the deficit can sometimes be undetectable (e.g., Holdstock et al., 2008). This variation depends on how much of the affected structure or circuit is disrupted. Some of the etiologies cause less selective or pure amnesia than others because they disrupt structures and circuits involved in cognitive functions other than aware memory. For example, Alzheimer's disease may initially manifest primarily as amnesia, but attentional and executive function deficits are often apparent early on.

It is now almost universally accepted that amnesia arises when the efficient working of at least two functional circuits that mediate slightly different memory-related functions are disrupted, although the nature of the disrupted functions is still disputed (e.g., Montaldi & Mayes, 2010; Wixted & Squire, 2011). In particular, there have long been rival views that AA-related memory functions are disrupted by dysfunction in neural circuits that link different parts of the MTL to structures in the midline diencephalon, retrosplenial cortex, and probably parts of the frontal and parietal cortices (for example, Brown et al., 2010; Wixted & Squire, 2011).

Before discussing the rival views, it is important to consider two factors that underlie the processing differences between structures. First, the processing differences depend on the kinds of inputs the structures receive. Second, they also depend on whether the structures process those inputs in different ways. Therefore, knowledge of neural inputs, outputs, and cytoarchitectonics constrains thinking about what each structure in a circuit does. This knowledge suggests that the MTL structures receive and presumably process distinct inputs, with the perirhinal cortex dealing primarily with *item-related inputs* (comprising all the components of items), the parahippocampal cortex primarily with *spatial-context-related inputs*, and the hippocampus primarily with associative *item-context-related inputs*. Hippocampal structure is archicortical, whereas parahippocampal and perirhinal cortices are neocortical structures, which strongly implies that they will process their inputs in different ways. Each of these MTL structures links into circuits comprising several extra-MTL structures, and each of these structures also receives specific inputs, has specific cytoarchitectonics, and has specific outputs. The function of each circuit depends on the integrated working of the processing of all its constituent structures.

The functional differences depend on the kinds of information and memory functions that underlie aware memory for personal events and facts. It is widely believed that performance on recognition tests is driven to variable degrees by two kinds of memory: recollection and familiarity (Migo et al., 2012). Recollection is a form of aware memory in which the test stimulus cues the recall of information that was associated with the stimulus when it was previously encountered. When such recall occurs during a recognition test, it helps diagnose the previous encounter of the stimulus and so enables its recognition. Given that all recall must involve some kind of cue, it is believed that other forms of recall share very similar neural bases to recollection, particularly as far as amnesia is concerned. Familiarity is an aware form of memory for an encoded stimulus that involves recall of nothing about the stimulus, including any associates of previous encounters. It is plausible to argue that these different kinds of retrieval are related to different kinds of memory representation (see discussion later in this chapter). There has been a long-running disagreement about whether the different MTL circuits, as they relate to familiarity and recollection, can be dissociated in amnesia by lesions selectively affecting different parts of the MTL and their connections (for reviews, see Montaldi & Mayes, 2010; Wixted & Squire, 2011).

One of the rival views is that recollection and stimulus familiarity depend on the same MTL-related neural circuits, but that different MTL-related circuits may mediate recall and recognition memory for *different kinds* of input (Wixted & Squire, 2011). This view also allows that the different circuits may process differently so as to create *different kinds of memory representations*, although these will not differentially support recollection and/or familiarity. For example, the hippocampus may create more "abstract" representations of its inputs. The second of the rival views is that damage to any of the different parts of a hippocampal circuit (including the fornix, mammillary bodies, anterior thalamus, and perhaps retrosplenial cortex) selectively disrupts recollection, whereas damage to circuits linked to the perirhinal cortex and perhaps parahippocampal cortex disrupts familiarity memory (e.g., Brown, Warburton, & Aggleton, 2010; Montaldi & Mayes, 2010). A version of this view also proposes that hippocampal recollection is typically of item-context associations, whereas perirhinal cortex mediates item familiarity, and para-hippocampal cortex mediates context familiarity (Montaldi & Mayes, 2010). The two rival views are sometimes inappropriately called "single process" and "dual process" views, respectively; the name is inappropriate because both views allow for multiple processes. They differ in the type of processing and memory representations that each utilizes. "Dual process" views postulate that there are two groups of processes, each producing a distinct kind of memory representation (hence these views are sometimes also described as "multiple trace" theories). "Single process" views postulate one group of processes that produce one *kind* of memory representation (hence these views are sometimes described as "single trace" theories). The two rival views predict different kinds of dissociation within amnesia, but disagreement about which of these predictions is best supported by lesion evidence persists because this evidence is inconsistent. For example, although hippocampal lesions have been found to disrupt recollection and familiarity equally, it has also been found that they can selectively disrupt recollection, whereas perirhinal cortex lesions selectively disrupt familiarity (see Montaldi & Mayes, 2010, for a review).

However, other (non-lesion) evidence supports the second of the rival views that the MTL is functionally heterogeneous with respect to recollection and familiarity. Thus, a neural network model supports the view that the hippocampus creates recall-supporting representations, whereas the MTL neocortical structures create familiarity-supporting memory representations (Norman, 2010; Norman & O'Reilly, 2003). The recall-supporting representations stress differences between similar inputs (pattern separation), whereas the familiarity-supporting representations stress similarities between inputs (pattern generalization). There is extensive fMRI and single-unit recording evidence for the hippocampal pattern separation and pattern completion/recall processes, and for the MTL neocortical role in pattern generalizing and familiarity-like memory (see LaRocque et al., 2013; Yassa & Stark, 2011). It therefore seems most likely that there is a hippocampal circuit that creates pattern-separated item-context associative memory representations that primarily support cued recall, whereas the perirhinal and parahippocampal complexes create pattern-generalized item and context memory representations, respectively, that primarily support familiarity memory.

Although most attention has been paid to arbitrating between the above two rival views, other kinds of functional heterogeneity have been suggested. For example, there are claims that AA and RA sometimes (albeit rarely) dissociate, although measurement and other problems (i.e., such as disagreement about the existence of a temporal gradient in RA, at least for episodic memories) mean that there is still not agreement about these claims. Evidence of a complete dissociation would need to compare similar kinds of memory for similar information experienced to a similar degree in the pre- versus post-morbid periods. Further, to be convincing, RA severity for memories acquired fairly close in time to trauma would need to be sampled because it is agreed (despite the controversy about the temporal gradient in RA) that these memories are at least as severely impaired as any older memories in RA when it is present.

Measuring the Severity of Amnesia

The continued disagreements about the nature of the memory-related functions that should sometimes partially or completely dissociate from each other have made it harder to reach agreement about what measures of amnesia severity are valid. For example, at present, AA severity is still measured by how much performance on the tests that mainly tap recall for any kind of information is impaired relative to what would be expected from a non-amnesic person matched on intelligence. If a version of the "dual process" view is correct, then, with certain lesions, impairments of recall should occur when item recognition of similar information is intact or nearly so. The view indicates that this pattern should be found even more strongly with recollection and item familiarity, as has been reported (see Montaldi & Mayes, 2010, for a review). Conversely, the view predicts that other lesions should leave recall/recollection intact but impair item recognition or familiarity, as has been reported (for example, see Barbeau et al., 2011). So, if the dual process view is right, global AA severity measures are inappropriate because a "moderate" AA might comprise a severe recollection impairment with intact item familiarity, a severe item familiarity impairment with intact recollection, or moderate impairments of both recollection and item familiarity. Similarly, if memory for different kinds of information dissociates (as some versions of the dual process view propose), then a distinct set of memory tests that allow for the proposed kinds of material specificity need to be used to tap the severity of amnesia. Also, given that AA and RA often seem to partially, if not fully, dissociate from each other (see Mayes et al., 1997), it seems wise to separate AA and RA tests from each other in order to tap severity in a safe way, but this needs to be done by tapping the appropriate memory functions. Thus, recall/recollection and item recognition/familiarity should be tapped for corresponding kinds of information in order to assess AA and RA separately. In practice, this means using tests that are matched for recall or recognition (or recollection and familiarity), and for the information tapped when AA severity and RA severity are being compared. This use of appropriate separate measures will help identify how severely impaired the different AA and RA memory functions are.

The *degree* to which the brain trauma disrupts functioning in one or more of the amnesia-related circuits determines the severity of the corresponding amnesic symptoms. For example, when Herpes simplex invades the brain, it usually causes more extensive damage in the MTL than hypoxia, and, when it does so, it causes a generally more severe amnesia. This seems to suggest that the more a given structure is destroyed, the more severely the underlying memory function to which it contributes through its interactions with a set of connected structures (the function's brain circuit or system) will be disrupted. However, the evidence for this claim is not great, and its interpretation is tricky, partly because there is often uncertainty about the function of the damaged structure. For example, with human hippocampal damage it is disputed whether damage selectively impairs recall/recollection of associative memory representations, or whether it impairs item familiarity equally. This is relevant to the interpretation of recognition deficits because recognition is believed to be often well supported by familiarity, although cued recall also provides a variable degree of support. This implies that only if hippocampal damage selectively impairs cued recall will this damage impair recognition less than recall. There is no clear evidence that the extent of hippocampal damage correlates with increasing recognition deficits in humans (for reviews, see Brown et al., 2010; Montaldi & Mayes, 2010) and the evidence from monkey lesion research is disputed. On the one hand, Baxter and Murray (2001a, b) have argued that, although larger rhinal cortex lesions in monkeys cause greater item recognition memory deficits (measured with a delayed non-matching-to-sample task), larger hippocampal lesions cause milder item recognition deficits than smaller lesions. On the other hand, Zola and Squire (2001) have argued that there is no correlation at all, although small hippocampal lesions do disrupt recognition.

Depending on which view of hippocampal function is correct, it is clearly more appropriate to relate the extent of hippocampal damage either to recollection and other kinds of recall or to general measures of recall and recognition that ignore any amnesia-related differences of recall from familiarity. Even if the measure is theoretically appropriate, it does not follow that performance should decline as a linear function of extent of damage. But, if the measure does not correspond to the correct functional theory, we should certainly not assume that the efficiency of the hippocampus or any other amnesia-related structure inevitably declines as a linear or even monotonic function of how much of it has been destroyed. For example, with the hippocampus, if it selectively mediates cued recall of a wide range of associations, it could be that small lesions disrupt item recognition more than large lesions because the remaining hippocampus works abnormally and disrupts function not only of other structures in the recall/recollection circuit, but also of structurally connected structures such as the perirhinal cortex, which, according to the "dual process" view, lies in another functional circuit that mediates item familiarity (see Mayes et al., 2007). With larger lesions, there is less residual hippocampus to wreak havoc on perirhinal cortex familiarity functioning, so recognition, which depends on familiarity as well as cued recall, is less disrupted. With a disruption mechanism like this, which involves pathological interaction between two functionally distinct and dissociable memory systems, the degree of impairment may paradoxically be an inverted U-shaped function of how much of a structure is damaged.

What Factors Influence Degree of Change in Amnesic Severity Across Time?

It is well known that different amnesic patients not only show amnesia of different severity at onset but also recover to markedly different degrees across time. Furthermore, marked variation in level of recovery is found even within single etiologies. For example, of a sample of 104 Korsakoff patients, who were observed over a period ranging from 3 months to 10 years following diagnosis, Victor et al. (1989) reported that 22 recovered until no memory or intellectual deficit was detectable, 26 recovered significantly, 29 recovered slightly, and 27 showed no measurable change in their memory and learning abilities. Much of this work was carried out before 1971, when memory testing was cruder, so the "no deficit" group would probably still have shown mild impairments with more sophisticated testing. Since their diagnosis, these patients were detoxified by ensuring that they were abstinent from alcohol. They were also given an adequate diet, often including high levels of thiamine. The thiamine and/or a full diet accelerated recovery from the symptoms of Wernicke's encephalopathy (e.g., ophthalmoplegia and confusion, with nystagmus and ataxia settling more slowly). These Wernicke symptoms often preceded and then accompanied the memory impairment. However, recovery of memory tended to be much slower than recovery from the symptoms of Wernicke's encephalopathy. It was not clear to what degree thiamine therapy accelerated and increased memory recovery. This is partly because there have been no control studies of thiamine treatment's effects on recovery of memory, as Korsakoff's syndrome is often preceded by Wernicke's encephalopathy, which is treated as a medical emergency, as its symptoms are life-threatening and respond well to thiamine. However, De Wardener and Lennox (1947) found differential memory outcome in a study of thiamine-deprived, starved, and amnesic prisoners of war, depending on whether thiamine was available or not. The key point is that about three-quarters of Korsakoff patients show some degree of recovery of memory over a period of 2 years or so when they abstain from alcohol and when their intake of multivitamins, including thiamine, is increased. It remains to be explored to what degree the recovery of memory relates to physiological/anatomical changes in the regions, such as the anterior thalamus and mammillary bodies, damage to which is believed to contribute to amnesia in Korsakoff's syndrome. A fortiori whether treatment with thiamine helps normalize these and other structures in parallel with improving memory needs to be investigated.

In a similar way, hypoxia (which often primarily disrupts the hippocampus) can cause severe global amnesia with equally impaired recall, recognition, and familiarity memory from which there is little or no recovery (Cipolotti et al., 2001), severe amnesia that recovers to a less severe form (sometimes with global disruption of recognition as well as recall and sometimes with only impaired recall; e.g., Henke et al., 1999), and occasionally there is what seems to be complete recovery (Holdstock et al., 2008).

With these two etiologies of amnesia (thiamine deficiency and hypoxia), it is far from fully understood what causes the great variation in degree of recovery of memory, and it should be borne in mind that measures of the severity of the memory disorder in Korsakoff syndrome have not always been very appropriate (see Aggleton & Shaw, 1996, for a discussion). The same uncertainty about the key factors underlying recovery applies to most etiologies of amnesia, although several factors seem plausible. The following paragraphs list the key factors that may play a role in recovery from amnesia.

The first factor involves the return of the disrupted system to its pretrauma state, which leads to restitution of the temporarily impaired memory-supporting processes. This factor is illustrated by transient global amnesia (TGA), which is by definition a largely reversible form of amnesia. This syndrome has a rapid onset, which is sometimes triggered by emotional events, in which an often dense and global AA is accompanied by an RA of variable severity and extent. The AA usually dissipates in a period of a few hours to about a day, and does not usually re-occur. Studies that have examined blood flow in the brain have found that flow is often reduced in the MTL and occasionally in the midline thalamus during an attack, but returns to normal following recovery (Guillery-Girard et al., 2004). It was previously claimed that structural MRI showed no evidence of brain damage following an attack. More recently, however, small punctate lesions have been identified in the hippocampus of some TGA patients that seem to be associated with a small degree of hardly detectable, residual memory impairment (Jager et al., 2009; Sander & Sander, 2005). Therefore, most of the memory impairment in TGA is reversible, and this impairment is not caused by the destruction of amnesia-related structures, but by some kind of temporary dysfunction. One plausible but still unproved suggestion is that it is caused by spreading depression, which produces periodic waves of neural overactivity that are followed by a period of inactivity (see Gorji, 2001, for a review). Recovery is simply a function of how long the physiological disturbance of the amnesia-related and still largely intact brain structures persists. If an amnesia is, to some extent, caused by a kind of disruptive physiological process, then recovery should partially relate to the reversal of this process, which usually occurs without any kind of intervention. This might apply to memory problems caused or worsened by electroconvulsive shock treatment, epileptic seizures, or closed head injury-related edema, although ultimately the distinction between this and the plastic changes that occur following structural damage may be slightly blurred. In summary, it is important to stress that the first factor's successful operation means that not only do the briefly impaired memory processes recover to their pretraumatic levels, but so do the neural processes within the structure(s) that supported these processes pretraumatically.

A second plausible factor underlying the degree of recovery from amnesia and impaired psychological functions in general is the degree to which the brain system supporting the impaired memory or any kind of function has been destroyed. Destruction includes neuronal death, which will include axonal loss, although this may occur on its own. It is plausible to assume that as destruction increases, the mediated function declines and also shows less recovery. However, the function that describes this recovery may not be linear, but might be a negative or positive asymptotic function of the proportion of the target structure destroyed. The recovery that does occur is likely to involve restitution of the initially lost memory processes, provided that the proportion of the system damaged is low. Unfortunately, assessment of the contribution of this factor is made very difficult by two problems: our inadequate knowledge of the precise extent of the neural systems that mediate the impaired memory functions, and our inability to measure in full detail the extent of damage to these systems with current techniques, such as structural MRI.

The problems in assessing the second factor are illustrated by the example of hippocampal damage. If hippocampal damage *selectively* disrupts all forms of recall but leaves item familiarity intact and item recognition largely intact, then only recall testing is appropriate to measure the severity of this kind of memory impairment, and some forms of recall may be more sensitive than others to the degree of hippocampal damage. Thus, there is evidence that hippocampal activity increases with amount recalled (for example, Qin et al., 2011), which suggests that a given lesion may disrupt the recall of large amounts of information (e.g., a whole paragraph) more severely than it will disrupt the recall of smaller amounts of information (e.g., a single fact). Presumably, recalling more information calls on more of the processing that is served by the hippocampus, so more of the structure needs to remain intact and potentially functional, that is, tests of rapid recall of large amounts of information are likely to be most sensitive to damage and hence should be used. Given that prefrontal cortex lesions may also disrupt recall and perhaps particularly recall of larger amounts of information because of disruption of executive functions (see Mayes, 1988, for a discussion), it is important to control for any such damage when trying to identify the relationship between hippocampal dysfunction measures and extent of recovery of recall. If the hippocampus does not mediate familiarity, then tests of recognition, which only partly depend on recollection, are going to be very insensitive measures of hippocampal damage, unless this causes abnormal functioning in intact structures mediating familiarity. As was discussed earlier, however, if the hippocampus is largely destroyed, then this will not happen, and familiarity will be intact in the face of severely impaired recall.

Assuming that hippocampal damage selectively disrupts recall (particularly rapid recall of large amounts of information), current MRI techniques provide the main means of determining how the reduction across time of this measured impairment relates to the proportion of hippocampus that remains functional. Some evidence suggests that at least one patient, who has 50% volume reduction of his hippocampus in a T1-weighted MRI scan, seems to have functional activity in his residual hippocampus, as shown with fMRI when scanned long after the triggering trauma (Maguire et al., 2001, 2005). If this finding is correct, then some of the "hippocampal" gray matter in the structural scan must include appropriately connected and working neurons. But Jeneson et al. (2010) have argued, on the basis of rare postmortem data from Rempel-Clower et al. (1996), that functional hippocampus is unlikely to be present when more than a third of the structure is shown to be missing on structural MRI. The problem in defining how much hippocampus is functional is that gray matter on T1-weighted images includes glial cells (that increase in response to a lesion), as well as residual neuronal cell bodies, and the images are not sensitive to the short-range, unmyelinated fibers that interconnect the different parts of the hippocampus.

In summary, these problems and the lack of research on the relationship between extent of brain damage and degree of recovery of memory across time mean that there is still no certain knowledge about whether the second factor (the proportion of a memory-mediating structure or circuit that has been destroyed) is important in explaining recovery from amnesia. There is an impression that there is less recovery from fairly dense post-encephalitic amnesia than there is from hypoxic amnesia, where damage is mainly focused on the hippocampus, and that this is due to more extensive damage (Kopelman, personal communication). However, in order to check whether this impression is correct with controlled studies, it may be critical to ensure that appropriately selective memory measures are used. This is because post-encephalitic amnesia may damage not only the hippocampus, so as to impair recall, but also the perirhinal and parahippocampal cortices, so as to impair familiarity. Thus, global AA severity measures, rather than more selective recall and familiarity measures, will fail to identify whether post-encephalitic cases show little recovery of familiarity as well as of recall and whether the levels shown relate to the amount of perirhinal/parahippocampal cortex and hippocampal damage, respectively.

A third plausible factor relates to the age at which damage to an amnesia-related structure occurs. If the Kennard principle that early lesions disrupt functions less or allow more recovery of function (which is a controversial claim and is clearly untrue of many functions) applies to early onset organic memory disorders, then greater recovery or less severe problems should follow early damage to, for example, the hippocampus. However, although plastic processes may differ in the young, it is not clear that this always provides an advantage following early brain damage (Schneider, 1979) or indeed whether it affects amnesia severity or degree of recovery at all. For many years, the apparent absence of early onset amnesia was seen as a puzzle, and researchers wondered whether this might mean that early lesions did not notably impair aware memory. Alternatively, it was speculated that early onset damage might impair aware memory and that this might lead to a failure to develop knowledge of verbal and other kinds of semantics. A person like this would be seen as intellectually impaired rather than amnesic. Indeed, precisely this proposal has been applied to people with low-functioning autism, who have impairments in recognizing as well as recalling recently studied information (Bigham et al., 2010).

The puzzle was partially resolved when Vargha-Khadem et al. (1997) reported three cases with selective hippocampal atrophy of very early onset. These cases had what was reported as relatively selective recall deficits because their item recognition was normal, although their recognition of associations between different kinds of information, such as faces and voices, and objects and locations, was not. It is believed that these kinds of associative recognition depend nearly entirely on recollection. Similar results have been reported in patients with adult onset hippocampal lesions (Mayes et al., 2002; 2004; see Montaldi & Mayes, 2010, for a review). However, Vargha-Khadem and her colleagues also reported that their early onset cases, who were teenagers at the time of testing, showed normal levels of semantic knowledge. They, therefore, suggested that acquisition of semantic information was preserved and only acquisition of episodic information was disrupted. This seemed to contrast with adult onset hippocampal amnesia, even when there were also relatively selective recall deficits, as in the early onset cases. In the adults' case, acquisition of semantic information was impaired when there were multiple learning trials and the task was made hard to avoid ceiling effects in controls (Holdstock et al., 2004). Ceiling confounds may have occurred in measuring semantic memory in the three cases of Vargha-Khadem and her colleagues because much semantic learning involves myriad repetitions and rehearsals. Even if the semantic memory acquisition rate of the early onset cases was slowed, their performance may still have seemed normal on relatively easy knowledge tests. Evidence now suggests that this may be true (Gardiner et al., 2008). There is, therefore, no convincing support for the idea that early onset hippocampal damage is less disruptive of aware memory acquisition than adult onset lesions. However, research has shown that *neonatal* hippocampal lesions in macaque monkeys, unlike adult onset lesions, spared learning of spatial associative tasks (for example, Lavenex et al., 2007). Therefore, it could be that differences only appear with very early lesions when functions may not have been fully assigned to the hippocampus (see Braun et al., 2008). To what extent this advantage relates to the possibly greater plasticity of the very young hippocampus, or to its supposedly slower development, remains uncertain.

A fourth factor that relates to "initial" severity of amnesia, as well as degree of recovery from it, is whether the triggering trauma is rapid or occurs progressively over a long period of time. There is direct evidence for this in humans for non-memory functions. For example, Desmurget et al. (2007) have compared the cognitive effects of surgically removing slow-growing gliomas with those of strokes that had produced similarly sized and cortically located lesions. The stroke patients showed severe verbal and motor impairments from which there was little recovery. In contrast, the glioma patients, in whom cortical damage had very slowly increased until surgery was performed, often showed no detectable cognitive consequences. This phenomenon has been neurocomputationally modeled by Keidel et al. (2010). Within a modular framework of brain processing, they argued that, when a module is slowly destroyed, it is possible for neighboring module(s) to undergo a period of guided training in which new connections are formed to enable the tuning of the processing that is gradually being lost. The trained neural modules are able to also maintain their original functions. This is made possible only if the lesion extends slowly. If it occurs rapidly, there is not time for guided training to occur and enable the necessary new connections to be formed.

An important point about this argument should be noted. It seems to allow that the guided training produces a modification more like restitution than compensation because, at least under some conditions, the processing may be very similar to how it was premorbidly, even though it must now be mediated by a distinct structure. This applies to motor and verbal functions where the slowly damaged and the slowly trained structures are both mainly neocortical and share a very architectonically similar six-layered structure. Therefore, provided the progressively damaged region has long enough time to guide formation of appropriate new connections in its neighbor(s), the neighboring structure(s) will become able to mediate the identical processes (same inputs that are processed in the same way). To the extent that amnesia involves disruption of circuits comprising subcortical and neocortical components, the guided training that slow onset lesions often allow may be less effective because of cytoarchitectonic differences between the training and to-be-trained structures. If correct, this would imply that aware memory disorders will benefit less from slow onset brain damage than will disorders of movement and language.

Possible evidence against this has been provided by Braun et al. (2008), who compared the effects of right temporal lobectomy in two groups of temporal lobe epilepsy patients. In one group, the epilepsy had been caused by a brain tumor. Both the tumor and the epilepsy had only been present on average for less than 2 years prior to surgery in the first group. In the other group, the epilepsy, which had been caused by sclerosis, had been present on average for nearly 17 years. The patients were given a test of memory for color-location associations. Surgical damage was measured with structural MRI, and both groups showed fairly similar damage to the right hippocampus, entorhinal cortex, and perirhinal cortex. There was hardly any damage more posteriorly to the parahippocampal cortex, as would be expected from this surgery, although (also as expected) there was some inferior temporal cortex damage that seemed to be greater in the sclerotic patients. Although both groups were equally impaired when tested immediately, only the tumor group forgot pathologically fast over a short delay. It was, therefore, argued that associative aware memory was more impaired in the tumor group because the MTL damage had developed more rapidly. However, it should be conceded that early age of onset of pathology in the sclerotic cases is also consistent with the pattern of deficit in the two patient groups. It remains unclear with the patients who had the history of slowly developing sclerosis whether the damaged MTL structures were able to reorganize because they were not extensively damaged or whether the contralateral MTL structures had undergone compensatory changes, as is often argued with temporal lobe epilepsy.

It has been noted by Robertson and Murre (1999) that cognitive deficits recover less well in patients who are under-aroused and who have problems controlling/maintaining their attention. Pure amnesia is not believed to involve arousal and attentional disorders, but many cases are impure, with some degree of arousal and attentional disruption. Such patients may have brain stem or frontal cortex dysfunction that may worsen the initial severity of the memory deficit caused by the pure amnesic disorder alone and also may reduce the likelihood of the pure amnesia disorder showing some recovery over time. *If amnesia resembles other cognitive impairments in this respect, then low arousal and poor attentional control should be a fifth factor that influences not only initial severity of the aware memory disorder but also the extent of recovery in amnesic patients, although possibly to different degrees.* This should be plausible provided that guided learning and plasticity play any role in retuning partially damaged memory-mediating brain systems (restitution) or in adaptively modifying undamaged structures that mediate new processes when the previously responsible structures have been effectively destroyed (compensation).

A sixth factor influencing recovery from amnesia that can be difficult to distinguish from the effects of low arousal and poor attentional controls is the modification, usually via drugs, of modulatory inputs into the structures damaged in amnesia. The MTL structures, in particular, are modulated by input from midbrain and brain stem structures that contain acetylcholine, dopamine, noradrenaline, and serotonin-releasing neurons (for example, Takahashi et al., 2008). It is well known that this modulation has effects on the acquisition of episodic and semantic memories (for example, see Bissonette et al., 2011; Duzel et al., 2008). Patients who are developing the typical form of Alzheimer's disease, in which early degeneration of cholinergic basal forebrain neurons is a sign, are treated with modest success with acetylcholinesterase inhibitors, such as donepezil and galantamine. There is evidence that treatments produce modest memory improvements (for example, Sahakian et al., 1993) and slow cognitive decline (Small et al., 2005), although these claims should be treated with caution because memory improvements are not found in all patients, and evidence of slowed cognitive decline in the immediate pre-diagnostic stage of the disease is conflicting (Raschetti et al., 2007).

However, there have been few studies of such treatment in more stable kinds of amnesia. There are two exceptions: post-encephalitic amnesia, and amnesia associated with ruptured and repaired aneurysms. Peters and Levin (1977) and Catsman-Berrevoets et al. (1986) examined the effects of the anticholinesterase physostigmine over a period of weeks or months, respectively, and found some evidence of memory improvement in several post-encephalitic amnesics. Unfortunately, these studies do not appear to have been followed up, and useful scan information was not yet easily obtainable. It is, therefore, unclear how extensive the MTL damage was in these patients and, therefore, how any recovery might have been mediated by boosting levels of acetylcholine. More recently, Benke et al. (2005) conducted an open-label pilot study of donepezil treatment on amnesics who had suffered rupture and repair of aneurysms, mainly of the anterior communicating artery, who probably had basal forebrain damage (Benke et al., 2005). The drug was given daily and was well tolerated, and the patients showed significant improvements in recall after short and longer delays, which were greater than the improvements shown by their controls. Importantly, because some or all of the effects on memory of cholinergic drugs are often ascribed to direct enhancement of attention, neither attention nor executive functions improved significantly.

Similar work has also been done with dopaminergic drugs. Recall memory, in particular, is known to decline in aging even when this is not associated with dementia. Duzel et al. (2008) primarily used MRI to obtain magnetization transfer ratio as a measure of structural integrity in the hippocampus, frontal white matter, and a combination of the substantia nigra and ventral tegmental area dopamine system. More of the variance in verbal learning and memory scores was explained by substantia nigra and ventral tegmental area magnetization transfer ratio than by hippocampal or frontal white matter magnetization transfer ratio. There was only a weak relationship to working memory performance. Chowdhury et al. (2012) examined the effects of L-DOPA treatment on memory for scenes in a group of elderly people using a double blind placebo controlled study. Scene recollection was improved in the elderly, but only at a middle level dose of the drug (there was an inverted U-function relating recollection to drug dose) and most robustly after a 6-hour delay following learning. The latter effect is consistent with evidence that dopamine enhances de novo protein synthesis-dependent consolidation in the hippocampus, which creates more stable and long-lasting memories (for example, Bethus et al., 2010). This was consistent with fMRI evidence from the study that the L-DOPA–driven improvement in recollection at the 6-hour delay was unrelated to hippocampal encoding activity, but was explained by a post-encoding dopamine-driven consolidation enhancement.

Some kinds of neuromodulatory drugs do seem to mildly improve memory in some amnesic patients or elderly people who probably have modest dysfunction of the same brain systems as amnesics. This effect is probably related to increasing the efficiency of episodic and semantic learning and memory brain structures directly. It is less clear whether these modulatory effects are also facilitating recovery of memory in a way that is independent of their effects on arousal and attention. This is very hard to establish in humans, but there is some evidence that at least cholinergic modulation facilitates recovery of function in monkeys who have suffered either fornix or mammillary body lesions (i.e., whose extended hippocampal system has been lesioned). Croxson et al.'s (2012) depletion of acetylcholine bilaterally from the perirhinal cortex, entorhinal cortex, and temporal pole had no effect on an object-in-place scene learning, which was disrupted by either fornix or mammillary body lesions. However, if these extended hippocampal system lesions were preceded by the cholinergic depletion, the memory disruption was exacerbated, whereas when the cholinergic depletion followed, there was no effect. The authors argued that this indicates that the cholinergic input helps recovery of memory in the animals given extended hippocampal system lesions. A similar effect in humans may explain how procholinergic drugs might slow the progression of Alzheimer's disease, as some evidence suggests they do. Determining whether dopaminergic, noradrenergic, and serotonergic modifications of amnesia-related structures also influence the degree of recovery of memory will require much more research, as will determining optimum dose levels for drugs.

Furthermore, it is still unclear whether memory recovery enhancement by procholinergic (or possibly other modulatory) drugs involves reorganization and partial restitution of processing within the extended hippocampal system, or whether it involves a compensatory change mediated by structures that previously mediated different memory processes. There is some interesting evidence that a different kind of drug, the anti-epileptic drug levetiracetam, may stimulate restoration of pattern separation in people with amnestic mild cognitive impairment (aMCI; Bakker et al., 2012). Pattern separation (the creation of distinctive representations that support recall) is mediated by the CA3 and dentate gyrus regions of the hippocampus. In aMCI, although mild hippocampal dysfunction has been associated with increased hippocampal activity (Dickerson & Sperling, 2008), which may disrupt pattern completion (see Yassa & Stark, 2011), this pattern of increased hippocampal activity has not always been found (for example, Hampstead et al., 2012). The discrepant findings may relate to the aMCI diagnostic criteria used, how early in the course of aMCI the measure is taken, and what method is used. For example, Westerberg et al. (2013) looked at very early aMCI patients and used arterial spin labeling to measure blood flow, and found insignificant hippocampal volume reduction, but increased blood flow in the hippocampus, whereas Hampstead et al. (2011) used fMRI during the encoding of object-location associations and found significant hippocampal hypoactivation in the aMCI patients. The truth is no doubt complex, but whatever it is, it seems that levetiracetam reduces hippocampal hyperactivity, and this may normalize pattern separation and improve recall memory. Bakker et al.'s (2012) study showed such an enhancement with the recognition of specific objects with highly similar lures, which depends mainly on recollection. This improvement did not, unfortunately, extend to more global measures of memory function. Nevertheless, the finding is exciting and points to the possibility that a variety of drugs may partially reverse amnesia, at least when damage is mild, by restituting function. It also suggests that not all plastic changes in slowly developing amnesia are adaptive because the hippocampal hyperactivity seems to be disruptive in aMCI.

However, the issue of whether high levels of hippocampal activity in aMCI are disruptive remains confused, particularly since Hampstead et al. (2012) found that memory strategy training in MCI produced increased hippocampal activity at encoding and retrieval not only in healthy elderly controls, but in patients who showed deficient hippocampal activity prior to training. The authors interpreted this finding as evidence that this increased activation was adaptive. One possibility is that aMCI activity was increased following training because more elaborative encoding and retrieval were engaged that boosted memory: increased top-down control from frontal regions controlling the elaboration may also have maximized residual hippocampal functioning so that improved memory reflected better frontally mediated encoding and retrieval and better hippocampally mediated associative consolidation and storage. Consistent with this, the study found a memory improvement for object-location associations that was greater in the aMCI patients than their controls. Interestingly, Hampstead et al. (2011) found that memory for object-location associations was correlated with activity in more posterior hippocampal regions in aMCI patients than in controls, perhaps reflective of an atrophic process that runs in an anterior to posterior direction.

Conclusions and Future Needs

Cases of organic amnesia differ markedly in severity and in how much recovery occurs over time, but there is little established and systematic knowledge about the detailed nature of these variations and even less is known about the factors that determine them, except where the pathology reverses spontaneously (for unknown reasons), as in TGA. However, severity is likely to be increased and recovery reduced when more memory-related systems are disrupted and the proportion of each that is damaged is greater. These phenomena may also be influenced by the age of onset of the pathology, the rate at which it develops, whether the amnesia is accompanied by any arousal or attention disorder, and factors that moderate the level of input into the damaged and undamaged memory-related structures from modulating brain regions, such as the cholinergic component of the basal forebrain. Various kinds of memory rehabilitation (such as strategy training) as a factor have been discussed by, for example, Robertson and Murre (1999), who also mention the negative impact of pathological inhibition of damaged structures by disinhibited structures. This inhibition perhaps arises most often from unilateral lesions, such as occur with amnesia that is associated with temporal lobe epilepsy. For example, with the Sprague effect that was identified first in cats, when left visual neglect, caused by a right posterior neocortex lesion, is followed by a second lesion to the left superior colliculus, the visual neglect largely disappears (Sprague, 1996). It is plausible to propose that the second lesion allows recovery because it prevents dysfunctional inhibition of the mirror image right superior colliculus. It is unknown whether a similar phenomenon influences recovery from material-specific amnesias that have been caused by an initial unilateral lesion.

All the above factors are likely to affect the degree to which damaged or undamaged memory-related brain structures and circuits can form adaptive, new connections following the triggering damage. Although such changes may lead to partial restitution of memory processes, they may also lead to new, compensatory processes being expressed. Price and Friston (2002) have provided a framework for understanding compensatory processes and have also indicated why very little is known about them. They argued that many cognitive tasks can be completed in multiple ways, that is, many functions can be completed using several different combinations of processes. Imaging studies cannot on their own identify the structure of this redundancy whenever more than one memory system, each mediating the same memory function in different ways, is active. Equally, when the most efficient memory system is active and the less efficient systems are inhibited, as has been suggested by Fanselow (2010), imaging will fail to detect these additional neural systems. Neuropsychological studies of amnesic patients on their own will also fail to identify the structure of this redundancy when only one of the redundant systems has been damaged, particularly if it is a less efficient system. Price and Friston, therefore, argue that understanding can only emerge from an iterative approach that examines the effects of lesions while also performing parallel fMRI studies of such patients, as well as healthy controls. This has not been done at all with organic amnesia in humans, and we remain ignorant of whether amnesia affects brain systems showing this kind of redundancy, although Fanselow (2010) has found evidence in rodents that there may be redundancy for some hippocampal functions. His argument was that less efficient systems are released from hippocampal inhibition following hippocampal damage. Whether this applies to humans remains unknown but should make an interesting focus of future research.

This research will need to use the iterative approach suggested by Price and Friston in order to explore the factors influencing initial amnesic severity and recovery. It will probably need to be done collaboratively across several research centers because large numbers of patients will be required. The research will help define a number of basic science issues, such as what the redundant brain systems are and how much their efficiencies vary. Large cross-center studies will also be needed to learn systematically about how amnesic severity varies and how much recovery varies in different etiologies. Such studies will help identify the importance of the "plausible factors" underlying recovery.

In parallel, interventional studies with suitably large patient groups should determine how the adaptive plastic changes underlying recovery can be enhanced. Such research should explore different interventional procedures that include treatment with growth factors, such as brain-derived neurotrophic factor, and deep brain stimulation.

Finally, while all this is going on, stem cell transplant research should be explored much more intensively. A very interesting start has been made to this work. For example, Bissonnette et al. (2011) have created methods for developing human embryonic stem cells into functional basal forebrain neurons. Stem cell transplantation work has advanced further with the hippocampus, where it has been applied successfully to the hippocampus in rodents and monkeys, producing functional growth of the transplant and recovery of memory (for example, Virley et al., 1999). It remains to be shown whether this approach will work with human hippocampal amnesics. There is already evidence from Virley and his colleagues that conditionally immortal neuroepithelial stem cell grafts are able to migrate to the CA1 region of the hippocampus after four-vessel occlusion in a damage-dependent way. This preference for regions of cell loss and their apparent ability to adopt appropriate neuronal and glial cell morphologies and presumably to form normal connections suggests that they provide a point-to-point repair mechanism, which enables them to restore previously lost hippocampal memory function (for example, see Hodges et al., 2000). At present, stem cell transplantation is the only potentially complete solution for treating severe and stable human organic amnesias, and its success may well depend on the operation of similar plastic processes to those underlying recovery from amnesia when this occurs.

References

Aggleton, J. P., & Shaw, C. (1996). Amnesia and recognition memory: A re-analysis of psychometric data. *Neuropsychologia, 34,* 51–62.

Bakker, A., Krauss, G. L., Albert, M. S., Speck, C. L., Jones, L. R., Stark, C. E., Yassa, M. A., Bassett, S. S., Shelton, A. L., & Gallagher, M. (2012). Reduction of hippocampal hyperactivity improves cognition in amnestic mild cognitive impairment. *Neuron, 74,* 467–474. doi10.1016/j.neuron.2012.03.023

Barbeau, E. J., Pariente, J., Felician, O., & Puel, M. (2011). Visual recognition memory: A double anatomo-functional dissociation. *Hippocampus, 21,* 929–934.

Baxter, M. G., & Murray, E. A. (2001a). Opposite relationship of hippocampal and rhinal cortex damage to delayed nonmatching-to-sample deficits in monkeys. *Hippocampus, 11,* 61–71.

Baxter, M. G., & Murray, E. A. (2001b). Effects of hippocampal lesions on delayed nonmatching-to-sample in monkeys: A reply to Zola and Squire (2001). *Hippocampus, 11,* 201–203.

Benke, T., Koylu, B., Delazer, M., Trinka, E., & Kemmler, G. (2005). Cholinergic treatment of amnesia following basal forebrain lesion due to aneurysm rupture: An open-label study. *Eur J Neurol, 12,* 791–786.

Bethus, I., Tse, D., & Morris, R. G. (2010). Dopamine and memory: Modulation of the persistence of memory for novel hippocampal NMDA receptor-dependent paired associates. *J Neurosc, 30,* 1610–1618.

Bigham, S., Boucher, J., Mayes, A., & Anns, S. (2010). Assessing recollection and familiarity in autistic spectrum disorders: Methods and findings. *J Autism Dev Disord, 40,* 878–889.

Bissonnette, C. J., Lyass, L., Bhattacharyya, B. J., Belmadni, A., Miller, R. J., & Kessler, J. A. (2011). The controlled generation of functional basal cholinergic neurons from human embryonic stem cells. *Stem Cells, 29,* 802–811.

Braun, M., Finke, C., Ostendorf, F., Lehmann, T.-N., Hoffmann, K.-T., & Ploner, C. J. (2008). Reorganization of associative memory in humans with long-standing hippocampal damage. *Brain, 131,* 2742–2750. doi: 10,1093/brain/awn191

Brown, M. W., Warburton, E. C., & Aggleton, J. P. (2010). Recognition memory: Material, processes, and substrates. *Hippocampus, 20*, 1228–1244.

Catsman-Berrevoets, C. E., Van Harskamp, F., & Appelhof, A. (1986). Beneficial effect of physostigmine on clinical amnesic behaviour and neuropsychological test results in a patient with a post-encephalitic amnesic syndrome. *J Neurol, Neurosur Ps, 49*, 1088–1090.

Chowdhury, R., Guitart-Masip, M., Bunzeck, N., Dolan, R. J., & Duzel, E. (2012). Dopamine modulates episodic memory persistence in old age. *J Neurosci, 32*, 14193–14204. doi: 101523/JNEUROSCI.1278-12.2012

Croxson, P. L., Browning, P. G. F., Gaffan, D., & Baxter, M. G. (2012). Acetylcholine facilitates recovery of episodic memory after brain damage. *J Neurosci, 32*, 13787–13795. doi: 10.1523/JNEUROSCI.294712.2012

Cipolotti, L, Shallice, T., Chan, D., Fox, N., Scahill, R., Harrison, G., Stevens, J., & Rudge, P. (2001). Long-term retrograde amnesia. . . the crucial role of the hippocampus. *Neuropsychologia, 39*, 151–172.

Desmurget, M., Bonnetblanc, F., & Duffau, H. (2007). Contrasting acute and slow-growing lesions: A new door to brain plasticity. *Brain, 130*, 898–914. doi: 10.1093/brain/awl300

De Wardener, H. E., & Lennox, B. (1947). Cerebral beriberi (Wernicke's encephalopathy): Review of 52 cases in a Singapore prisoner-of-war hospital. *Lancet, 1*, 11–17.

Dickerson, B. C., & Sperling, R. A. (2008). Functional abnormalities of the medial temporal lobe memory system in mild cognitive impairment and Alzheimer's disease: Insights from functional MRI studies. *Neuropsychologia, 46*, 1624–1635.

Duzel, S., Schutze, H., Stallforth, S., Kaufmann, J., Bodammer, N., Heinze, H-J., & Duzel, E. (2008). A close relationship between verbal memory and SN/VTA integrity in young and older adults. *Neuropsychologia, 46*, 3042–3052.

Fanselow, M. S. (2010). From contextual fear to a dynamic view of memory systems. *Trends Cognitive Sci, 14*, 7–15.

Gardiner, J. M., Brandt, K. R., Baddeley, A. D., Vargha-Khadem, F., & Mishkin, M. (2008). Charting the acquisition of semantic knowledge in a case of developmental amnesia. *Neuropsychologia, 46*, 2865–2868. doi: 10.1016/j.neuropsychologia.2008.05.021

Gorji, A. (2001). Spreading depression: A review of the clinical evidence. *Brain Res Rev, 31*, 33–60.

Guillery-Girard, B., Desgranges, B., Urban, C., Piolino, P., de la Sayette, V., & Eustache, E. (2004). The dynamic time course of memory recovery in transient global amnesia. *J Neurol, Neurosur Ps, 75*, 1532–1540.

Hampstead, B. M., Stringer, A. Y., Stilla, R. F., Amaraneni, A., & Sathian, K. (2011). Where did I put that? Patients with amnestic mild cognitive impairment demonstrate widespread reductions in activity during the encoding of ecologically relevant object-location associations. *Neuropsychologia, 49*, 2349–2361.

Hampstead, B. M., Stringer, A. Y., Stilla, R. F., Giddens, M., & Sathian, K. (2012). Mnemonic strategy training partially restores hippocampal activity in patients with mild cognitive impairment. *Hippocampus, 22*, 1652–1658.

Henke, K. (2010). A model of memory systems based on processing modes rather than consciousness. *Nature Rev Neurosci, 11*, 523–532.

Henke, K., Kroll, N. E. A., Behniea, H., Amaral, D. G., Miller, M. B., Rafal, R., & Gazzaniga, M. S. (1999). Memory lost and memory regained following bilateral hippocampal damage. *J Cognitive Neurosci, 11*, 682–697.

Hampstead, B. J., Stringer, A. Y., Stilla, R. F., Giddens, M., & Sathian, K. (2012). Mnemonic strategy training partially restores hippocampal activity in patients with mild cognitive impairment. *Hippocampus, 22*, 1652–1658.

Hodges, H., Sowinski, P., Virley, D., Nelson, A., Watson, W. P., Veizovic, T., Patel, S., Mora, A., Rashid, T., French, S. J., Chadwick, A., Gray, J. A., & Sinden, J. D. (2000). Functional reconstruction of the hippocampus: Fetal versus conditionally immortal neuroepithelial stem cell grafts. *Novart Fdn Symp, 231*, 53–65; discussion 65–69.

Holdstock, J. S., Mayes, A. R., Isaac, C. L., & Roberts, J. N. (2004). Differential involvement of the hippocampus and temporal cortices in rapid and slow learning of new semantic information. *Neuropsychologia, 40*, 748–768

Holdstock, J. S., Parslow, D. M., Morris, R. G., Fleminger, S., Abrahams, S., Denby, C., Montaldi, D., & Mayes, A. R. (2008). Two case studies illustrating how relatively selective hippocampal lesions in humans can have quite different effects on memory. *Hippocampus, 18*, 679–691.

Inostroza, M., & Born, J. (2013). Sleep for preserving and transforming episodic memory. *Ann Rev Neurosci*, *36*, 79–102.

Jager. T., Szabo, K., Griebe, M., Bazner, H., Moller, J., & Hennerici, M. G. (2009). Selective disruption of hippocampus-mediated recognition memory processes after episodes of transient global amnesia. *Neuropsychologia*, *47*, 70–76.

Jeneson, A., Kirwan, C. B., Hopkins, R. O., Wixted, J. T., & Squire, L. R. (2010). Recognition memory and the hippocampus: A test of the hippocampal contribution to recollection and familiarity. *Learn Memory*, *17*, 63–70.

Jeneson, A., & Squire, L. R. (2012). Working memory, long-term memory, and medial temporal lobe function. *Learn Memory*, *19*, 15–25.

Keidel, J. L., Welbourne, S. R., & Lambon Ralph, M. A. (2010). Solving the paradox of the equipotential and modular brain: A neurocomputational model of stroke vs slow-growing glioma. *Neuropsychologia*, *48*, 1716–1724.

LaRocque, K., Smith, M., Carr, V., Witthoft, N., Grill-Spector, K., & Wagner, A. (2013) Global similarity and pattern separation in the medial temporal lobe predict subsequent memory. *J Neurosci*, *33*, 5466–5499.

Lavenex, P., Banta Lavenex, P., & Amaral, D. G. (2007). Spatial relational learning persists following neonatal hippocampal lesions in macaque monkeys. *Nature Neurosci*, *10*, 234–239.

Lee, A. C. H., Yeung, L.-K., & Barense, M. D. (2012). The hippocampus and visual perception. *Front Human Neurosci*, *6*, 1–17.

Maguire, E. A., Frith, C. D., Rudge, P., & Cipolotti, L. (2005). The effect of adult-acquired hippocampal damage on memory retrieval: An fMRI study. *NeuroImage*, *27*, 146–152.

Maguire, E. A., Vargha-Khadem, F., & Mishkin, M. (2001). The effects of bilateral hippocampal damage on fMRI regional activations and interactions during memory retrieval. *Brain*, *124*, 1156–1170.

Mayes, A. R. (1988). *Human organic memory disorders*. Cambridge; Cambridge University Press.

Mayes, A. R., Daum, I., Markowitsch, H., & Sauter, W. (1997). The relationship between retrograde and antero-grade amnesia in patients with typical global amnesia. *Cortex*, *33*, 197–217.

Mayes, A. R., Holdstock, J. S., Isaac, C. L., Hunkin, N. M., & Roberts, N. (2002). Relative sparing of item recognition memory in a patient with adult-onset damage limited to the hippocampus. *Hippocampus*, *12*, 325–340.

Mayes, A. R., Holdstock, J. S., Isaac, C. L., Montaldi, D., Grigor, J., Gummer, A., . . . Norman, K. A. (2004). Associative recognition in a patient with selective hippocampal lesions and relatively normal item recognition. *Hippocampus*, *14*, 763–784.

Mayes, A. R., Montaldi, D., & Migo, E. (2007). Associative memory and the medial temporal lobes. *Trends Cognitive Sci*, *11*, 126–135.

Migo, E. M., Mayes, A. R., & Montaldi, D. (2012). Measuring recollection and familiarity: Improving the remember/know procedure. *Conscious Cogn*, *21*, 1435–1455.

Montaldi, D., & Mayes, A. R. (2010). The role of recollection and familiarity in the functional differentiation of the medial temporal lobes. *Hippocampus*, *20*, 1291–1314.

Moscovitch, M., & Nadel, L. (1998). Consolidation and the hippocampal complex revisited: In defense of the multiple-trace model. *Curr Opin Neurobiol*, *8*, 297–300.

Norman, K. A. (2010). How hippocampus and cortex contribute to recognition memory: Revisiting the complementary learning systems model. *Hippocampus*, *20*, 1217–1227.

Norman, K. A., & O'Reilly, R. C. (2003). Modelling hippocampal and neocortical contributions to recognition memory: A complementary learning systems account. *Psychol Rev*, *110*, 611–646.

Pertzov, Y., Miller, T. D., Gorgoraptis, N., Caine, D., Schott, J. M., Butler, C., & Husain, M. (2013). Binding deficits in memory following medial temporal lobe damage in patients with voltage-gated potassium channel complex antibody-associated limbic encephalitis. *Brain*, *136*, 2474–2485. doi: 10.1093/brain/awt129

Peters, B. H., & Levin, H. S. (1977). Memory enhancement after physostigmine treatment in the amnesic syndrome. *Arch Neurology*, *34*, 215–219.

Poldrack, R. A., & Packard, M. G. (2003). Competition among multiple memory systems: Converging evidence from animal and human brain studies. *Neuropsychologia*, *41*, 245–251.

Price, C. J., & Friston, K. J. (2002). Degeneracy and cognitive anatomy. *Trends Cognitive Sci*, *6*, 416–421.

Qin, S., van Marle, H. J. F., Hermans, E. J., & Fernandez, G. (2011). Subjective sense of memory strength and the objective amount of information accurately remembered are related to distinct neural correlates at encoding. *J Neurosci*, *31*, 8920–8927.

Rempel-Clower, N. L., Zola, S. M., Squire, L. R., & Amaral, D. G. (1996). Three cases of enduring memory impairment after bilateral damage limited to the hippocampal formation. *J Neurosci, 16*, 5233–5255.

Robertson, I. H., & Murre, J. M. J. (1999). Rehabilitation of brain damage: Brain plasticity and principles of guided recovery. *Psychol Bull, 125*, 544–575.

Raschetti, R., Albanese, E., Vanacore, N., & Maggini, M. (2007). Cholinesterase inhibitors in mild cognitive impairment: A systematic review of randomised trials. *PLOS Med 4*, 1818–1828. doi: 10.1371/journal.pmed.0040338. PMC 2082649. PMID 18044984.

Sander, K., & Sander, D. (2005). New insights into transient global amnesia: Recent imaging and clinical findings. *Lancet Neurol, 4*, 437. doi: 10.1016/S1474-4422(05)70121-6

Schneider, G. E. (1979). Is it really better to have your brain lesion early? A revision of the "Kennard principle." *Neuropsychologia, 17*, 557–583.

Snaphaan, L., Rijpkema, M., van Uden, I., Fernandez, G., & de Leeuw, F-E. (2009). Reduced medial temporal lobe functionality in stroke patients: A functional magnetic resonance imaging study. *Brain, 132*, 1882–1888.

Sahakian, B. J., Owen, A. M., Morant, N. J., Eagger, S. A., Boddington, S., Crayton, L., Crockford, H. A., Crooks, M., Hill, K., & Levy, R. (1993). Further analysis of the cognitive effects of tetrahydroaminoacridine (THA) in Alzheimer's disease: Assessment of attentional and mnemonic function using CANTAB. *Psychopharmacol (Berlin), 110*, 395–401.

Small, G. W., Kaufer, D., Mendiondo, M. S., Quarg, P., & Spiegel, R. (2005). Cognitive performance in Alzheimer's disease patients receiving rivastigmine for up to 5 years. *Int J Clin Pract, 59*, 473–477.

Sprague, J. M. (1996). Neural mechanisms of visual orienting responses. *Prog Brain Res, 112*, 1–15.

Squire, L. R., & Zola, S. M. (1998) Episodic memory, semantic memory and amnesia. *Hippocampus, 8*, 205–211.

Takahashi, H., Kato, M., Takano, H., Arakawa, R., Okumura, M., Otsuka, T., Kodaka, F., Hayashi, M., Okubo, Y., Ito, H., & Suhara, T. (2008). Differential contribution of prefrontal and hippocampal dopamine D1 and D2 receptors in human cognitive functions. *J Neurosci, 28*, 12032–12038.

Vargha-Khadem, F., Gadian, D. G., Watkins, K. E., Connelly, A., Van Paesschen, W., & Mishkin, M. (1997). Developmental amnesia: Effect of early hippocampal pathology on episodic and semantic memory. *Science, 277*, 376–380.

Victor, M., Adams, R. D., & Collins, G. H. (1989). *The Wernicke-Korsakoff syndrome and related neurologic disorders due to alcoholism and malnutrition (2nd ed.).* Philadelphia: F. A. Davis.

Virley, D., Ridley, R. M., Sinden, J. D., Kershaw, T. R., Harland, S., Rashid, T., French, S., Sowinski, P., Gray, J. A., Lantos, P. L., & Hodges, H. (1999). Primary CA1 and conditionally immortal MHP36 cell grafts restore conditional discrimination learning and recall in marmosets after excitoxic lesions of the hippocampal CA1 field. *Brain, 122*, 2321–2335.

Westerberg, C., Mayes, A., Florczak, S. M., Zufen, C., Creery, J., Parrish, T., Weintraub, S. M., Mesulam, M., Reber, P. J., & Paller, K. A. (2013). Distinct medial temporal contributions to different forms of recognition in amnestic mild cognitive impairment and Alzheimer's disease. *Neuropsychologia, 51*, 2450–2461.

Wilson, B. A. (2009). *Memory rehabilitation: Integrating, theory and practice.* London: Guilford Press.

Wixted, J. T., & Squire, L. R. (2011). The medial temporal lobe and the attributes of memory. *Trends Cognitive Sci, 15*, 210–217.

Yassa, M. A., & Stark, C. E. L. (2011) Pattern separation in the hippocampus. *Trends Cognitive Sci, 34*, 515–525.

Zola, S. M., & Squire, L. R. (2001) Relationship between magnitude of damage to the hippocampus and impaired recognition memory in monkeys. *Hippocampus, 11*, 92–98.

12

Aging-Related Changes in Neural Substrates of Motor and Cognitive Systems

Bruce Crosson and Keith M. McGregor

Introduction

Profound alterations in brain activity underlying motor and cognitive functions occur as we age. We are only beginning to understand just how these changes affect behavior. Some evidence indicates that brain activity unique to older persons is compensatory for decreases in cognitive functions (e.g., Cabeza, Anderson, Locantore, & McIntosh, 2002); yet other evidence suggests that, in at least some instances, it could interfere with cognitive functions (e.g., Meinzer et al., 2009; Meinzer, Seeds, et al., 2012). What causes shifts in brain activity patterns as we age? Mounting evidence indicates that decreases in inhibitory mechanisms play a role in aging-related behavioral change (McGregor, Heilman, et al., 2012; McGregor et al., 2011). However, recent studies also indicate an association between amyloid burden and decreased cognitive function in cognitively "normal" older adults (Sperling et al., 2009). Research indicates that aging-related patterns of behavior and their underlying neural substrates can be mitigated by a history of high physical activity (e.g., Liang et al., 2010; McGregor, Heilman, et al., 2012; McGregor et al., 2011, 2013; Zlatar et al., 2013). Further, exercise interventions in previously sedentary older persons have been shown to reverse some aging-related changes (e.g., Colcombe et al., 2004; Voss et al., 2010).

Given this potential to mitigate aging-related patterns of behavior and brain activity, understanding neural and behavioral changes in aging should be given a high priority. Reducing such changes can increase independence and quality of life for older persons as they continue to age. Evidence also indicates that interventions like exercise may be able to delay the onset of dementia (e.g., Liang et al., 2010), potentially saving millions of healthcare dollars. Although activity and behavioral differences from younger adults are most profound over the age of 70, McGregor et al. (2013) have shown that they can occur in midlife (40–60 years of age), suggesting that interventions should begin at least as early as age 40.

This chapter focuses on aging-related changes in brain function. It will begin by reviewing changes in the motor system that occur in aging because we are closer to understanding the neural mechanisms for some aging-related changes in the motor system than in other systems. Further, our preliminary data indicates that it is possible to use these aging-related motor phenomena as a template for understanding some changes in cognitive systems. Hence, the motor system is a good place to begin our discussion. Subsequently, we will turn to changes in cognitive systems. Some provocative literature has recently been published by our research group on neural substrates for language changes in aging. For this reason, we will focus particularly on recent findings regarding the language system and what they mean for aging, discussing other cognitive systems as needed to round out our understanding of neural and cognitive changes in older adults. Finally, we will conclude this chapter by addressing implications for neural plasticity and rehabilitation in aging related diseases, the possibility of mitigating aging-relating changes, and future research directions.

The Motor System and Aging

Older adults frequently complain of increased clumsiness and slowed reaction times in the upper extremity. Motor performance measures such as reaction time (Salthouse, 1984), psychomotor speed (finger tapping) (Cullum et al., 1989; Salthouse, 1996), fine dexterity (Carmeli et al., 2003) and reach accuracy (Christou, 2011; Kornatz et al., 2005; Sarlegna, 2006) all show decreases with advancing age. While some individuals find such loss of function a mere annoyance or slight embarrassment, many individuals suffer more severe consequences, including loss of job responsibilities or social withdrawal. Mechanical problems certainly account for some alteration of function, as older adults are more likely to exhibit muscle atrophy, degradation of connective tissue, and degenerative joint disease, which all impair upper extremity motor performance. However, there is strong evidence that these factors do not explain the majority of the variance when comparing dexterity between older and younger adults (Christou, 2011; Latash & Zatsiorsky, 2009).

Recent research has indicated that upper extremity performance declines in older age and may be related to changes in levels of interhemispheric inhibition of the primary motor cortices (Bernard, Taylor, & Seidler, 2011; Fling, Peltier, Bo, Welsh, & Seidler, 2011; Langan et al., 2010). During volitional movement of a single upper extremity, the contralateral primary motor cortex (cM1) exhibits an increase in metabolic activity consistent with increased synaptic function. In functional magnetic resonance imaging (fMRI), this increased synaptic activity results in a positive blood oxygenation level dependent response (BOLD), a gamma-variate function that roughly resembles a bell curve (Ogawa et al., 1990). In our lab and others, numerous studies have shown that during unimanual activity, there is a difference in the pattern of interhemispheric BOLD activity in M1 when comparing older and younger adults. Sedentary older adults (50+ years who engage in voluntary exercise less than 45 minutes per week) show a positive BOLD signal bilaterally in primary motor cortex (M1) during unimanual task performance, indicating that they are recruiting cortical activity in both hemispheres. However, in younger adults, the activity level of the ipsilateral primary motor (iM1) area (ipsilateral to the moving hand—i.e., right hand movement - right M1) tends to decrease as compared to baseline levels (rest). This phenomenon results in a negative BOLD signal during fMRI and is essentially an inverted bell curve (gamma-variate). The negative BOLD response (NBR) has been a topic of considerable study in recent years, particularly with respect to the finding that a sedentary lifestyle is associated with a positive BOLD response, rather than an NBR, in iM1 (McGregor et al., 2009, 2011; Naccarato et al., 2006; Riecker et al., 2006).

While there has been some debate over whether the NBR represents a respiratory-induced statistical anti-correlation (Birn et al., 2006), new evidence shows that when accounting for physiological parameters, the NBR in sensorimotor areas (M1S1), specifically, represents active neural processes (Bright et al., 2014). In aggregate, the work to date on the physiological origin of the NBR has resulted in the prevailing opinion that the NBR represents an active inhibition of cortical activity (Bright et al., 2013; Goense et al., 2012; Lenzi et al., 2007; McGregor et al., 2013; Northoff et al., 2007; Stefanovic et al., 2004, 2005; Shmuel et al., 2006). Very recent work has now indicated that the likely origin of the NBR is through increased levels of gamma-amino butyric acid (GABA), which is the primary inhibitory neurotransmitter system in the human cerebral cortex. Using magnetic resonance spectroscopy (MRS), Northoff et al. (2007) first showed the relationship between GABA levels and the NBR when investigating the so-called default mode network in the resting state. It is well known that, during most active states, retrosplenial cortical areas show an NBR relative to a resting state in younger adults (Buckner; Grecius et al., 2003; Raichle et al., 2001). Northoff et al. (2007) employed MRS to quantify changes in GABA in retrosplenial voxels and found significantly greater GABA concentrations in subjects with greater task-related NBRs, a finding replicated by Hu, Chen, Gu, and Yang (2013). MRS has also been used to quantify the amount of GABA in the primary motor cortex during motor learning involving anodal transcranial direct stimulation (tDCS) (Stagg et al., 2011). In a group of younger adults, application of anodal tDCS applied to the left motor cortex showed a corresponding decrease in left M1 GABA concentrations as assessed by MRS. Moreover, this decrease in GABA concentration on the left side predicted improved motor performance during right-hand tasks. However, it has yet to be shown if MRS can be used to quantify GABA changes across age groups in interhemispheric M1S1 activity.

The behavioral relevance of the aging-related loss of the NBR in iM1 to motor performance has been a matter of debate, however. The neurophysiological and imaging studies to date have bred three lines of thought. The first is that aging-related alteration of patterns of cortical activity may be epiphenomenal and may not interact with the function of the motor system. A wealth of evidence, however, has shown that alterations of motor function are associated with changes in the levels of interhemispheric inhibition (Bernard & Seidler, 2012; Fling et al., 2011; Fling & Seidler, 2011; Giovannelli et al., 2009; Langan et al., 2010; McGregor, Carpenter, et al., 2012; McGregor et al., 2011; Talelli, Ewas, Waddingham, Rothwell, & Ward, 2008; Talelli, Waddingham, Ewas, Rothwell, & Ward, 2008).

A second interpretation of aging-related loss of inhibition in M1S1 involves the notion of aging-related cortical compensation. Largely driven by reports using fMRI, this view argues that the higher positive BOLD responses observed bilaterally in the motor cortex of aging adults acts in a compensatory manner to assist task completion (Heuninckx, Wenderoth, Debaere, Peeters, & Swinnen, 2005; Mattay et al., 2002; Wu & Hallett, 2005; Zimerman, Heise, Gerloff, Cohen, & Hummel, 2012). The critical assumption in this opinion is that the aging brain loses the capacity (via gray or white matter dysfunction) to complete tasks without the intervention of additional neural substrates. This, in turn, argues for a hierarchical pattern of activity across hemispheres whereby more difficult tasks require the intervention of the ipsilateral motor cortex. While related literature has shown some support for this hierarchical recruitment hypothesis (Hutchinson et al., 2002; Stippich, Blatow, Durst, Dreyhaupt, & Sartor, 2007; Verstynen, Diedrichsen, Albert, Aparicio, & Ivry, 2005), it is challenged by other studies that do not show increased bilaterality of M1 recruitment with greater task demands (McGregor, Craggs, Benjamin, Crosson, & White, 2009; McGregor et al., 2011, 2012; Riecker et al., 2006; Wu & Hallett, 2005; Van Impe, Coxon, Goble, Wenderoth, & Swinnen, 2009).

The third interpretation of aging-related change in interhemispheric inhibition and motor function is that increased recruitment of the ipsilateral motor cortex during unimanual movements exerts a deleterious effect on motor performance. Recent work from our laboratory lends support to this interpretation, as sedentary middle-aged adults who had less interhemispheric inhibition during unimanual tasks performed worse on tests of psychomotor speed and dexterity (McGregor et al., 2011, 2012, 2013). Further, as described in McGregor et al. (2012), the engagement of the ipsilateral motor cortex during a bimanual task (coin rotation) eliminates the dexterity advantage enjoyed by individuals with intact interhemispheric inhibition. It is likely that trancallosal communication during unimanual tasks is inhibitory in nature (Giovannelli et al., 2009; Lenzi et al., 2007; Llufriu et al., 2012; Manson, Palace, Frank, & Matthews, 2006; Manson et al., 2008; Meyer, Roricht, & Woiciechowsky, 1998; Stefanovic, Warnking, & Pike, 2004) within healthy individuals, and its reduction in older adults (and in instances of frank pathology) hinders proper task performance. This is of note from a neurophysiological perspective also because most transcallosal fibers are glutamatergic and have synapses with excitatory receptors (Berlucchi, 1990). Therefore, intervening inhibitory interneurons are the likely origin of the inhibition shown in the ipsilateral cortex. There are numerous studies showing that increasing excitability in the contralateral motor cortex via anodal transcranial direct stimulation results in improved unimanual motor learning capacity and better motor performance (Furuya, Nitsche, Paulus, & Altenmuller, 2013; Hummel et al., 2010; Saucedo Marquez, Zhang, Swinnen, Meesen, & Wenderoth, 2013; Zimerman et al., 2013).

While fMRI has been used to probe patterns of motor cortical recruitment during unimanual activity, its use in this context is somewhat novel. Over the past 20 years, the standard technique for motor systems inquiry has been the use of transcranial magnetic stimulation (TMS), which offers excellent temporal resolution. Interestingly, aging-related studies of interhemispheric communication have employed this modality and have yielded analogous findings to investigations involving fMRI. For example, using a paired-pulse TMS (consisting of two TMS coils presented over each primary motor cortex) paradigm, Peinemann et al. (2001) reported decreases in levels of interhemispheric inhibition with increasing age, a finding later replicated by Talelli et al. (2008a, 2008b). Using a separate, but related measure called the ipsilateral silent period (a brief, involuntary cessation of muscle activity shortly after stimulation of the ipsilateral M1), Sale and Semmler (2005) reported that their elderly volunteers showed a significantly shorter duration of ipsilateral inhibition—a finding recently replicated by others (Fujiyama, Garry, Levin, Swinnen, & Summers, 2009; Fujiyama, Hinder, Schmidt, Garry, & Summers, 2012) and in our work (McGregor et al., 2011). In aging adults, recent studies have shown that the decline in unimanual motor performance in older adults is associated with a shorter duration of the ipsilateral silent period (Fling et al, 2011; McGregor et al., 2011, 2013) and differences in excitability of the ipsilateral hemisphere (Fling, Peltier, Bo, Welsh, & Seidler, 2011; Langan et al., 2010). The implication of these findings is that aging is associated with decreased interhemispheric inhibition that may be driving declines in motor performance.

While this section has commented on aging-related changes, it is relevant to note that recent work from our laboratory and others suggests that chronological age may not be the ultimate cause of the aforementioned changes in interhemispheric inhibition (Manson et al., 2006; McGregor, Carpenter, et al., 2012; McGregor et al., 2011, 2013; Talelli, Ewas, et al., 2008; see also Irlbacher et al., 2007). We have shown that while sedentary aging is associated with loss of interhemispheric inhibition, the regular and long-term engagement in aerobic activity slows or even reverses this loss. As reported by McGregor et al. (2013), even adults at the age of 40 show changes in interhemispheric communication that are associated with motor decline. That is, in fMRI, sedentary aging adults tend to show higher levels of bilateral positive BOLD and a lower duration of the ipsilateral silent period as compared to physically active and younger adults. Importantly, both of these measures correlated with poorer motor performance as compared to physically active age cohorts. However, highly fit individuals of a similar age cohort showed activity typically associated with younger adults (18–30 years), specifically negative BOLD in ipsilateral M1S1 and longer TMS silent periods. As such, the aging-related changes in motor activity and upper extremity performance described above may not be inevitable consequences of age, and, importantly, may be modifiable in sedentary older individuals.

Language, Cognition, and Aging

The work of McGregor and colleagues (see discussion earlier in this chapter) has been an important stimulus for our research group to re-evaluate data that we have collected about language and aging. Indeed, a re-examination of Wierenga and colleagues' (2008) fMRI data indicated some similarities to McGregor and colleagues' motor-system findings discussed above. Wierenga et al. (2008) examined BOLD responses to single trials of visually presented picture naming in younger (20–34 years of age) and older adults (68–84 years of age). They found that in the right pars triangularis, the anterior division of the right-hemisphere homolog to Broca's area, there was a significant activity difference between younger and older adults. This activity difference was characterized by a largely negative BOLD signal in younger adults and a positive BOLD signal in older adults (Figure 12.1). It is of interest that in high-performing older adults, performance accuracy was positively correlated with BOLD signal in the right pars triangularis; that is, greater positive BOLD response was associated with greater performance accuracy. However, in low-performing older adults, greater BOLD signal was associated with decreased performance accuracy. Hence, for picture naming, older adults whose performance is higher may be able to use right pars triangularis activity to enhance performance, while the opposite is true for lower performing older adults.

Meinzer et al. (2009) followed up on the results of Wierenga et al. (2008), asking if spoken generation of category members (semantic fluency) would demonstrate a similar pattern of results to picture naming. In this study, the investigators used blocks of 10 trials per category, paced to accommodate sparse temporal sampling (Hall et al., 1999). (Sparse temporal sampling allows for the collection of images after subjects have finished

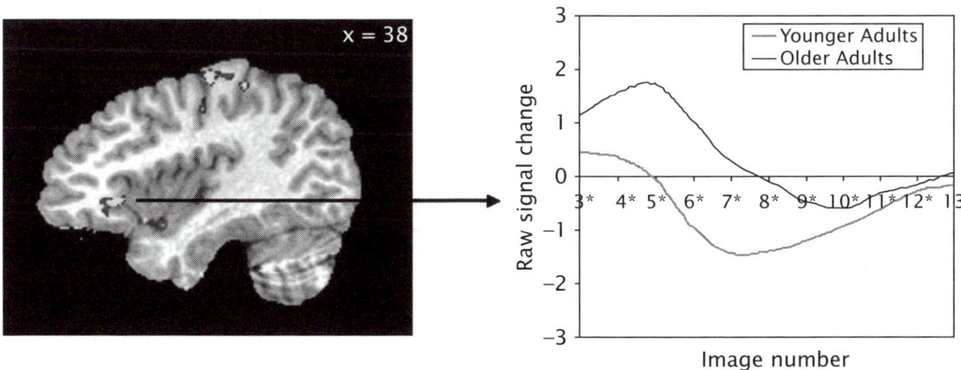

FIGURE 12.1 A significant difference in BOLD response between younger and older adults during picture naming is due largely to the decrease in activity in younger adults and the increase of activity in older adults. Reprinted from *Neurobiology of Aging*, Volume 29, C. E. Wierenga, M. Benjamin, K. Gopinath, W. M. Perlstein, C. M. Leonard, L. J. Gonzalez Rothi, T. Conway, M. A. Cato, R. Briggs, & B. Crosson, Age-related changes in word retrieval: Role of bilateral frontal and subcortical networks, pp. 436–451, Copyright 2008, with permission from Elsevier.

speaking to avoid the large signal artifacts occurring when subjects speak in the scanner.) The control task was repeating the word "pause" (German for "rest") for a block of 10 trials at a similar pace to word generation blocks. Meinzer et al. (2009) found two areas of right frontal cortex in which older adults (64–88 years of age) demonstrated greater activity relative to the control task than younger adults (20–33 years of age), one in pars triangularis, similar to the Wierenga et al. (2008) study, and the other in the middle frontal gyrus. In both areas, for older persons, there was a significant negative correlation between category-member-generation accuracy and BOLD signal: the more negative the BOLD response was, the higher was the subject's accuracy, and the more positive the BOLD response was, the lower was the subject's accuracy. Subjects also generated words that began with specific letters (phonemic fluency), but this task did not demonstrate age-related differences in activity. Two aspects of these findings deserve comment. First, there was no bimodal response, as there was in Wierenga et al.'s (2008) study, where the relationship between performance accuracy and BOLD response changed with the performance level. This difference between the studies could relate to differences between category-member generation and picture naming. The former is less determined by the external stimulus than the latter. We have previously shown differences in medial and lateral frontal cortex for word generation depending on the level of external versus internal determination of responses (Crosson et al., 2001). It is also possible that the necessity to generate 10 items from relatively discrete categories made Meinzer et al.'s (2009) task more difficult than picture naming. The second aspect deserving comment is that the negative relationship between task accuracy and BOLD response in the right frontal cortex of older adults raises the possibility that right frontal activity may actually hamper, rather than help, word retrieval in aging. This interpretation is the opposite of the canonical interpretation that right frontal activity assists left frontal regions that become less capable with aging. It is worth noting in this regard that there are cognitive paradigms in which increased non-dominant-hemisphere activity with aging is associated with better performance (e.g., Cabeza et al., 2002). It also should be mentioned that Meinzer et al. (2009) did not address brain regions dominated by negative BOLD response.

This latter problem was addressed in a subsequent study by Meinzer et al. (2012). The experimental and control tasks were similar to those mentioned above, except that there were more blocks of each, and the native language of participants was English as opposed to German. This study was confirmatory of the previous findings in that regions of significant activity differences (older > younger) in multiple right frontal areas showed negative correlations between BOLD response and accuracy of category-member generation, though activity differences were in somewhat different right frontal locations than in the previous study. However, the novel finding from this study was that several regions in younger adults (19–32 years of age) demonstrated greater negative BOLD responses than older adults (61–80 years of age). The regions exhibiting negative BOLD are interesting because they are consistently associated with the default mode network (DMN), which may undergo aging-related changes in cortical recruitment. In Meinzer et al. (2012), there were significant negative correlations between BOLD response and accuracy of performance such that more negative BOLD responses were associated with better performance in the older group. These two regions were in the posterior cingulate/precuneus and anterior, inferior parietal regions. Subjects also performed a phonemic fluency task compared to the repetition baseline, and there were no aging-related differences in positive BOLD signal, although there was a similar loss of negative BOLD signal in aging during the semantic fluency task. The importance of the loss of negative BOLD signal in the older adults has yet to be unraveled. An important question is whether or not this loss of negative BOLD in aging is related to loss of inhibition in aging or to some other substrate. Animal model studies have demonstrated a loss of GABA projection neurons and interneurons (Madhusudan, Sidler, & Knuesel, 2009; McQuail, Banuelos, LaSarge, Nicolle, & Bizon, 2012; Schmidt, Redecker, Bruehl, & Witte, 2010; Stanley, Fadel, & Mott, 2012) and that GABA and $GABA_A$ agonists can normalize activity in the visual cortex of older primates (Leventhal, Wang, Pu, Zhou, & Ma, 2003). Hence, GABA activity appears to be a good target for future aging research.

Meinzer et al. (2012) used similar tasks to the two previous experiments, except that they varied task difficulty (easy vs. difficult). For *left* inferior frontal gyrus activity, difficulty modulated BOLD responses to both the semantic and phonemic fluency tasks such that activity was more positive in the more difficult tasks. This modulation was similar in both younger (19–32 years of age) and older (61–80 years of age) groups; that is, there was no age-by-difficulty interaction for either phonemic or semantic fluency. Responses in the *right* inferior frontal gyrus were rather different. For category-member generation in this part of cortex, BOLD responses were negative relative to the repetition baseline for the younger group and not different between difficulty levels. In the older group, BOLD responses for semantic fluency were negative in the easy condition, positive in the difficult condition, and significantly different between the two conditions. This significant age-by-difficulty interaction indicates that only the older adults modulated their BOLD responses from the easy to the difficult semantic fluency condition. Although there was no age-by-difficulty interaction for the phonemic fluency task in the right inferior frontal gyrus, it is worth noting that the younger subjects went from a negative BOLD response for the easy task to no response for the difficult task, while the older subjects went from no response for the easy task to a positive BOLD response for the difficult task. This modulation of activity from the easy to the difficult task was significant for both groups. But the important point for the right inferior frontal gyrus is that only the older subjects showed a positive BOLD response in either the easy or the difficult semantic fluency task. Although it could be claimed that right inferior frontal gyrus activity for phonemic fluency appears to be modulated by task difficulty, it is not certain that any level of difficulty would have evoked a positive response for the younger group, as it did for the older group. Further, the data do not support a claim that difficulty is the only factor involved for semantic fluency. The age-by-difficulty indicates that age plays a role in increasing the BOLD response to difficult semantic items. The behavioral data support this conclusion.

Although the effect is greater for the older than the younger group in the semantic task, the difficult tasks produced reduced accuracy relative to the easy tasks for both ages in both conditions.

Exercise, Aging, and Cortical Inhibition

As noted above, McGregor et al. (2011, 2013) found that a recent history of regular moderate to strenuous physical activity mitigates the effects of age by improving motor performance, mitigating the reduction of the ipsilateral silent period, and preserving some degree of negative BOLD in iM1. Correlations between motor performance and the ipsilateral silent period (McGregor, Heilman, et al., 2012) and correlations between the ipsilateral silent period and negative BOLD (McGregor et al., 2011) suggest a common substrate underlying these phenomena, perhaps a reduction of GABAergic activity in aging.

We have also wondered whether changes in the language system would show a similar response to a recent history of exercise. Zlatar et al. (2013) studied younger (19–37 years of age), sedentary older (63–81 years of age), and physically active older (60–85 years of age) groups of adults. They used a silent category-member generation task compared to visual fixation. In our experience, this task-baseline combination has yielded similar findings to the spoken versions used in the Meinzer et al. studies (2009, 2012, 2012), except that basal ganglia activity are more robust in silent generation (Crosson et al., 2003). As predicted, sedentary older adults showed more positive BOLD responses than either physically active older adults or younger adults, indicating some effects of a history of greater physical activity. However, the effects of exercise history did not appear to be as robust or as specific as they were in the motor system (McGregor et al., 2011). Ipsilateral silent periods were measured in these participants using single-pulse stimulation of the dominant M1. As the reader will recall, the ipsilateral silent period is one measure of cortical inhibition. For the entire sample across groups, the duration of the ipsilateral silent period was negatively correlated with BOLD signal magnitude in the left and right posterior perisylvian cortices and in the left and right thalami. In other words, shorter ipsilateral silent periods were associated with greater BOLD responses. These latter data raise the question of whether decreased inhibition plays a role in increased cortical activity during cognitive tasks in aging. Another interesting facet of these latter correlations is that posterior perisylvian activity often is associated with the default network, yet there was no correlation between ipsilateral silent period and BOLD activity in the medial portions of this network (i.e., the posterior cingulate/precuneus region).

Clearly, further research is necessary to define the physiological substrates of changes in BOLD activity in older adults. Our findings suggest that changes in cortical inhibition should be further investigated as one potential substrate of the aging-related changes that we see in our fMRI studies of BOLD activity. However, there are other known (and likely unknown) aging-related changes that affect BOLD responses and cognition. For example, in a meta-analysis, Rowe et al. (2010) showed that the incidence of a high beta-amyloid burden positively accelerates as a function of age after the age of 60. On the average, it is present in about 30% of cognitively unimpaired adults in this age range. Beta-amyloid is a biomarker for Alzheimer's disease and may play some role in the cascade of physiological events leading to cognitive decline in this disease. The posterior cingulate/precuneus region is one of the first sites where beta-amyloid accumulates (e.g., Aizenstein et al., 2008). Sperling et al. (2009) showed that a high beta-amyloid burden in the posterior cingulate/precuneus region of cognitively "normal" older adults was associated with loss of negative BOLD in this area during memory encoding. The centrality of the posterior cingulate/precuneus region to the default network suggests that cognitive functions showing a relationship to changes in this region are good candidates for further exploration. It seems likely that amyloid burden contributes to the loss of either negative (Meinzer, Seeds, et al., 2012) or positive (Moffat, Elkins, & Resnick, 2006) BOLD responses in this region as age increases.

Up to this point, we have focused primarily on recent evidence regarding aging-related changes in the language system. A main theme in both frontal cortex and the default network is the transformation of negative BOLD in younger adults to either a positive BOLD response in iM1 during movement or in right inferior frontal cortex during word finding, or to a lack of a BOLD response in the default network during word finding. The relationship of GABA with negative BOLD responses in posterior cingulate cortex and the precuneus for younger subjects (Hu et al., 2013; Northoff et al., 2007) and indications of loss of GABA neurons and activity with aging (Madhusudan et al., 2009; McQuail et al., 2012; Schmidt et al., 2010; Stanley et al., 2012) suggest that loss of negative BOLD in aging may be related to reduction in GABAergic inhibition. This proposition deserves further research attention. However, not every aging-related change in brain activity is reflective of a shift from a negative toward a positive BOLD response.

Hence, a few words should be said about the diversity of findings regarding brain activity in aging. For example, we have already pointed out that increased activity in the non-dominant hemisphere of older adults does not always have a negative relationship with performance. As a case in point, in a source memory task, left (non-dominant) frontal activity was characteristic of high- but not low-performing older adults (Cabeza et al., 2002). An important question is, in what instances is greater activity in older adults is helpful, and when does it interfere with performance? An important cue to answer this question may be the actual hemodynamic responses of the older and younger subjects. An interesting study by Cabeza et al. (2004) explored frontal responses of younger and older adults to three tasks: verbal working memory, visual attention, and retrieval of episodic memories. For visual attention and episodic retrieval, significant frontal differences between groups were characterized by negative BOLD responses in younger participants and positive BOLD responses in older participants, similar to word-finding tasks from our laboratory, as discussed earlier. However, significant differences in frontal responses for the working memory task were characterized by positive BOLD responses in younger adults, but even larger positive BOLD responses in older adults. On the other hand, Moffat et al. (2006) also showed a reduction in positive BOLD response from younger to older adults in the retrosplenial cortex during a spatial navigation task. As we have already noted, we find ourselves wondering if a change from a negative to a positive BOLD response with aging connotes a loss of inhibition, which in turn can lead to interference with cognition by irrelevant activity. Such a phenomenon could explain changes in attention with aging. However, we also wonder if a change from a positive BOLD response to an even greater positive BOLD response is a sign of compensatory activity. As just noted, reduction of positive BOLD responses also can occur with aging. It is possible that the loss of positive BOLD responses weakens the cognitive activity that it supports, but it is also possible that older adults find different neural routes by which to accomplish tasks in which such changes occur. If we can gain a greater understanding of what these neural patterns represent in terms of underlying neural substrates, we will be in a better position to mitigate the resulting aging-related deficits in cognitive and motor functions.

To summarize, we have studied aging-related changes in neural activity underlying word production. Several interesting findings have emerged from this work. Primary among them is that increased right frontal activity during word finding often is associated with decreased performance. This raises the possibility that right frontal activity hinders, rather than facilitates, word retrieval. This hypothesis is bolstered by the fact that activity signatures change from negative to positive BOLD with aging. In other words, it appears that activity in right frontal regions during word finding is suppressed in younger participants but is increased in older participants. However, more research will be necessary to test this hypothesis.

We also have shown that negative BOLD activity during word finding in the medial posterior portion of the default network (posterior cingulate/precuneus) disappears with aging, and its disappearance is associated with lower performance in word-finding tasks. The nature of this negative activity in younger participants needs to be investigated further, but we hypothesize that it involves suppression of attentional mechanisms, allowing participants to focus on the generation of words, as opposed to task-irrelevant information. Changes in attentional networks with aging are well known.

It is possible that loss of GABAergic activity affecting frontal cortex accounts for changes in frontal cortex. However, there are likely to be other factors that also affect the loss of negative BOLD, especially in the posterior cingulate cortex and precuneus. In particular, this is an area where amyloid burden accumulates early in many older adults and may interact with other aging-related changes in neural substrates. Again, these are hypotheses requiring further investigation.

Change from negative to positive or neutral BOLD activity with aging is not a universal finding. Some studies have shown an increase in an already positive BOLD signal with aging, and others have shown a decrease in a positive BOLD signal. These findings indicate that activity changes during cognitive tasks in aging are complex phenomena, which are not amenable to a monolithic explanation. Many factors are likely to contribute to the diversity of findings, including the nature of the neural substrate and which aging-related change(s) is(are) affecting them, whether older persons perform tasks using different cognitive resources than younger persons, the nature of the experimental and baseline tasks, and so on. Nonetheless, understanding these changes is important and will be briefly addressed in the next section.

Implications for Neural Plasticity and Rehabilitation in Aging-Related Diseases

We will conclude this chapter by asking two important questions. First, what are the implications of aging-related changes in the neural substrates for plasticity in older adults? Neural plasticity is important for learning at all ages. Recent work has suggested that GABAergic inhibition through $GABA_A$ receptors may play a role in the competitive selection of dendritic spines during learning in pyramidal cells in the CA1 sector of the rat hippocampus (Hayama et al., 2013). As noted earlier, the idea that the loss of negative BOLD signal in aging may be related to decreased GABAergic activity is intriguing. Important questions in this regard are how widespread the loss of GABAergic activity in aging is, and what its effects on plasticity are. For example, does competitive selection of synapses during learning extend beyond the hippocampus, and if so, what are the effects of loss of GABAergic activity in aging on this competitive selection? As noted earlier, our recent work indicates that exercise may mitigate loss of negative BOLD signal in older adults. Could this effect be related to preservation of GABAergic activity with exercise? Obviously, there are many questions to be answered about how aging affects neural plasticity and whether these effects can be mitigated. This is an important area for future research.

The second question is, what are the effects of aging-related changes on plasticity during rehabilitation? As one example, stroke is a condition frequently requiring rehabilitation, and it is a disease primarily of older persons. Thus, aging-related changes in neural plasticity are likely to affect stroke rehabilitation. If changes from negative to positive BOLD responses in motor and language systems represent a loss of suppression of one area of cortex by another, what are the consequences of this loss of suppression for the learning processes that support motor or aphasia rehabilitation? Is the presence of such changes predictive of rehabilitation outcome? If so, what are the underlying neural mechanisms? For example, would the presence of amyloid burden or decline of transcallosal inhibition in stroke patients predict recovery or rehabilitation outcome? We believe that rehabilitation for aging-related conditions must take into account aging-related changes in brain functions. As the reader has probably already surmised, at this point in time, we have more questions than answers about aging-related changes in brain function.

In closing, figures from the US Census Bureau indicate that in 2010, almost 57 million Americans (18.4% of the population) were 60 years of age or older. By 2050, the number of Americans of this age will nearly double to approximately 112 million (25.5% of the population; Administration on Aging, 2010). Aging-related changes in cognition and motor functions limit independence and detract from the quality of life in older persons. Further, in all likelihood, aging-related changes in brain function affect rehabilitation in aging-related diseases. Healthcare costs and productivity implications of caring for older adults with limited independence are staggering. Yet, we have much to learn about the neural substrates of aging-related changes in cognition and behavior, and we know even less about how to mitigate these changes. Thus, making progress in understanding aging-related changes and mitigating them has enormous economic implications, as well as implications for quality of life in an aging population. From this viewpoint, research on aging-related phenomena is urgent. We have illustrated a few novel findings in the realm of neural changes in aging. Even with this progress, however, we currently have more questions than answers. The sooner we find answers to these questions, the better our lives ultimately will be.

Acknowledgments

The contents do not represent the views of the Department of Veterans Affairs or the United States Government. This work was supported by the following Department of Veteran Affairs Rehabilitation Research and Development Grants: Center of Excellence (# C9246C), Career Development Award Level-2 (KMM: # E0956W), Senior Research Career Scientist (BC: #B6364L), Merit Review Pilot (BC: # IRX000994A).

References

Administration on Aging, Department of Health and Human Services. (2010). Projected future growth of loder pobulation: By age: 1900–2050. Retrieved, May 15, 2014 from http://www.aoa.gov/Aging_Statistics/future_growth/future_growth.aspx

Aizenstein, H. J., Nebes, R. D., Saxton, J. A., Price, J. C., Mathis, C. A., Tsopelas, N. D., . . . Klunk, W. E. (2008). Frequent amyloid deposition without significant cognitive impairment among the elderly. *Arch Neurol*, 65(11), 1509–1517. doi: 10.1001/archneur.65.11.1509

Berlucchi, G. (1990). Commisurotomy studies in animals. In F. Boller & J. Grafman (Eds.), *Handbook of neurophysiology* (Vol. 4, pp. 9–47). Amsterdam: Elsevier.

Bernard, J. A., & Seidler, R. D. (2012). Evidence for motor cortex dedifferentiation in older adults. *Neurobiol Aging*, 33(9), 1890–1899. doi: 10.1016/j.neurobiolaging.2011.06.021

Birn, R. M., Diamond, J. B., Smith, M. A., & Bandettini, P. A. (2006). Separating respiratory-variation-related fluctuations from neuronal-activity-related fluctuations in fMRI. *Neuroimage*, 31(4), 1536–1548.

Bernard, J. A., Taylor, S. F., & Seidler, R. D. (2011). Handedness, dexterity, and motor cortical representations. *J Neurophysiol*, 105(1), 88–99. doi: 10.1152/jn.00512.2010

Bright, M. G., Bianciardi, M., de Zwart, J. A., Murphy, K., & Duyn, J. H. (2014). Early anti-correlated BOLD signal changes of physiologic origin. *Neuroimage*, 87, 287–296.

Cabeza, R., Anderson, N. D., Locantore, J. K., & McIntosh, A. R. (2002). Aging gracefully: Compensatory brain activity in high-performing older adults. *Neuroimage*, 17(3), 1394–1402.

Cabeza, R., Daselaar, S. M., Dolcos, F., Prince, S. E., Budde, M., & Nyberg, L. (2004). Task-independent and task-specific age effects on brain activity during working memory, visual attention and episodic retrieval. *Cereb Cortex*, 14(4), 364–375.

Carmeli, E., Patish, H., & Coleman, R. (2003). The aging hand. *J Gerontol A Biol Sci Med Sci*, 58(2), 146–152.

Christou, E. A. (2011). Aging and variability of voluntary contractions. *Exerc Sport Sci Rev, 39*(2), 77–84. doi: 10.1097/JES.0b013e31820b85ab

Colcombe, S. J., Kramer, A. F., Erickson, K. I., Scalf, P., McAuley, E., Cohen, N. J., . . . Elavsky, S. (2004). Cardiovascular fitness, cortical plasticity, and aging. *P Natl Acad Sci USA, 101*(9), 3316–3321. doi: 10.1073/pnas.0400266101

Crosson, B., Benefield, H., Cato, M. A., Sadek, J. R., Moore, A. B., Wierenga, C. E., . . . Briggs, R. W. (2003). Left and right basal ganglia and frontal activity during language generation: Contributions to lexical, semantic, and phonological processes. *J Int Neuropsychol Soc, 9*(7), 1061–1077. doi: 10.1017/S135561770397010X

Crosson, B., Sadek, J. R., Maron, L., Gokcay, D., Mohr, C. M., Auerbach, E. J., . . . Briggs, R. W. (2001). Relative shift in activity from medial to lateral frontal cortex during internally versus externally guided word generation. *J Cogn Neurosci, 13*(2), 272–283.

Cullum, C. M., Thompson, L. L., & Heaton, R. K. (1989). The use of the Halstead-Reitan test battery with older adults. *Clin Geriatr Med, 5*(3), 595–610.

Fling, B. W., Peltier, S. J., Bo, J., Welsh, R. C., & Seidler, R. D. (2011). Age differences in interhemispheric interactions: Callosal structure, physiological function, and behavior. *Front Neurosci, 5*, 38. doi: 10.3389/fnins.2011.00038

Fling, B. W., & Seidler, R. D. (2011). Fundamental differences in callosal structure, neurophysiologic function, and bimanual control in young and older adults. *Cereb Cortex.* doi: 10.1093/cercor/bhr349

Fujiyama, H., Garry, M. I., Levin, O., Swinnen, S. P., & Summers, J. J. (2009). Age-related differences in inhibitory processes during interlimb coordination. [Research Support, Non-U.S. Gov't]. *Brain Res, 1262*, 38–47. doi: 10.1016/j.brainres.2009.01.023

Fujiyama, H., Hinder, M. R., Schmidt, M. W., Garry, M. I., & Summers, J. J. (2012). Age-related differences in corticospinal excitability and inhibition during coordination of upper and lower limbs. [Research Support, Non-U.S. Gov't]. *Neurobiol Aging, 33*(7), 1484 e1481–1414. doi: 10.1016/j.neurobiolaging.2011.12.019

Furuya, S., Nitsche, M. A., Paulus, W., & Altenmuller, E. (2013). Early optimization in finger dexterity of skilled pianists: Implication of transcranial stimulation. *BMC Neurosci, 14*, 35. doi: 10.1186/1471-2202-14-35

Giovannelli, F., Borgheresi, A., Balestrieri, F., Zaccara, G., Viggiano, M. P., Cincotta, M., & Ziemann, U. (2009). Modulation of interhemispheric inhibition by volitional motor activity: An ipsilateral silent period study. *J Physiol, 587*(Pt 22), 5393–5410. doi: 10.1113/jphysiol.2009.175885

Goense, J., Merkle, H., & Logothetis, N. K. (2012). High-resolution fMRI reveals laminar differences in neurovascular coupling between positive and negative BOLD responses. *Neuron, 76*(3), 629–639.

Greicius, M. D., Krasnow, B., Reiss, A. L., & Menon V. (2003). Functional connectivity in the resting brain: a network analysis of the default mode hypothesis. *Proc Natl Acad Sci U S A*, Jan 7;*100*(1), 253–258.

Hall, D. A., Haggard, M. P., Akeroyd, M. A., Palmer, A. R., Summerfield, A. Q., Elliott, M. R., . . . Bowtell, R. W. (1999). "Sparse" temporal sampling in auditory fMRI. *Hum Brain Mapp, 7*(3), 213–223.

Hayama, T., Noguchi, J., Watanabe, S., Takahashi, N., Hayashi-Takagi, A., Ellis-Davies, G. C., . . . Kasai, H. (2013). GABA promotes the competitive selection of dendritic spines by controlling local Ca2+ signaling. *Nat Neurosci, 16*(10), 1409–1416. doi: 10.1038/nn.3496

Heuninckx, S., Wenderoth, N., Debaere, F., Peeters, R., & Swinnen, S. P. (2005). Neural basis of aging: the penetration of cognition into action control. *J Neurosci, 25*(29), 6787–6796. doi: 10.1523/JNEUROSCI.1263-05.2005

Hu, Y., Chen, X., Gu, H., & Yang, Y. (2013). Resting-state glutamate and GABA concentrations predict task-induced deactivation in the default mode network. *J Neurosci, 33*(47), 18566–18573. doi: 10.1523/JNEUROSCI.1973-13.2013

Hummel, F. C., Heise, K., Celnik, P., Floel, A., Gerloff, C., & Cohen, L. G. (2010). Facilitating skilled right hand motor function in older subjects by anodal polarization over the left primary motor cortex. *Neurobiol Aging, 31*(12), 2160–2168. doi: 10.1016/j.neurobiolaging.2008.12.008

Hutchinson, S., Kobayashi, M., Horkan, C. M., Pascual-Leone, A., Alexander, M. P., & Schlaug, G. (2002). Age-related differences in movement representation. *NeuroImage, 17*(4), 1720–1728.

Irlbacher, K., Brocke, J., Mechow, J. V., & Brandt, S. A. (2007). Effects of GABA(A) and GABA(B) agonists on interhemispheric inhibition in man. *Clin Neurophysiol, 118*(2), 308–316. doi: 10.1016/j.clinph.2006.09.023

Kornatz, K. W., Christou, E. A., & Enoka, R. M. (2005). Practice reduces motor unit discharge variability in a hand muscle and improves manual dexterity in old adults. *J Appl Physiol, 98*(6), 2072–2080.

Langan, J., Peltier, S. J., Bo, J., Fling, B. W., Welsh, R. C., & Seidler, R. D. (2010). Functional implications of age differences in motor system connectivity. *Front Syst Neurosci, 4*, 17. doi: 10.3389/fnsys.2010.00017

Latash, M. L., & Zatsiorsky, V. M. (2009). Multi-finger prehension: Control of a redundant mechanical system. *Adv Exp Med Biol, 629*, 597–618. doi: 10.1007/978-0-387-77064-2_32

Lenzi, D., Conte, A., Mainero, C., Frasca, V., Fubelli, F., Totaro, P., . . . Pantano, P. (2007). Effect of corpus callosum damage on ipsilateral motor activation in patients with multiple sclerosis: A functional and anatomical study. *Hum Brain Mapp, 28*(7), 636–644.

Leventhal, A. G., Wang, Y., Pu, M., Zhou, Y., & Ma, Y. (2003). GABA and its agonists improved visual cortical function in senescent monkeys. [Research Support, U.S. Gov't, P.H.S.]. *Science, 300*(5620), 812–815. doi: 10.1126/science.1082874

Liang, K. Y., Mintun, M. A., Fagan, A. M., Goate, A. M., Bugg, J. M., Holtzman, D. M., . . . Head, D. (2010). Exercise and Alzheimer's disease biomarkers in cognitively normal older adults. [Research Support, N.I.H., Extramural]. *Ann Neurol, 68*(3), 311–318. doi: 10.1002/ana.22096

Llufriu, S., Blanco, Y., Martinez-Heras, E., Casanova-Molla, J., Gabilondo, I., Sepulveda, M., . . . Saiz, A. (2012). Influence of corpus callosum damage on cognition and physical disability in multiple sclerosis: A multimodal study. *PLoS One, 7*(5), e37167. doi: 10.1371/journal.pone.0037167

Madhusudan, A., Sidler, C., & Knuesel, I. (2009). Accumulation of reelin-positive plaques is accompanied by a decline in basal forebrain projection neurons during normal aging. *Eur J Neurosci, 30*(6), 1064–1076. doi: 1 0.1111/j.1460-9568.2009.06884.x

Manson, S. C., Palace, J., Frank, J. A., & Matthews, P. M. (2006). Loss of interhemispheric inhibition in patients with multiple sclerosis is related to corpus callosum atrophy. *Exp Brain Res, 174*(4), 728–733.

Manson, S. C., Wegner, C., Filippi, M., Barkhof, F., Beckmann, C., Ciccarelli, O., . . . Matthews, P. M. (2008). Impairment of movement-associated brain deactivation in multiple sclerosis: Further evidence for a functional pathology of interhemispheric neuronal inhibition. *Exp Brain Res, 187*(1), 25–31.

Mattay, V. S., Fera, F., Tessitore, A., Hariri, A. R., Das, S., Callicott, J. H., & Weinberger, D. R. (2002). Neurophysiological correlates of age-related changes in human motor function. *Neurology, 58*(4), 630–635.

McGregor, K. M, Craggs, J., Benjamin, M., Crosson, B., & White, K. (2009). Age-related changes in motor control during unimanual movements. *Brain Imaging Behav, 3*(4), 317–331. doi: 10.1007/s11682-009-9074-3

McGregor, K. M., Carpenter, H., Kleim, E., Sudhyadhom, A., White, K. D., Butler, A. J., . . . Crosson, B. (2012). Motor map reliability and aging: A TMS/fMRI study. *Exp Brain Res, 219*(1), 97–106. doi: 10.1007/s00221-012-3070-3

McGregor, K. M., Heilman, K. M., Nocera, J. R., Patten, C., Manini, T. M., Crosson, B., & Butler, A. J. (2012). Aging, aerobic activity and interhemispheric communication. *Brain Sciences, 2*, 634–648.

McGregor, K. M., Nocera, J. R., Sudhyadhom, A., Patten, C., Manini, T., Kleim, J. A., . . . Butler, A. J. (2013). Effects of aerobic fitness on aging-related changes of interhemispheric inhibition and motor performance. *Front Aging Neurosci, 5*. doi: 10.3389/fnagi.2013.00066

McGregor, K. M., Zlatar, Z., Kleim, E., Sudhyadhom, A., Bauer, A., Phan, S., . . . Crosson, B. (2011). Physical activity and neural correlates of aging: A combined TMS/fMRI study. *Behav Brain Res, 222*(1), 158–168. doi: 10.1016/j.bbr.2011.03.042

McQuail, J. A., Banuelos, C., LaSarge, C. L., Nicolle, M. M., & Bizon, J. L. (2012). GABA(B) receptor GTP-binding is decreased in the prefrontal cortex but not the hippocampus of aged rats. *Neurobiol Aging, 33*(6), 1124 e1121–1112. doi: 10.1016/j.neurobiolaging.2011.11.011

Meinzer, M., Flaisch, T., Seeds, L., Harnish, S., Antonenko, D., Witte, V., . . . Crosson, B. (2012). Same modulation but different starting points: Performance modulates age differences in inferior frontal cortex activity during word-retrieval. *PLoS One, 7*(3), e33631. doi: 10.1371/journal.pone.0033631

Meinzer, M., Flaisch, T., Wilser, L., Eulitz, C., Rockstroh, B., Conway, T., . . . Crosson, B. (2009). Neural signatures of semantic and phonemic fluency in young and old adults. *J Cogn Neurosci, 21*(10), 2007–2018. doi: 10.1162/jocn.2009.21219

Meinzer, M., Seeds, L., Flaisch, T., Harnish, S., Cohen, M. L., McGregor, K., . . . Crosson, B. (2012). Impact of changed positive and negative task-related brain activity on word-retrieval in aging. *Neurobiol Aging, 33*(4), 656–669. doi: 10.1016/j.neurobiolaging.2010.06.020

Meyer, B. U., Roricht, S., & Woiciechowsky, C. (1998). Topography of fibers in the human corpus callosum mediating interhemispheric inhibition between the motor cortices. *Ann Neurol, 43*(3), 360–369.

Moffat, S. D., Elkins, W., & Resnick, S. M. (2006). Age differences in the neural systems supporting human allocentric spatial navigation. *Neurobiol Aging, 27*(7), 965–972. doi: 10.1016/j.neurobiolaging. 2005.05.011

Naccarato, M., Calautti, C., Jones, P. S., Day, D. J., Carpenter, T. A., & Baron, J. C. (2006). Does healthy aging affect the hemispheric activation balance during paced index-to-thumb opposition task? An fMRI study. *Neuroimage, 32*(3), 1250–1256.

Northoff, G., Walter, M., Schulte, R. F., Beck, J., Dydak, U., Henning, A., . . . Boesiger, P. (2007). GABA concentrations in the human anterior cingulate cortex predict negative BOLD responses in fMRI. *Nat Neurosci, 10*(12), 1515–1517. doi: 10.1038/nn2001

Ogawa, S., Lee, T., Kay, A., & Tank, S. D. (1990). Brain magnetic resonance imaging with contrast dependent on blood oxygenation. *Proc Natl Acad Sci U S A, 87*(24), 9868–9872.

Peinemann, A., Lehner, C., Conrad, B., & Siebner, H. R. (2001). Age-related decrease in paired-pulse intracortical inhibition in the human primary motor cortex. *Neurosci Lett, 313*(1–2), 33–36.

Raichle, M. E., MacLeod, A. M., Snyder, A. Z., Powers, W. J., Gusnard, D. A., & Shulman, G. L. (2001). A default mode of brain function. *P Natl Acad Sci USA, 98*(2), 676–682. doi: 10.1073/pnas.98.2.676

Riecker, A., Groschel, K., Ackermann, H., Steinbrink, C., Witte, O., & Kastrup, A. (2006). Functional significance of age-related differences in motor activation patterns. *NeuroImage, 32*(3), 1345–1354.

Rowe, C. C., Ellis, K. A., Rimajova, M., Bourgeat, P., Pike, K. E., Jones, G., . . . Villemagne, V. L. (2010). Amyloid imaging results from the Australian Imaging, Biomarkers and Lifestyle (AIBL) study of aging. *Neurobiol Aging, 31*(8), 1275–1283. doi: 10.1016/j.neurobiolaging.2010.04.007, *22*(2), 771–778.

Sale, M. V., & Semmler, J. G. (2005). Age-related differences in corticospinal control during functional isometric contractions in left and right hands. *Journal of Applied Physiology, 99*, 1483–1493.

Salthouse, T. A. (1984). Effects of age and skill in typing. *Journal of Experimental Psychology: General, 113*(3), 345–371.

Salthouse, T. A. (1996). The processing-speed theory of adult age differences in cognition. *Psychol Rev, 103*(3), 403–428.

Sarlegna, F. R. (2006). Impairment of online control of reaching movements with aging: a double-step study. *Neurosci Lett. 403*(3):309-14.

Saucedo Marquez, C. M., Zhang, X., Swinnen, S. P., Meesen, R., & Wenderoth, N. (2013). Task-specific effect of transcranial direct current stimulation on motor learning. *Front Hum Neurosci, 7*, 333. doi: 10.3389/fnhum.2013.00333

Schmidt, S., Redecker, C., Bruehl, C., & Witte, O. W. (2010). Age-related decline of functional inhibition in rat cortex. *Neurobiol Aging, 31*(3), 504–511. doi: 10.1016/j.neurobiolaging.2008.04.006

Shmuel, A., Augath, M., Oeltermann, A., & Logothetis, N. K. (2006). Negative functional MRI response correlates with decreases in neuronal activity in monkey visual area V1. *Nat Neurosci, 9*(4), 569–577.

Sperling, R. A., Laviolette, P. S., O'Keefe, K., O'Brien, J., Rentz, D. M., Pihlajamaki, M., . . . Johnson, K. A. (2009). Amyloid deposition is associated with impaired default network function in older persons without dementia. *Neuron, 63*(2), 178–188. doi: 10.1016/j.neuron.2009.07.003

Stagg, C. J., Jayaram, G., Pastor, D., Kincses, Z. T., Matthews, P. M., & Johansen-Berg, H. (2011). Polarity and timing-dependent effects of transcranial direct current stimulation in explicit motor learning. *Neuropsychologia, 49*(5), 800–804.

Stanley, E. M., Fadel, J. R., & Mott, D. D. (2012). Interneuron loss reduces dendritic inhibition and GABA release in hippocampus of aged rats. *Neurobiol Aging, 33*(2), 431 e431–413. doi: 10.1016/j.neurobiolaging.2010.12.014

Stefanovic, B., Warnking, J. M., & Pike, G. B. (2004). Hemodynamic and metabolic responses to neuronal inhibition. *NeuroImage, 22*(2), 771–778.

Stippich, C., Blatow, M., Durst, A., Dreyhaupt, J., & Sartor, K. (2007). Global activation of primary motor cortex during voluntary movements in man. *NeuroImage, 34*(3), 1227–1237. doi: 10.1016/j.neuroimage.2006.08.046

Talelli, P., Ewas, A., Waddingham, W., Rothwell, J. C., & Ward, N. S. (2008a). Neural correlates of age-related changes in cortical neurophysiology. *Neuroimage, 40*(4), 1772–1781.

Talelli, P., Waddingham, W., Ewas, A., Rothwell, J. C., & Ward, N. S. (2008b). The effect of age on task-related modulation of interhemispheric balance. *Exp Brain Res, 186*(1), 59–66.

Van Impe, A., Coxon, J. P., Goble, D. J., Wenderoth, N., & Swinnen, S. P. (2009). Ipsilateral coordination at preferred rate: Effects of age, body side and task complexity. *NeuroImage, 47*(4), 1854–1862. doi: 10.1016/j.neuroimage.2009.06.027

Verstynen, T., Diedrichsen, J., Albert, N., Aparicio, P., & Ivry, R. B. (2005). Ipsilateral motor cortex activity during unimanual hand movements relates to task complexity. *J Neurophysiol, 93*(3), 1209–1222. doi: 10.1152/jn.00720.2004

Voss, M. W., Erickson, K. I., Prakash, R. S., Chaddock, L., Malkowski, E., Alves, H., . . . Kramer, A. F. (2010). Functional connectivity: A source of variance in the association between cardiorespiratory fitness and cognition? *Neuropsychologia, 48*(5), 1394–1406. doi: 10.1016/j.neuropsychologia.2010.01.005

Wierenga, C. E., Benjamin, M., Gopinath, K., Perlstein, W. M., Leonard, C. M., Rothi, L. J., . . . Crosson, B. (2008). Age-related changes in word retrieval: Role of bilateral frontal and subcortical networks. *Neurobiol Aging, 29*(3), 436–451. doi: 10.1016/j.neurobiolaging.2006.10.024

Wu, T., & Hallett, M. (2005). The influence of normal human ageing on automatic movements. *J Physiol, 562*(Pt 2), 605–615. doi: 10.1113/jphysiol.2004.076042

Zimerman, M., Heise, K. F., Gerloff, C., Cohen, L. G., & Hummel, F. C. (2012). Disrupting the ipsilateral motor cortex interferes with training of a complex motor task in older adults. *Cereb Cortex.* doi: 10.1093/cercor/bhs385

Zimerman, M., Nitsch, M., Giraux, P., Gerloff, C., Cohen, L. G., & Hummel, F. C. (2013). Neuroenhancement of the aging brain: Restoring skill acquisition in old subjects. *Ann Neurol, 73*(1), 10–5. doi: 10.1002/ana.23761.

Zlatar, Z. Z., Towler, S., McGregor, K. M., Dzierzewski, J. M., Bauer, A., Phan, S., . . . Crosson, B. (2013). Functional language networks in sedentary and physically active older adults. *J Int Neuropsychol Soc, 19*(6), 625–634. doi: 10.1017/S1355617713000246

13

Spatially Biased Decisions: Toward a Dynamic Interactive Model of Visual Neglect

Paolo Bartolomeo

Introduction

In our everyday life, we have the impression of being fully aware of the world around us. In fact, this is a powerful illusion, which often has dire consequences, for example in terms of street accidents. In fact, we fully experience only a tiny fraction of the enormous amount of information that reaches our senses, which is unmanageable for our limited processing capacities. Thus, we are aware of only a restricted portion of our environment. If we don't pay attention, we can easily miss perceptually very salient objects (Mack & Rock, 1998) or major changes in the visual scene (Beck, Rees, Frith, & Lavie, 2001; O'Regan, Rensink, & Clark, 1999). For example, when normal people see displays such as that shown in Figure 13.1, focusing their attention on the cross in order to state whether or not its arms are equal in length, they are likely to fail to report having seen a salient but unexpected black square presented on some of the trials (Mack & Rock, 1998).

In another well-known experiment (Simons & Chabris, 1999), normal participants looked at two groups of people wearing black or white T-shirts and making basketball passes. Participants had to count ball passes made by members of one of the teams while ignoring those made by the other team. Unexpectedly, a character dressed up as a gorilla crossed the visual scene during the ball passes. Around half of the participants typically failed to see the gorilla. Presumably, their attention prevented them from noticing the strange and perceptually conspicuous event because it was fully engaged in the difficult task of actively following a dynamic scene (the ball passes performed by one team) while selecting out another (the ball passes made by the other team). Thus, attention seems crucial to our awareness of the external world (Boxes 13.1 and 13.2).

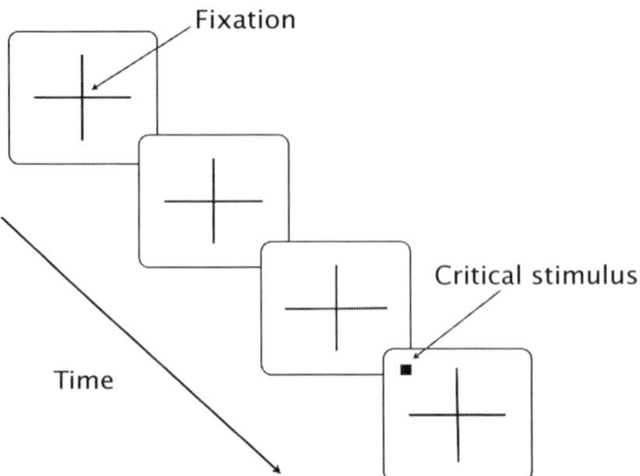

FIGURE 13.1 The inattentional blindness task used by Mack and Rock (1998). A substantial proportion of normal participants who were trying to establish whether the two arms of the cross were equal failed to notice the presence of the square (critical stimulus) on the fourth trial.

The Neglect Syndrome

Hemispheric damage involving the networks described in Box 13.2 often induces signs of lateralized spatial bias, whereby patients show a preference for responding to events occurring on the side of space ipsilateral to the lesion, as compared to events occurring on the other, contralesional side. Spatial bias can range from a mild asymmetry of response latencies to lateralized events, to situations in which patients seem to act as if the contralesional half of the world no longer exists (Bartolomeo & Chokron, 2001). In this extreme but frequent case (approximately half of right-brain-damaged patients; Azouvi et al., 2002), patients demonstrate a dramatic lack of awareness for events occurring in the part of space contralateral to their brain lesion, which most often occurs in the right hemisphere. The resulting peculiar patterns of performance in everyday life and on paper-and-pencil tests are collectively described as visual neglect (Bartolomeo, 2007, 2014; Heilman, Watson, & Valenstein, 2003; Parton, Malhotra, & Husain, 2004).

The cause of neglect is most often vascular strokes, but signs of neglect may also be observed as a consequence of brain tumors (Hughlings Jackson, [1876] 1932), or of neurodegenerative conditions, such as Alzheimer's disease (Bartolomeo et al., 1998) and posterior cortical atrophy (Andrade, et al., 2010; Andrade, Kas, Samri, et al., 2012; Andrade, Kas, Valabrègue, et al., 2012). Given the growing prevalence of neurodegenerative conditions with increasing life expectancy in Western countries, these causes of neglect are likely to progressively become more of a clinical concern.

Neglect patients are unaware of events occurring in a portion (usually the left half) of their environment. They also display a tendency to look to right-sided details as soon as a visual scene deploys, as if their attention were "magnetically" attracted by these details (Gainotti, D'Erme, & Bartolomeo, 1991). They are usually unaware of their deficits (anosognosia), and often obstinately deny being hemiplegic. Patients with left brain

---

BOX 13.1 Attention and Awareness

Experiments such as those reported by Mack and Rock (1998) and by Simons and Chabris (1999) dramatically demonstrate that distracting attention can prevent highly salient items from entering awareness in normal individuals. These counterintuitive findings, along with many others (reviewed by Chica & Bartolomeo, 2012), stress the crucial importance of spatial attention, and its modulation, for the building of our conscious experience.

These phenomena are dependent upon the anatomical architecture of the visual system. Photoreceptors in the retina are disposed in a spatially inhomogeneous structure. A small (1-mm in diameter) central fovea contains the highest density of photoreceptors, and is surrounded by a low-resolution peripheral receptor surface. Only stimuli falling on the fovea are processed in full resolution, and as such they have increased probability of being perceptually identified and of accessing visual awareness. In order to align a peripheral stimulus with the fovea, organisms orient toward important stimuli by turning their gaze, head and trunk toward them (Sokolov, 1963). This allows further perceptual processing of the detected stimulus, such as its classification as a useful or dangerous object. Orienting movements are thus a typical form of "embodied" cognition (Ballard, Hayhoe, Pook, & Rao, 1997), or a process in which body movements are necessary for the processing of information. Indeed, orienting movements facilitate the optimization of processing resources by segregating mechanisms dedicated to simple detection, which mainly require frontoparietal cortical networks (see Box 13.2), from resources responsible for more complex identification tasks based on object shape, color, and texture, which depend on more ventral cortical pathways in the occipital and temporal lobes (Goodale & Milner, 1992; Mishkin, Ungerleider, & Macko, 1983). This dorsal/ventral segregation must have important computational advantages, because it emerges even in very simple artificial systems designed to simulate basic visual behaviors (Di Ferdinando, Parisi, & Bartolomeo, 2007; Rueckl, Cave, & Kosslyn, 1989).

---

damage may also show signs of right-sided neglect, albeit more rarely and usually in a less severe form (Bartolomeo, Chokron, & Gainotti, 2001; Beis, et al., 2004). Neglect is a substantial source of handicap and disability for patients, and entails a poor functional outcome in stroke patients (Malhotra, Coulthard, & Husain, 2006). Diagnosis is important, because effective rehabilitation strategies are available (Pisella, Rode, Farne, Tilikete, & Rossetti, 2006), and there are promising possibilities for pharmacological treatments (Gorgoraptis et al., 2012). Furthermore, in many cases the "negative" nature of neglect deficits (impaired active exploration of a part of space) renders the diagnosis difficult or impossible if signs of neglect are not actively searched for by clinicians. This

BOX 13.2 The Architecture of Attentional Circuits in the Brain

Selective attention must allow an organism to successfully cope with a continuously changing environment while maintaining its goals. This flexibility calls for mechanisms that (a) allow for the processing of novel, unexpected events in order to respond with appropriate behavior (e.g., approaching, avoidance, or other actions tailored to the specific situation); and (b) allow for the maintenance of finalized behavior in spite of distracting events (Allport, 1989). For example, attention can be directed to an object in space either in a relatively reflexive way (e.g., when a honking car attracts the attention of a pedestrian) or in a more controlled mode (e.g., when the pedestrian monitors the traffic light, waiting for the "go" signal to appear). It is therefore plausible that different attentional processes serve these two partially conflicting goals. A traditional distinction in experimental psychology refers to more exogenous processes for orienting attention to novel events (Yantis, 1995), as opposed to more endogenous orienting processes, which would be responsible for directing the organism's attention toward relevant targets despite the presence of distractors in the environment (LaBerge, Auclair, & Siéroff, 2000).

Today, we have a fair amount of detailed information regarding the anatomy, function, dynamics, and pathology of the human brain networks that subserve the orienting of gaze and attention. Important components of these networks include the dorsolateral prefrontal cortex (PFC) and the posterior parietal cortex (PPC). Physiological studies indicate that these two structures show interdependence of neural activity. In the monkey, analogous PPC and PFC areas do not act independently of one another, but show coordinated activity when the animal selects a visual stimulus as a saccade target (Buschman & Miller, 2007). Importantly, PFC and PPC show distinctive dynamics and seem to use two different "languages" when attention is selected reflexively in response to the stimulus (bottom-up or exogenous orienting), as opposed to more top-down (or endogenous) goals. In particular, bottom-up signals appear first in the parietal cortex and are characterized by an increase of frontoparietal oscillations in the gamma band (25–100 Hz), whereas top-down signals emerge first in the frontal cortex and tend to synchronize in the beta band (12–30 Hz; Buschman & Miller, 2007).

Functional MRI studies in healthy human participants (reviewed by Corbetta & Shulman, 2002) indicate the existence of multiple frontoparietal networks for spatial attention (see Figure 13.2, at right).

A dorsal attentional network (DAN), composed of cortex of the intraparietal sulcus/superior parietal lobule and the frontal eye field/dorsolateral prefrontal region, shows increased blood oxygenation level dependent (BOLD) responses during the orienting period. Functional magnetic resonance imaging (fMRI) also demonstrates

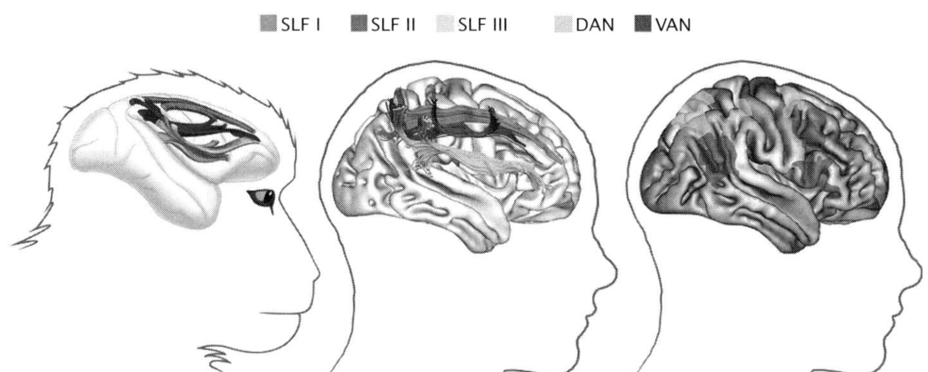

FIGURE 13.2 Frontoparietal networks in the monkey (left, from Schmahmann & Pandya, 2006) and in the human right hemisphere (middle, from Thiebaut de Schotten et al., 2011). Right: attentional networks in the right hemisphere according to Corbetta and Shulman (2002). Figure as originally published in *Frontiers in Human Neuroscience 6*, 110, 2012 "Brain networks of visuospatial attention and their disruption in visual neglect", by Paolo Bartolomeo, Michel Thiebaut de Schotten, Ana B. Chica. (see color insert)

a more a ventral attentional network (VAN), which includes the temporoparietal junction and the ventral PFC (inferior and middle frontal gyri), and shows increased BOLD responses when participants have to respond to targets presented in unexpected locations. Thus, the VAN is considered important for detecting unexpected but behaviorally relevant events. Importantly, the DAN is bilateral and symmetric, whereas the VAN is strongly lateralized to the right hemisphere.

Not surprisingly, given this fMRI evidence on frontoparietal attentional networks, PFC and PPC are directly and extensively interconnected by three major white matter pathways. These pathways were first identified in the monkey brain, as SLF I (dorsal), SLF II (intermediate), and SLF III (ventral) (Petrides & Pandya, 1984; Schmahmann & Pandya, 2006) (see Figure 13.2, at left). Recent evidence from advanced in vivo tractography techniques and postmortem dissections suggests that a similar architecture exists in the human brain (Thiebaut de Schotten et al., 2011) (see Figure 13.2, middle). In humans, the most dorsal branch (SLF I) originates in Brodmann's areas (BAs) 5 and 7 and projects to BAs 8, 9, and 32. The middle pathway (SLF II) originates in BAs 39 and 40 within the inferior parietal lobule (IPL) and reaches prefrontal BAs 8 and 9. The most ventral pathway (SLF III) originates in BA 40 and terminates in BAs 44, 45 and 47. These results are consistent with the fMRI evidence on attentional networks mentioned earlier. In particular, the SLF III connects the cortical nodes of the VAN, whereas the DAN is connected by the SLF I. The SLF II connects the parietal component of the VAN to the prefrontal component of the DAN, thus allowing direct communication between ventral and dorsal attentional networks. Importantly, the SLF III (connecting VAN nodes) is anatomically

(Continued)

> **BOX 13.2** (*Continued*)
>
> larger in the right hemisphere than in the left hemisphere, whereas the SLF I (connecting DAN nodes) is more symmetrically organized (Thiebaut de Schotten et al., 2011). This result is in good agreement with asymmetries of BOLD responses during fMRI, with larger right-hemisphere responses for the VAN and more symmetrical activity for the DAN (Corbetta & Shulman, 2002). Also, the SLF II demonstrates some asymmetry in favor of the right hemisphere, but not in all individuals; Thiebaut de Schotten et al. (2011) showed that right lateralization of SLF II is strongly correlated to behavioral signs of right-hemisphere specialization for visuospatial attention, such as pseudo-neglect in line bisection (i.e., small leftward deviations of the subjective midline produced by normal individuals; Bowers & Heilman, 1980; Jewell & McCourt, 2000; Toba, Cavanagh, & Bartolomeo, 2011), and asymmetries in the speed of detection of events presented in the right or left hemifield.

is unfortunate, because simple paper-and-pencil tests can easily establish the diagnosis at the patient's bedside (Figure 13.3).

Visual neglect is not a homogeneous condition. Different patients may exhibit distinct patterns of performance (Bartolomeo & Chokron, 2001), depending on damage to distinct brain modules (Verdon, Schwartz, Lovblad, Hauert, & Vuilleumier, 2010) or networks (Bartolomeo, Thiebaut de Schotten, & Doricchi, 2007). For example, patients may neglect left-sided targets on cancellation tasks but may accurately bisect horizontal lines, or they may explore the whole cancellation sheet but deviate rightward on line bisection (Binder, Marshall, Lazar, Benjamin, & Mohr, 1992). However, attentional deficits are often prominent in neglect patients, who characteristically show a bias in spatial orienting, favoring ipsilesional (typically right-sided) events over contralesional (left-sided) events (Bartolomeo & Chokron, 2002), as well as deficits in non-spatial forms of attention such as alerting (Chica, Thiebaut de Schotten, et al., 2012; Robertson, Mattingley, Rorden, & Driver, 1998).

Attention and Neglect

In addition to its clinical importance, neglect also raises important issues concerning the brain mechanisms of consciousness, perception, and attention. In particular, the study of patients with visual neglect has made a substantial contribution to the analysis of attentional processes and their neural substrates (Bartolomeo & Chokron, 2002; Corbetta & Shulman, 2011). Neglect is characterized, among other symptoms, by severe problems in orienting attention toward left-sided objects (Bartolomeo & Chokron, 2002; Rastelli, Funes, Lupiáñez, Duret, & Bartolomeo, 2008). Typically, however, neglect patients' deficits of spatial attention are not generalized, but concern first and foremost exogenous, or

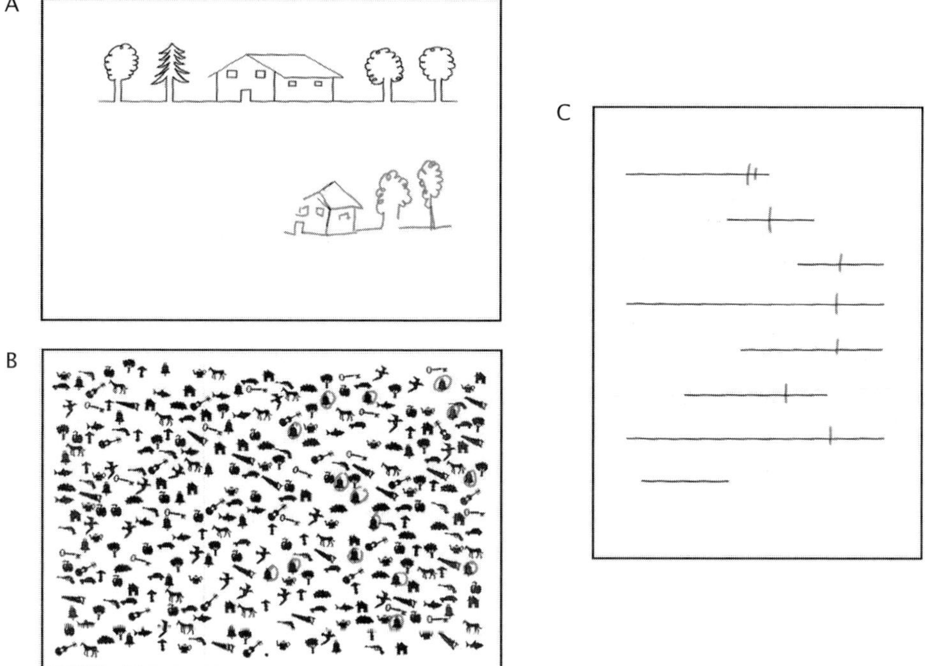

FIGURE 13.3 Performance of a patient with left spatial neglect on paper-and-pencil tests. A: A copy of a linear drawing with omission of left-sided elements. B: Target cancellation task; the patient was asked to circle all the bells; she omitted all the targets situated on the left half of the sheet, plus a few right-sided targets. C: Bisection of horizontal lines; note the rightward deviation of the bisection mark and the complete omission of one left-sided line. Figure as originally published in *Frontiers in Human Neuroscience 6*, 110, 2012 "Brain networks of visuospatial attention and their disruption in visual neglect", by Paolo Bartolomeo, Michel Thiebaut de Schotten, Ana B. Chica.

stimulus-related, orienting (see Bartolomeo & Chokron, 2002, for review), with a relative sparing of more endogenous, or voluntary, forms of orienting (Bartolomeo, Siéroff, Decaix, & Chokron, 2001; Siéroff, Decaix, Chokron, & Bartolomeo, 2007). For example, Rastelli et al. (2008) demonstrated that the attention-capturing onset, but not the offset, of right-sided visual objects was able to induce a pathological attentional bias in neglect patients (see also D'Erme, Robertson, Bartolomeo, Daniele, & Gainotti, 1992). Thus, it is right-sided objects (and not spatial regions) that tend to capture patients' attention, consistent with the peculiar relationships between object-based and exogenous forms of attention (Macquistan, 1997).

Importantly, recent accumulating evidence from behavioral, neurophysiologic, neuropsychological, and neuroimaging experiments in normal participants (reviewed by Chica & Bartolomeo, 2012) indicate that while endogenous attention may have weak influence on subsequent conscious perception of near-threshold stimuli, exogenous attention appears to be a necessary, although not sufficient, step in the development of reportable visual experiences. Thus, there is an impressive convergence of findings between the striking spatial unawareness shown by neglect patients, their severe impairment of exogenous orienting of attention, and the importance of exogenous attention for conscious visual perception in normal individuals (Bartolomeo, 2008; see Box 13.1).

Consistent with these notions and with localization of attentional networks (Box 13.2), direct evidence in a neurosurgical patient demonstrated that temporary inactivation of the SLF II in the human right hemisphere impairs the symmetrical distribution of visual attention and produces signs of severe left neglect (Thiebaut de Schotten et al., 2005). Indeed, damage to SLF networks in the right hemisphere (Figure 13.4) is the typical lesional correlate of left visual neglect, not only in neurosurgical patients (Shinoura et al., 2009), but also in patients with vascular (Bartolomeo, 2006; Bartolomeo et al., 2007; Ciaraffa, Castelli, Parati, Bartolomeo, & Bizzi, 2012; Corbetta, Kincade, Lewis, Snyder, & Sapir, 2005; Corbetta & Shulman, 2011; Doricchi, Thiebaut de Schotten, Tomaiuolo, & Bartolomeo, 2008; He et al., 2007) and neurodegenerative conditions (Andrade, Kas, Samri, et al., 2012; Andrade, Kas, Valabrègue, et al., 2012). Signs of left neglect after right hemisphere damage have often been attributed to inappropriate activity of the left, unimpaired hemisphere (see Boxes 13.3–5).

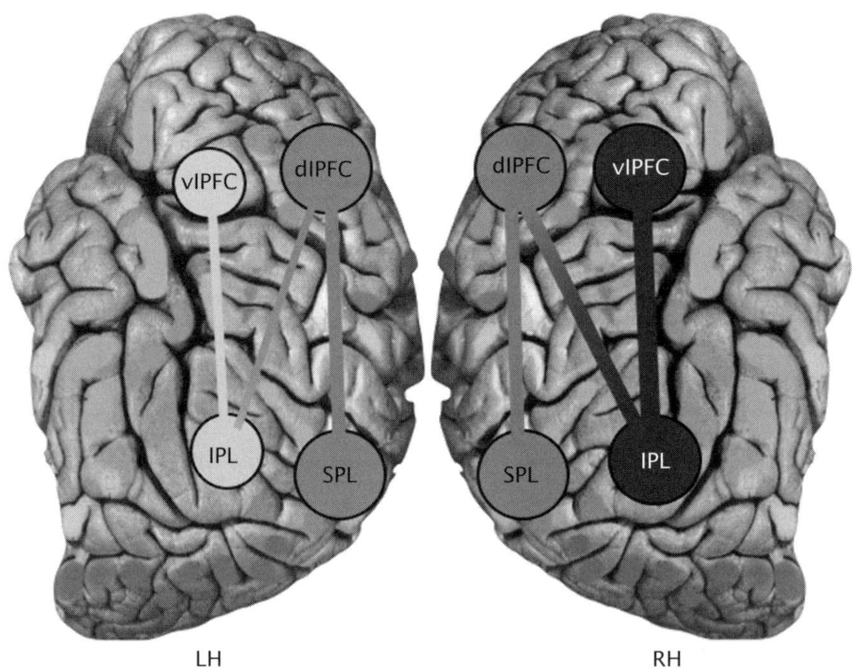

FIGURE 13.4 Schematic depiction of frontoparietal attentional networks for visuospatial processing in the two hemispheres, based on Corbetta and Shulman (2002) and Thiebaut de Schotten et al. (2011). The size of the cortical nodes and of their connections symbolizes their putative importance in visuospatial processing. IPL: inferior parietal lobule; SPL: superior parietal lobule; dlPFC: dorsolateral prefrontal cortex; vlPFC: ventrolateral prefrontal cortex.

Historically, Kinsbourne's opponent processor model (Kinsbourne, 1970, 1977, 1987, 1993) was the first articulated explanation of neglect signs based on the orienting of attention that took into account the hemispheric asymmetry of neglect: contralesional neglect is more frequent, severe, and durable after right hemisphere lesions than after left brain damage. The opponent processor model draws upon the very general biological evidence that reciprocally inhibiting opponent systems are an evolutionarily advantageous way of solving the problem of deciding whether to turn right or left. The dominant system would achieve its goal of turning the organism by progressively inhibiting its contralateral counterpart. According to the model, each hemisphere shifts attention toward the contralateral hemispace by inhibiting the other hemisphere. Moreover, in the normal brain there is a tendency to rightward orienting, supported by the left hemisphere, which has a stronger orienting tendency than the right hemisphere. Right hemisphere lesions, by disinhibiting the left hemisphere, exaggerate this physiological rightward bias, thus giving rise to left neglect (Figure 13.5).

Left neglect would not reflect an attentional deficit, but an attentional bias consisting of enhanced attention to the right. The verbal interaction between patient and examiner would further enhance left neglect by further activating the already disinhibited left hemisphere (Kinsbourne, 1970). Additionally, left neglect patients would suffer from an abnormally narrow window of attention, which would deprive them of the possibility of a more general overview of the visual scene (Kinsbourne, 1993). Right neglect would rarely be observed because much larger lesions of the left hemisphere are needed to overcome its stronger tendency to rightward

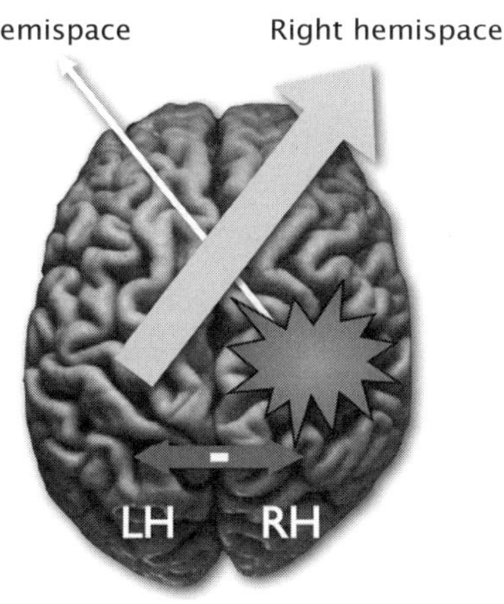

FIGURE 13.5 The opponent processor model of neglect. Right hemisphere damage would decrease interhemispheric inhibition and consequently enhance the left hemisphere physiological tendency to orient attention toward the right side of space, thereby producing right hyperattention and left hypoattention.

(Continued)

orienting, and because the verbal exchanges with the examiner would now work in the opposite direction, thus minimizing right neglect.

The opponent processor model has attractive explanatory power for several features of neglect behavior, such as the magnetic attraction of attention toward right-sided items typical of these patients (De Renzi, Gentilini, Faglioni, & Barbieri, 1989; Gainotti et al., 1991; Mark, Kooistra, & Heilman, 1988), which may well depend on relative hyperactivity of attentional networks in the left hemisphere (Corbetta et al., 2005). Also consistent with the model, a patient who showed a severe left neglect following a first right-sided parietal infarct abruptly recovered from neglect 10 days later, when he suffered from a second, left-sided infarct in the dorsolateral PFC (Vuilleumier, Hester, Assal, & Regli, 1996). However, several aspects of the model have been questioned. For example, engagement in verbal behavior does not seem to have a special role in triggering or increasing signs of neglect, which in clinical settings can easily be observed in everyday situations, even when no verbal exchange takes place. Moreover, Gainotti et al. (2002) had neglect patients perform cancellation tests with targets consisting either of letters or of shapes, and found that patients' pattern of omissions was independent of the verbal or nonverbal nature of the task, again contrary to the assumption of the opponent processor model. Also, the postulated dominance of the left hemisphere for spatial orienting has been challenged by abundant evidence consistent with the opposite notion of a greater importance of right-hemisphere structures for this ability. In particular, while the left hemisphere is mostly concerned with events occurring on the contralateral, right hemispace, the right hemisphere has a more bilateral competence (Corbetta & Shulman, 2002; Gitelman et al., 1999; Heilman & Van Den Abell, 1980). Finally, Bartolomeo and Chokron (1999) obtained evidence against the opponent processor model. With increasing severity of neglect, the model would predict a progressive decrease of response times to right-sided stimuli, because they would be processed by a more and more disinhibited left hemisphere. However, the result was the opposite. Not only response times to left targets, but also those to right targets increased with increasing neglect, contrary to the predictions of the opponent processor model. The two regression lines were not, however, parallel. With increasing neglect, responses to left targets increased more steeply than those to right targets did, suggesting that a rightward attentional bias participates in left neglect. However, this rightward bias seems one of defective, and not enhanced, attention, perhaps because of additional non-lateralized impairments resulting from right hemisphere damage (see discussion later in this chapter). Also, functional neuroimaging studies of neglect and neglect recovery have provided evidence against the hypothesis that neglect results from a hyperactive left hemisphere (see Box 13.4).

Despite these problems with the general assumptions of the opponent processor model, some of its aspects have been confirmed by subsequent evidence. A recent model of intra- and interhemispheric interactions in neglect, based on fMRI evidence in neglect patients (Corbetta et al., 2005; He et al., 2007), stipulates that damage to the right-hemisphere VAN causes a functional imbalance between the left and right DANs, with a relative hyperactivity of the left dorsal frontoparietal network, which would provoke an attentional bias toward right-sided objects and neglect of left-sided items. Consistent with this hypothesis, suppressive transcranial magnetic stimulation (TMS) over left frontoparietal regions correlated with an improvement of patients' performance on cancellation tests (Koch et al., 2008). Moreover, a recent study of magneto-encephalographic activity in neglect patients (Rastelli et al., 2013) found evidence for activity in the left frontal cortex selectively preceding episodes of unawareness for left-sided targets. Rastelli et al. (2013) directly compared brain regional synchrony in relation to detected and omitted left-sided targets. Results showed that *before* stimulus presentation, low beta synchronization activity was specifically increased within left frontal areas before pathological omissions of response to left-sided targets. No beta oscillations were found in this pre-stimulus period when patients correctly detected target presence, or for target-absent trials. It is thus possible that inappropriate left prefrontal activity in neglect patients contributes to their lack of exploration/detection of left-sided events, especially when the left frontal lobe does not receive appropriate input from more posterior or contralateral regions (Bartolomeo et al., 2007). To conclude, the available evidence is not consistent with, and in many cases deviates considerably from, the assumptions of the opponent processor model. However, some aspects of the model might still be valid in explaining neglect behavior. Thus, activity in the left, unaffected hemisphere can be either adaptative or maladaptative in neglect compensation. The reasons for this paradoxical situation are still unclear (see Box 13.5).

BOX 13.4 Functional Neuroimaging Studies of Neglect and Neglect Recovery

Functional neuroimaging has provided important evidence on the network-based nature of neglect signs, and on the adaptive and maladaptive evolution of functional changes in the brain. Studies of diaschisis in left neglect (Fiorelli, Blin, Bakchine, Laplane, & Baron, 1991; Pantano, et al., 1992; Perani, Vallar, Paulesu, Alberoni, & Fazio, 1993) have demonstrated a widespread hypometabolism in both the lesioned and the intact hemisphere. A study of resting state functional connectivity in acute neglect patients (Carter et al., 2010) found that disruption of interhemispheric connectivity

(Continued)

between attentional networks was correlated with impaired contralesional detection, whereas the mutual inhibition assumption of the opponent processor model would have predicted the opposite result. A recent fMRI study in the monkey (Wilke, Kagan, & Andersen, 2012) provided further important evidence on interhemispheric interactions in neglect-like behavior. In different trials, monkeys had either to produce saccades to peripheral targets that were individually presented, or to choose one of two bilateral stimuli as a saccade target. Reversible pharmacological inactivation of the lateral intraparietal area (LIP) resulted in a choice bias favoring ipsilesional over contralesional targets, similar to neglect/extinction behavior. Functional MRI demonstrated decreased BOLD response in nearby regions in the inactivated hemisphere for single contralesional targets. On bilateral presentations, however, when the monkey chose the contralesional target, thus countering the pharmacologically induced choice bias, there was increased activity in several frontal and parietotemporal areas in both hemispheres. These results seem in sharp contrast with the opponent processor model, which would instead have predicted increased activation for ipsilesional, not contralesional, targets in the intact hemisphere. According to Wilke et al. (2012), the bihemispheric activity pattern may indicate additional recruitment of contralesionally tuned neuronal populations because of increased effort. As the authors note, however, BOLD response in fMRI does not always immediately correspond to functional activations, but is a global signal that pools together inhibitory and excitatory, contra- and ipsilaterally tuned neuronal populations. Thus, caution is needed when interpreting these and other fMRI results. Despite these caveats, in human patients as well, recovery from neglect seems to correlate with restoration of normal metabolism not only in the unaffected regions of the right hemisphere, but also in the left hemisphere (Pantano et al., 1992; Perani et al., 1993). More generally, an increase of neural activity, metabolism, and perfusion in the unaffected hemisphere seems to be a general mechanism of prolonged recovery from neurological and neuropsychological impairments after unilateral strokes (Meyer, Obara, & Muramatsu, 1993). On the other hand, cortical hypoperfusion in regions distant from the lesion can be an important correlate of neuropsychological deficits after subcortical strokes (Hillis et al., 2002), and restoration of normal perfusion in specific regions correlates well with recovery from distinct forms of neglect (Khurshid et al., 2012). Unfortunately, while post-stroke plastic reorganization in the affected and in the healthy hemisphere has been well explored for sensorimotor functions (O'Shea, Johansen-Berg, Trief, Göbel, & Rushworth, 2007; Rossini, Calautti, Pauri, & Baron, 2003), less is known concerning cognitive abilities. Most research in this field concerns aphasic disorders; only a handful of studies explored the neuroimaging correlates of spontaneous or rehabilitation-induced recovery from neglect (Cappa & Perani, 2010).

BOX 13.5 The Paradox of the Left Hemisphere

The evidence reviewed in this chapter appears to suggest contradictory roles in left neglect for attentional networks in the left hemisphere. Left neglect has been shown to decrease with either acute vascular lesion of the healthy left hemisphere (Vuilleumier et al., 1996) or TMS interference with the left parietal lobe (Koch et al., 2008, 2012; Oliveri et al., 2001). This is consistent with evidence correlating neglect with a hyperactivity of these networks relative to their right hemisphere homologues (Corbetta et al., 2005; Koch et al., 2008; see also Box 13.1). However, in other cases, neglect recovery seems to correlate with an increase in functioning of left hemisphere attention networks (Pantano et al., 1992; Perani et al., 1993). Thus, left hemisphere attentional network activity seems to be maladaptive in some cases, but adaptive in others.

To explain these discrepancies, we need more articulated models of intra- and interhemispheric functioning of attentional networks in neglect. First, the opponent processor model may be a plausible model for functioning of subcortical structures such as the superior colliculi (Rushmore, Valero-Cabre, Lomber, Hilgetag, & Payne, 2006; Sprague, 1966), but understanding callosal interhemispheric interactions as being exclusively inhibitory is clearly an oversimplification (see, e.g., Doty, 2003). Callosal connections are likely to exert both excitatory and inhibitory effects (mostly through interneurons) on the opposite hemisphere, much as intrahemispheric long-range connections serve to integrate the activity of cortical nodes in brain networks. Second, the left hemisphere might well assume different roles in neglect, depending on its ability to take into account information coming from the left hemispace. As originally suggested by Norman Geschwind (1965), an isolated left hemisphere might in some cases take over the control of performance, with consequent rightward attentional bias (Bartolomeo et al., 2007; Berlucchi, Aglioti, & Tassinari, 1997). Consistent with these notions, anterior callosal damage (genu and trunk) may determine response-related left neglect for tasks performed with the right hand (Kashiwagi, Kashiwagi, Nishikawa, Tanabe, & Okuda, 1990; Pouget, Pradat-Diehl, Rivaud-Pechoux, Wattiez, & Gaymard, 2011). Otherwise, damage to the callosal splenium, when occurring together with damage to the visual cortex or visual pathways in the right hemisphere, may determine left neglect signs through a deafferentation, as such lesions would completely deprive the left hemisphere of visual information coming from the left visual field. This has been documented both in monkeys (Gaffan & Hornak, 1997) and in human patients (Park et al., 2006; Tomaiuolo et al., 2010). Although surgical section of the corpus callosum does not typically cause signs of neglect (Berlucchi et al., 1997; but see Corballis, Corballis, Fabri, Paggi, & Manzoni, 2005), it may do so in patients with previous right hemisphere damage (Heilman & Adams, 2003). In the latter case,

(Continued)

BOX 13.5 (*Continued*)

callosal disconnection presumably prevents the left hemisphere from compensating for the deficits induced by right hemisphere damage by taking charge of left-sided events (Bartolomeo et al., 2007). In agreement with these notions, microstructural damage of the posterior corpus callosum has been shown to correlate with the clinical severity of neglect, as expressed by patients' scores on a paper-and-pencil test battery (Bozzali et al., 2012).

If these considerations are valid, then there might be the possibility of triggering recovery or ameliorating neglect in patients with right brain damage by improving the quality of interhemispheric communication. For example, it is well known that prism adaptation, which acts through a realignment of visuomotor coordinates processed by the cerebellum (Luauté et al., 2006), can ameliorate left neglect (Rossetti et al., 1998). On the basis of the previous considerations, we might hypothesize that prism-induced benefits might partly rely on improved communication through cortico-ponto-cerebellar connections, which are among the quantitatively most important connections across the midline, after the corpus callosum (Glickstein & Berlucchi, 2008). The positron emission tomographic (PET) results collected by Luauté et al. (2006) on five patients treated with prism adaptation seem consistent with this hypothesis, because behavioral recovery was correlated with increased blood flow in several left hemispheric regions (thalamus, temporo-occipital cortex, medial temporal lobe) and in the right cerebellum, with a paradoxical decrease in the right posterior parietal cortex. If confirmed, prism-induced trans-midline integration would be an example of network-based plasticity, with dramatic behavioral consequences induced by a simple sensorimotor manipulation.

The Genesis of Neglect Behavior

Visual neglect is a multiform disorder, likely to result from the interaction of distinct mechanisms, whose identity and patterns of interaction may vary across patients (Bartolomeo, 2007, 2014; Husain, 2008). However, a defining characteristic of neglect is impaired attention and awareness for contralesional events. Attention and visual awareness deficits are presumably closely linked in neglect, both from functional and anatomical points of view (Bartolomeo, Thiebaut de Schotten, & Chica, 2012). We propose that key aspects of neglect behavior result from a cascade of events originating in an inappropriate decision to orient gaze and attention toward ipsilesional visual items as soon as the visual scene develops. Right hemisphere damage may also determine non-spatial attentional deficits (Husain & Rorden, 2003), such as impaired sustained attention (Robertson, 2001) and arousal (Robertson et al., 1998). These deficits likely contribute to neglect behavior by hindering reorienting toward contralesional stimuli, which may compensate for neglect signs

(Bartolomeo, 1997; Bartolomeo, Siéroff, et al., 2001). Recovery from non-spatial attentional deficits may thus permit neglect compensation, by allowing contralesional reorienting after the initial ipsilesional bias. If so, then patients who recovered from neglect should show residual forms of spatial bias toward ipsilesional stimuli under stringent (e.g., time-constrained) test conditions. This prediction has repeatedly been confirmed (Bartolomeo, 1997, 2000; Bonato, Priftis, Marenzi, Umiltà, & Zorzi, 2010; Mattingley, Bradshaw, Bradshaw, & Nettleton, 1994). Indeed, patients with right hemisphere damage and normal performance on paper-and-pencil testing can show signs of spatial attentional bias, such as early orienting toward ipsilesional, right-sided stimuli (Bartolomeo, 1997; Gainotti et al., 1991; Mattingley et al., 1994). Thus, in the absence of such compensatory mechanisms, the initial ipsilesional orienting can be followed by other similar orienting movements, in a vicious circle that confines the patient's behavior to the ipsilesional sector of space and prevents the patient from exploring and taking cognizance of contralesional objects (Bartolomeo & Chokron, 2002).

Neglect Behavior and "Wrong" Exploratory Decisions

An increasingly popular way to look at complex behaviors is to employ conceptualizations based on decision-making. Decisions reflect the commitment to act in a particular way, on the basis of the accumulation of evidence favoring one option over another in a noisy environment (Gold & Shadlen, 2007; Schall, 2001). Even with high-contrast visual targets, saccade production needs a decision step distinct from contrast-dependent detection (Carpenter, 2004). In this framework, choices depend on sampling mechanisms that collect and integrate evidence about the target until a criterion level of certainty is reached and a response is produced (Summerfield & Tsetson, 2012). Bayesian models of visual perception (Kersten, Mamassian, & Yuille, 2004) and visual search (Cain, Vul, Clark, & Mitroff, 2012) refer to similar ideas.

A key aspect of neglect behavior is that patients show a definite preference for making exploratory movements with their eyes and head toward events occurring on their right, ipsilesional side. Orienting movements are motor activities that cannot be executed in more than one direction at a time. They are thus a typical example of processes that, at some time, must involve a decision. The concept of perceptual decisions in noisy visual environments (e.g., varying percentages of random dots moving toward a specific direction; see Gold & Shadlen, 2007) can be readily extended to the much more common decision concerning which side to orient gaze/attention when exploring a visual scene with left- and right-sided stimuli competing for attention. Given that the visual field mainly deploys horizontally, when a visual scene unfolds in natural settings, agents often face a binary choice concerning whether to look at left-sided or at right-sided items.

As proposed by Bartolomeo and Chokron (2002), a unilateral brain lesion may generally delay the processing of information coming from the contralateral field. This may especially be true when brain damage generates a dysfunction of frontoparietal attentional networks, whose activity modulates the progression of perceptual processing in the ventral visual stream (Moran & Desimone, 1985; Roe et al., 2012). Thus, activity in the ventral visual stream may be unilaterally impaired by a dysfunction of more dorsal, frontoparietal networks in the same hemisphere. An additional, non-lateralized slowing of attentional operations, depending on right brain damage, might further hold back the processing of left-sided stimuli, to the point of exceeding a deadline after which this information can no longer affect behavior (Bartolomeo & Chokron, 2002). For example, these added delays might render the time needed to decide whether a left target is in fact present (Carpenter & Williams, 1995) too long to react to it (e.g., by programming a saccade). Thus, increased processing time might be a crucial factor underlying spatial deficits.

Accumulating evidence suggests that several nodes of the brain attentional networks described in Box 13.2 are important for reaching perceptual decisions. Neurophysiological studies in nonhuman primates (reviewed by Gold & Shadlen, 2007) and functional neuroimaging evidence in humans (Kayser, Buchsbaum, Erickson, & D'Esposito, 2009) indicate the lateral intraparietal area (LIP) in the intraparietal sulcus as a candidate region for the accumulation of sensory evidence. In addition, LIP neurons code for the behavioral relevance of stimuli (Gottlieb, Kusunoki, & Goldberg, 1998), another function that may be crucial for exploration choices. Consistent with the important connections that the LIP has with the frontal eye field (FEF), this prefrontal structure has also been associated with the accumulation of sensory evidence. When monkeys have to make saccades to a target with some degree of perceptual uncertainty, there is a pre-saccadic growth of activity in the FEF (Gold & Shadlen, 2007). The dorsolateral PFC (especially in the left hemisphere; Heekeren, Marrett, & Ungerleider, 2008), along with its neighboring motor and premotor regions (including the FEF), has been proposed to be important in accumulating sensory evidence to compute a decision variable (Heekeren et al., 2008). Neurons in the PFC can actively encode perceptual decisions not only about the presence, but also about the absence of a stimulus (Merten & Nieder, 2012). Inappropriate activation of a left-hemisphere "absence" system, which might receive inconsistent or degraded information from the lesioned right hemisphere in response to left-sided stimuli, might account for the paradoxical behavior shown by some neglect patients. Such patients, when asked to press a button when a visual stimulus is presented and another one when no stimulus occurs, may be faster to produce erroneous "absent" responses for stimuli presented on the left side than correct judgments of absence when no stimulus is presented (Mijovic'-Prelec, Shin, Chabris, & Kosslyn, 1994). It is thus possible that inappropriate activity of left PFC in neglect patients partly explains their lack of exploration/detection of left-sided events (Rastelli et al., 2013), especially when the left PFC does not receive appropriate input from more posterior or contralateral regions. This hypothesis is consistent with the clinical observation of regression of left neglect signs in a patient after a second lesion occurred in the left PFC (Vuilleumier et al., 1996).

Besides the dorsolateral regions that compose the DAN, other prefrontal regions such as the middle frontal gyrus (MFG) may also participate in control over parietal accumulation activity (Kayser et al., 2009), thus establishing complex frontoparietal networks with dorsal (LIP-FEF) and ventral components (MFG and inferior frontal gyrus), connected by distinct branches of the SLF (Thiebaut de Schotten et al., 2008, 2011). Also, medial prefrontal areas such as the anterior cingulate cortex/supplementary motor area (ACC/SMA) are likely to contribute to the evidence accumulator process at the basis of perceptual decisions (Kayser et al., 2009), perhaps by checking for errors or by implementing a "waiting" signal delaying motor response until accumulated evidence is deemed sufficient. The right IFG, which can be directly damaged in some neglect patients (Husain & Kennard, 1996), or disconnected from more posterior regions in other patients (Urbanski et al., 2008), might be part of an evaluation circuit that determines whether the task needs more attentional resources, due to its perceptual uncertainty or difficulty (Heekeren et al., 2008). The right IFG might also cooperate with the medial prefrontal cortex in signaling the system to hold on the motor response, for example because the accumulator has not yet reached sufficient levels of evidence. Note that the capacity of the right IFG to inhibit prepotent but inappropriate responses (Aron, Robbins, & Poldrack, 2004) may in fact be just an instance of its more general ability to maintain a task set against distractions, or in sustaining/focusing attention on the task-relevant items (Hampshire, Chamberlain, Monti, Duncan, & Owen, 2010). This role would be shared with the heavily and directly connected IPL (Singh-Curry & Husain, 2009). Recall that the IFG and IPL are cortical endpoints of the VAN in the right hemisphere (Corbetta & Shulman, 2002) (see Box 13.2). Moreover, as mentioned earlier, neurons in the LIP code for the behavioral relevance of stimuli (Gottlieb et al., 1998). Thus, a prominent role of the right-hemisphere VAN could be the identification of task-relevant items worthy of being the target of persisting attentional focusing. A relatively efficient left-hemisphere homologue of the VAN, if receiving adequate input from the right hemisphere, might ensure that left-sided stimuli are still deemed worthy of attentional focusing by the ipsilateral DAN, thus leading to partial compensation of neglect signs (Bartolomeo et al., 2012).

Thus, several nodes of the frontoparietal attentional networks are implicated in steps leading to decisions. Specifically, dysfunction of frontoparietal networks in the right hemisphere, which is a key pathophysiological factor in neglect (Bartolomeo, 2006; Bartolomeo et al., 2007; Ciaraffa et al., 2012; Corbetta et al., 2005; Corbetta & Shulman, 2011; Doricchi et al., 2008; He et al., 2007), may interfere with the accumulation of sensory evidence that generates exploratory behavior toward the neglected side, or with the labeling of left-sided items as being behaviorally relevant and thus worthy of attentional focusing. An inappropriate decision threshold might thus be reached by homologous left-hemisphere networks or structures, such as the left FEF or neighboring PFC, and may trigger neglect behavior by orienting attention and gaze toward the right side. The left hemisphere FEF and adjacent regions in the dorsolateral PFC may thus represent a critical node in triggering inappropriate rightward orienting behavior, with consequent neglect for left-sided events, which do not get adequate exploration.

A key factor in the production of spatially biased exploratory decisions may be inappropriate neural communication within the attentional networks (see Figure 13.4), both within and between the hemispheres (Bartolomeo et al., 2007). We propose that brain damage may give rise to peculiar patterns of performance as a result of the isolation of processes that were previously integrated in large-scale networks. This *lesion-induced modularity* can be the result of damage to long-range white matter pathways, whose disconnection may act as the "isolating" mechanisms in human neuropsychology in general (Catani & ffytche, 2005; Geschwind, 1965), and in neglect in particular (Bartolomeo et al., 2007; Doricchi et al., 2008). Pathological isolation of cortical modules in neglect may eventually disrupt the large-scale broadcasting of information that, according to current models (Chica, Paz-Alonso, Valero-Cabré, & Bartolomeo, 2012; Dehaene, Changeux, Naccache, Sackur, & Sergent, 2006), sets the neural conditions for our conscious experience.

Conclusions and Perspectives

Neglect behavior, with its important clinical consequences, is likely to result from a complex interplay of maladaptive neural activities both in the lesioned and in the intact hemisphere, resulting from damage to the attentional networks in the right hemisphere. The fact that spatial attention is an essential factor in the active exploration of space, which is itself at the basis of our visual experience (Box 13.1), should not come as a surprise to neurologists and neuropsychologists who are familiar with neglect patients suffering from severe impairments of these processes. Recently, much progress has been made in our knowledge of how attentional systems are organized in a distributed manner within and between the hemispheres (Box 13.2), and how dysfunctional nodes and connections of the relevant brain networks may give rise to signs of spatial neglect. Converging evidence from anatomical and brain-imaging studies indicates that neglect signs depend on a complex interplay of intrahemispheric and interhemispheric network dysfunctions (Boxes 13.3–5). The network-based nature of attentional disturbances in neglect, however, leaves open the possibility of influencing the activity of intact nodes through external intervention. As a consequence, various methods have been devised to modulate neglect signs (Bartolomeo, Siéroff, et al., 2001; Chokron, Dupierrix, Tabert, & Bartolomeo, 2007), such as prism adaptation and TMS, by acting on nodes or connections of the attentional networks not directly damaged by the lesion. Unfortunately, most of these modes of intervention appear to have a short-term effect. The challenge is now to find ways to induce long-term plasticity in the attentional networks, for example by "teaching" intact left-hemisphere structures to take into account information coming from the left side of space. Although our knowledge of the modes of action of these procedures is still far from being exhaustive, the accumulating evidence on the activity of dynamic networks in attention and neglect raises hopes that methods of neglect rehabilitation tailored to the specific neurocognitive deficits of patients with specific lesions in different brain localizations will eventually be developed.

References

Allport, D. A. (1989). Visual attention. In M. I. Posner (Ed.), *Foundations of cognitive science* (pp. 631–687). Cambridge, MA: MIT Press.

Andrade, K., Kas, A., Samri, D., Sarazin, M., Dubois, B., Habert, M. O., et al. (2012). Visuospatial deficits and hemispheric perfusion asymmetries in posterior cortical atrophy. *Cortex, 49*(4), 940–947.

Andrade, K., Kas, A., Valabrègue, R., Samri, D., Sarazin, M., Habert, M. O., et al. (2012). Visuospatial deficits in posterior cortical atrophy: structural and functional correlates. *J Neurol Neurosurg Psychiatry, 83*(9), 860–863.

Andrade, K., Samri, D., Sarazin, M., Cruz De Souza, L., Cohen, L., Thiebaut de Schotten, M., et al. (2010). Visual neglect in posterior cortical atrophy. *BMC Neurology, 10*, 68.

Aron, A. R., Robbins, T. W., & Poldrack, R. A. (2004). Inhibition and the right inferior frontal cortex. [Review]. *Trends Cognitive Sci, 8*(4), 170–177.

Azouvi, P., Samuel, C., Louis-Dreyfus, A., Bernati, T., Bartolomeo, P., Beis, J.-M., et al. (2002). Sensitivity of clinical and behavioural tests of spatial neglect after right hemisphere stroke. *J Neurol Neurosurg Psychiatry, 73*(2), 160–166.

Ballard, D. H., Hayhoe, M. M., Pook, P. K., & Rao, R. P. N. (1997). Deictic codes for the embodiment of cognition. *Behav Brain Sci, 20*(4), 723–767.

Bartolomeo, P. (1997). The novelty effect in recovered hemineglect. *Cortex, 33*(2), 323–332.

Bartolomeo, P. (2000). Inhibitory processes and compensation for spatial bias after right hemisphere damage. *Neuropsychol Rehabil, 10*(5), 511–526.

Bartolomeo, P. (2006). A parieto-frontal network for spatial awareness in the right hemisphere of the human brain. *Arch Neurology, 63*, 1238–1241.

Bartolomeo, P. (2007). Visual neglect. [Review]. *Curr Opin Neurol, 20*(4), 381–386.

Bartolomeo, P. (2008). Varieties of attention and of consciousness: Evidence from neuropsychology. [Review]. *Psyche, 14*(1), http://www.theassc.org/vol_14_2008.

Bartolomeo, P. (2014). *Attention disorders after right brain damage: Living in halved worlds.* London: Springer-Verlag.

Bartolomeo, P., & Chokron, S. (1999). Left unilateral neglect or right hyperattention? *Neurology, 53*(9), 2023–2027.

Bartolomeo, P., & Chokron, S. (2001). Levels of impairment in unilateral neglect. In F. Boller & J. Grafman (Eds.), *Handbook of neuropsychology* (2nd ed., Vol. 4, pp. 67–98). Amsterdam: Elsevier Science Publishers.

Bartolomeo, P., & Chokron, S. (2002). Orienting of attention in left unilateral neglect. *Neurosci Biobehav Rev, 26*(2), 217–234.

Bartolomeo, P., Chokron, S., & Gainotti, G. (2001). Laterally directed arm movements and right unilateral neglect after left hemisphere damage. *Neuropsychologia, 39*(10), 1013–1021.

Bartolomeo, P., Dalla Barba, G., Boissé, M. T., Bachoud-Lévi, A. C., Degos, J. D., & Boller, F. (1998). Right-side neglect in Alzheimer's disease. *Neurology, 51*(4), 1207–1209.

Bartolomeo, P., Siéroff, E., Decaix, C., & Chokron, S. (2001). Modulating the attentional bias in unilateral neglect: The effects of the strategic set. *Exp Brain Res, 137*(3/4), 424–431.

Bartolomeo, P., Thiebaut de Schotten, M., & Chica, A. B. (2012). Brain networks of visuospatial attention and their disruption in visual neglect. *Front Human Neurosci, 6*, 110.

Bartolomeo, P., Thiebaut de Schotten, M., & Doricchi, F. (2007). Left unilateral neglect as a disconnection syndrome. *Cerebral Cortex, 45*(14), 3127–3148.

Beck, D. M., Rees, G., Frith, C. D., & Lavie, N. (2001). Neural correlates of change detection and change blindness. *Nat Neurosci, 4*(6), 645–650.

Beis, J. M., Keller, C., Morin, N., Bartolomeo, P., Bernati, T., Chokron, S., et al. (2004). Right spatial neglect after left hemisphere stroke: Qualitative and quantitative study. *Neurology, 63*(9), 1600–1605.

Berlucchi, G., Aglioti, S., & Tassinari, G. (1997). Rightward attentional bias and left hemisphere dominance in a cue-target light detection task in a callosotomy patient. *Neuropsychologia, 35*(7), 941–952.

Binder, J., Marshall, R., Lazar, R., Benjamin, J., & Mohr, J. P. (1992). Distinct syndromes of hemineglect. *Arch Neurol, 49*(11), 1187–1194.

Bonato, M., Priftis, K., Marenzi, R., Umiltà, C., & Zorzi, M. (2010). Increased attentional demands impair contralesional space awareness following stroke. *Neuropsychologia, 48*(13), 3934–3940.

Bowers, D., & Heilman, K. M. (1980). Pseudoneglect: Effects of hemispace on a tactile line bisection task. *Neuropsychologia, 18*, 491–498.

Bozzali, M., Mastropasqua, C., Cercignani, M., Giulietti, G., Bonni, S., Caltagirone, C., et al. (2012). Microstructural damage of the posterior corpus callosum contributes to the clinical severity of neglect. *PLoS One, 7*(10), e48079.

Buschman, T. J., & Miller, E. K. (2007). Top-down versus bottom-up control of attention in the prefrontal and posterior parietal cortices. *Science, 315*(5820), 1860–1862.

Cain, M. S., Vul, E., Clark, K., & Mitroff, S. R. (2012). A bayesian optimal foraging model of human visual search. *Psychol Sci, 23*(9), 1047–1054.

Cappa, S. F., & Perani, D. (2010). Imaging studies of recovery from unilateral neglect. [Review]. *Exp Brain Res, 206*(2), 237–241.

Carpenter, R. H. S. (2004). Contrast, probability, and saccadic latency: Evidence for independence of detection and decision. *Curr Biol, 14*(17), 1576–1580.

Carpenter, R. H. S., & Williams, M. L. L. (1995). Neural computation of log likelihood in control of saccadic eye movements. *Nature, 377*(6544), 59–62.

Carter, A. R., Astafiev, S. V., Lang, C. E., Connor, L. T., Rengachary, J., Strube, M. J., et al. (2010). Resting interhemispheric functional magnetic resonance imaging connectivity predicts performance after stroke. *Ann Neurol, 67*(3), 365–375.

Catani, M., & ffytche, D. H. (2005). The rises and falls of disconnection syndromes. *Brain, 128*(Pt 10), 2224–2239.

Chica, A. B., & Bartolomeo, P. (2012). Attentional routes to conscious perception. [Review]. *Front Psychol, 3*(1), 1–12.

Chica, A. B., Paz-Alonso, P. M., Valero-Cabré, A., & Bartolomeo, P. (2012). Neural bases of the interactions between spatial attention and conscious perception. *Cerebral Cortex, 23*(6), 1269–1279.

Chica, A. B., Thiebaut de Schotten, M., Toba, M. N., Malhotra, P., Lupiáñez, J., & Bartolomeo, P. (2012). Attention networks and their interactions after right-hemisphere damage. *Cortex, 48*(6), 654–663.

Chokron, S., Dupierrix, E., Tabert, M., & Bartolomeo, P. (2007). Experimental remission of unilateral spatial neglect. *Neuropsychologia, 45*(14), 3127–3148.

Ciaraffa, F., Castelli, G., Parati, E. A., Bartolomeo, P., & Bizzi, A. (2012). Visual neglect as a disconnection syndrome? A confirmatory case report. *Neurocase, 19*(4), 351–359.

Corballis, M. C., Corballis, P. M., Fabri, M., Paggi, A., & Manzoni, T. (2005). Now you see it, now you don't: Variable hemineglect in a commissurotomized man. *Cogn Brain Res, 25*(2), 521–530.

Corbetta, M., Kincade, M. J., Lewis, C., Snyder, A. Z., & Sapir, A. (2005). Neural basis and recovery of spatial attention deficits in spatial neglect. *Nat Neurosci, 8*(11), 1603–1610.

Corbetta, M., & Shulman, G. L. (2002). Control of goal-directed and stimulus-driven attention in the brain. *Nat Rev Neurosci, 3*(3), 201–215.

Corbetta, M., & Shulman, G. L. (2011). Spatial neglect and attention networks. *Annu Rev Neurosci, 34*, 569–599.

D'Erme, P., Robertson, I., Bartolomeo, P., Daniele, A., & Gainotti, G. (1992). Early rightwards orienting of attention on simple reaction time performance in patients with left-sided neglect. *Neuropsychologia, 30*(11), 989–1000.

De Renzi, E., Gentilini, M., Faglioni, P., & Barbieri, C. (1989). Attentional shifts toward the rightmost stimuli in patients with left visual neglect. *Cortex, 25*, 231–237.

Dehaene, S., Changeux, J. P., Naccache, L., Sackur, J., & Sergent, C. (2006). Conscious, preconscious, and subliminal processing: A testable taxonomy. *Trends Cogn Sci, 10*(5), 204–211.

Di Ferdinando, A., Parisi, D., & Bartolomeo, P. (2007). Modeling orienting behavior and its disorders with "ecological" neural networks. *J Cogn Neurosci, 19*(6), 1033–1049.

Doricchi, F., Thiebaut de Schotten, M., Tomaiuolo, F., & Bartolomeo, P. (2008). White matter (dis)connections and gray matter (dys)functions in visual neglect: Gaining insights into the brain networks of spatial awareness. *Cortex, 44*(8), 983–995.

Doty, R. (2003). Forebrain commissures: Glimpses of neurons producing mind. In E. Zaidel & M. Iacoboni (Eds.), *The parallel brain: The cognitive neuroscience of the corpus callosum* (pp. 157–165). Cambridge, MA: The MIT Press.

Fiorelli, M., Blin, J., Bakchine, S., Laplane, D., & Baron, J. C. (1991). PET studies of cortical diaschisis in patients with motor hemineglect. *J Neurol Sci, 104*, 135–142.

Gaffan, D., & Hornak, J. (1997). Visual neglect in the monkey. Representation and disconnection. *Brain, 120*(Pt 9), 1647–1657.

Gainotti, G., D'Erme, P., & Bartolomeo, P. (1991). Early orientation of attention toward the half space ipsilateral to the lesion in patients with unilateral brain damage. *J Neurol Neurosurg Psychiatry, 54,* 1082–1089.

Gainotti, G., Perri, R., & Cappa, A. (2002). Left hand movements and right hemisphere activation in unilateral spatial neglect: A test of the interhemispheric imbalance hypothesis. *Neuropsychologia, 40*(8), 1350–1355.

Geschwind, N. (1965). Disconnexion syndromes in animals and man: Part I. *Brain, 88,* 237–294.

Gitelman, D. R., Nobre, A. C., Parrish, T. B., LaBar, K. S., Kim, Y.-H., Meyer, J. R., et al. (1999). A large-scale distributed network for covert spatial attention: Further anatomical delineation based on stringent behavioural and cognitive controls. *Brain, 122*(6), 1093–1106.

Glickstein, M., & Berlucchi, G. (2008). Classical disconnection studies of the corpus callosum. *Cortex, 44*(8), 914–927.

Gold, J. I., & Shadlen, M. N. (2007). The neural basis of decision making. [Review]. *Ann Rev Neurosci, 30,* 535–574.

Goodale, M. A., & Milner, A. D. (1992). Separate visual pathways for perception and action. *Trends Neurosci, 15*(1), 20–25.

Gorgoraptis, N., Mah, Y. H., Machner, B., Singh-Curry, V., Malhotra, P., Hadji-Michael, M., et al. (2012). The effects of the dopamine agonist rotigotine on hemispatial neglect following stroke. *Brain, 135*(Pt 8), 2478–2491.

Gottlieb, J. P., Kusunoki, M., & Goldberg, M. E. (1998). The representation of visual salience in monkey parietal cortex. *Nature, 391*(6666), 481–484.

Hampshire, A., Chamberlain, S. R., Monti, M. M., Duncan, J., & Owen, A. M. (2010). The role of the right inferior frontal gyrus: Inhibition and attentional control. *NeuroImage, 50*(3), 1313–1319.

He, B. J., Snyder, A. Z., Vincent, J. L., Epstein, A., Shulman, G. L., & Corbetta, M. (2007). Breakdown of functional connectivity in frontoparietal networks underlies behavioral deficits in spatial neglect. *Neuron, 53*(6), 905–918.

Heekeren, H. R., Marrett, S., & Ungerleider, L. G. (2008). The neural systems that mediate human perceptual decision making. *Nat Rev Neurosci, 9*(6), 467–479.

Heilman, K. M., & Adams, D. J. (2003). Callosal neglect. *Arch Neurol, 60*(2), 276–279.

Heilman, K. M., & Van Den Abell, T. (1980). Right hemisphere dominance for attention: The mechanism underlying hemispheric asymmetries of inattention (neglect). *Neurology, 30*(3), 327–330.

Heilman, K. M., Watson, R. T., & Valenstein, E. (2003). Neglect and related disorders. In K. M. Heilman & E. Valenstein (Eds.), *Clinical neuropsychology* (4th ed., pp. 296–346). New York: Oxford University Press.

Hillis, A. E., Wityk, R. J., Barker, P. B., Beauchamp, N. J., Gailloud, P., Murphy, K., et al. (2002). Subcortical aphasia and neglect in acute stroke: The role of cortical hypoperfusion. *Brain, 125*(Pt 5), 1094–1104.

Hughlings Jackson, J. [1876] (1932). Case of large cerebral tumour without optic neuritis and with left hemiplegia and imperception. In J. Taylor (Ed.), *Selected writings of John Hughlings Jackson* (Vol. 2, pp. 146–152). London: Hodden and Stoughton.

Husain, M. (2008). Hemineglect. *Scholarpedia, 3*(2), 3681.

Husain, M., & Kennard, C. (1996). Visual neglect associated with frontal lobe infarction. *J Neurol, 243*(9), 652–657.

Husain, M., & Rorden, C. (2003). Non-spatially lateralized mechanisms in hemispatial neglect. *Nat Rev Neurosci, 4*(1), 26–36.

Jewell, G., & McCourt, M. E. (2000). Pseudoneglect: A review and meta-analysis of performance factors in line bisection tasks. *Neuropsychologia, 38*(1), 93–110.

Kashiwagi, A., Kashiwagi, T., Nishikawa, T., Tanabe, H., & Okuda, J. (1990). Hemispatial neglect in a patient with callosal infarction. *Brain, 113*(Pt 4), 1005–1023.

Kayser, A. S., Buchsbaum, B. R., Erickson, D. T., & D'Esposito, M. (2009). The functional anatomy of a perceptual decision in the human brain. *J Neurophysiology, 103*(3), 1179–1194.

Kersten, D., Mamassian, P., & Yuille, A. (2004). Object perception as Bayesian inference. *Ann Rev Psychol, 55*(1), 271–304.

Khurshid, S., Trupe, L. A., Newhart, M., Davis, C., Molitoris, J. J., Medina, J., et al. (2012). Reperfusion of specific cortical areas is associated with improvement in distinct forms of hemispatial neglect. *Cortex, 48*(5), 530–539.

Kinsbourne, M. (1970). A model for the mechanism of unilateral neglect of space. *Trans Am Neurol Assoc, 95,* 143–146.

Kinsbourne, M. (1977). Hemi-neglect and hemisphere rivalry. In E. A. Weinstein & R. P. Friedland (Eds.), *Hemi-inattention and hemisphere specialization* (Vol. 18, pp. 41–49). New York: Raven Press.

Kinsbourne, M. (1987). Mechanisms of unilateral neglect. In M. Jeannerod (Ed.), *Neurophysiological and neuropsychological aspects of spatial neglect* (pp. 69–86). Amsterdam: Elsevier Science Publishers.

Kinsbourne, M. (1993). Orientational bias model of unilateral neglect: Evidence from attentional gradients within hemispace. In I. H. Robertson & J. C. Marshall (Eds.), *Unilateral neglect: Clinical and experimental studies* (pp. 63–86). Hove, UK: Lawrence Erlbaum Associates.

Koch, G., Bonni, S., Giacobbe, V., Bucchi, G., Basile, B., Lupo, F., et al. (2012). Theta-burst stimulation of the left hemisphere accelerates recovery of hemispatial neglect. *Neurology, 78*(1), 24–30.

Koch, G., Oliveri, M., Cheeran, B., Ruge, D., Lo Gerfo, E., Salerno, S., et al. (2008). Hyperexcitability of parietal-motor functional connections in the intact left-hemisphere of patients with neglect. *Brain, 131*(Pt 12), 3147–3155.

LaBerge, D., Auclair, L., & Siéroff, E. (2000). Preparatory attention: Experiment and theory. *Conscious Cogn, 9,* 396–434.

Luaute, J., Michel, C., Rode, G., Pisella, L., Jacquin-Courtois, S., Costes, N., et al. (2006). Functional anatomy of the therapeutic effects of prism adaptation on left neglect. *Neurology, 66*(12), 1859–1867.

Mack, A., & Rock, I. (1998). *Inattentional blindness.* Cambridge, MA: The MIT Press.

Macquistan, A. D. (1997). Object-based allocation of visual attention in response to exogenous, but not endogenous, spatial precues. *Psychonom Bull Rev, 4*(4), 512–515.

Malhotra, P., Coulthard, E., & Husain, M. (2006). Hemispatial neglect, balance and eye-movement control. *Curr Opin Neurol, 19*(1), 14–20.

Mark, V. W., Kooistra, C. A., & Heilman, K. M. (1988). Hemispatial neglect affected by non-neglected stimuli. *Neurology, 38*(8), 1207–1211.

Mattingley, J. B., Bradshaw, J. L., Bradshaw, J. A., & Nettleton, N. C. (1994). Residual rightward attentional bias after apparent recovery from right hemisphere damage: Implications for a multicomponent model of neglect. *J Neurol Neurosurg Psychiatry, 57,* 597–604.

Merten, K., & Nieder, A. (2012). Active encoding of decisions about stimulus absence in primate prefrontal cortex neurons. *Proc Natl Acad Sci U S A, 109*(16), 6289–6294.

Meyer, J. S., Obara, K., & Muramatsu, K. (1993). Diaschisis. *Neurol Res, 15*(6), 362–366.

Mijovic'-Prelec, D., Shin, L. M., Chabris, C. F., & Kosslyn, S. M. (1994). When does "no" really mean "yes"? A case study in unilateral visual neglect. *Neuropsychologia, 32,* 151–158.

Mishkin, M., Ungerleider, L. G., & Macko, K. A. (1983). Object vision and spatial vision: Two cortical pathways. *Trends Neurosci, 6,* 414–417.

Moran, J., & Desimone, R. (1985). Selective attention gates visual processing in the extrastriate cortex. *Science, 229*(4715), 782–784.

O'Regan, J. K., Rensink, R. A., & Clark, J. J. (1999). Change-blindness as a result of "mudsplashes." *Nature, 398*(6722), 34.

O'Shea, J., Johansen-Berg, H., Trief, D., Göbel, S., & Rushworth, M. F. S. (2007). Functionally specific reorganization in human premotor cortex. *Neuron, 54*(3), 479–490.

Oliveri, M., Bisiach, E., Brighina, F., Piazza, A., La Bua, V., Buffa, D., et al. (2001). rTMS of the unaffected hemisphere transiently reduces contralesional visuospatial hemineglect. *Neurology, 57*(7), 1338–1340.

Pantano, P., Di Piero, V., Fieschi, C., Judica, A., Guariglia, C., & Pizzamiglio, L. (1992). Pattern of CBF in the rehabilitation of visual spatial neglect. *Int J Neurosci, 66,* 153–161.

Park, K. C., Lee, B. H., Kim, E. J., Shin, M. H., Choi, K. M., Yoon, S. S., et al. (2006). Deafferentation-disconnection neglect induced by posterior cerebral artery infarction. *Neurology, 66*(1), 56–61.

Parton, A., Malhotra, P., & Husain, M. (2004). Hemispatial neglect. *J Neurol Neurosurg Psychiatry, 75*(1), 13–21.

Perani, D., Vallar, G., Paulesu, E., Alberoni, M., & Fazio, F. (1993). Left and right hemisphere contribution to recovery from neglect after right hemisphere damage: An [18F]FDG PET study of two cases. *Neuropsychologia*, *31*(2), 115–125.

Petrides, M., & Pandya, D. N. (1984). Projections to the frontal cortex from the posterior parietal region in the rhesus monkey. *J Compar Neurol*, *228*(1), 105–116.

Pisella, L., Rode, G., Farne, A., Tilikete, C., & Rossetti, Y. (2006). Prism adaptation in the rehabilitation of patients with visuo-spatial cognitive disorders. *Curr Opin Neurol*, *19*(6), 534–542.

Pouget, P., Pradat-Diehl, P., Rivaud-Pechoux, S., Wattiez, N., & Gaymard, B. (2011). An oculomotor and computational study of a patient with diagonistic dyspraxia. *Cortex*, *47*(4), 473–483.

Rastelli, F., Funes, M. J., Lupiáñez, J., Duret, C., & Bartolomeo, P. (2008). Left neglect: Is the disengage deficit space- or object-based? *Exp Brain Res*, *187*(3), 439–446.

Rastelli, F., Tallon-Baudry, C., Migliaccio, R., Toba, M. N., Ducorps, A., Pradat-Diehl, P., et al. (2013). Neural dynamics of neglected targets in patients with right hemisphere damage. *Cortex*, *49*(7), 1989–1996.

Robertson, I. H. (2001). Do we need the "lateral" in unilateral neglect? Spatially nonselective attention deficits in unilateral neglect and their implications for rehabilitation. *NeuroImage*, *14*(1), S85–S90.

Robertson, I. H., Mattingley, J. B., Rorden, C., & Driver, J. (1998). Phasic alerting of neglect patients overcomes their spatial deficit in visual awareness. *Nature*, *395*(6698), 169–172.

Roe, A. W., Chelazzi, L., Connor, C. E., Conway, B. R., Fujita, I., Gallant, J. L., et al. (2012). Toward a unified theory of visual area V4. [Review]. *Neuron*, *74*(1), 12–29.

Rossetti, Y., Rode, G., Pisella, L., Farnè, A., Li, L., Boisson, D., et al. (1998). Prism adaptation to a rightward optical deviation rehabilitates left hemispatial neglect. *Nature*, *395*, 166–169.

Rossini, P. M., Calautti, C., Pauri, F., & Baron, J.-C. (2003). Post-stroke plastic reorganisation in the adult brain. *Lancet Neurol*, *2*(8), 493–502.

Rueckl, J. G., Cave, K. R., & Kosslyn, S. M. (1989). Why are "what" and "where" processed by separate cortical visual systems? A computational investigation. *J Cogn Neurosci*, *1*, 171–186.

Rushmore, R. J., Valero-Cabre, A., Lomber, S. G., Hilgetag, C. C., & Payne, B. R. (2006). Functional circuitry underlying visual neglect. *Brain*, *129*(Pt 7), 1803–1821.

Schall, J. D. (2001). Neural basis of deciding, choosing and acting. *Nat Rev Neurosci*, *2*(1), 33.

Schmahmann, J. D., & Pandya, D. N. (2006). *Fiber pathways of the brain*. New York: Oxford University Press.

Shinoura, N., Suzuki, Y., Yamada, R., Tabei, Y., Saito, K., & Yagi, K. (2009). Damage to the right superior longitudinal fasciculus in the inferior parietal lobe plays a role in spatial neglect. *Neuropsychologia*, *47*(12), 2600–2603.

Siéroff, E., Decaix, C., Chokron, S., & Bartolomeo, P. (2007). Impaired orienting of attention in left unilateral neglect: A componential analysis. *Neuropsychology*, *21*(1), 94–113.

Simons, D. J., & Chabris, C. F. (1999). Gorillas in our midst: Sustained inattentional blindness for dynamic events. *Perception*, *28*(9), 1059–1074.

Singh-Curry, V., & Husain, M. (2009). The functional role of the inferior parietal lobe in the dorsal and ventral stream dichotomy. *Neuropsychologia*, *47*(6), 1434–1448.

Sokolov, E. N. (1963). Higher nervous functions: the orienting reflex. *Ann Rev Physiol*, *25*, 545–580.

Sprague, J. M. (1966). Interaction of cortex and superior colliculus in mediation of visually guided behavior in the cat. *Science*, *153*(743), 1544–1547.

Summerfield C., & Tsetsos K. (2012). Building Bridges between Perceptual and Economic Decision-Making: Neural and Computational Mechanisms. *Front Neurosci*, *6*, 70.

Thiebaut de Schotten, M., Dell'Acqua, F., Forkel, S. J., Simmons, A., Vergani, F., Murphy, D. G. M., et al. (2011). A lateralized brain network for visuospatial attention. *Nat Neurosci*, *14*(10), 1245–1246.

Thiebaut de Schotten, M., Kinkingnéhun, S. R., Delmaire, C., Lehéricy, S., Duffau, H., Thivard, L., et al. (2008). Visualization of disconnection syndromes in humans. *Cortex*, *44*(8), 1097–1103.

Thiebaut de Schotten, M., Urbanski, M., Duffau, H., Volle, E., Levy, R., Dubois, B., et al. (2005). Direct evidence for a parietal-frontal pathway subserving spatial awareness in humans. *Science*, *309*(5744), 2226–2228.

Toba M. N., Cavanagh, P., & Bartolomeo, P. (2011) Attention biases the perceived midpoint of horizontal lines. *Neuropsychologia*, *49*(2), 238–346.

Tomaiuolo, F., Voci, L., Bresci, M., Cozza, S., Posteraro, F., Oliva, M., et al. (2010). Selective visual neglect in right brain damaged patients with splenial interhemispheric disconnection. *Exp Brain Res*, *206*(2), 209–217.

Urbanski, M., Thiebaut de Schotten, M., Rodrigo, S., Catani, M., Oppenheim, C., Touzé, E., et al. (2008). Brain networks of spatial awareness: Evidence from diffusion tensor imaging tractography. *J Neurol Neurosurg Psychiatry, 79*(5), 598–601.

Verdon, V., Schwartz, S., Lovblad, K. O., Hauert, C. A., & Vuilleumier, P. (2010). Neuroanatomy of hemispatial neglect and its functional components: A study using voxel-based lesion-symptom mapping. *Brain, 133*(Pt 3), 880–894.

Vuilleumier, P., Hester, D., Assal, G., & Regli, F. (1996). Unilateral spatial neglect recovery after sequential strokes. *Neurology, 46*, 184–189.

Wilke, M., Kagan, I., & Andersen, R. A. (2012). Functional imaging reveals rapid reorganization of cortical activity after parietal inactivation in monkeys. *P Natl Acad Sci, 109*(21), 8274–8279.

Yantis, S. (1995). Attentional capture in vision. In A. F. Kramer, G. H. Coles & G. D. Logan (Eds.), *Converging operations in the study of visual selective attention* (pp. 45–76). Washington, DC: American Psychological Association.

14

Neuroplasticity in Apraxia Recovery

Lewis A. Wheaton

Introduction

Apraxia is traditionally identified as a disorder of planning and/or execution of skilled movements (praxis). For necessity of clear diagnosis, the deficits seen in apraxia cannot be attributable to other elemental motor (e.g., paresis) or cognitive impairments (e.g., diminished awareness). Problems with praxis will manifest as motor action and/or conceptual deficits related to tool use and/or communicative gestures. Commonly, the clinical manifestations of apraxia may be dismissed as clumsiness or confusion, despite these clear error patterns. Of the several forms of apraxia, ideomotor is the most commonly studied form, perhaps because of its unique and characteristic deficits. Ideomotor apraxia is associated with skilled movements that have temporal and/or spatial errors, including perseverations, incorrect actions, and occasionally no movement (Schnider et al., 1997; Goldenberg & Hagmann, 1998; Leiguarda & Marsden, 2000; Hanna-Pladdy et al., 2001b; Buxbaum & Saffran, 2002; Buxbaum et al., 2003). These deficits are commonly seen in pantomime in the clinical setting, but also during daily living outside the clinic (Dovern et al., 2012; Heilman & Gonzalez Rothi, 2003). Several other forms of apraxia exist, which have been summarized (Wheaton & Hallett, 2007). Notably, conceptual apraxia results in deficits of selecting the appropriate tools to conduct the task that is to be performed. Thus, the deficit in conceptual apraxia occurs not in the motor act per se, but at the cognitive level in understanding tool-object associations and perhaps task outcomes (Heilman et al., 1997). Research in our laboratory has proposed a potential dissociation of conceptual from ideomotor deficits, as conceptual knowledge of tool usage appears to involve ventral areas, namely superior temporal areas and the insula (Mizelle & Wheaton, 2010a, 2010b; Mizelle et al., 2013). Lesions associated with ideomotor apraxia will be discussed in more detail later. Patients with apraxia have been shown to have impairments of activities of daily living (Foundas et al., 1995; Hanna-Pladdy et al., 2001a, 2001b, 2003).

The prevalence of apraxia as an outcome of neural damage has been the subject of a long-standing debate. Unfortunately, the high prevalence of the disorder has been masked by the concern that a definitive diagnosis requires exclusion of numerous other conditions that may coexist. Despite this, apraxia has been clearly shown in numerous neurological disorders. While commonly studied and identified in stroke, apraxia has been reported in conditions such as Parkinson's disease (Leiguarda et al., 1997), Huntington's disease (Hamilton et al., 2003), corticobasal degeneration (Cordato et al., 2001; Chainay & Humphreys, 2003; Salter et al., 2004), Alzheimer's disease (Ochipa et al., 1992; Derouesne et al., 2000), and multiple sclerosis (Kamm et al., 2012). In the case of stroke, apraxia is prevalent in one-third to 75% of left hemisphere stroke survivors (Donkervoort et al., 2000; Vanbellingen et al., 2010). These estimates and observations are largely based on the occurrence of the ideomotor form of apraxia. Vital to rehabilitation considerations, apraxia severity is strongly related to day-to-day functional impairment and recovery after stroke (Chestnut & Haaland, 2008).

Due to the prevalence of apraxia, its effects on activities of daily living, and its relevance to motor improvement after stroke, understanding how people can recover from apraxia is of vital concern. However, as several review articles have pointed out, there remains a void in empirical knowledge on rehabilitation strategies in apraxia (Buxbaum, 2001; Buxbaum et al., 2008; Vanbellingen & Bohlhalter, 2011). There is also limited understanding of the neurophysiological and neuroplastic changes that can accompany or enhance recovery (Wheaton & Hallett, 2007).

The underlying goal of this chapter will be to consider the neuroanatomy, neurophysiology, and neuroplasticity of apraxia, with a focus on how these topics impact rehabilitation research efforts. In order to achieve this goal, this chapter will focus on what research has shown us about the clinico-anatomical correlations of apraxia and the consideration of possible neurophysiological mechanisms that may relate to neuroplasticity. Finally, selected lingering questions with relevance to apraxia neurorehabilitation will be discussed. Unless specifically mentioned, focus is placed on the ideomotor form of apraxia.

Neuroanatomy of Apraxia

The localization of apraxia has been a tremendous challenge, in part because of the complexity of the cognitive architecture devoted to intact praxis function (Goldenberg, 2003). In general terms, lesion studies agree that apraxia is commonly related to left parietofrontal lesions (Haaland et al., 2000; Leiguarda & Marsden, 2000; Grafton & Hamilton, 2007; Buxbaum & Kalenine, 2010). Apraxia is largely considered a "disconnection" disorder resulting from damaged connectivity of posterior brain regions, encoding conceptual knowledge of tools, from anterior, action-encoding areas. Such a disconnection may arise from parietal cortical, frontal cortical, or subcortical white matter damage. Human neuroimaging has largely confirmed this parietofrontal localization for intact praxis using functional magnetic resonance imaging (fMRI) (Chaminade et al., 2005; Johnson-Frey et al., 2003, 2005; Bohlhalter et al., 2009) and electroencephalography (EEG; Wheaton et al., 2005a, 2005b, 2005c, 2009).

Lesion Localization

There are many discrepancies in the literature regarding what lesion localizations are common in the apraxias, and even within a single form of apraxia. One of the more classic studies of lesion overlap in patients with apraxia found a large degree of overlap in both parietal and frontal areas, suggesting that both are vital in leading to apraxia (Haaland et al., 2000). In one of the first studies of its kind, Kertesz and Ferro (1984) considered that lesions of the deep parieto- and occipitofrontal and anterior callosal fibers seem to be crucial in apraxia (Kertesz & Ferro, 1984). Going along the lines of the original theory of apraxia (Liepmann, 1900, 1905, 1907), the parietal cortex has long been regarded as the vital brain area for encoding representations of tool use and gesture tasks, and thus is of prominent importance for lesions leading to ideomotor apraxia (Heilman et al., 1982). However, lesion studies have begun to suggest that the frontal cortex is most commonly implicated in apraxia (Goldenberg et al., 2007; Huey et al., 2009).

There is experimental support of the crucial role of the frontal lobe. A recent study using transcranial magnetic stimulation (TMS), specifically, theta burst stimulation (TBS), over parietal and frontal areas may enhance our understanding of lesion localization and symptom variability in apraxia (Bohlhalter et al., 2011). In this study, healthy participants received TBS over parietal or frontal cortex while producing gestures that were assessed using the Test of Upper Limb Apraxia (TULIA; Vanbellingen et al., 2011). The authors found that stimulation over the inferior frontal gyrus resulted in deficits in gesture reproduction, notably as "body-part-as-object" errors. This was mainly attributed to extra distal movements and omissions (see Figure 14.1). Stimulation of the inferior parietal lobule did not have a significant effect on TULIA scores.

Using TBS over the inferior frontal gyrus may lead to a particular disruption of a network responsible for selecting or translating movements of tools into the body schema in a normal way, but not content errors (perseverations, substitutions) or spatial errors (Bohlhalter et al., 2011). However, the deficit pattern induced by Bohlhalter and colleagues (2011) is not common to all patients with apraxia (Hanna-Pladdy et al., 2001b).

There are reports of apraxia arising from right hemisphere damage, though the occurrence of apraxia after right hemisphere stroke remains controversial. Comparing left- and right-hemisphere damaged patients, left-hemisphere damaged patients were more impaired in pantomime of tool use, but there was no difference in deficits of gestures, suggesting that both the left and right hemispheres may store gesture representations (Roy et al., 2000). Recent findings suggest why praxis errors may occur in right-hemisphere damaged patients. A study of left- and right-hemisphere damaged patients showed common impairment in daily task performance (Poole et al., 2009). However, impairments in left-hemisphere patients were largely due to ideomotor apraxia, while impairments in right-hemisphere patients were mainly due to spatial deficits. It is perhaps the case that

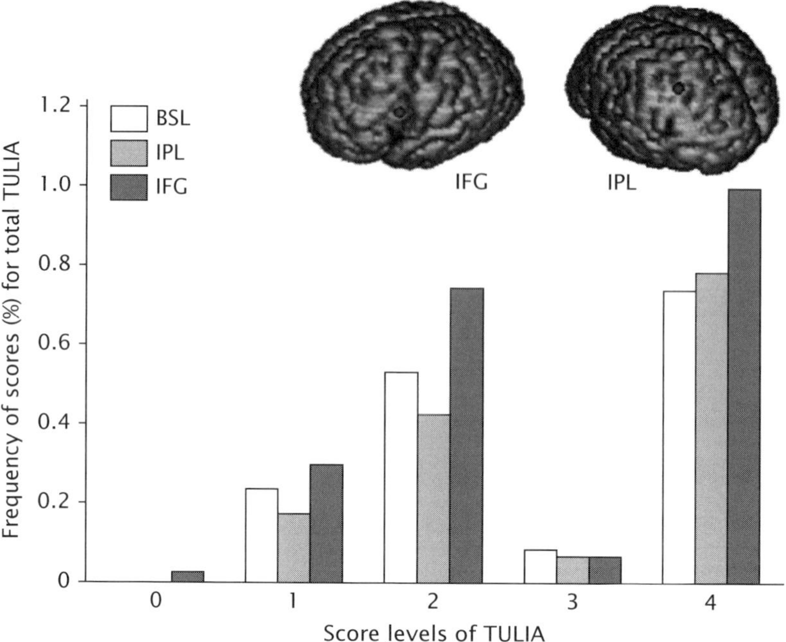

FIGURE 14.1 Frequency distribution of TULIA scores at abnormal levels 0–4 between the different experimental conditions for pantomime gestures over all 14 participants (0, no movement; 1, final position is false, major errors in spatial orientation; 2, uncorrected body-part-as-object errors, extra movements, and omissions; 3, extra movements and omissions that were corrected; 4, movement is too slow, hesitating, robot-like). Higher frequencies of score level 2 and 4 largely account for the inferior frontal TBS effect on TULIA subscores. IFG, inferior frontal gyrus; IPL, inferior parietal lobule; BSL, baseline) Caption text and figure reprinted with permission from Bohlhalter et al. (2011), Elsevier.

patients with apraxia from right-hemisphere damage may typically have deficits more related to right dominance of visuospatial processing, rather than skillful motor control processes directly (Goldenberg et al., 2001). Overall, apraxia seen after right hemisphere damage appears to be rare, and less severe compared to left hemisphere damage (Hanna-Pladdy et al., 2001a, Vanbellingen et al., 2010).

Disconnection and Clinico-Anatomical Correlations

As apraxia has long been regarded as a deficit that arises via disconnection of parietal and frontal lobes (from either direct damage to the relevant cortical areas or to the white matter connecting them), proposals considering remodeled connectivity of praxis function are valuable. Understanding the physiology resultant from such a disconnection is necessary. This concept extends to appreciating network modifications beyond localized lesion profiles. In one proposal (Catani & ffytche, 2005), a focus is placed on the role of hodological mechanisms, in which dysfunctional *pathways* play a role beyond purely topological damage (where a *local brain area* is affected). This is seen in Figure 14.2, where brain lesions can cause extensive damage to more widespread pathways and subsequent cortical dysfunction through cortical or white matter damage. Through hodological mechanisms, it becomes possible to consider that local cortical lesions may result in vast deficit profiles based on the physiological outcome of damaged pathways (ffytche & Catani, 2005). By considering the function of damaged pathways, it is possible that lesions to one cortical location can result in hyper- or hypofunction, which may affect remote regions (such as through diaschisis). A classical topological view would suggest that damage to a local brain area (Figure 14.2C) would result in dysfunction of that local brain area (red arrow), and those adjacent to it (yellow arrows). A hodological

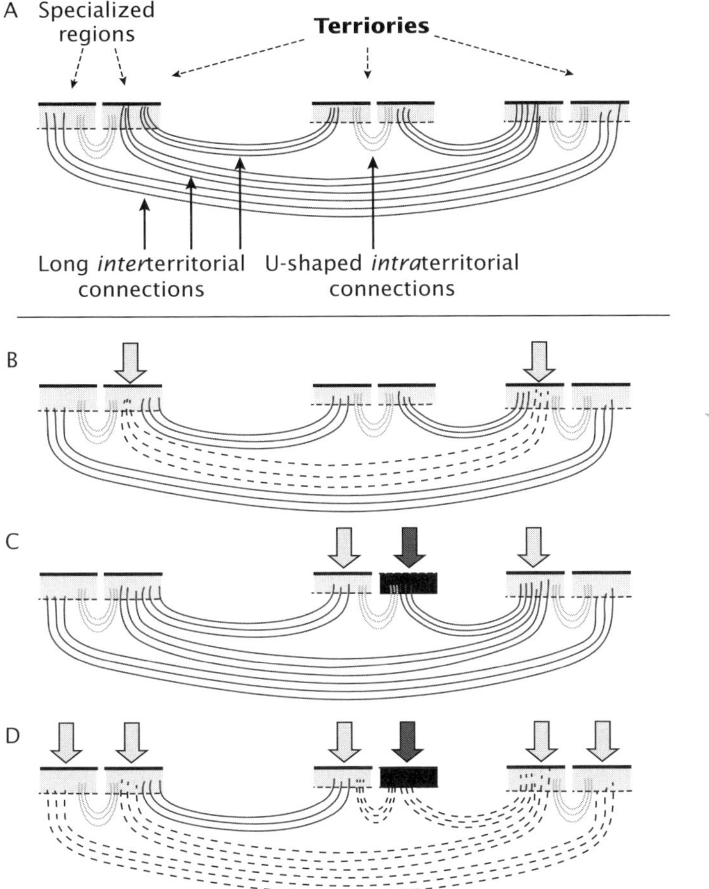

FIGURE 14.2 A hodotopic framework for clinicopathological correlations. A: The contemporary view of the cortex and its connections. Different regions of specialized cortex (gray rectangles) are connected by U-shaped fibers (green) to form extended territories, themselves connected by long, interterritorial fibers (red). B: The consequence of white matter pathology. The dashed pathway is either hyper- or hypofunctional. Yellow arrows indicate dysfunctional cortical regions, in this case through a hodological mechanism. C: The consequence of cortical pathology. The black region of cortex is hyper- or hypofunctional. The red arrow indicates cortex dysfunctional through a topological mechanism. For some tasks, distant cortical regions may be dysfunctional through a secondary hodological mechanism (yellow arrows). D: The consequence of combined white matter and cortical pathology. The black area of cortex and dashed pathways are hyper- or hypofunctional. Yellow arrows indicate widespread cortical regions affected by a hodological mechanism, while the red arrow indicates a region of topological dysfunction. Caption text and figure reprinted with permission from Catani and ffytche (2005), Oxford University Press.

perspective (Figure 14.2D) would argue that the lesion to the same local brain area would result in dysfunction at multiple cortical areas due to damage at connecting adjacent areas (intraterritorial) and widespread (interterritorial) cortical regions through dysfunctional white matter. Under hodology, subtle differences in tract damage can result in unique clinicopathological outcomes. As these authors propose, considering purely parietofrontal circuitry, the hodological theory would anticipate that the form of apraxia developing after restricted lesions to the parietal lobe (e.g., superior parietal cortex) may depend on what the damaged area controls, as well as its connectivity. This idea has been elaborated to demonstrate the physiological mechanisms (such as coherent networks) that can strengthen clinico-anatomical correlations (Catani & Thiebaut de Schotten, 2012).

The disagreement about lesion localization in apraxia (parietal versus frontal) could obscure valuable information concerning common network impairment resulting from varying lesions. Classic work in monkeys has demonstrated clinical outcomes of hand-shaping deficits that are similar for parietal (Gallese et al., 1994) and premotor (Fogassi et al., 2001) lesions, implicating damage to a common physiological network despite differing lesion localizations. Methods that evaluate anatomical connectivity variations, using diffusion tensor imaging (DTI), in stroke survivors with and without apraxia with diverse lesion profiles would be beneficial to elaborating on this idea (Weiss & Fink, 2010). Work using DTI has been helpful in identifying white matter projections that have reduced density in apraxia. Using DTI, white matter pathways were studied in patients with corticobasal syndrome, revealing that apraxia was correlated with decreases in dorsolateral parietofrontal association fiber and intraparietal fiber density (Borroni et al., 2008). This work also demonstrated that commissural projections at the body and splenium of the corpus callosum may help explain the bilateral appearance of apraxia. The potential role of interhemispheric connectivity has been demonstrated in a case study of left-hand apraxia in a right-handed patient with posterior cortical atrophy, who showed decreases in posterior corpus callosum fiber density (Migliaccio et al., 2012). This finding suggests that disconnection of the left parietal lobe from the right hemisphere specifically caused this unusual apraxia pattern, in line with original theories of unilateral apraxia (Goldenberg, 2003).

Connectivity and Neuroplasticity

How does neural connectivity in apraxia relate to neuroplasticity? Isolation of neural networks may initially seem superfluous to that point, but understanding neuroanatomical correlates allows for understanding the location of neuroplastic responses that may arise through natural processes or rehabilitation efforts (Hummel & Cohen, 2005). As will be discussed, more detailed knowledge of the neural networks (and not just lesion locations) engaged in apraxia can drive specific neurorehabilitation interventions aimed at improving apraxia, such as specific therapeutic or brain stimulation protocols to modulate intact networks, thus enhancing outcomes.

Neurophysiology of Apraxia Recovery

Much work needs to be done to understand the neuroplastic mechanisms underpinning rehabilitation and recovery in apraxia. Ideally, studies can identify mechanisms of neuroplastic reorganization (whether maladaptive or beneficial) from the acute to the chronic phase, gathering information about natural recovery, or understanding which patients might benefit from neurorehabilitation. The convergence of clinical, behavioral, and neuroimaging evidence has led to specific proposals on the mechanism of neuroplasticity, which should inform and refine research efforts in the future. In our discussion of the neuroplastic mechanisms of apraxia, we will focus on clinical studies with a strong neuroanatomical and neurophysiological emphasis.

Apraxia Recovery

It is clear that recovery from apraxia can occur. Research has shown significant improvements in apraxia after stroke (for a review, see Buxbaum et al., 2008). Using hierarchical linear modeling, patient outcomes have been assessed at the "acute-subacute" and "chronic" phases to assess natural recovery of apraxia by evaluating motor (pantomime, pantomime by picture, concurrent imitation, delayed imitation, and tool use) and conceptual (action identification, tool naming by action, tool identification, and tool naming) knowledge of tools in left- and right-hemisphere damaged patients (Stamenova et al., 2011). Tool identification showed the strongest recovery over time, along with tool naming, in both acute-subacute and chronic patients. Subacute patients had significantly higher rates of recovery than chronic patients in pantomime to verbal command and pictures. These patterns seem to fit well with the idea that recovery is greatest in the time period 15–30 days following injury (Basso et al., 1987).

While chronicity from stroke plays a role, the hemisphere of damage may also play a strong role in apraxia signs and recovery. Stamenova, Roy, and Black (2010) performed a study to assess performance differences on transitive and intransitive gesture impairment in left- and right-hemisphere damaged patients. Left-hemisphere damaged patients were more impaired with transitive or intransitive gestures, confirming the concept that the left hemisphere is vital to praxis functions (Stamenova et al., 2010). Chronic patients showed more accuracy at praxis testing than acute patients (perhaps through acute neuroplasticity), and right-hemisphere damaged patients over time improved close to cutoff scores (Figure 14.3). From these data, chronic patients with right hemisphere damage may be the most likely to recover from deficits (as their apraxia is mild), with the greatest *degree of recovery* possible after left hemisphere damage.

Underlying Neuroplasticity?

The data from the stroke literature suggesting that apraxia recovery may occur in the acute phase may imply that neuroplastic change is occurring naturally to restore praxis functions. However, as apraxia persists into the chronic stage, this recovery is often incomplete,

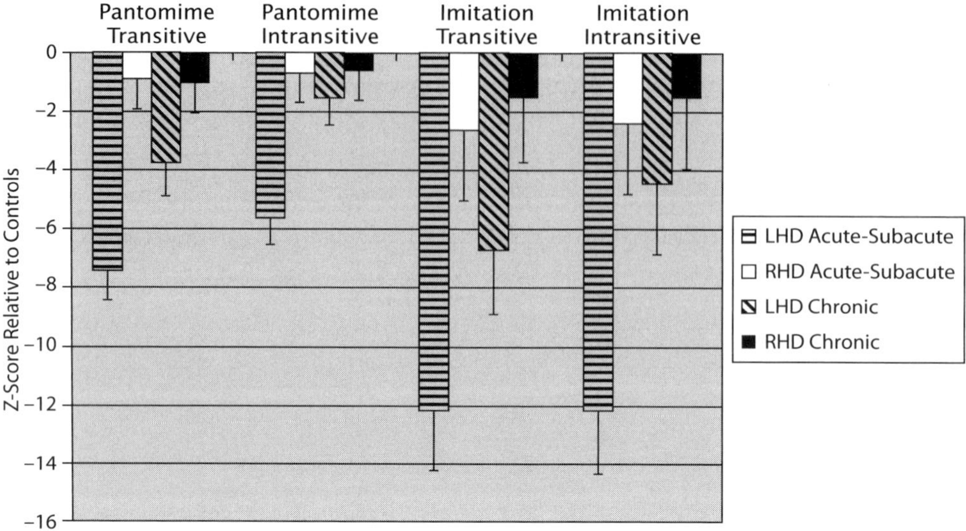

FIGURE 14.3 Average performance in Z-scores for the four patient groups on each task modality. Error bars represent standard errors. Caption text and figure reprinted with permission from Stamenova et al. (2010), Elsevier.

potentially requiring therapeutic intervention to drive restorative neuroplasticity. Several ideas have been proposed as to how this may occur, but unfortunately few studies have actually been performed to index this recovery using neuroimaging or neural stimulation to verify neuroplasticity proposals. Therapeutic interventions aimed at triggering neuroplasticity (potentially involving the right hemisphere) have been long proposed to enhance praxis motor control, and are discussed in the next section.

A Role for the Right Hemisphere in Recovery?

Since the earliest discussions of apraxia, it has been proposed that the right hemisphere plays a significant role in recovery (Liepmann, 1905; Geschwind, 1965). The importance of integrity of the right hemisphere was posited in an early lesion localization study (Kertesz & Ferro, 1984). In this study, 177 right-handed patients with single left hemispheric stroke were assessed for lesion profiles with apraxia. A core finding was that many persons with apraxia due to small lesions had damage to the anterior periventricular white matter, damaging cortical connections (namely, the occipitofrontal fasciculus). Imitation deficits were seen bilaterally, and were proposed to be due to damage to the anterior callosal projections that connect premotor areas. Several patients with left hemisphere lesions (left parietal and/or parietofrontal) did not have apraxia. Because the right hemisphere was intact, and some patients with left hemisphere lesions did not show apraxia at the time of evaluation, Kertesz and Ferro (1984) explicitly posited that right hemispheric representations may allow for praxis performance in the context of left hemisphere lesions.

An additional early investigation proposing a role for the right hemisphere in apraxia recovery came in 1993 by way of a case study of a right-handed man with a left hemispheric stroke (Rapcsak et al., 1993). The patient, a 62-year-old man, suffered a massive left hemispheric stroke that resulted in apraxia along with other deficits (including aphasia, alexia, and agraphia). MRI confirmed a near complete destruction of the left hemisphere cortex and white matter, along with basal ganglia and thalamic lesions. The right hemisphere appeared intact. He was tested on the ability to perform transitive, intransitive, and multistep tool-based movements upon command, along with non-symbolic hand postures, and gesture recognition and discrimination. Performance of transitive gestures was strongly impaired, with spatial errors, but the correct content of the movement was typically apparent. He showed no perseverative errors. Further, his performance was near that of healthy controls on object use and multistep tool movements. Because this patient suffered nearly a left hemisphere ablation, it was proposed that the patient's right hemisphere was now mediating skilled hand movements with tools.

The case study of Rapcsak and colleagues (1993) argues for the importance of kinesthetic-tactile feedback (as tool pantomime was affected, while tool use was not). It remains unclear why such a deficit pattern may emerge. Research has suggested that in patients with apraxia, transformation of visual information into intrinsic motor commands can result in spatially inaccurate initiation of non-praxis movements (Mutha et al., 2010). Here, comparisons of biomechanical data were made in survivors of left parietofrontal stroke (with and without apraxia) who had largely overlapping damage. Mutha et al. (2010) proposed that the spatial deficits in the apraxic group resulted from specific impairment of feed-forward control in the initial phases of the movement, whereas the patients were able to utilize the right hemisphere for final position accuracy. The relevance to the above-mentioned findings of Rapcsak and colleagues (1993) can be seen, as object-based actions may heavily rely on final position accuracy, and perhaps may utilize right hemispheric representation of actions. In the case of pantomime errors, final target accuracy is more vague and thus less capable of utilizing right hemispheric representations to establish final position accuracy, leading to continued spatial errors upon movement (Heilman et al., 1982; Hermsdorfer et al., 2006). Actual tool use may engage increased capacity to utilize right hemispheric motor control strategies to rely on final position sense instead of predictive feed-forward control (Yadav & Sainburg, 2011). However, not all apraxia patients demonstrate this behavioral benefit of object use. It has been suggested that incorporation of a tool into the body schema can be difficult in apraxia patients, a function possibly regulated by premotor (Rushworth et al., 2003) or parietal (Iriki et al., 1996) areas.

Because of the expanse of the injury seen in the case study of Rapcsak and colleagues (1993), it is perhaps unlikely that "neuroplasticity" per se was the mechanism underlying proposed right hemispheric engagement for certain praxis functions, but that the right hemisphere was capable of engaging "context-dependent execution of familiar, well-established action routines. . .," (p. 195), based on the patient's marked inability to perform unfamiliar actions. In this case, right hemisphere representations could presumably be recalled when necessary, enabling the performance of tasks learned prior to stroke.

Similar concepts have emerged from study of right-handed patients who have undergone callosotomy and are capable of performing tool use actions with the left hand (which would require right hemispheric operation; Lausberg et al., 2003a, 2003b).

Recent neuroimaging research has considered neuroplasticity in apraxia, emphasizing a role of the right hemisphere in recovery. The left parietal cortex has connectivity to right parietal and frontal areas (Cavada & Goldman-Rakic, 1989a, 1989b; McGuire et al., 1991), making it possible for right hemisphere parietal and/or premotor networks to engage in familiar praxis skills. The right premotor cortex also has descending connectivity to promote bilateral engagement of motor circuits (Brinkman & Kuypers, 1973). With these anatomical pathways in place, it is possible for the right hemisphere to be uniquely positioned to engage in adaptive neuroplasticity. In prior work, we explicitly sought to evaluate how functional neural networks might circumvent lesioned cortex in patients with ideomotor apraxia to promote normal tool use behaviors (Wheaton et al., 2008). Using EEG, patients with ideomotor apraxia resulting from stroke or corticobasal degeneration were assessed before and after relearning how to conduct correct pantomimes upon command. We evaluated cortical connectivity using coherence between electrodes overlying specific neural regions (Nunez et al., 1997). All findings were relative to healthy subjects, who showed the expected patterns of strong left parietofrontal network activation (Figure 14.4, top). The stroke patients (with left parietofrontal injury) showed significant increases in right parietofrontal network activity during pantomime after learning (Figure 14.4, middle). Patients with corticobasal degeneration showed marked increases in left parietal–right premotor networks (Figure 14.4, bottom). This finding strongly suggests that non-dominant right hemisphere networks may be engaged during the planning of tool use pantomimes as a result of learning how to perform pantomimes correctly. Though the goal of this study was not to formulate a specific training paradigm, it does demonstrate that right hemispheric neural networks may promote correct tool use behaviors in apraxia patients. Further longitudinal studies can build upon this proposal to validate the role of right hemispheric connectivity in long-term neuroplastic mechanisms and functional recovery.

Approaches From Outside the Apraxia Field

While findings of potential right hemisphere engagement during recovery are encouraging, there is little in identification of the *mechanism* of improvement. In other words, it is unclear how right hemispheric networks may operate to improve praxis function.

To improve our understanding of the basis of beneficial therapies, stronger proposals of the physiology of the systems damaged in apraxia are vital. This can help in identifying what rehabilitation protocols are effective and how they cause lasting changes in neural function. An example of this is seen in interhemispheric interactions in paresis resulting from stroke (Hoyer & Celnik, 2011). In rehabilitation of hemiparesis, some proposals place emphasis on the integrity of ipsilesional motor pathways and balance of ipsi-/contralesional hemispheric connectivity. Extended periods of brain stimulation to inhibit

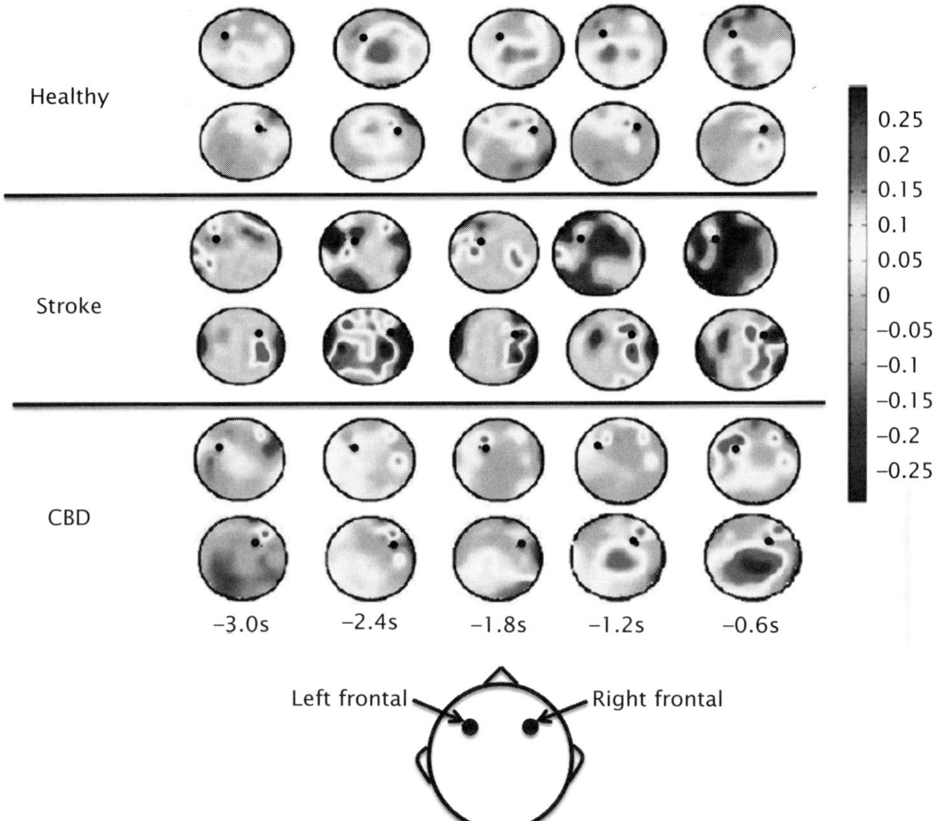

FIGURE 14.4 Head plots of a top-down view of the head (see inset for orientation) of whole brain EEG coherence relative to electrodes over left and right premotor cortex (as indicated by black dots) during motor planning (from 3 seconds before to 0.6 seconds before execution). Top shows coherence patterns in normal subjects, a stroke patient (middle), and corticobasal degeneration (CBD) patient (bottom). Coherence increases are shown in red; decreases in blue. Reprinted with permission from Wheaton et al. (2008), Elsevier. (see color insert)

one motor cortex can increase the excitability of the opposite motor cortex (Schambra et al., 2003), which is explained using a "disinhibition" model. Several studies since have illustrated the beneficial effects of inhibition of the contralesional hemisphere on promoting excitability of the ipsilesional hemisphere (Takeuchi et al., 2005; Fregni et al., 2006; Takeuchi et al., 2008). This work collectively would suggest a "maladaptive" role of the contralesional hemisphere in the functional changes occurring after paresis. Correcting this imbalance could result in improved therapeutic outcomes.

An interesting contrast to the maladaptive role of the contralateral hemisphere is in the emphasis of beneficial contralesional involvement. In capsular stroke, the contralesional hemisphere may promote higher-order mechanisms of recovery via contralesional pathways (Gerloff et al., 2006). Similar findings have been shown in highly affected stroke patients whose contralesional pre-motor cortices exert influence on the ipsilesional sensorimotor network to enhance motor function (Bestmann et al., 2010) and help support improved motor skill outcomes in well-recovered patients (Schaechter & Perdue, 2008).

While these findings are not conclusive or exclusive of other mechanisms, they do provide evidence that positive rehabilitation outcomes for apraxia after stroke can clearly be achieved. In the case of apraxia, it remains unclear if contralesional right hemisphere involvement would relate to enhanced or diminished function of damaged networks in the left hemisphere. As well, there is no evidence on whether affecting cortical excitability can be beneficial to apraxia. Asymmetric interhemispheric inhibition may be a principal physiological outcome of limb-kinetic apraxia (Okuma et al., 2000), which may be affected by patterns of hemispheric dominance (Heilman et al., 2000). In the case of ideomotor apraxia, one mechanism related to this might be in "releasing" motor plans in cases of absent, slow, or multistep movement sequences in which motor plans demonstrate decreased fluidity. However, left-hemisphere damaged patients with apraxia may develop a right premotor cortex that is capable of planning motor control for both the left and right limbs (Rushworth et al., 2003).

Brain stimulation protocols have shown motor planning effects via interhemispheric pathways. Using a paired-pulse TMS protocol, stimulation of the right caudal intraparietal sulcus can facilitate contralateral motor cortex (Koch et al., 2007, 2009). Such a modulation may be particularly robust for movements requiring visual feedback and spatial organization, which is modulated by right parietal areas (Rushworth et al., 2001; Chaminade et al., 2005). Similar networks could be beneficial in enhancing motor organization and planning in apraxia while undergoing therapeutic interventions, an option yet to be ruled out in the literature. Indeed, promising evidence has demonstrated that transcranial direct current stimulation of the inferior parietal lobule facilitates matching of hand gestures in healthy subjects (Weiss et al., 2013). Such evidence opens a window into future studies using stimulation to improve praxis performance in patients with apraxia.

In cognitive-motor functions, research has demonstrated benefits of contralesional- and ipsilesional-driven therapies to enhance outcomes in aphasia (for a review, see Schlaug et al., 2011). Therapies designed to promote improved speech production by shifting lateralization of speech from the left to the right hemisphere have shown promise (Crosson et al., 2007, 2009). Findings of potential right hemisphere engagement during recovery in aphasia are promising for the potential success of similar approaches in apraxia. Utilizing brain stimulation protocols alongside therapy has shown promising results (Barwood et al., 2012; Naeser et al., 2011, 2012). Sadly, in apraxia research, efforts in establishing stronger clinico-anatomical correlates while evaluating promising neuroplasticity-driven therapies (such as stated above) are still immature.

Future Directions in Neuroplasticity and Recovery

The Influence of Motor Learning and/or Recall

While apraxia remains a deficit of skilled use of the upper extremities, there is room to discuss the nature and mechanisms of the deficits in clearer terms. One concept that is being explored is the role of motor learning and recall. As far back as 1975, studies revealed that left-hemisphere lesioned patients with apraxia (compared to left-hemisphere lesioned non-apraxics) show a diminished rate of learning and notably diminished recall of a novel motor task (Heilman et al., 1975). Consideration of motor recall is an area that should be further developed. Recent research has begun to develop this topic (Dovern et al., 2011). In this study, investigators utilized a serial reaction time task, which showed incidental learning over repeated sessions in patients with and without apraxia, but patients with apraxia showed diminished explicit recall of the incidentally learned task (Figure 14.5). Diminished recall was associated with lesions involving the left dorsal premotor cortex. The suggestion is that incidental motor learning training may be beneficial and that automatic retrieval (rather than intentional retrieval) of skilled action may improve recall of developed action representations after injury. One of the core difficulties in apraxia is in developing therapies that will enable recall of specific skilled actions and concepts that one has developed over the life span (Buxbaum et al., 2008). As was proposed in the review by Buxbaum and colleagues (2008), implicit skillful motor learning of praxis could enhance praxis function and become a route to parietofrontal mechanisms of automatic retrieval of action sequences. Research has shown that patients with apraxia are impaired at motor control (anticipatory fingertip force during a lift) of familiar objects, but could develop proper motor control for novel object movements comparable to healthy subjects without verbal instruction (Dawson et al., 2010). Similarly, patients with apraxia may have impaired habitual actions to familiar tools, as novel actions to familiar tools can be

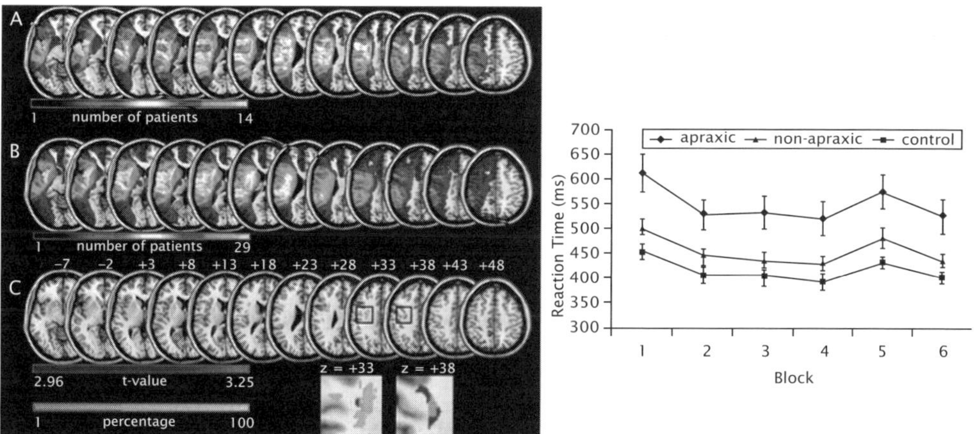

FIGURE 14.5 Left: Lesion patterns of apraxic and non-apraxic patients and their relation to the area in the dorsal premotor cortex associated with impaired intentional retrieval of sequence items (in patients with unimpaired incidental sequence-specific learning). A, B: Lesion overlays of the patients with apraxia ($n = 14$, A) and without apraxia ($n = 29$, B). Color bars indicate the number of patients with a lesion in the region that is colored, respectively. C: A region within the dorsal premotor cortex was shown to be affected more often in apraxic compared with non-apraxic patients (areas marked with orange). Right: Average group RTs for the six blocks of the SRT paradigm. Average RT data with standard error bars for the apraxic patients (black diamonds), non-apraxic patients (dark gray triangles), and healthy control subjects (light gray squares) across the SRT paradigm. Blocks 1–4 and 6 contain the sequence to be learned, while block 5 (transfer block) contains another similar complex sequence. Reprinted with permission from Dovern et al. (2011), Society for Neuroscience.

successfully developed (Sunderland et al., 2013). Such findings relate well to the work suggesting that internal models of action are damaged in familiar object-related actions in patients with apraxia (Buxbaum et al., 2005). Ongoing studies should carefully address how motor learning may develop in apraxia, and how generalizable these findings are to enhance functional rehabilitation outcomes.

Prior work may indicate mechanisms involved during implicit learning of motor sequences. Honda and colleagues (1998) developed a serial reaction time task that assessed for implicit learning of a motor sequence, followed by an explicit learning phase (Honda et al., 1998). While both implicit and explicit learning were recognized, a core neuroanatomical finding (using positron emission tomography) showed involvement of the bilateral parietofrontal network during explicit recall. This differs from the lesion-based analysis of Dovern et al. (2011), which related impairments of explicit recall in apraxia to left dorsal premotor cortex. At any rate, this may suggest a mechanism of a left-hemispheric apraxia patient utilizing non-lesioned (right hemispheric) brain areas using explicit recall (Wheaton et al., 2008). Paradigms could be developed to take advantage of how action encoding could utilize intact brain areas to recall actions that are similar to seen actions in an effort to automatically retrieve action subsets (Costantini et al., 2008). It should be borne in mind, however, that priming action subsets as a tool to engage action planning circuits in patients with apraxia may be detrimental to action production and identification for new tools, by promoting action interference (Desmarais et al., 2007). Thus, further investigation of potential differences in the effects of implicit priming versus explicit recall is warranted.

The Role of Right Hemisphere in Action Learning and Recall

Several studies have considered the involvement of learning the use of novel tools in order to isolate a possible role for the right hemisphere in acquiring and storing tool knowledge. One such study involved the use of multiple novel tools that subjects had to learn over several days of training, with pre- and post-training fMRI (Weisberg et al., 2007). The fMRI findings not only demonstrated an increased parietofrontal response pre- to post-training, but also a diminished response in the bilateral lateral fusiform gyri. While one interpretation of these findings may be related to the effects of repetition suppression, they might also relate to skilled task retrieval. Our laboratory sought to elaborate more on this point. In an EEG experiment, subjects were trained on the use of a new tool that was learned either through visual demonstration or motor practice (Figure 14.6). When performing pantomimes of the new tool after visual learning, strong right temporo-parieto-occipital activation was seen, compared to largely left parietal activity for new tools learned with motor practice (Mizelle et al., 2011). This suggests that the learning (or recall) of tool function that is not based in kinematics utilizes right hemispheric representations of action. Importantly, while all subjects showed correct pantomime to the tools, these activations were seen during motor planning, which underscores that right temporoparietal areas

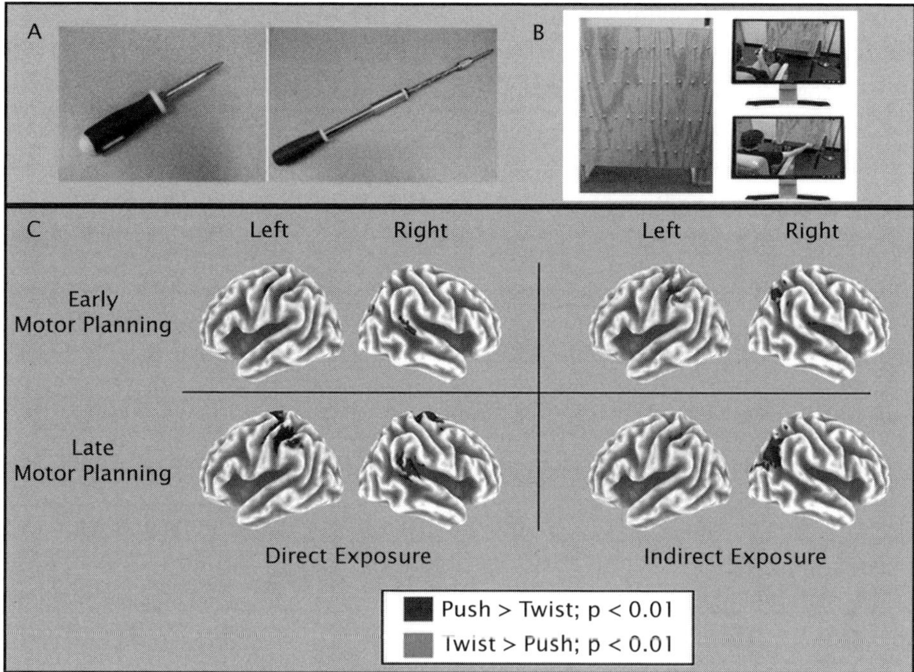

FIGURE 14.6 A: Two screwdrivers used in the present study, familiar twist (left) and novel push (right). B: The practice board for direct exposure (left) and video presentations for both tools (right). C: Significant (*p* <.01) activation differences for the comparison of familiar versus novel screwdrivers for each exposure type. In all panels, greater activation for the push screwdriver is shown in blue and for the twist screwdriver in red. Reprinted with permission from Mizelle et al. (2011), MIT Press.

perhaps encode action goals in skill development (Quallo et al., 2009; Van Overwalle & Baetens, 2009), and could play a significant role in performance of praxis and possibly recovery.

Similarly, studies have shown that tools which are unfamiliar or rarely used are encoded in similar right hemispheric areas (Vingerhoets et al., 2011). Utilization of right hemispheric stored concepts of action may be a neural process involved in task performance in patients with apraxia who have learned how to perform skilled praxis movements through practice (Wheaton and Hallett, 2007; Wheaton et al., 2008).

A Role for the Cerebellum?

A review of neural substrates of motor learning considers that widespread parietofrontal neural networks also coordinate with basal ganglia and cerebellum. Data strongly implicate the importance of the cerebellum in apraxia (Higuchi et al., 2007), and the cerebellum likely is a strong candidate for utilizing learned motor strategies in apraxia recovery (Steele & Penhune, 2010). This is rooted in the observation that the cerebellum (and basal ganglia) play vital roles in coordinating spatial and motor parameters necessary in motor sequence learning (Hikosaka et al., 2002). Explicit retrieval of a motor skill during actual use more readily relies on cerebellar activation compared to pantomime or imagined use

(Imamizu et al., 2007; Imamizu & Kawato, 2009). Interestingly, actual use of a tool compared to pantomime (and logically imagination) does require a differential level of motor skill (Senkfor, 2008; Hermsdorfer et al., 2012, 2013). It is possible that internal model formation (through implicit learning) could additionally involve cerebellar mechanisms to optimize behaviors based on contextual action goals (Imamizu et al., 2003, 2007; Imamizu & Kawato, 2009). If indeed the cerebellum is needed in recalling optimized motor strategies, therapy that emphasizes highly developed cerebellar representations of action may be beneficial to promoting motor strategies lost in cortical strokes that cause apraxia. Consideration of the influence that the cerebellum has on cortical neuroplastic processes in patients with apraxia remains to be, and should be, established.

Conclusions

Due to the spectrum of deficits in higher-order motor function, apraxia remains a compelling area of research. Much work has been done in the field of apraxia; however, a true knowledge of the mechanisms of neuroplasticity remains enigmatic. Unlike other deficits after stroke that have better developed proposals that can relate to rehabilitation efforts, much work remains in the field of apraxia. As research progresses, careful consideration of how recovery occurs on a neural systems level can help in guiding therapies and in developing a deeper understanding of the neural processes that lead to functional improvements, whether natural or through rehabilitation. This necessitates a broader understanding of functional, physiological, and anatomical studies to develop a stronger understanding of the potential for neuroplasticity in apraxia. Of special interest should be the careful examination of the impact of motor learning mechanisms on rehabilitation, which could tie together issues of neuroplasticity and right hemispheric involvement in recovery. Developing stronger clinico-anatomical correlates and neurophysiology of recovery will be essential in advancing the field.

Acknowledgment

Special thanks to Kenneth M. Heilman, MD, FAAN, for assistance in writing this chapter and to Mark Hallett, MD, for introducing me to the field of apraxia many years ago.

References

Barwood, C. H., Murdoch, B. E., Whelan, B. M., Lloyd, D., Riek, S., O'Sullivan, J. D., Coulthard, A., & Wong, A. (2012). Improved receptive and expressive language abilities in nonfluent aphasic stroke patients after application of rTMS: An open protocol case series. *Brain Stimul, 5*, 274–286.

Basso, A., Capitani, E., Della Sala, S., Laiacona, M., & Spinnler, H. (1987). Ideomotor apraxia: A study of initial severity. *Acta Neurol Scand, 76*, 142–146.

Bestmann, S., Swayne, O., Blankenburg, F., Ruff, C. C., Teo, J., Weiskopf, N., Driver, J., Rothwell, J. C., & Ward, N. S. (2010). The role of contralesional dorsal premotor cortex after stroke as studied with concurrent TMS-fMRI. *J Neurosci, 30*, 11926–11937.

Bohlhalter, S., Hattori, N., Wheaton, L., Fridman, E., Shamim, E. A., Garraux, G., & Hallett, M. (2009). Gesture subtype-dependent left lateralization of praxis planning: an event-related fMRI study. *Cereb Cortex*, 19, 1256–1262.

Bohlhalter, S., Vanbellingen, T., Bertschi, M., Wurtz, P., Cazzoli, D., Nyffeler, T., Hess, C. W., & Muri, R. (2011). Interference with gesture production by theta burst stimulation over left inferior frontal cortex. *Clin Neurophysiol*, 122, 1197–1202.

Borroni, B., Garibotto, V., Agosti, C., Brambati, S.M., Bellelli, G., Gasparotti, R., Padovani, A., & Perani, D. (2008). White matter changes in corticobasal degeneration syndrome and correlation with limb apraxia. *Arch Neurol*, 65, 796–801.

Brinkman, J., & Kuypers, H. G (1973). Cerebral control of contralateral and ipsilateral arm, hand and finger movements in the split-brain rhesus monkey. *Brain*, 96, 653–674.

Buxbaum, L. J. (2001). Ideomotor apraxia: A call to action. *Neurocase*, 7, 445–458.

Buxbaum, L. J., Haaland, K. Y., Hallett, M., Wheaton, L., Heilman, K. M., Rodriguez, A., & Gonzalez Rothi, L. J. (2008). Treatment of limb apraxia: Moving forward to improved action. *Am J Phys Med Rehabil*, 87, 149–161.

Buxbaum, L. J., Johnson-Frey, S. H., & Bartlett-Williams, M. (2005). Deficient internal models for planning hand-object interactions in apraxia. *Neuropsychologia*, 43, 917–929.

Buxbaum, L. J., & Kalenine, S. (2010). Action knowledge, visuomotor activation, and embodiment in the two action systems. *Ann NY Acad Sci*, 1191, 201–218.

Buxbaum, L. J., & Saffran, E. M. (2002). Knowledge of object manipulation and object function: Dissociations in apraxic and nonapraxic subjects. *Brain Lang*, 82, 179–199.

Buxbaum, L. J., Sirigu, A., Schwartz, M. F., & Klatzky, R. (2003). Cognitive representations of hand posture in ideomotor apraxia. *Neuropsychologia*, 41, 1091–1113.

Catani, M., & ffytche, D. H. (2005). The rises and falls of disconnection syndromes. *Brain*, 128, 2224–2239.

Catani, M., & Thiebaut de Schotten, M. (2012). The clinicoanatomical correlational method. In M. Catani & M. Thiebaut de Schotten (Eds.), *Atlas of human brain connections* (pp 55–65). Oxford: Oxford University Press.

Cavada, C., & Goldman-Rakic, P. S. (1989a). Posterior parietal cortex in rhesus monkey: I. Parcellation of areas based on distinctive limbic and sensory corticocortical connections. *J Comp Neurol*, 287, 393–421.

Cavada, C., & Goldman-Rakic, P. S. (1989b). Posterior parietal cortex in rhesus monkey: II. Evidence for segregated corticocortical networks linking sensory and limbic areas with the frontal lobe. *J Comp Neurol* 287, 422–445.

Chainay, H., & Humphreys, G. W. (2003). Ideomotor and ideational apraxia in corticobasal degeneration: A case study. *Neurocase*, 9, 177–186.

Chaminade, T., Meltzoff, A. N., & Decety, J. (2005). An fMRI study of imitation: Action representation and body schema. *Neuropsychologia*, 43, 115–127.

Chestnut, C., & Haaland, K. Y. (2008) Functional significance of ipsilesional motor deficits after unilateral stroke. *Arch Phys Med Rehabil*, 89, 62–68.

Cordato, N. J., Halliday, G. M., McCann, H., Davies, L., Williamson, P., Fulham, M., & Morris, J. G. (2001). Corticobasal syndrome with tau pathology. *Mov Disord*, 16, 656–667.

Costantini, M., Committeri, G., & Galati, G. (2008). Effector- and target-independent representation of observed actions: Evidence from incidental repetition priming. *Exp Brain Res*, 188, 341–351.

Crosson, B., Fabrizio, K. S., Singletary, F., Cato, M. A., Wierenga, C. E., Parkinson, R. B., Sherod, M. E., Moore, A. B., Ciampitti, M., Holiway, B., Leon, S., Rodriguez, A., Kendall, D. L., Levy, I. F., & Rothi, L. J. (2007). Treatment of naming in nonfluent aphasia through manipulation of intention and attention: A phase 1 comparison of two novel treatments. *J Int Neuropsychol Soc*, 13, 582–594.

Crosson, B., Moore, A. B., McGregor, K. M., Chang, Y. L., Benjamin, M., Gopinath, K., Sherod, M. E., Wierenga, C. E., Peck, K. K., Briggs, R. W., Rothi, L. J., & White, K. D. (2009). Regional changes in word-production laterality after a naming treatment designed to produce a rightward shift in frontal activity. *Brain Lang*, 111, 73–85.

Dawson, A. M., Buxbaum, L. J., & Duff, S. V. (2010). The impact of left hemisphere stroke on force control with familiar and novel objects: Neuroanatomic substrates and relationship to apraxia. *Brain Res*, 1317, 124–136.

Derouesne, C., Lagha-Pierucci, S., Thibault, S., Baudouin-Madec, V., & Lacomblez, L. (2000). Apraxic disturbances in patients with mild to moderate Alzheimer's disease. *Neuropsychologia*, 38, 1760–1769.

Desmarais, G., Pensa, M. C., Dixon, M. J., & Roy, E. A. (2007). The importance of object similarity in the production and identification of actions associated with objects. *J Int Neuropsychol Soc*, 13, 1021–1034.

Donkervoort, M., Dekker, J., van den Ende, E., Stehmann-Saris, J. C., & Deelman, B. G. (2000). Prevalence of apraxia among patients with a first left hemisphere stroke in rehabilitation centres and nursing homes. *Clin Rehabil*, 14, 130–136.

Dovern, A., Fink, G. R., Saliger, J., Karbe, H., Koch, I., & Weiss, P. H. (2011) Apraxia impairs intentional retrieval of incidentally acquired motor knowledge. *J Neurosci*, 31, 8102–8108.

Dovern, A., Fink, G. R., & Weiss, P. H. (2012). Diagnosis and treatment of upper limb apraxia. *J Neurol*, 259, 1269–1283.

ffytche, D. H., & Catani, M. (2005) Beyond localization: From hodology to function. *Phil Trans Roy Soc London B*, 360, 767–779.

Fogassi, L., Gallese, V., Buccino, G., Craighero. L., Fadiga, L., & Rizzolatti, G. (2001). Cortical mechanism for the visual guidance of hand grasping movements in the monkey: A reversible inactivation study. *Brain* 124, 571–586.

Foundas, A. L., Macauley, B. L., Raymer, A. M., Maher, L. M., Heilman, K. M., & Gonzalez Rothi, L. J. (1995). Ecological implications of limb apraxia: Evidence from mealtime behavior. *J Int Neuropsychol Soc*, 1, 62–66.

Fregni, F., Boggio, P. S., Valle, A. C., Rocha, R. R., Duarte, J., Ferreira, M. J., Wagner, T., Fecteau, S., Rigonatti, S. P., Riberto, M., Freedman, S. D., & Pascual-Leone, A. (2006). A sham-controlled trial of a 5-day course of repetitive transcranial magnetic stimulation of the unaffected hemisphere in stroke patients. *Stroke*, 37, 2115–2122.

Gallese, V., Murata, A., Kaseda, M., Niki, N., & Sakata, H. (1994) Deficit of hand preshaping after muscimol injection in monkey parietal cortex. *Neuroreport* 5, 1525–1529.

Gerloff, C., Bushara, K., Sailer, A., Wassermann, E. M., Chen, R., Matsuoka, T., Waldvogel, D., Wittenberg, G. F., Ishii, K., Cohen, L. G., & Hallett, M. (2006). Multimodal imaging of brain reorganization in motor areas of the contralesional hemisphere of well recovered patients after capsular stroke. *Brain*, 129, 791–808.

Geschwind, N. (1965). Disconnexion syndromes in animals and man. II. *Brain*, 88, 585–644.

Goldenberg, G. (2003). Pantomime of object use: A challenge to cerebral localization of cognitive function. *NeuroImage*, 20(Suppl 1), S101–106.

Goldenberg, G., & Hagmann, S. (1998). Tool use and mechanical problem solving in apraxia. *Neuropsychologia*, 36, 581–589.

Goldenberg, G., Hermsdorfer, J., Glindemann, R., Rorden, C., & Karnath, H. O. (2007). Pantomime of tool use depends on integrity of left inferior frontal cortex. *Cereb Cortex*, 17, 2769–2776.

Goldenberg, G., Laimgruber, K., & Hermsdorfer, J. (2001). Imitation of gestures by disconnected hemispheres. *Neuropsychologia*, 39, 1432–1443.

Grafton, S. T., & Hamilton, A. F. (2007). Evidence for a distributed hierarchy of action representation in the brain. *Hum Mov Sci*, 26, 590–616.

Haaland, K. Y., Harrington, D. L., & Knight, R. T. (2000). Neural representations of skilled movement. *Brain*, 123(Pt 11), 2306–2313.

Hamilton, J. M., Haaland, K. Y., Adair, J. C., & Brandt, J. (2003). Ideomotor limb apraxia in Huntington's disease: Implications for corticostriate involvement. *Neuropsychologia*, 41, 614–621.

Hanna-Pladdy, B., Daniels, S. K., Fieselman, M. A., Thompson, K., Vasterling, J. J., Heilman, K. M., & Foundas, A. L. (2001a). Praxis lateralization: Errors in right and left hemisphere stroke. *Cortex*, 37, 219–230.

Hanna-Pladdy, B., Heilman, K. M., & Foundas, A. L. (2001b). Cortical and subcortical contributions to ideomotor apraxia: Analysis of task demands and error types. *Brain*, 124, 2513–2527.

Hanna-Pladdy, B., Heilman, K. M., & Foundas, A. L. (2003). Ecological implications of ideomotor apraxia: Evidence from physical activities of daily living. *Neurology*, 60, 487–490.

Heilman, K. M., & Gonzalez Rothi, L. J. (2003). Apraxia. In K. M. Heilman & E. Valenstein (Eds.), *Clinical neurophysiology* (pp. 215–235). New York: Oxford University Press.

Heilman, K. M., Maher, L. M., Greenwald, M. L., & Rothi, L. J. (1997). Conceptual apraxia from lateralized lesions. *Neurology*, 49, 457–464.

Heilman, K. M., Meador, K. J., & Loring, D. W. (2000). Hemispheric asymmetries of limb-kinetic apraxia: A loss of deftness. *Neurology*, 55, 523–526.

Heilman, K. M., Rothi, L. J., & Valenstein, E. (1982). Two forms of ideomotor apraxia. *Neurology*, 32, 342–346.

Heilman, K. M., Schwartz, H. D., & Geschwind, N. (1975). Defective motor learning in ideomotor apraxia. *Neurology*, 25, 1018–1020.

Hermsdorfer, J., Hentze, S., & Goldenberg, G. (2006). Spatial and kinematic features of apraxic movement depend on the mode of execution. *Neuropsychologia*, 44, 1642–1652.

Hermsdorfer, J., Li, Y., Randerath, J., Goldenberg, G., & Johannsen, L. (2012). Tool use without a tool: Kinematic characteristics of pantomiming as compared to actual use and the effect of brain damage. *Exp Brain Res*, 218, 201–214.

Hermsdorfer, J., Li, Y., Randerath, J., Roby-Brami, A., & Goldenberg, G. (2013). Tool use kinematics across different modes of execution: Implications for action representation and apraxia. *Cortex*, 49, 184–199.

Higuchi, S., Imamizu, H., & Kawato, M. (2007). Cerebellar activity evoked by common tool-use execution and imagery tasks: An fMRI study. *Cortex*, 43, 350–358.

Hikosaka, O., Nakamura, K., Sakai, K., & Nakahara, H. (2002). Central mechanisms of motor skill learning. *Curr Opin Neurobiol*, 12, 217–222.

Honda, M., Deiber, M. P., Ibanez, V., Pascual-Leone, A., Zhuang, P., & Hallett, M. (1998). Dynamic cortical involvement in implicit and explicit motor sequence learning: A PET study. *Brain*, 121(Pt 11), 2159–2173.

Hoyer, E. H., & Celnik, P. A. (2011). Understanding and enhancing motor recovery after stroke using transcranial magnetic stimulation: *Restor Neurol Neurosc*, 29, 395–409.

Huey, E. D., Pardini, M., Cavanagh, A., Wassermann, E. M., Kapogiannis, D., Spina, S., Ghetti, B., & Grafman, J. (2009). Association of ideomotor apraxia with frontal gray matter volume loss in corticobasal syndrome. *Arch Neurol*, 66, 1274–1280.

Hummel, F. C., & Cohen, L.G. (2005). Drivers of brain plasticity. *Curr Opin Neurol*, 18, 667–674.

Imamizu, H., & Kawato, M. (2009) Brain mechanisms for predictive control by switching internal models: Implications for higher-order cognitive functions. *Psychological Res*, 73, 527–544.

Imamizu, H., Kuroda, T., Miyauchi, S., Yoshioka, T., & Kawato, M. (2003). Modular organization of internal models of tools in the human cerebellum. *P Natl Acad Sci USA* 100, 5461–5466.

Imamizu, H., Sugimoto, N., Osu, R., Tsutsui, K., Sugiyama, K., Wada, Y., & Kawato, M. (2007). Explicit contextual information selectively contributes to predictive switching of internal models. *Exp Brain Res*, 181, 395–408.

Imazu, S., Sugio, T., Tanaka, S., & Inui, T. (2007). Differences between actual and imagined usage of chopsticks: an fMRI study. *Cortex*, 43, 301–307.

Iriki, A., Tanaka, M., & Iwamura, Y. (1996). Coding of modified body schema during tool use by macaque postcentral neurones. *Neuroreport* 7, 2325–2330.

Johnson-Frey, S. H., Maloof, F. R., Newman-Norlund, R., Farrer, C., Inati, S., & Grafton, S. T. (2003). Actions or hand-object interactions? Human inferior frontal cortex and action observation. *Neuron*, 39, 1053–1058.

Johnson-Frey, S. H., Newman-Norlund, R., & Grafton, S. T. (2005). A distributed left hemisphere network active during planning of everyday tool use skills. *Cereb Cortex*, 15, 681–695.

Kamm, C. P., Heldner, M. R., Vanbellingen, T., Mattle, H. P., Muri, R., & Bohlhalter, S. (2012). Limb apraxia in multiple sclerosis: Prevalence and impact on manual dexterity and activities of daily living. *Arch Phys Med Rehabil*, 93, 1081–1085.

Kertesz, A., & Ferro, J. M. (1984). Lesion size and location in ideomotor apraxia. *Brain* 107(Pt 3), 921–933.

Koch, G., Fernandez Del Olmo, M., Cheeran, B., Ruge, D., Schippling, S., Caltagirone, C., & Rothwell, J. C. (2007). Focal stimulation of the posterior parietal cortex increases the excitability of the ipsilateral motor cortex. *J Neurosci*, 27, 6815–6822.

Koch, G., Ruge, D., Cheeran, B., Fernandez Del Olmo, M., Pecchioli, C., Marconi, B., Versace, V., Lo Gerfo, E., Torriero, S., Oliveri, M., Caltagirone, C., & Rothwell, J. C. (2009). TMS activation of interhemispheric pathways between the posterior parietal cortex and the contralateral motor cortex. *J Physiol*, 587, 4281–4292.

Lausberg, H., Cruz, R. F., Kita, S., Zaidel, E., & Ptito, A. (2003a). Pantomime to visual presentation of objects: Left hand dyspraxia in patients with complete callosotomy. *Brain* 126, 343–360.

Lausberg, H., Kita, S., Zaidel, E., & Ptito, A. (2003b). Split-brain patients neglect left personal space during right-handed gestures. *Neuropsychologia*, 41, 1317–1329.

Leiguarda, R. C., & Marsden, C. D. (2000) Limb apraxias: Higher-order disorders of sensorimotor integration. *Brain*, 123(Pt 5), 860–879.

Leiguarda, R. C., Pramstaller, P. P., Merello, M., Starkstein, S., Lees, A. J., & Marsden, C. D. (1997). Apraxia in Parkinson's disease, progressive supranuclear palsy, multiple system atrophy and neuroleptic-induced parkinsonism. *Brain*, 120(Pt 1), 75–90.

Liepmann, H. (1900). Das Krankheitsbild der Apraxie (motorischen/Asymbolie). *Mon Psychiatr Neurol*, 8, 15–44.

Liepmann, H. (1905). Die linke Hemisphare und das Handeln. *Munchen Med Wochen*, 49, 2322–2326, 2365–2378.

Liepmann, H. (1907). Ein Fall von linksseitiger Agraphie und Apraxie bei reshtsseitiger Lahmung. *J Psychol Neurol*, 10, 214–227.

McGuire, P. K., Bates, J. F., & Goldman-Rakic, P. S. (1991). Interhemispheric integration: I. Symmetry and convergence of the corticocortical connections of the left and the right principal sulcus (PS) and the left and the right supplementary motor area (SMA) in the rhesus monkey. *Cereb Cortex*, 1, 390–407.

Migliaccio, R., Agosta, F., Toba, M. N., Samri, D., Corlier, F., de Souza, L. C., Chupin, M., Sharman, M., Gorno-Tempini, M. L., Dubois, B., Filippi, M., & Bartolomeo, P. (2012). Brain networks in posterior cortical atrophy: A single case tractography study and literature review. *Cortex*, 48, 1298–1309.

Mizelle, J. C., Kelly, R. L., & Wheaton, L. A. (2013). Ventral encoding of functional affordances: A neural pathway for identifying errors in action. *Brain Cogn*, 82, 274–282.

Mizelle, J. C., Tang, T., Pirouz, N., & Wheaton, L. A. (2011). Forming tool use representations: A neurophysiological investigation into tool exposure. *J Cogn Neurosci*, 23, 2920–2934.

Mizelle, J. C., & Wheaton, L. A. (2010a). Neural activation for conceptual identification of correct versus incorrect tool-object pairs. *Brain Res*, 1354, 100–112.

Mizelle, J. C., & Wheaton, L. A. (2010b). Why is that hammer in my coffee: A multimodal imaging investigation of contextually-based tool understanding. *Front Human Neurosci* 4, 10.3389/fnhum.2010.00233.

Mutha, P. K., Sainburg, R. L., & Haaland, K. Y. (2010). Coordination deficits in ideomotor apraxia during visually targeted reaching reflect impaired visuomotor transformations. *Neuropsychologia*, 48, 3855–3867.

Naeser, M. A., Martin, P. I., Ho, M., Treglia, E., Kaplan, E., Bashir, S., & Pascual-Leone, A. (2012). Transcranial magnetic stimulation and aphasia rehabilitation. *Arch Phys Med Rehabil*, 93, S26–34.

Naeser, M. A., Martin, P. I., Theoret, H., Kobayashi, M., Fregni, F., Nicholas, M., Tormos, J. M., Steven, M. S., Baker, E. H., & Pascual-Leone, A. (2011). TMS suppression of right pars triangularis, but not pars opercularis, improves naming in aphasia. *Brain Lang*, 119, 206–213.

Nunez, P. L., Srinivasan, R., Westdorp, A. F., Wijesinghe, R. S., Tucker, D. M., Silberstein, R. B., & Cadusch, P. J. (1997). EEG coherency. I: Statistics, reference electrode, volume conduction, Laplacians, cortical imaging, and interpretation at multiple scales. *Electroencephalogr Clin Neurophysiol*, 103, 499–515.

Ochipa, C., Rothi, L. J., & Heilman, K. M. (1992). Conceptual apraxia in Alzheimer's disease. *Brain*, 115(Pt 4), 1061–1071.

Okuma, Y., Urabe, T., Mochizuki, H., Miwa, H., Shimo, Y., Mori, H., & Mizuno, Y. (2000). Asymmetric cortico-cortical inhibition in patients with progressive limb-kinetic apraxia. *Acta neurologica Scandinavica*, 102, 244–248.

Poole, J. L., Sadek, J., & Haaland, K. Y. (2009). Ipsilateral deficits in 1-handed shoe tying after left or right hemisphere stroke. *Arch Phys Med Rehabil* 90, 1800–1805.

Quallo, M. M., Price, C. J., Ueno, K., Asamizuya, T., Cheng, K., Lemon, R. N., & Iriki, A. (2009). Gray and white matter changes associated with tool-use learning in macaque monkeys. *Proc Natl Acad Sci USA*, 106, 18379–18384.

Rapcsak, S. Z., Ochipa, C., Beeson, P. M., & Rubens, A. B. (1993). Praxis and the right hemisphere. *Brain Cogn*, 23, 181–202.

Roy, E. A., Heath, M., Westwood, D., Schweizer, T. A., Dixon, M. J., Black, S. E., Kalbfleisch, L., Barbour, K., & Square, P. A. (2000). Task demands and limb apraxia in stroke. *Brain Cogn*, 44, 253–279.

Rushworth, M. F., Johansen-Berg, H., Gobel, S. M., & Devlin, J. T. (2003). The left parietal and premotor cortices: Motor attention and selection. *Neuroimage*, 20(Suppl 1), S89–100.

Rushworth, M. F., Krams, M., & Passingham, R. E. (2001). The attentional role of the left parietal cortex: The distinct lateralization and localization of motor attention in the human brain. *J Cogn Neurosci*, 13, 698–710.

Salter, J. E., Roy, E. A., Black, S. E., Joshi, A., & Almeida, Q. (2004). Gestural imitation and limb apraxia in corticobasal degeneration. *Brain Cogn*, 55, 400–402.

Schaechter, J. D., & Perdue, K.L. (2008). Enhanced cortical activation in the contralesional hemisphere of chronic stroke patients in response to motor skill challenge. *Cerebral cortex*, 18, 638–647.

Schambra, H. M., Sawaki, L., & Cohen, L. G. (2003). Modulation of excitability of human motor cortex (M1) by 1 Hz transcranial magnetic stimulation of the contralateral M1. *Clinical Neurophysiol*, 114, 130–133.

Schlaug, G., Marchina, S., & Wan, C. Y. (2011). The use of non-invasive brain stimulation techniques to facilitate recovery from post-stroke aphasia. *Neuropsychol Rev*, 21, 288–301.

Schnider, A., Hanlon, R. E., Alexander, D. N., & Benson, D. F. (1997). Ideomotor apraxia: behavioral dimensions and neuroanatomical basis. *Brain Lang*, 58, 125–136.

Senkfor, A. J. (2008). Memory for pantomimed actions versus actions with real objects. *Cortex*, 44, 820–833.

Stamenova, V., Black, S. E., & Roy, E. A. (2011). A model-based approach to long-term recovery of limb apraxia after stroke. *J Clin Exp Neuropsyc*, 33, 954–971.

Stamenova, V., Roy, E. A., & Black, S. E. (2010). Associations and dissociations of transitive and intransitive gestures in left and right hemisphere stroke patients. *Brain Cognition*, 72, 483–490.

Steele, C. J., & Penhune, V. B. (2010). Specific increases within global decreases: A functional magnetic resonance imaging investigation of five days of motor sequence learning. *J Neurosci*, 30, 8332–8341.

Sunderland, A., Wilkins, L., Dineen, R., & Dawson, S. E. (2013). Tool-use and the left hemisphere: What is lost in ideomotor apraxia? *Brain Cogn*, 81, 183–192.

Takeuchi, N., Chuma, T., Matsuo, Y., Watanabe, I., & Ikoma, K. (2005). Repetitive transcranial magnetic stimulation of contralesional primary motor cortex improves hand function after stroke. *Stroke*, 36, 2681–2686.

Takeuchi, N., Tada, T., Toshima, M., Chuma, T., Matsuo, Y., & Ikoma, K. (2008). Inhibition of the unaffected motor cortex by 1 Hz repetitive transcranical magnetic stimulation enhances motor performance and training effect of the paretic hand in patients with chronic stroke. *J Rehabil Med*, 40, 298–303.

Van Overwalle, F., & Baetens, K. (2009). Understanding others' actions and goals by mirror and mentalizing systems: a meta-analysis. *NeuroImage*, 48, 564–584.

Vanbellingen, T., & Bohlhalter, S. (2011). Apraxia in neurorehabilitation: Classification, assessment and treatment. *NeuroRehabilitation*, 28, 91–98.

Vanbellingen, T., Kersten, B., Van de Winckel, A., Bellion, M., Baronti, F., Muri, R., & Bohlhalter, S. (2011). A new bedside test of gestures in stroke: The apraxia screen of TULIA (AST). *J Neurol Neurosur Ps*, 82, 389–392.

Vanbellingen, T., Kersten, B., Van Hemelrijk, B., Van de Winckel, A., Bertschi, M., Muri, R., De Weerdt, W., & Bohlhalter, S. (2010). Comprehensive assessment of gesture production: A new test of upper limb apraxia (TULIA). *Eur J Neurol*, 17(1), 59–66.

Vingerhoets, G., Vandekerckhove, E., Honore, P., Vandemaele, P., & Achten, E. (2011). Neural correlates of pantomiming familiar and unfamiliar tools: action semantics versus mechanical problem solving? *Hum Brain Mapp*, 32, 905–918.

Weisberg, J., van Turennout, M., & Martin, A. (2007). A neural system for learning about object function. *Cereb Cortex*, 17, 513–521.

Weiss, P. H., Achilles, E. I., Moos, K., Hesse, M. D., Sparing, R., & Fink, G. R. (2013). Transcranial direct current stimulation (tDCS) of left parietal cortex facilitates gesture processing in healthy subjects. *J Neurosci*, 33, 19205–19211.

Weiss, P. H., & Fink, G. R. (2010). [Structural and functional neuroimaging of the pathophysiology of apraxia]. *Nervenarzt*, 81, 1444–1449.

Wheaton, L., Fridman, E., Bohlhalter, S., Vorbach, S., & Hallett, M. (2009). Left parietal activation related to planning, executing and suppressing praxis hand movements. *Clin Neurophysiol*, 120, 980–986.

Wheaton, L. A., Bohlhalter, S., Nolte, G., Shibasaki, H., Hattori, N., Fridman, E., Vorbach, S., Grafman, J., & Hallett, M. (2008.) Cortico-cortical networks in patients with ideomotor apraxia as revealed by EEG coherence analysis. *Neurosci Lett*, 433, 87–92.

Wheaton, L. A., & Hallett, M. (2007). Ideomotor apraxia: a review. *J Neurol Sci*, 260, 1–10.

Wheaton, L. A., Nolte, G., Bohlhalter, S., Fridman, E., & Hallett, M. (2005a). Synchronization of parietal and premotor areas during preparation and execution of praxis hand movements. *Clin Neurophysiol*, 116, 1382–1390.

Wheaton, L. A., Shibasaki, H., & Hallett, M. (2005b). Temporal activation pattern of parietal and premotor areas related to praxis movements. *Clin Neurophysiol*, 116, 1201–1212.

Wheaton, L. A., Yakota, S., & Hallett, M. (2005c). Posterior parietal negativity preceding self-paced praxis movements. *Exp Brain Res*, 163, 535–539.

Yadav, V., & Sainburg, R. L. (2011). Motor lateralization is characterized by a serial hybrid control scheme. *Neuroscience*, 196, 153–167.

Plasticity of Cognition and the New Emerging Technologies

15

Clinical Brain-Machine Interfaces

Surjo R. Soekadar, Leonardo G. Cohen,
and Niels Birbaumer

Introduction

Since the invention of electroencephalography (EEG) by Hans Berger (1929) in a quest for the substrates of mental activity, the idea of deciphering the underlying code to read out thoughts from brain activity has inspired numerous novelists and science-fiction writers. Berger's early observation that, for instance, modulations of occipital alpha oscillations (8–12 Hz) relate to visual perception (Chatrian et al., 1959) supported the idea of a modular architecture of the brain (Broca, 1861; Brodmann, 1913; Gall, 1835). Such topographic specificity was also found in the motor domain, where performance, imagination, and/or imitation of movements were found to be associated with modulations of brain oscillations, termed "sensorimotor rhythms" (SMRs, 8–15 Hz) (Pfurtscheller & Aranibar, 1979). These findings encouraged the assumption that in the future, the precise detection of mental processes across different domains would be possible, once the underlying codes were found and once the exact modules for each function were located. This would not only be important to test core hypotheses related to the principles and mechanisms of brain function, but also would open new doors to diagnose and treat neurological and/or mental disorders. Today, after almost 100 years of brain research, some remarkable progress toward this goal has been made; at the same time, many new and yet unanswered questions have evolved.

The development of real-time systems that can translate brain events into control signals of external devices, known today as brain-computer or brain-machine interfaces (BCI/BMI), is closely related to the evolution of computers capable of performing a large number of arithmetic operations and transformations in a short time. Besides such application, large-scale analysis and modeling of the functioning brain (Eliasmith et al., 2012; Hipp et al., 2012) became important frontiers in neuroscience where high-performance computers are indispensable. A few years after William Grey Walter and his colleagues developed the first automatic EEG frequency analyser in the 1960s (Walter, 1963; Walter et al., 1964), Barry Sterman's laboratory used this technique to train cats to produce SMR through operant (instrumental) conditioning (Wyrwicka & Sterman, 1968). In this experiment, production of SMR became continuously translated into sensory feedback, and increases were contingently rewarded. The finding that operant conditioning of brain activity, even of single cerebral cortical neurons (Fetz, 1969), was possible became the key principle on which the majority of current BCI/BMI systems are based, and this finding initiated extensive research efforts investigating the link between brain physiology and behavior. In 1973, Jacques Vidal presented a first system that was capable of translating brain events into computer control signals, naming it "brain-computer interface" (BCI; Vidal, 1973).

After Sterman and his colleagues found that operant training of SMRs can increase seizure thresholds in cats (Sterman et al., 1969), studies involving humans with epilepsy demonstrated a significant reduction of grand-mal seizures (Sterman & Macdonald, 1978). This motivated a large body of clinical trials evaluating the relevance of such "neurofeedback" training in the treatment of various disorders. Treatment studies of children diagnosed with attention deficit-hyperactivity disorder (ADHD; Lubar & Shouse, 1976) were particularly promising. However, only a few years later, the entire field of neurofeedback fell into disrepute, as many premature claims based on successes in single patients diagnosed with various disorders could not be validated in larger, controlled clinical trials. Nevertheless, and despite incomplete understanding of the mechanisms underlying neurofeedback-related behavioral effects, a number of well-controlled studies have now provided evidence that operant conditioning of brain activity can influence brain function and behavior (Monastra et al., 2005; Fuchs et al., 2003; Kotchoubey et al., 2001), a principle that later was revived in the context of clinical BCI/BMI applications aimed at the restoration of brain function (Birbaumer et al., 2009).

Besides SMR, other neurophysiological signals were also used in neurofeedback to treat epilepsy, for example, slow cortical potentials (SCPs). SCPs are negative or positive polarizations of the EEG that last from 300 ms to several seconds (Birbaumer, 1999a) and relate to depolarizations of the apical dendritic tree in the upper cortical layers caused by synchronous firing, mainly from thalamocortical afferents. Functionally, SCPs are thought to be associated with a threshold regulation mechanism (involving glial cells) for local excitatory mobilization (recorded as negativity) or inhibition (recorded as positivity) of cortical networks. When some epileptic patients exhibited almost 100% accuracy in the control of SCPs, the last author of the present chapter suggested using this learnable skill to enable completely paralyzed patients to communicate. Successful demonstration of such direct brain communication in two patients suffering from locked-in syndrome (LIS; Birbaumer et al., 1999b) created notable enthusiasm and led to considerable efforts to increase the speed of communication using other brain signals or advanced methods for rapid classification (the latter issue has been the subject of most scientific papers in the area of BCI/BMI research).

As the detectability of a particular brain event depends on the signal-to-noise ratio, that is, the certainty of information in a given time period, most BCIs/BMIs use event- or task-related brain signals in which the exact onset of a task or stimulus is known. Moreover, another advantage of using brain signals related to the perceptual or motor domain relates to the accessibility of the relevant primary cortical areas, in contrast to other domains, especially cognitive and affective domains, where the critical areas turned out to be difficult to identify and often included structures in the depth of the brain (Guillory & Bujarski, 2014), which are particularly challenging to assess non-invasively. Only recently have methods like functional magnetic resonance imaging (fMRI) or deep brain stimulation (DBS) opened the door for real-time BCI/BMI applications based on brain activity in these areas (Benabid et al., 2011). It is foreseeable that in the coming decades, clinical applications of BCI/BMI will increasingly expand into cognitive and affective domains as knowledge on their neurophysiological correlates increases and technology advances. Assuming that population codes of neural cell assemblies constitute the substrate for behaviorally relevant information, represented in the firing patterns of the constituent single neurons, local field potentials (LFPs) and large-scale oscillations, it is plausible that a BCI/BMI that includes the activity of all or many relevant cell assemblies, and the relevant population codes, will provide the largest degrees of freedom and the strongest basis for advancing the field.

In non-invasive BCI research, mainly six types of brain signals have been tested so far: (1) slow cortical potentials (SCPs), (2) sensorimotor rhythms (SMR, 8–15 Hz, also termed "rolandic alpha" or "mu-rhythm," depending on the context) and motor-related beta rhythms (13–30 Hz), (3) event-related potentials (ERPs), (4) steady-state visual or auditory evoked potentials (SSVEP/SSAEP), (5) blood oxygenation level dependent (BOLD) imaging using fMRI, and (6) concentration changes of oxy/deoxy hemoglobin using near-infrared spectroscopy (NIRS). Implantation of epicortical electrode grids or multi-electrode arrays (MEAs), on the other hand, allows online translation of (1) local field potentials (LFPs), (2) single-unit activity (SUA), or (3) multi-unit activity (MUA). As these systems require a surgical procedure for implantations of sensors or electrodes, they became termed *invasive* BCI/BMI (Hochberg et al., 2006).

While the SMR seems functionally related to an inhibitory mode of the cortico-basal ganglia loop (Sterman & Clemente, 1962), reflecting motor quiescence, SCPs were ascribed an active role in the preparatory distribution of sensory, motor, and attentional resources (Birbaumer et al., 1990) linked to a cortico-striatal-reticular thalamic feedback loop. The intactness of this cortical-subcortical loop seems critical for successful acquisition of operant brain control (Hinterberger et al., 2005), a finding important for the use of these measures in patient populations with brain lesions.

In contrast, control of an ERP-based BCI/BMI, for example the P300-based BCI, does not require any operant learning, and exploits the fact that perception of an unexpected, rare sensory stimulus is associated with a positive deflection in the EEG occurring approximately 300 ms after stimulus presentation. Accordingly, detection of a P300 allows inferences about the stimulus to which a subject is attending (Farwell & Donchin, 1988). Similarly, in SSVEP BCI/BMI systems, multiple visual stimuli or objects are presented on a display, each flickering at a particular frequency (Zhu et al., 2010). In such paradigms the BCI/BMI user can select one of these objects by fixating it with the eyes, resulting in time-locked sensory-evoked potentials (SEP) recorded over occipital brain areas. Analysis of the SSVEP's frequencies allows inferring which object was selected (Sakurada et al., 2013). Both P300 and SSVEP/SSAEP are mainly used for BCI-based systems allowing for letter or symbol selection to spell words or give specific commands. These BCI spellers can reach considerable information transfer rates (ITR) (over 100 bit/min; Spüler et al., 2012), and it was found that the neural substrates of the ERPs used in such systems include generators in a widespread network involving the primary sensory and particularly parieto-occipital areas linked to selective attention (Kiss et al., 1989).

Due to the dependency on sensory stimulation, these systems were subsumed as *reactive* BCI/BMI, in contrast to *active* BCI/BMI, in which translation of brain activity does not depend on constant sensory stimulation. To increase the signal-to-noise ratio, that is, to reduce uncertainty of information, most active BCI/BMI systems contrast brain activity between two different time windows in which the presence or absence of a specific brain signal is known to exist in one of them (often defined as the baseline or reference condition; Soekadar et al., 2011). If the onset and end of the second time window follow a predetermined cue (externally paced), such a system is defined as a *synchronous* BCI/BMI. As the presence of a brain signal or brain state is known in one of the windows, the majority of synchronous BCI/BMI utilize this window to recalibrate or readapt the system and thereby account for the non-stationary nature of EEG signals (McFarland et al., 2011). While this continuous adaptation provides high classification accuracy in discriminating between two different brain signals or brain states, it has obvious practical limitations, as it does not allow self-paced BCI/BMI control, which is desirable, for example, when operating a hand exoskeleton. Recently, *asynchronous* BCIs/BMIs were developed (Müller-Putz et al., 2006) that allow self-paced or asynchronous control, for example for voluntary grasping with an orthotic device (Ortner et al., 2011). As the classification accuracy of these systems is often lower compared with synchronous BCI/BMI, it was suggested that neurophysiological and other bio-signals, for example electromyography (EMG) and electrooculography (EOG), should be merged in order to increase usability and reliability in daily life (Ribeiro et al., 2013).

A decade ago, BCI/BMI systems were developed that use metabolic brain signals assessed by real-time fMRI (deCharms et al., 2004;Weiskopf et al., 2003; Yoo et al., 2004). Human volunteers learned to up- or down-regulate BOLD signals even in deep brain structures, for instance, the insular cortex or the amygdala (Caria et al., 2007). It was found that repeated training was associated with increased functional connectivity between various brain regions functionally linked to the trained area (Zotev et al., 2011). Similarly, functional near-infrared spectroscopy (fNIRS) can be used to quantify the metabolic activity of cortical brain areas at a depth of 1–3 cm relative to the surface of the skull. Multiple channels of light sources and detectors placed over the skull, operating at wavelengths near the infrared range (700–1,000 nm) allow quantification of cerebral oxygenation and blood flow in localized cortical regions. Compared to an immovable and expensive MRI-based metabolic BCI/BMI, an fNIRS-based BCI/BMI is portable and can be used in daily-life environments (Sitaram et al., 2007a).

In contrast to the described non-invasive BCI/BMI approaches, invasive BCI/BMIs require opening of the skull and insertion of implantable electrodes, entailing the risk of infection or bleeding (Walcott et al., 2012). However, due to the proximity of the electrodes to the neural tissue, signal-to-noise ratios of the recorded brain signals are higher compared to non-invasive recordings and are less contaminated by signals related to muscle activity or motions (Leuthardt et al., 2004). The motivation to develop invasive BCI/BMI was mainly driven by the finding that decoding of different movement directions from single neurons is possible (Georgopoulos et al., 1986). Since then, reconstruction of complex movements from neuronal activity was pursued, using both non-invasive (Waldert et al., 2008) and invasive methods (Hochberg et al., 2006). Firing patterns acquired through single-neuron recordings from the motor cortex (Nicolelis et al., 2003) or parietal neuronal pools (Scherberger et al., 2005) enabled monkeys to learn to control a cursor toward moving targets on a computer display. A total of 32 neurons were sufficient to move an artificial arm enabling a monkey to feed himself (Velliste et al., 2008). More recently, intracortical recordings of speech-related neural activity allowed classification of different vowels and speech intentions (Brumberg et al., 2011; Pei et al., 2011) or the spatial goals of movements (Hwang & Andersen, 2012), indicating that intracortical recordings can also be used in non-motor, cognitive domains.

Epicortical electrodes that do not penetrate the cortical tissue provide fewer degrees of freedom than multiple single-unit recordings, but avoid many risks associated with intracortical recordings (Schalk & Leuthardt, 2011). Offline decoding of electrocorticographic (ECoG) signals reached up to 80% classification accuracy for correct identification of five isometric hand postures (Chestek et al., 2013), but such high accuracy could not be achieved in online applications. Nevertheless, results are promising, and they suggest that ECoG will play an important role in applications where high signal-to-noise ratios are desired, but fewer degrees-of-freedom compared to intracortical recordings are sufficient.

Given that operant conditioning represents a key aspect of BMI learning, structural and functional plasticity within neural circuits relevant to control the specific physiological feature used for BMI control is important. Once it became clear that many, if not all, neurological and psychiatric disorders are associated with abnormal activity of specific neural circuits, it was suggested that BMI might be a useful tool to harness neuroplasticity (Wang et al., 2010) and improve clinical outcomes, for example in neurological rehabilitation (Dobkin, 2007), continuing and advancing the research tradition of neurofeedback.

Clinical Applications of Brain-Machine Interfaces

BMIs used in clinical environments follow two different strategies. While *assistive* or *biomimetic* BMI systems strive to substitute lost functions, for example communication (Birbaumer et al., 1999b), or to achieve continuous, high-dimensional control of robotic devices, or rely on functional electric stimulation (FES; Pfurtscheller et al., 2003) to assist in daily life environments, *rehabilitative* BMI systems (also termed *restorative* or *biofeedback* BMIs), in contrast, aim at the normalization of neurophysiologic activity to facilitate the restoration of brain function (Birbaumer & Cohen, 2007; Ramos-Murguialday et al., 2013; Soekadar et al., 2011). In other words, assistive or biomimetic BMI systems usually aim at high decoding accuracies and ITR, while rehabilitative BCIs/BMIs are designed as "training tools" to induce use-dependent brain plasticity (Wang et al., 2010) toward improved brain function; high classification accuracy, ITR, or the number of degrees of freedom in reconstruction of motor function are secondary, while feedback quality and reward contingency are more important in this form of BMI application (Soekadar et al., 2011).

The first clinically relevant BCI/BMI was used for restoration of communication in severe paralysis (Birbaumer et al., 1999b). Whereas the speed of communication possible with BCI/BMI technology has improved substantially (Spüler et al., 2012), these systems have not completely achieved what direct brain-computer communication once promised: reliable communication in complete paralysis, for example after onset of complete locked-in syndrome (CLIS; Birbaumer et al., 2014; Kübler & Birbaumer, 2008). The reason for this failure of direct brain communication in patients diagnosed with complete paralysis remains unclear, but it has led to the hypothesis that loss of the contingency between a voluntary response and its feedback or loss of subsequent reward in individuals who are completely paralyzed prevents operant learning, even if afferent input and cognitive processing (attention, memory, imagery) remain intact (Kübler & Birbaumer, 2008). If the voluntary response is only cognitive, such as in covert goal-oriented imagery in the locked-in state, feedback or reward does not follow a reliable environmental or internal change and consequently becomes extinguished. Psychophysical studies demonstrate that if the behavioral response is elicited independently of a conscious decision and intention, the conscious awareness of the contingency and the conscious experience of the decision ("will") vanishes (Haggard et al., 2002). In CLIS, all contingencies between goal-directed thinking and intentions are lost because there is no environmental response to the particular intention. Such "extinction of goal-directed thinking" or "extinction of thought" would make any attempts to reinstate communication using BCI technology obsolete (Birbaumer et al., 2014). However, it is conceivable that CLIS patients use internal imagined response-effect contingencies that allow maintenance of goal-directed thinking, an issue that is still under investigation. Classical conditioning, however, does not need associations between responses and reward contingencies (Pavlov, 1927), and allows basic yes-no communication in a novel BCI/BMI paradigm using semantic classical conditioning (De Massari et al., 2012; Gallegos-Ayala et al., 2014).

Another extensively explored direction in clinical BCI/BMI applications deals with the restoration of movement in paralysis. Using a non-invasive system, the Graz BCI group was the first to demonstrate volitional SMR modulation for control of FES of a quadriplegic patient's paralyzed hand (Pfurtscheller et al., 2003). While the patient imagined a movement, the associated modulation of the SMR was translated into FES control signals, resulting in grasping motions of his paralyzed hand. After this proof-of-concept study, numerous publications addressed the different aspects that are important to allow intuitive control of biomimetic devices or FES in a daily life environment.

In 2006, successful implantation of densely packed microelectrode arrays in the primary motor cortex of two quadriplegic human patients enabled them to use LFPs to control a computer cursor in various directions (Hochberg et al., 2006). Recently, a study using two 96-channel intracortical microelectrodes placed in the motor cortex of a 52-year-old woman with tetraplegia demonstrated robust movements of a prosthetic limb along seven dimensions for orientation and grasping (Collinger et al., 2013; 3D translation of the prosthetic limb's endpoint coordinates, 3D orientation of the wrist, and 1D performance of grasping motions). These demonstrations are impressive and suggest that invasive BCI/BMI will become a realistic option to improve the living conditions of patients with tetraplegia for whom other assistive technologies are not applicable or do not reach such high degrees of freedom. However, the completion of larger clinical trials currently pursued (ClinicalTrials.gov Identifier: NCT00912041) is necessary to evaluate the long-term stability and risks related to permanently implanted intracortical BCI/BMI electrodes. Also, thus far, some basic issues have not been resolved that relate, for example, to the day-to-day volatility of decoding accuracies that might be a consequence of biological responses to implanted foreign bodies and the instability of neural representations (Rokni et al., 2007), resulting in non-stationarity of individual neurons' activity (Andersen et al., 2004).

In contrast to this work aiming at assistive use of invasive and non-invasive BCI/BMI technology, the development of rehabilitative BCI/BMI systems goes back to early work pursued in a collaborative research effort between the University of Tübingen and the National Institutes of Neurological Disorders and Stroke (NINDS). Based on previous reports on potentially beneficial effects of neurofeedback in stroke (e.g. Rozelle & Budzynski, 1995) and data indicating that stroke patients with the best motor recovery are the ones in whom ipsilesional cortical function is closer to that found in healthy controls (Calautti et al., 2010; Platz et al., 2002), Birbaumer & Cohen (2007) developed an SMR-based BCI/BMI system to enable severely affected stroke patients to control an orthotic device opening and closing their paralyzed hand, thus providing immediate sensory feedback contingent upon their ipsilesional brain activity. A first study indicated that the majority of chronic stroke patients can indeed learn to control this system by modulating the ipsilesional SMR or mu-rhythm (Buch et al., 2008, 2012), but a few weeks of training did not result in any significant motor function improvement. However, when daily

BCI/BMI training was coupled with goal-directed behavioral physical therapy and was repeatedly applied for 3 months over the time of 1 year, remarkable improvements of motor and cognitive capacities were reported (Broetz et al., 2010). In this study, a 67-year-old hemiparetic patient suffering from chronic stroke after a right-sided thalamic bleed, who was unable to use his hand or arm for any relevant daily living activity and was dependent on assistance for personal hygiene and dressing, fully regained the ability to extend his fingers and became independent of any walking aid or assistance for personal hygiene. Remarkably, concentration and attentiveness also improved significantly, demonstrated, for instance, by his capacity to drive a car again. Analysis of brain activation during attempted motions with his affected arm indicated an activation increase toward the ipsilesional hemisphere (Caria et al., 2011). This promising case study motivated a larger clinical trial involving over 30 chronic stroke patients with severe paralysis who were unable to grasp. The study showed that 1 month of daily ipsilesional BMI training, combined with goal-directed behavioral physiotherapy, resulted in significant motor improvements in these patients, while random BMI-feedback did not (Ramos-Murguialday et al., 2013). Further analysis of neurophysiological parameters indicated that motor evoked potentials (MEPs) from the ipsilesional hemisphere, reflecting the integrity of the descending corticospinal tract, could predict motor recovery of the trained patients (Brasil et al., 2012). While the integrity of the ascending sensory pathways was not assessed in this study, their importance for successful BCI/BMI control and learning was recently demonstrated (Shaikhouni et al., 2013). Given the heterogeneity of stroke patients, these results are remarkable and underline the capacity of chronic stroke patients with severe motor deficits to regain their function under effective learning paradigms. They further suggest that BMI-related neurorehabilitation can improve brain function across different domains.

Following the same principle, real-time fMRI (rt-fMRI) was also used to train ipsilesional motor cortical areas, with one study reporting an improvement of motor function (Sitaram et al., 2012). In this context, a study that showed successful regulation of dopaminergic mid-brain regions, including the substantia nigra and ventral tegmentum, is of particular interest for BCI/BMI training protocols targeting the motor domain, for example in stroke or Parkinson's disease (Sulzer et al., 2013). It is conceivable that multisite rt-fMRI BMI feedback training allowing synchronized upregulation of task-related brain regions disconnected due to a brain lesion can increase impaired brain connectivity and thus enhance brain function.

As rt-fMRI allows online interpretation of metabolic brain activity in deeper brain structures, shown to be involved in the regulation of emotion and motivation, several studies investigated the applicability of rt-fMRI in patient populations, targeting the activation of dysfunctional brain circuits. In a proof-of-concept study, Linden et al. used rt-fMRI to train eight patients diagnosed with unipolar major depressive disorder (MDD) to upregulate brain regions of emotional control (such as the ventrolateral prefrontal cortex [VLPFC] and insula; Linden et al., 2012). All patients gained control and reported significant improvement of their mood, which did not occur in a control group receiving placebo feedback. Similar results were reported in a recent study in which unmedicated MDD patients learned to increase amygdala activation during recall of happy autobiographical memories (Young et al., 2014). In another study, six criminal psychopaths, who showed reduced or absent activation in the fear circuit, were trained to upregulate their anterior insula. In line with previous work indicating deficient fear conditioning in psychopathy (Birbaumer et al., 2005), participants scoring high on psychopathy scales were less successful in learning brain self-regulation of their fear circuit than those with lower scores and showed increased effective connectivity between brain regions related to emotion control after the training (Sitaram et al., 2007b). However, insula training did not result in any behavioral modifications outside the laboratory.

The pre-clinical and phase 1 trials described here corroborate earlier findings in animals and healthy human volunteers that the use of BCI/BMI systems can result in structural and functional plasticity within neural circuits engaged in BCI/BMI learning and control. However, larger and well-controlled clinical studies are necessary to evaluate the efficacy of these novel tools in the treatment of neurological and mental disorders. This, however, presents the field with many challenges that require special attention.

Current Challenges and Future Clinical Applications

While most attention so far has been directed toward invasive BMI applications aiming at the skillful control of robotic limbs, controlled studies are required that investigate the necessity of taking the risk associated with invasive procedures for any therapeutic or assistive BMI application. Also, the risk-benefit ratio in long-term studies needs to be thoroughly assessed. It is unclear which patient groups and which individual patients benefit the most from invasive BMI. Also, the relevance of invasive BMI for restoration of communication in complete paralysis, for example CLIS, remains uncertain (Birbaumer et al., 2014). While major efforts in the BCI/BMI field are focused toward improving the accuracy and speed of the online detection and classification of specific brain signals, only very limited data are available testing these novel mathematical algorithms and methods in patient populations in whom normal neurophysiology is altered and learning impeded (Soekadar et al., 2011). Furthermore, the availability of new technologies that can improve patients' quality of life often impacts many ethical dimensions, including social, medical, or legal issues, and, in particular, raises questions about the accessibility of these new technologies that require more validation, and intensive interdisciplinary discourse (Soekadar & Birbaumer, 2014a).

Successful development and application of rehabilitative BCI/BMI systems critically depend on understanding the relationship between a brain physiological feature and a disturbed brain function. Despite considerable research efforts, this relationship is still poorly understood. In this context, correlations of multimodal assessments, for example, combining intra- and epicortical recordings (Bansal et al., 2012) with EEG, magnetoencephalographic (MEG) measures, targeting specific brain functions, may be of particular value. Besides linear brain signal analysis, nonlinear measures capturing more complex brain dynamics (Robinson et al., 2013) promise important neurophysiological insights, but their implementation in online BCI/BMI systems is currently difficult due to excessive computational demands. Nevertheless, successful identification of linear and nonlinear measures related to brain function deficits would not only be important for the development of new treatment strategies that involve BMI systems, but such neurophysiological "biomarkers" could also improve the specificity of neuropharmacological or other forms of treatments.

Despite a large body of studies suggesting that cognitive plasticity occurs as a result of BMI use, this area is still in its infancy, and was largely neglected in the earlier stages of BMI/BCI development. As our knowledge increases about the neurophysiology of higher cognitive function and the technical means of directly interacting with these processes, BMI targeting cognitive plasticity will come into reach, and will likely improve our understanding of the fundamental basis of cognition. An example of a brain disorder that allows for investigation of the relationship between cognitive plasticity and specific neurophysiological measures is Alzheimer's disease (AD). For instance, AD patients compared to healthy controls exhibit a general slowing of task-free brain oscillatory activity (Berendse et al., 2000), specifically showing significant changes in delta (2–4 Hz) and beta (16–28 Hz) band frequencies (De Haan et al., 2008; Fernandez et al., 2006). An increase of frontal and central delta and theta signal power was found, whereas higher frequencies showed decreased power in posterior temporal and occipital areas (Berendse et al., 2000). In line with a previously described association between the level of cholinergic activity and increased delta power (Riekkinen et al., 1991), a correlation between cognitive decline and an increase in the magnetic dipole density of temporo-parietal delta and theta activity was found in AD (Fernandez et al., 2005). The described findings allowed discriminating individuals with AD from healthy controls at high precision (>80%; Poza et al., 2008). Quantification of magnetic dipole density during a memory task resulted in sensitivity of 90% and specificity of 100% when combined with MRI spectroscopy (myoinositol/N-acetyl aspartate; Fernandez et al., 2005). In order to investigate the value of whole-head MEG recordings to assess in vivo biomarkers for AD, a recent study evaluated delta current density (DCD) across the posterior parietal, occipital, pre-rolandic, and precuneus cortices, and compared individuals with mild cognitive impairment (MCI), AD patients with different severity scores, and healthy controls (Fernández et al., 2013). The transition from MCI to mild dementia and from mild to more severe dementia could be reliably indexed by an increase in DCD of the right parietal cortex and precuneus. These studies show that the cognitive functions related to specific neurophysiological measures can, indeed, be assessed and quantified. While most approaches transform and average brain signals, leading to a loss of information related to dynamically and rapidly changing brain states, the development of tools capable of assessing this information will substantially improve the sensitivity and specificity of potential biomarkers, which, in a second step, can be used as targets for BMI training aimed at normalizing neural dynamics in disturbed brain circuits.

Whereas some basic mechanisms and neural substrates related to abstract learning of BMI control have been identified (Koralek et al., 2012; Soekadar et al., 2014b), the role of brain plasticity in the success or failure of BMI applications is still widely under-investigated. Similar to the challenge of evaluating the efficacy of neuro- and psychopharmacological substances in the treatment of patient groups who receive a specific diagnosis even though there may be considerable variability in the underlying causes of their symptoms, clinical trials that investigate the efficacy of specific interventions, like BCI/BMI training, should use dimensional approaches that integrate different neurophysiological, psychophysical, genetic, and psychopathological measures to characterize the patient population, as proposed in the Research Domain Criteria (RDoC) framework (Cuthbert, 2014).

While cognitive restoration using BCI/BMI technology is relatively unexplored, many other techniques and devices have shown to be highly useful, including behavioral techniques or invasive and non-invasive attempts at modulating brain activity. Here, non-invasive and invasive electric brain stimulation play an increasingly important role (Dayan et al., 2013). Recently, a new strategy for in vivo assessment of neuromagnetic brain activity during transcranial electric stimulation (TES) was introduced (Soekadar et al., 2013a). This novel method allows purposeful modulation of brain oscillations during performance of cognitive or motor tasks while whole-brain neuromagnetic activity is being recorded, thus opening the door to systematic investigation of the link between dynamic plasticity of neuromagnetic activity and brain functions attributable to large-scale networks. The first studies that have successfully combined electric brain stimulation and BCI/BMI technology (Soekadar et al., 2013b; Soekadar & Birbaumer, 2014c; Soekadar et al., 2014d) promise to provide clinicians with a greater selection of options in the future to facilitate the restoration of motor and cognitive brain functions.

Conclusions

The technological advances of the last years in the BCI/BMI field, which were mainly driven by the exponential growth and availability of computational capacities and improved sensor technology, now promise substantial progress toward clinical applications of assistive and/or rehabilitative BCI/BMI systems in the coming decades. While BCI/BMI technology can be used as a powerful tool in basic neuroscience to investigate motor, affective, and cognitive plasticity, BCI/BMI technology will also play an increasingly important role in the diagnostics and treatment of many neurological and psychiatric disorders.

Acknowledgments

This work was supported by the Intramural Research Program (IRP) of the National Institute of Neurological Disorders and Stroke (NINDS), United States; the German Federal Ministry of Education and Research (BMBF, grant number 01GQ0831, 16SV5838K to SRS and NB); the BMBF to the German Center for Diabetes Research (DZD e.V., grand number 01GI0925); the Deutsche Forschungsgemeinschaft (DFG, grant number SO932-2 to SRS and Reinhart Koselleck Project support to NB); the European Commission under the project WAY and BNCI 2020 (grant number 288551 and 609593, respectively, to SRS and NB); the Volkswagenstiftung (VW) and the Baden-Württemberg Stiftung, Germany.

References

Andersen, R. A., Musallam, S., Pesaran, B. (2004). Selecting the signals for a brain–machine interface. *Curr Opin Neurobiol, 14*, 720–726.

Bansal, A. K., Truccolo, W., Vargas-Irwin, C. E. & Donoghue, J. P. (2012). Decoding 3D reach and grasp from hybrid signals in motor and premotor cortices: Spikes, multiunit activity, and local field potentials. *J Neurophysiol, 107*, 1337–1355.

Benabid, A. L., Costecalde, T., Torres, N., Moro, C., Aksenova, T., Eliseyev, A., Charvet, G., Sauter, F., Ratel, D., Mestais, C., Pollak, P. & Chabardes, S. (2011). Deep brain stimulation: BCI at large, where are we going to? *Prog Brain Res, 194*, 71–82.

Berendse, H. W., Verbunt, J. P. A., Scheltens, Ph., van Dijk, B. W., & Jonkman E. J. (2000). Magnetoencephalographic analysis of cortical activity in Alzheimer's disease: A pilot study. *Clin Neurophysiol, 111*, 604–612.

Berger, H. (1929). Über das Elektrenkephalogramm des Menschen. *Arch Psychiat Nerven, 87*, 527–570.

Birbaumer, N. (1999a). Slow cortical potentials: Plasticity, operant control, and behavioral effects. *Neuroscientist, 5*, 74–78.

Birbaumer, N., Ghanayim, N., Hinterberger, T., Iversen, I., Kotchoubey, B., Kübler, A., Perelmouter, J., Taub, E., & Flor, H. (1999b). A spelling device for the paralysed. *Nature, 398*, 297–298.

Birbaumer, N., Ramos Murguialday, A., Weber, C., & Montoya, P. (2009). Neurofeedback and brain-computer interface clinical applications. *Int Rev Neurobiol, 86*, 107–117.

Birbaumer, N., Veit, R., Lotze, M., Erb, M., Hermann, C., Grodd, W., & Flor, H. (2005). Deficient fear conditioning in psychopathy: A functional magnetic resonance imaging study. *Arch Gen Psychiat, 62*, 799–805.

Birbaumer, N., Elbert, T., Canavan, A. & Rockstroh, B. (1990). Slow potentials of the cerebral cortex and behavior. *Physiol Rev, 70*, 1–41.

Birbaumer, N., & Cohen, L. G. (2007). Brain-computer interfaces: Communication and restoration of movement in paralysis. *J Physiol, 579*, 621–636.

Birbaumer. N., Gallegos-Ayala, G., Wildgruber, M., Silvoni, S., & Soekadar, S. R. (2014). Direct brain control and communication in paralysis. *Brain Topog, 27*, 4–11.

Brasil, F., Curado, M. R., Witkowski, M., Garcia, E., Broetz, D., Birbaumer, N., & Soekadar, S. R. (2012). *MEP predicts motor recovery in chronic stroke patients undergoing 4-weeks of daily physical therapy*. Human Brain Mapping Annual Meeting, Beijing, 33WTh.

Broca, P. (1861). Remarks on the seat of the faculty of articulated language, following an observation of aphemia (loss of speech)." *B Soc Anat, 36*, 330–357.

Brodmann, K. (1913). Neue Forschungsergebnisse der Großhirnrindenanatomie. *Ver Ges DN, 85*, 200–240.

Broetz, D., Braun, C., Weber, C., Soekadar, S. R., Caria, A., & Birbaumer, N. (2010). Combination of brain-computer interface training and goal-directed physical therapy in chronic stroke: A case report. *Neurorehab Neural Re, 24*, 674–679.

Brumberg, J. S., Wright, E. J., Andreasen, D. S., Guenther, F. H., & Kennedy, P. R. (2011). Classification of intended phoneme production from chronic intracortical microelectrode recordings in speech-motor cortex. *Front Neurosci, 5*, 65.

Buch, E., Weber, C., Cohen, L. G., Braun, C., Dimyan, M. A., Ard, T., Mellinger, J., Caria, A., Soekadar, S. R., Fourkas, A., & Birbaumer, N. (2008). Think to move: A neuromagnetic brain-computer interface (BCI) system for chronic stroke. *Stroke, 39*, 910–917.

Buch, E. R., Modir Shanechi, A., Fourkas, A. D., Weber, C., Birbaumer, N., Cohen, L. G. (2012). Parietofrontal integrity determines neural modulation associated with grasping imagery after stroke. *Brain, 135*, 596–614.

Calautti, C., Jones, P. S., Naccarato, M., Sharma, N., Day, D. J., Bullmore, E. T., Warburton, E. A., & Baron, J. C. (2010). The relationship between motor deficit and primary motor cortex hemispheric activation balance after stroke: Longitudinal fMRI study. *J Neurol Neurosur Ps, 81*, 788–792.

Caria, A., Veit, R., Sitaram, R., Lotze, M., Weiskopf, N., Grodd, W., & Birbaumer, N. (2007). Regulation of anterior insular cortex activity using real-time fMRI. *NeuroImage, 35*, 1238–1246.

Caria, A., Weber, C., Brötz, D., Ramos, A., Ticini, L. F., Gharabaghi, A., Braun, C., & Birbaumer, N. (2011). Chronic stroke recovery after combined BCI training and physiotherapy: A case report. *J Psychophysiol, 48*, 578–582.

Chatrian, G. E., Petersen, M. C., & Lazarte, J. A. (1959). The blocking of the rolandic wicket rhythm and some central changes related to movement. *Electroen Clin Neuro, 11*, 497–510.

Chestek, C. A., Gilja, V., Blabe, C. H., Foster, B. L., Shenoy, K. V., Parvizi, J., & Henderson, J. M. (2013). Hand posture classification using electrocorticography signals in the gamma band over human sensorimotor brain areas. *J Neural Eng, 10*, 026002.

Collinger, J. L., Wodlinger, B., Downey, J. E., Wang, W., Tyler-Kabara, E. C., Weber, D. J., McMorland, A. J., Velliste, M., Boninger, M. L. & Schwartz, A. B. (2013). High-performance neuroprosthetic control by an individual with tetraplegia. *Lancet, 381*, 557–564.

Cuthbert, B. N. (2014). The RDoC framework: Facilitating transition from ICD/DSM to dimensional approaches that integrate neuroscience and psychopathology. *World Psychiat, 13*, 28–35.

Dayan, E., Censor, N., Buch, E. R., Sandrini, M., & Cohen, L. G. (2013). Noninvasive brain stimulation: From physiology to network dynamics and back. *Nat Neurosci, 16*, 838–844.

De Haan, W., Stam, C. J., Jones, B. F., Zuiderwijk, I. M., van Dijk, B. W., & Scheltens, Ph. (2008). Restingstate oscillatory brain dynamics in Alzheimer Disease. *J Clin Neurophysiol, 25*, 187–193.

deCharms, R. C, Christoff, K., Glover, G. H., Pauly, J. M., Whitfield, S., & Gabrieli, J. D. (2004). Learned regulation of spatially localized brain activation using real-time fMRI. *NeuroImage, 21*, 436–443.

De Massari, D., Matuz, T., Furdea, A., Ruf, C. A., Halder, S., Birbaumer, N. (2012). Brain-computer interface and semantic classical conditioning of communication in paralysis. *Biol Psychol, 92*, 267–274.

Dobkin, B. H. (2007). Brain-computer interface technology as a tool to augment plasticity and outcomes for neurological rehabilitation. *J Physiol, 579*, 637–642.

Eliasmith, C., Stewart, T. C., Choo, X., Bekolay, T., DeWolf, T., Tang, Y., & Rasmussen, D. (2012). A large-scale model of the functioning brain. *Science, 338*, 1202–1205.

Farwell, L. A., & Donchin, E. (1988). Talking off the top of your head: Toward a mental prosthesis utilizing event-related brain potentials. *Electroen Clin Neuro, 70*, 510–523.

Fernandez, A., Garcia-Seguria, J. M., Ortiz, T., Montoya, J., Maestu, F., Gil-Gregorio, P, Campo, P., & Viaño, J. (2005). Proton magnetic resonance spectroscopy and magnetoencephalographic estimation of delta dipole density: A combination of techniques that may contribute to the diagnosis of Alzheimer's disease. *Dement Geriatr Cogn, 20*, 169–177.

Fernandez, A., Hornero, R., Mayo, A., Poza, J., Maestu, F. & Ortiz, T. (2006). Quantitative magnetoencephalography of spontaneous brain activity in Alzheimer's disease. *Alz Dis Assoc Dis, 20*, 153–159.

Fernández, A., Turrero, A., Zuluaga, P., Gil-Gregorio, P., del Pozo, F., Maestu, F., & Moratti, S. (2013). MEG delta mapping along the healthy aging-Alzheimer's disease continuum: diagnostic implications. *J Alzheimers Dis, 35*, 495–507.

Fetz, E. E. (1969). Operant conditioning of cortical unit activity. *Science, 163*, 955–958.

Fuchs, T., Birbaumer, N., Lutzenberger, W., Gruzelier, J. H., & Kaiser, J. (2003). Neurofeedback treatment for attention-deficit/hyperactivity disorder in children: A comparison with methylphenidate. *Appl Psychophys Biof, 28*, 1–12.

Gall, F. J. (1835). On the functions of the brain and of each of its parts: with observations on the possibility of determining the instincts, propensities, and talents, or the moral and intellectual dispositions of men and animals, by the configuration of the brain and head. Translated from the French by Winslow Lewis, *Marsh, Capen & Lyon, Boston, 2*, 47–177.

Gallegos-Ayala, G., Furdea, A., Takano, K., Ruf, C. A., Flor, H., & Birbaumer, N. (2014). Brain communication in a completely locked-in patient using bedside near-infrared spectroscopy. *Neurology, 82*, 1930–1932.

Georgopoulos, A. P., Schwartz, A. B., & Kettner, R. E. (1986). Neuronal population coding of movement direction. *Science, 233*, 1416–1419.

Guillory, S. A., & Bujarski, K. A. (2014). Exploring emotions using invasive methods: review of 60 years of human intracranial electrophysiology. *Soc Cogn Affect Neur*, (in press).

Haggard, P., Clark, S. & Kalogeras, J. (2002). Voluntary action and conscious awareness. *Nat Neurosci, 4*, 382–385.

Hinterberger, T., Veit, R., Wilhelm, B., Weiskopf, N., Vatine, J. J., & Birbaumer, N. (2005). Neuronal mechanisms underlying control of a brain-computer interface. *Eur J Neurosci, 21*, 3169–3181.

Hipp, J. F., Hawellek, D. J., Corbetta, M., Siegel, M., & Engel, A. K. (2012). Large-scale cortical correlation structure of spontaneous oscillatory activity. *Nat Neurosci, 15*, 884–890.

Hochberg, L. R., Serruya, M. D., Friehs, G. M., Mukand, J. A., Saleh, M., Caplan, A. H., Branner, A., Chen, D., Penn, R. D., & Donoghue, J. P. (2006). Neuronal ensemble control of prosthetic devices by a human with tetraplegia. *Nature, 442*, 164–171.

Hwang, E. J., & Andersen, R. A. (2012). Spiking and LFP activity in PRR during symbolically instructed reaches. *J Neurophysiol, 107*, 836–849.

Kiss, I., Dashieff, R. M., & Lordeon, P. (1989). A parieto-occipital generator for P300: Evidence from human intracranial recordings. *Int J Neurosci, 49*, 133–139.

Kotchoubey, B., Strehl, U., Uhlmann, C., Holzapfel, S., König, M., Fröscher, W., Blankenhorn, V., & Birbaumer, N. (2001). Modification of slow cortical potentials in patients with refractory epilepsy: A controlled outcome study. *Epilepsia, 42*, 406–416.

Koralek, A. C., Jin X., Long, J. D., II, Costa, R. M., & Carmena, J. M. (2012). Corticostriatal plasticity is necessary for learning intentional neuroprosthetic skills. *Nature, 483*, 331–335.

Kübler, A., & Birbaumer, N. (2008). Brain-computer interfaces and communication in paralysis: Extinction of goal directed thinking in completely paralysed patients? *Clin Neurophysiol, 119*, 2658–2666.

Leuthardt, E. C., Schalk, G., Wolpaw, J. R., Ojemann, J. G., & Moran, D. W. (2004). A brain-computer interface using electrocorticographic signals in humans. *J Neural Eng, 1*, 63–71.

Linden, D. E., Habes, I., Johnston, S. J., Linden, S., Tatineni, R., Subramanian, L., Sorger, B., Healy, D., & Goebel, R. (2012). Real-time self-regulation of emotion networks in patients with depression. *PLoS One, 7*, e38115.

Lubar, J. F., & Shouse, M. N. (1976). EEG and behavioral changes in a hyperkinetic child concurrent with training of the sensorimotor rhythm (SMR): A preliminary report. *Biofeedback Self-Reg, 1*, 293–306.

McFarland, D. J., Sarnacki, W. A., Wolpaw, J. R. (2011). Should the parameters of a BCI translation algorithm be continually adapted? *J Neurosci Methods, 199*, 103–107.

Monastra, V. J., Lynn, S., Linden, M., Lubar, J. F., Gruzelier, J., & LaVaque, T. J. (2005). Electroencephalographic biofeedback in the treatment of attention-deficit/hyperactivity disorder. *Appl Psychophys Biof, 30*, 95–114.

Müller-Putz, G. R., Scherer, R., Pfurtscheller, G., & Rupp, R. (2006). Brain-computer interfaces for control of neuroprostheses: From synchronous to asynchronous mode of operation. *Biomedizinische Technik (Berl), 51*, 57–63.

Nicolelis, M. A., Dimitrov, D., Carmena, J. M., Crist, R., Lehew, G., Kralik, J. D., & Wise, S. P. (2003). Chronic, multisite, multielectrode recordings in macaque monkeys. *P Natl Acad Sci USA, 100*, 11041–11046.

Ortner, R., Allison, B. Z., Korisek, G., Gaggl, H., & Pfurtscheller, G. (2011). An SSVEP BCI to control a hand orthosis for persons with tetraplegia. *IEEE T Neur Sys Reh, 19*, 1–5.

Pavlov, I. P. (1927). *Conditioned reflexes: An investigation of the physiological activity of the cerebral cortex.* Translated and Edited by G. V. Anrep. London: Oxford University Press.

Pei, X., Barbour, D. L., Leuthardt, E. C., & Schalk, G. (2011). Decoding vowels and consonants in spoken and imagined words using electrocorticographic signals in humans. *J Neural Eng, 8*, 046028.

Pfurtscheller, G., Müller, G. R., Pfurtscheller, J., Gerner, H. J., & Rupp, R. (2003). "Thought"–control of functional electrical stimulation to restore hand grasp in a patient with tetraplegia. *Neurosci Lett, 351*, 33–36.

Pfurtscheller, G., & Aranibar, A. (1979). Evaluation of event-related desynchronization (ERD) preceding and following self-paced movement. *Electroen Clin Neuro, 46*, 138–146.

Platz, T., Kim, I. H., Engel, U., Kieselbach, A., & Mauritz, K.-H. (2002). Brain activation pattern as assessed with multi-modal EEG analysis predict motor recovery among stroke patients with mild arm paresis who receive the Arm Ability Training. *Restor Neurol Neuros, 20,* 21–35.

Poza, J., Hornero, R., Escudero, J., Fernandez, A., & Sanchez, C. I. (2008). Regional analysis of spontaneous MEG rhythms in patients with Alzheimer's disease using spectral entropies. *Ann Biomed Eng, 36,* 141–152.

Ramos-Murguialday, A., Broetz, D., Rea, M., Läer, L., Yilmaz, O., Brasil, F. L., Liberati, G., Curado, M. R., Garcia-Cossio, E., Vyziotis, A., Cho, W., Agostini, M., Soares, E., Soekadar, S. R., Caria, A., Cohen, L. G., & Birbaumer, N. (2013). Brain-machine interface in chronic stroke rehabilitation: A controlled study. *Ann Neurol, 74,* 100–108.

Ribeiro, P. R. A., Brasil, F., Witkowski, M., Shiman, F., Cipriani, C., Vitiello, N., & Soekadar, S. R. (2013). Controlling assistive machines in paralysis using brain waves and other biosignals. *Adv Human-Computer Interact,* Article ID: 369425, 1–9.

Riekkinen, P., Buzsaki, G., Riekkinen, P., Jr., Soininen, H., & Partanen, J. (1991). The cholinergic system and EEG slow waves. *Electroen Clin Neuro, 78,* 89–96.

Robinson, S. E., Mandell, A. J., & Coppola, R. (2013). Spatiotemporal imaging of complexity. *Front Comp Neurosci, 6,* 101.

Rokni, U., Richardson, A. G., Bizzi, E., & Seung, H. S. (2007). Motor learning with unstable neural representations. *Neuron, 54,* 653–666.

Rozelle, G. R., & Budzynski, T. H. (1995). Neurotherapy for stroke rehabilitation: A single case study. *Biofeedback Self-Reg, 20,* 211–228.

Sakurada, T., Kawase, T., Takano, K., Komatsu, T. & Kansaku, K. (2013). A BMI-based occupational therapy assist suit: Asynchronous control by SSVEP. *Front Neurosci, 7,* 172.

Schalk, G., & Leuthardt, E. C. (2011). Brain-computer interfaces using electrocorticographic signals. *IEEE Rev Biomed Eng, 4,* 140–154.

Scherberger, H., Jarvis, M. R. & Andersen, R. A. (2005). Cortical local field potential encodes movement intentions in the posterior parietal cortex. *Neuron, 46,* 347–354.

Shaikhouni, A., Donoghue, J. P., & Hochberg, L. R. (2013). Somatosensory responses in a human motor cortex. *J Neurophysiol, 109,* 2192–2204.

Sitaram, R., Veit, R., Stevens, B., Caria, A., Gerloff, C., Birbaumer, N., & Hummel, F. (2012). Acquired control of ventral premotor cortex activity by feedback training: an exploratory real-time fMRI and TMS study. *Neurorehab Neural Re, 26,* 256–265.

Sitaram, R., Zhang, H., Guan, C., Thulasidas, M., Hoshi, Y., Ishikawa, A., Shimizu, K., & Birbaumer, N. (2007a). Temporal classification of multichannel near-infrared spectroscopy signals of motor imagery for developing a brain-computer interface. *NeuroImage, 34,* 1416–1427.

Sitaram, R., Caria, A., Veit, R., Gaber, T., Rota, G., Kübler, A., & Birbaumer, N. (2007b). FMRI brain-computer interface: A tool for neuroscientific research and treatment. *Comp Intell Neurosci, 25487.*

Soekadar, S. R., Witkowski, M., Mellinger, J., Ramos, A., Birbaumer, N., & Cohen, L. G. (2011). ERD-based online brain-machine interfaces (BMI) in the context of neurorehabilitation: Optimizing BMI learning and performance. *IEEE T Neur Sys Reh, 19,* 542–549.

Soekadar, S. R., Witkowski, M., Garcia-Cossio, E., Birbaumer, N., Robinson, S. E., & Cohen, L. G. (2013a). In vivo assessment of human brain oscillations during application of transcranial electric currents. *Nat Communic, 4,* 2032.

Soekadar, S. R., Witkowski, M., Robinson, S. E., & Birbaumer, N. (2013b). Combining electric brain stimulation and source-based brain-machine interface (BMI) training in neurorehabilitation of chronic stroke. *J Neurol Sci, 333,* e542.

Soekadar, S. R., & Birbaumer, N. (2014a). Brain-machine interfaces (BMI) for communication in complete paralysis: Ethical implications and challenges. Chapter 41. In J. Clausen & N. Levy (Eds.). *Handbook of neuroethics.* Springer Verlag, Dordrecht, Netherlands..

Soekadar, S., Witkowski, M., Birbaumer, N., & Cohen, L. G. (2014b). Enhancing Hebbian learning to control oscillatory activity *Cereb Cortex,* (in press).

Soekadar, S. R., & Birbaumer, N. (2014c). Improving the efficacy of ipsilesional brain-computer interface training in neurorehabilitation of chronic stroke. In C. Guger, B. Allison, and E. C. Leuthardt (Eds.), *Biosystems & Biorobotics.* Springer Verlag Berlin Heidelberg, 6, 75–84.

Soekadar, S., Witkowski, M., Garcia-Cossio, E., Birbaumer, N. & Cohen, L. G. (2014d). Learned EEG-based brain self-regulation of motor-related oscillations during application of transcranial electric brain stimulation: Feasibility and limitations. *Front Behav Neurosci.*, *8*, 93

Spüler, M., Rosenstiel, W., & Bogdan, M. (2012). Online adaptation of a c-VEP Brain-computer Interface (BCI) based on error-related potentials and unsupervised learning. *PLoS One*, *7*, e51077.

Sterman, M. B., & Clemente, C. D. (1962). Forebrain inhibitory mechanisms: cortical synchronization induced by basal forebrain stimulation. *Experimental Neurology*, *6*, 91–102.

Sterman, M. B., LoPresti, R. W., & Fairchild, M. D. (1969). *Electroencephalographic and behavioral studies of monomethyl hydrazinc toxicity in the cat.* Technical Report AMRL-TR-69-3, Air Systems Command, Wright-Patterson Air Force Base, Ohio.

Sterman, M. B., & Macdonald, L. R. (1978). Effects of central cortical EEG feedback training on incidence of poorly controlled seizures. *Epilepsia*, *19*, 207–222.

Sulzer, J., Sitaram, R., Blefari, M. L., Kollias, S., Birbaumer, N., Stephan, K. E., Luft, A., & Gassert, R. (2013). Neurofeedback-mediated self-regulation of the dopaminergic midbrain. *NeuroImage*, *83*, 817–825.

Velliste, M., Perel, S., Spalding, M. C., Whitford, A. S., & Schwartz, A. B. (2008). Cortical control of a prosthetic arm for self-feeding. *Nature*, *453*, 1098–1101.

Vidal, J. J. (1973). Toward direct brain-computer communication. *Annu Rev Biophys Bio*, *2*, 157–180.

Walcott, B. P., Redjal, N., & Coumans, J. V. (2012). Infection following operations on the central nervous system: Deconstructing the myth of the sterile field. *Neurosurg Focus*, *33*, E8.

Waldert, S., Preissl, H., Demandt, E., Braun, C., Birbaumer, N., Aertsen, A., & Mehring, C. (2008). Hand movement direction decoded from MEG and EEG. *J Neurosci*, *28*, 1000–1008.

Walter, W. G. (1963). Technique-interpretation. In D. Hill & G. Parr (Eds.), *Electroencephalography: A symposium on its various aspects.* New York: Macmillan.

Walter, W. G., Cooper, R., Aldridge, V. J., McCallum, W. C., & Winter, A. L. (1964). The contingent negative variation: An electrical sign of significance of association in the human brain. *Science*, *146*, 434.

Wang, W., Collinger, J. L., Perez, M. A., Tyler-Kabara, E. C., Cohen, L. G., Birbaumer, N., Brose, S. W., Schwartz, A. B., Boninger, M. L., & Weber, D. J. (2010). Neural interface technology for rehabilitation: Exploiting and promoting neuroplasticity. *Phys Med Rehabil Cli*, *21*, 157–178.

Weiskopf, N., Veit, R., Erb, M., Mathiak, K., Grodd, W., Goebel, R., & Birbaumer, N. (2003). Physiological self-regulation of regional brain activity using real-time functional magnetic resonance imaging (fMRI): Methodology and exemplary data. *NeuroImage*, *19*, 577–586.

Wyrwicka, W., & Sterman, M.B. (1968). Instrumental conditioning of sensorimotor cortex EEG spindles in the waking cat. *Physiol Behav*, *3*, 703–707.

Yoo, S. S., Fairneny, T., Chen, N. K., Choo, S. E., Panych, L. P., Park, H., Lee, S. Y., & Jolesz, F. A. (2004). Braincomputer interface using fMRI: Spatial navigation by thoughts. *NeuroReport*, *15*, 1591–1595.

Young, K. D., Zotev, V., Phillips, R., Misaki, M., Yuan, H., Drevets, W. C., & Bodurka, J. (2014). Real-time fMRI neurofeedback training of amygdala activity in patients with major depressive disorder. *PLoS One*, *9*, e88785.

Zhu, D., Bieger, J., Garcia Molina, G., & Aarts, R. M. (2010). A survey of stimulation methods used in SSVEP-based BCIs. *Comp IntellNeurosci*, 702357.

Zotev, V., Krueger, F., Phillips, R., Alvarez, R. P, Simmons, W. K., Bellgowan, P., Drevets, W. C., & Bodurka, J. (2011). Self-regulation of amygdala activation using real-time fMRI neurofeedback. *PLoS One*, *6*, e24522.

16

Assessment and Enhancement of Human Brain Plasticity Using Electromagnetic Stimulation

Dylan J. Edwards, Ana H. Medeiros, Mar Cortes, and Alvaro Pascual-Leone

Introduction

In a historical context, the concept of brain plasticity is new. The extent to which brain plasticity underlies human adaptive behavior and cognition, in both health and disease, has emerged as a field at the forefront of scientific discovery. At least 50 years of exploration in this area, together with progressively advancing technology, have enabled the rapid advancement of, and innovative approaches to, the examination and treatment of human neurological disorders. One of the most promising and contemporary tools in the field is electromagnetic stimulation. While the concept of this is not new, the exquisite refinement of stimulation techniques in the last several decades, particularly the use of non-invasive stimulation, has provided notable insight into human cognition and brain function, and has generated a promising new treatment approach. This chapter describes the historical and current understanding of brain plasticity and the effects of electromagnetic stimulation, and discusses the ways in which electromagnetic stimulation is used to understand brain function, as well as to promote adaptive brain plasticity. This potential for this exciting and rapidly expanding field is discussed together with limitations and ethical considerations. Human electromagnetic stimulation is presently one of the most heavily investigated and advanced interventions in cognitive neuroscience, psychiatry, and restorative neurology.

Historical Perspective of the Brain

The Brain as an Electrical Organ and Dynamic Structure

The use of electricity in physiological investigations of the brain, and later for therapeutic purposes, was facilitated in the middle of the eighteenth century by the advent of the first electricity storage device. Modern electrophysiology was founded by Italian medical doctor and physiologist Luigi Galvani (1737–1798), who described for the first time that neural tissues were electrically excitable. The observation of the muscle contraction as a consequence of such stimulation in frogs' nervous system led to the theory about the electricity intrinsic to the body. However, Italian physicist Alessandro Volta (1745–1827) proved that the external electrical stimulus was, actually, what generated the movement. Volta's investigations also led to discoveries about sensory systems, as the induced visual sensation by stimulating the eye, and his particular interest in electricity culminated in the development of the Voltaic pile—which opened a path to remarkable progress in electromagnetism, electrochemistry, and related fields (Piccolino, 1998). Giovanni Aldini (1762–1834), Galvani's nephew, also made a prominent contribution by using direct electric current stimulation in the brain to show the sensitivity of different cerebral areas in animals, as well as postmortem motor responses in humans (Parent, 2004).

In the early nineteenth century, Italian anatomist Luigi Rolando (1773–1831) pioneered in vivo brain electrical stimulation. In addition to his noteworthy contributions to brain anatomy and neurology, Rolando first showed an anatomical and functional correlation by removing the skull and directly stimulating an animal's motor cortex and cerebellum (Walsh & Pascual-Leone, 2005). Continuous improvements in investigative methods using electrical stimulation afforded more accuracy and quicker progress in learning more about brain functioning. In this sense, a new therapeutic approach to intractable epilepsy led to an impressive discovery in the 1950s: by performing a craniotomy in anesthetized, but conscious patients in order to locate and remove the source of seizures, Wilder Graves Penfield (1891–1976), a Canadian neurosurgeon, explored the cerebral cortex with small electrodes, and noticed different responses according to the brain area that was being stimulated. This allowed him to go even further by not only correlating brain anatomy and function, but also mapping cortical language, somatosensory, and motor areas. Nonetheless, the brain was thought as a static structure up to the early twentieth century (Penfield, 1952).

Based on his own morphological studies, Santiago Ramon y Cajal (1852–1934), Spanish histologist and physician, postulated that the brain had a defined number of individual and distinct cells after the critical period of development (Rakic, 2007). In that sense, if the brain remained immutable from early childhood to death, a brain injury or disease would lead to irreversible anatomical changes and permanent functional impairment. Nevertheless, Romanian neuroscientist Ioan Minea (1878–1941) confirmed the theories of his mentor, Gheorghe Marinesco (1864–1938), and introduced the concept of plasticity (Jones, 2000). Since then, structural and functional changes were not limited to the developing brain, but could also happen according to lifelong experience, training, environment, and even after a brain injury.

Further investigations led to an extensive comprehension of how relevant electrical potential was to the cellular physiology and how it seemed to play a complex role in critical processes, from embryonic events to adaptive responses and tissue repair processes in mature organisms, including plasticity. Currently, it is well established that neuroplasticity happens throughout the central nervous system (CNS) at molecular, cytoarchitectonic, and network levels, and embodies synaptic and non-synaptic mechanisms in both neural and non-neural/glial cells. One of the most well-studied and relevant components of plasticity in relation to brain stimulation is synaptic plasticity. This concept was described most prominently by Canadian psychologist Donald Hebb (1904–1985) around 1935, then later confirmed experimentally in the 1960s. The concept describes strengthening (or weakening) of synapses according to pre- and post-synaptic cell firing in relation to each other, and was the origin of the phrase: "cells that fire together, wired together" (Hebb, 2002). This form of plasticity is thought to underlie learning and memory processes, as well as sustained changes brought about by electromagnetic (EM) stimulation paradigms. Recognizing that such a theory does not fully account for plasticity because synaptic reinforcement can lead to network instability if not regulated, in the 1980s a theory was proposed that synaptic plasticity is heavily influenced by synaptic history. Through a series of processes—among them, long-term potentiation (LTP) and long-term depression (LTD)—synaptic plasticity is regulated by a process now called metaplasticity, or homeostatic plasticity.

The concept of metaplasticity becomes important for brain stimulation for several reasons. Not only might the effects of neuromodulation be regulated by these homeostatic mechanisms, but special consideration might need to be given according to brain state during stimulation, and if occurring in conjunction with other therapies. Moreover, the development of various stimulation and neuroimaging techniques has shown another very important functional aspect of plasticity. By interrupting endogenous processes or probing behavioral networks by eliciting a specific response, it has been demonstrated that such adjustments can occur in either adaptive or maladaptive directions. In this sense, modulation of sensory-motor information, motor learning and coordination, language skills, emotional responses, and cognition, including memory acquisition and formation, are examples of positive/adaptive plastic changes. On the other hand, maladaptive/negative plasticity (e.g., chronic pain, spasticity, drug tolerance and addiction, anxiety and depression), which has been thought to occur via similar processes, represents a challenge to clinicians and scientists who attempt to develop methods to limit, reverse, or even prevent such plasticity. Perhaps the most important new investigative approaches and theories about the effects of electrical stimulation in the nervous system, and the proper application of this tool for therapeutic purposes, are based on the concept and neurobiological mechanisms of neuroplasticity.

The Development and Current State of Electromagnetic Stimulation

In the late nineteenth century, electromagnetism, the field of science which establishes the relationship between electricity and magnetic phenomena, was consolidated by three physicists: Hans Christian Oersted (1777–1851), Michael Faraday (1791–1867), and James Clerk Maxwell (1831–1879). Oersted first observed this interaction and postulated that the polarity of the electric current induces changes in the magnetic field. Faraday discovered that magnetic flux can generate an electric current, and he created concepts of magnetic and electric field lines—which were mathematically proven by Maxwell's equations years later. In 1896, Jaques-Arsène d'Arsonval (1851–1940), French physician and physicist, used a magnetic field applied not only to the head, but also to the back and limbs directly, that did not produce sensory or motor responses in his volunteers' limbs. Instead, d'Arsonval's subjects reported visual events, like lights flashing in their eyes, which were called magnetophosphenes. Since then, others have worked on the development of coils in order to gain more focality and have explored how electromagnetism affects the central and peripheral nervous systems. In 1985 Anthony T. Barker and colleagues introduced transcranial magnetic stimulation (TMS), and the characteristic stimulus was used as it is today: a high-intensity magnetic field delivered painlessly by a coil placed upon the scalp of an awake seated human subject, leading to a neuronal depolarization. Since Barker and colleagues stimulated the hand motor area, a muscle twitch was observed as a consequence of the TMS pulse. Barker's experiment launched and shaped subsequent investigations in the field about the mechanisms underlying the TMS-induced muscle activation: a better understanding of motor cortical representation, the effects of voluntary movement on the brain excitability and vice versa, and the source of descending activity.

Well into the third decade of NIBS experimentation in humans, continuing engineering refinements of electromagnetic devices, together with improved understanding of cortical and corticospinal physiology and pathology, have proven TMS to be a useful, safe, and painless tool for examining and promoting human brain plasticity. Early studies typically used single pulse stimulation for mapping cortical motor regions and examining neurophysiological aspects of motor conductivity. With the demonstration that a transiently sustained change in brain excitability (outlasting the stimulation period for up to ~90 min) could be induced by a train of pulses (repetitive TMS, rTMS), the focus largely turned to development of stimulators and coils for repetitive stimulation for potential therapeutic benefit, especially with data supporting not only a change in brain excitability, but changes in human behavior. Machines became more powerful (higher capacitance), and pulse shape changed, thus enabling greater recruitment of brain tissue, as well as better spatial resolution according to coil geometry. At a later time, coils were designed specifically for inducing electrical currents in deeper targets in the brain, and a cooling system was developed to allow a better performance of stimulators when a greater number and duration of pulses were required. Concomitantly, a substantial effort to understand the behavioral effects of pulsed waveform shape and duration are now being explored in more detail.

Modern devices have conjugated their temporal resolution with good spatial resolution using structural magnetic resonance imaging (MRI), providing more anatomical accuracy to brain mapping strategies. The experimenter biofeedback, using a neuronavigation system, allows more precision not only in target, but also in consistency of stimulus trajectory. The conventional approach is still practiced in many laboratories worldwide and consists of scalp markings (either directly or on a swimming cap), usually with reference to the electroencephalography (EEG) 10–20 scalp reference system to provide position information, but this method yields no trajectory information. Furthermore, the underlying anatomical region is inferred by response (if motor), but is otherwise not known. Moreover, the subtle movements of both the head and coil that invariably occur during a treatment/experimental session may be best avoided not by head/coil manual restraint, but rather by a robotic coil holder that makes exquisitely sensitive adjustments in real time; such systems are now being developed and tested experimentally. Likely due to the consistency of targeting for the clinician/experimenter, rather than the vision of underlying anatomy, TMS using neuronavigation is reported to produce less variability of motor evoked potential (MEP) amplitude when compared to without navigation, providing, therefore, more reliable physiological information (see Figure 16.1). In addition, there is emerging evidence that the use of navigated rTMS may lead to more robust excitability modulation (Bashir et al., 2011)—in other words, more favorable to promote plastic events.

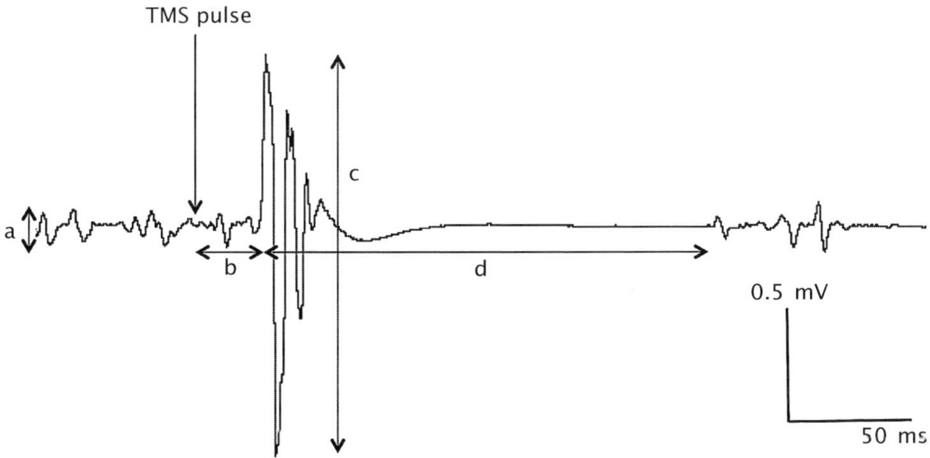

FIGURE 16.1 Diagram of experimental setup used for neuronavigation guided TMS.

State of the Art of Electromagnetic Stimulation

To this day, the term "brain stimulation" instills a variety of images in the minds of different people. It has been reported in the popular media (e.g., *Nature* magazine, *The Guardian* newspaper, and books such as Shorter and Healy's *Shock Therapy: A History of Electroconvulsive Treatment in Mental Illness*), and is the subject of scientific journals (e.g., *Brain Stimulation, Neuromodulation*) and dedicated national and international conferences. Despite the large non-clinical and experimental controlled environment work in the field, only some of the electromagnetic devices/techniques are currently practiced clinically—with a strict criteria for use sanctioned by the US Food and Drug Administration (FDA). On the other hand, there is a public perception of benefit, and commercial online products or home device development (including online do-it-yourself video, e.g., YouTube) are readily available.

While some argue that all electromagnetic therapy techniques are derivatives of the same thing, affecting higher brain function in the same way, physiology experiments show that according to the stimulation type (e.g., rTMS versus transcranial direct current stimulation, tDCS) and parameters (e.g., dose/frequency), the local and network consequence can be quite different. It may be possible that relationships between stimulation-induced physiological changes and functional/behavioral changes are not always causal or directly related, or that outcome measures do not capture the real effects, but rather are secondary effects or epiphenomena. Nevertheless, modeling, physiology, and behavioral data show that (1) electromagnetic fields (TMS or transcranial electrical stimulation, TES) can result in brain currents (Edwards et al., 2013; Yang et al., 2006); (2) these brain currents can alter local and often distributed physiology (Gratton et al., 2013; Kuo et al., 2013; Park et al., 2013); and (3) this can affect brain function and alter observable behavior (Edwards & Fregni, 2008; Giacobbe et al., 2013). Depending on the characteristics of stimulation, the effects may or may not be immediately observable, and may or may not be sustained. The most obvious effect is with EM stimulation of corticomotor areas resulting in motor system effects, such as muscle twitch, seizure, or even tremor reduction in the case of deep brain stimulation.

Existing treatments range from very mild, such as tDCS that only weakly affects the cortex, to very strong, resulting in seizure and transient loss of consciousness, such as electroconvulsive therapy (ECT) or the more recent magnetic seizure therapy. In addition to the continued use of ECT, the two EM stimulation methods that have dominated over the last couple of decades in the literature are TMS, activating cortical interneurons and secondarily projection neurons by short pulses; and tDCS, which does not cause overt activation of neurons, but changes neuronal firing probability. Numerous elegant studies exist describing physiologic insight as well as behavioral/clinical effects with suitable experimental control or sham. Questions that are presently being addressed scientifically include the following: To what extent does brain stimulation affect local versus anatomically distributed networks? Concerning local networks, does brain stimulation affect all neurons or only those with certain orientations and thresholds? Can we bias stimulation to certain networks by changing physiologic threshold, thus making them more permissive/susceptible/responsive, using drugs or behavioral interventions?

In this last regard, there is clearly an immediate interaction between cognitive processes and EM stimulation, with MEPs the most poignant example. When people concentrate on muscle relaxation, MEP amplitude can be reduced for a given stimulus intensity. Conversely, when people imagine movement or action, MEP amplitude can be raised. These and other experiments have identified that brain state is important for neuromodulation protocols, where brain state alters the effect of neuromodulation, enhancing or suppressing it, depending on conditions of the interaction. Indeed, physiologic studies of EM stimulation demonstrate homeostatic plasticity effects, where the aftereffects of one type of stimulation protocol can be disrupted or augmented by a second protocol (Doeltgen & Ridding, 2011). Stated differently, the aftereffects of a given EM neuromodulatory protocol can be influenced (increased or decreased) because of the brain state induced by a preceding protocol. This can even be the same protocol, but this interaction has typically been shown with different protocols. One example of this is the use of tDCS to increase (anodal) or decrease (cathodal) brain excitability prior to the application of synaptic activity—where the synaptic activity can be induced using rTMS. When anodal tDCS increase in excitability is followed by motor training in stroke patients with hemiparesis, for example, the physiologic interaction is positive, allowing a sustained elevation of corticospinal excitability, and is associated with improved voluntary motor control (Edwards et al., 2009; Giacobbe et al., 2013). These interactions need to be fully explored and reproduced, so that therapeutic protocols can be optimized and negative or null effects can be avoided. If homeostatic plasticity exists as current data suggest, it is plausible that merely increasing stimulation dose to achieve superior effects could be counterproductive (Batsikadze et al., 2013). As previously defined, homeostatic plasticity or metaplasticity is a process of maintaining homeostasis of the system in the face of important experience-related changes. This allows synaptic connections to become stronger or weaker without making the system unstable and has been described earlier in this chapter. Homeostatic plasticity can also influence the effect of neuromodulation protocols (Iyer et al., 2003). That is, forces acting to maintain network stability interact with excitability changes resulting from NIBS. In some cases (discussed elsewhere in this chapter), the interaction can be synergistic/complementary, while in others it can be antagonistic.

While scientists are eagerly attempting to identify rules of this interaction to maximize effect/benefit of NIBS in individuals, the interaction likely involves a host of factors, each one carrying various weights for influence. Therefore, subtle manipulation of the same variable might result in quite a different response. Similarly, subtle environmental or biological difference around the time of stimulation could have the same effect. At best, stable environmental conditions, including biological (e.g., not eating, time of day), intensity (relative to individual motor threshold), and position (coil placement), are parameters well-considered and adjusted appropriately. Rather than systematically developing stimulation rules for fluctuating biological conditions (a moving target), it may be wiser to acknowledge that various known and unknown factors contribute to the response, then to record in real time the individual response, and terminate stimulation accordingly (for instance, when a certain excitability threshold is crossed). The challenge is for scientists to identify meaningful biological signatures (e.g., MEP changes, EEG changes) and relate these to meaningful/functional changes in the network.

As well, the effect of dose might be important, not only within stimulation sessions, which have acute/immediate brain responses, but repeating the session after a period of rest/consolidation (+/– involving sleep) in a single day or across multiple days. Furthermore, how many sessions are optimal, and at what point does one plateau in positive response? Even before this, does a previous session make one more or less susceptible to respond to a subsequent session? When should someone start a maintenance program, and what is the optimal structure (e.g., according to presentation/resumption of symptoms, or prior to this as a prophylactic)? The nature and efficacy of maintenance programs are being tried experimentally and empirically in clinics and laboratory settings. With the (to-date) low-risk profile and with successful reduction of symptoms in patients, it may be argued that ongoing and potentially indefinite (controlled and monitored) treatment is warranted. But like many drugs, the long-term effects (positive or adverse), habituation, and even addiction need to be considered.

Finally, the potential for EM stimulation to alter genetics, to favor genetic transcription, or to interact with genetic therapies is only beginning to be fully explored (Elder et al., 2013; Jayasekeran et al., 2011). At the most basic level, EM neuromodulation protocols might be biased toward people with a specific genetic profile (e.g., brain-derived neurotrophic factor polymorphisms), and therefore a genetic screen may be useful to determine patients for whom these therapies might work (Cheeran et al., 2008; Jayasekeran et al., 2011; Lee et al., 2013). Separately, EM stimulation might augment transcription associated with favorable outcome, and there is early evidence of this (Ma et al., 2013). Finally, EM stimulation might also help focally/preferentially deliver a cerebral acting genetic agent to a brain region of interest, or might make tissue more susceptible to genetic therapy.

Assessing Brain Function Using Electromagnetic Stimulation

Current Methods of Electromagnetic Stimulation to Assess Brain Function

Powerful clinical tools have been largely used to assess how a population of neurons behaves, and to understand the different brain states and how they represent or interact with physiological and pathological processes. However, each method is limited by either spatial or temporal resolution and has to be complemented or substituted by 2- and 3-D brain imaging techniques in order to better correlate brain structure and function.

Therefore, radioactive markers (i.e., positron emission tomography, PET), magnetic fields and radio waves (i.e., functional MRI, fMRI) have been used by clinicians and neuroscientists for localizing changes in cerebral blood flow while particular tasks are addressed in order to understand and confirm cognitive processes and functional circuits. Also, current brain imaging methods have limitations and, perhaps most important, they are unable to show causality. In parallel, there are numerous neurobiological techniques (e.g., immunohistochemistry and brain plasticity biomarker analysis) that have provided substantial understanding of several mechanisms underlying specific clinical presentations. Nonetheless, these investigational tools have not filled the large gap in knowledge yet.

Available assessment tools can be placed on a "biology-function continuum" (see Figure 16.2), in which tools that describe the function indicate little about the biology or dysfunction mechanism, and vice versa. For example, clinical scales can accurately inform one of the voluntary motor control deficits while providing a nonspecific result of potential biological causes. On the contrary, a structural MRI provides clear indications of disrupted anatomy, though predictions of influence of voluntary control based on the given images are not always accurate. A stronger understanding of both the functional and biological is necessary to facilitate well-defined interventions in which sensitivity (the degree of precision to detect change afforded by a measurement instrument), reliability (confidence to rule out equipment, technique, or rater error when a change is detected),

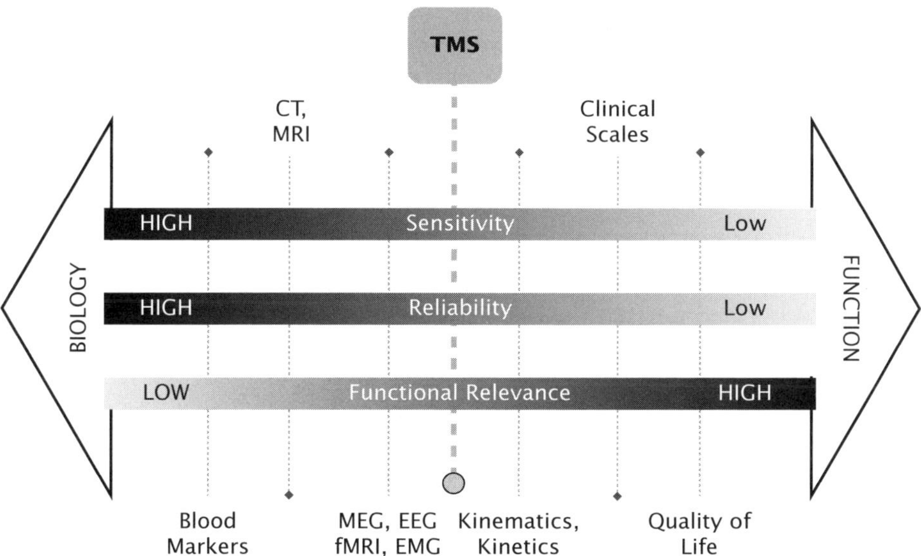

FIGURE 16.2 The biology-function continuum for assessment tools in stroke motor recovery. Following stroke, investigative tools and clinical evaluations are selected, depending on many factors, to inform clinical status, prognosis, treatment planning, recovery, and treatment outcome. The selection of a single tool may compromise on sensitivity, reliability, or functional relevance, but in combination they can provide power insight into function and mechanism. In our opinion, TMS falls in a mid-point, having aspects of biological and functional insight. When used in conjunction with other measures, it can be an important complement to enhance our understanding of motor recovery.

and functional relevance are evident. For these reasons, the combination of these methods provides powerful insight in most instances.

TMS is a diagnostic tool similar to fMRI and EEG, although different information is gathered, and with clear advantages since it can be used to selectively and temporarily introduce "noise" into targeted brain areas and show some sort of causality. TMS can also be identified in a manner similar to quantitative assessments of limb/body motions, forces, and muscle activity (i.e., Rehabilitation robotics). Moreover, these measures represent highly quantitative assessments of voluntary motor control that are sensitive, reliable, and relevant. Most significant is the sensitivity of the measurement tool, especially when testing minor changes in function (i.e., recovery over small amount of inpatient time, short exposure to novel training intervention). In these cases, it is not practical to launch into clinical training studies with gross yet relevant outcome measures without assurance that small clinical changes can be detected with a small dose. Another great relevance for TMS is the ability to uncover remaining functional pathways, even when clinical scales and/or functional tests cannot detect them, potentially providing biological substrates for TMS-guided treatment and rehabilitation (Edwards et al., 2013). In sum, TMS allows scientists to conduct experiments that enable them to form and test hypotheses regarding the function of specific brain regions. Such valuable information can lead to the development of treatments and possibly cures for diseases. In other instances, it may also help to further our understanding of the nature of intelligence and consciousness.

The integration and/or simultaneous use of the aforementioned techniques can serve as powerful complements in order to facilitate a greater understanding of cognitive functions. If specific excitability deficits can be identified, and it is known that the deficits are correlated with a deficit in functional outputs, then it can be presumed that interventions that are able to alter specific aspects of physiology can be targeted. Consequently, physiology can be restored and behavior improved. TMS can also be used to identify physiological effects of modern interventions in order to refine and develop therapies that result in the desired effect. Nonetheless, the longitudinal study approach is an alternate method in which TMS is used to track the course of recovery during conventional standard of care in which it acts as a probe to disrupted and changing physiology in the living human.

Eliciting a Response by Stimulating a Functional Area

The most robust evidence of the activation of brain circuits in awake humans is the fact that a single TMS pulse can elicit an observable (i.e., MEP) or perceptible (i.e., phospene) response. In addition, a single TMS pulse can elicit responses in remote brain areas, as assessed by EEG or fMRI, and will capture brain activation changes in those functionally related areas. In addition, anatomical and functional connections can be proved by conditioning a single pulse in one area, then observing the effect on a test pulse in another area (i.e., interhemispheric inhibition). Therefore, TMS not only provides information about the excitability of the motor cortex (measured by the MEP amplitude), but also the functional integrity of intracortical neuronal structures and the conduction of the corticospinal, corticonuclear, and transcallosal fibers. The results obtained after a TMS evaluation help to localize the lesion, predict the functional motor outcome after an injury, and distinguish between axonal or demyelinating lesions in the motor tracts, depending on the preservation of the conduction time. Some of the most relevant TMS parameters, as well as the invaluable application of TMS as a co-adjuvant diagnostic tool in select neurological disorders, will be explored in this section. Even so, the neurophysiological findings are not disease-specific, and such results need to be carefully interpreted in conjunction with the clinical data and other functional evaluations (Kobayashi & Pascual-Leone, 2003).

The resting motor threshold (RMT) is one of the most commonly assessed TMS parameters, since individual stimulation intensity is set relative to this, both experimentally (typically, a percentage of RMT; e.g., 120% of RMT), as well as therapeutically (including stimulation of non-motor areas). This parameter represents the lowest TMS intensity needed to elicit MEP with single-pulse stimuli. It is thought to largely represent the membrane excitability of cortical interneurons. Most significantly, it provides an understanding of the effectiveness of a chain of synapses from presynaptic cortical neurons to muscles. Furthermore, the motor threshold generally increases in corticospinal tract diseases, such as multiple sclerosis, stroke, and brain or spinal cord injury, magnifying the importance of TMS targeting. In patients with amyotrophic lateral sclerosis (ALS), for example, motor threshold is lower in the hand motor area compared with healthy subjects, and it increases during the advancement of the diseases (Hanajima & Ugawa, 1998; Mills & Nithi, 1997). So this parameter may help the diagnosis and progression of this challenging disorder. Similar to the motor threshold, a "phospene threshold" can be elicited when stimulating the occipital cortex with a single pulse. In patients with migraine, for example, phosphene thresholds are significantly lower than in healthy subjects. Mulleners and colleagues have suggested that the phosphene thresholds may prove useful in the monitoring of anti-migraine-medication efficacy (Mulleners, Chronicle, Vredeveld, & Koehler, 2002).

For the assessment of conduction velocity, such as with central motor conduction time (CMCT), the latency of the response from the spinal motor root is subtracted from the response to primary motor cortex stimulation. Differences in the normal range of CMCT may advocate for specific diseases. For instance, a marked length of CMCT may suggest demyelination of corticospinal path, while low amplitude responses may indicate loss of neurons or axons. This parameter has also shown high correlation with the presence of spinal cord MRI lesions and disease activity in progressive multiple sclerosis. In this particular disease, some TMS findings can be quite useful for an early diagnosis, as well as for prognosis prediction (Boniface et al., 1991; Haug & Kukowski, 1994; Hess et al., 1987).

Correlations of neurophysiological measures with therapeutic outcomes have been the focus of research studies for many different neurological conditions. To index cortical excitability, TMS responses over the motor area are measured by MEPs (see Figure 16.3). MEP amplitude studies both the integrity of the corticospinal tract and the excitability of the motor cortex and nerve roots. The presence of MEP has been used to investigate

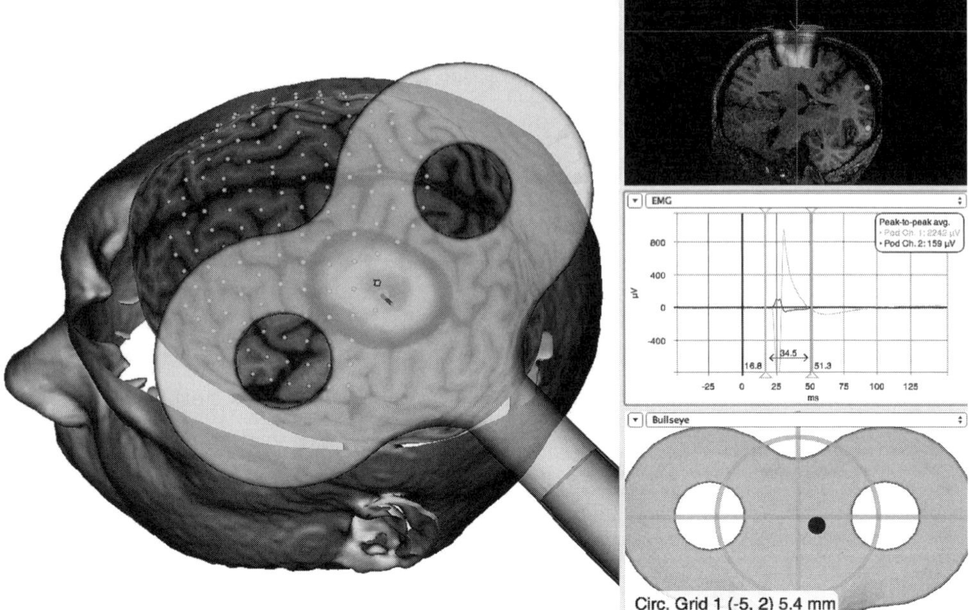

FIGURE 16.3 Transcranial magnetic stimulation mapping. Clockwise from left: 3D reconstruction from MRI, peeled to the level of the cortex where the hand-knob is evident on the pre-central gyrus. The TMS coil is held over this region, then systematically moved to grid-site targets, while the amplitude of the evoked muscle response from single TMS pulses is recorded and assigned a color gradient according to MEP amplitude (below). From multiple sites a motor map is produced and visualized on the image.

The real-time coil position and motor map as viewed in the coronal plane.

The motor evoked potential (MEP) from which the latency (conduction time from brain to muscle) and peak-to-peak amplitude (corticospinal excitability measure) are established.

The coil position with respect to the grid target. Real-time biofeedback is provided to the experimenter about location and coil tilt in order to have precision and consistency with targeting.

the integrity of the corticospinal pathway (i.e., in SCI, stroke), as a diagnostic tool, and also as a prognostic tool, since the presence of MEP in the very early stages after stroke relates to a more favorable recovery, while the absence of MEP suggests a poorer outcome (Escudero et al., 1998). In other conditions, such as OCD, the enhancement of cortical inhibition by the neuromodulation of the supplementary motor area (SMA) is correlated with beneficial therapeutic outcome, supporting the role of SMA in the modulation of OCD symptoms (Greenberg et al., 2000; Mantovani et al., 2013).

In order to study intracortical inhibitory and facilitatory mechanisms, various methods have been developed whereby the principal TMS pulse (the test pulse) may be conditioned by an earlier pulse (the conditioning pulse). The conditioning pulse is delivered in the order of one to several hundred milliseconds prior, and generates physiologic activity that influences the test pulse. The conditioning pulse can be in the same cortical location, a different cortical location (using a separate coil) that projects to the primary motor cortex where the test pulse is delivered, or from a peripheral nerve (delivered by peripheral electrical stimulation). The location of the conditioning pulse (i.e., same or different location as test pulse), the intensity of stimulation, and the interval between the pulses have a signature effect on the test stimulus response (known as the "conditioned MEP"). A change in the conditioned MEP amplitude can be examined during motor recovery after neurologic injury, or in relation to a well-controlled intervention to identify corresponding changes in interhemispheric or intracortical excitability. For example, patients with ALS often present an impairment of intracortical inhibition (with shorter silent periods) that can be reversed with antiglutamatergic drugs; thus this measure can provide great insight into the pathophysiology of the disease (Caramia et al., 2000; Desiato et al., 1999).

The interhemispheric interactions and transcallosal conduction times can also be studied by paired-pulse stimulation, when the single stimuli are applied to two different brain regions. For example, a first conditioning stimulus is given to one motor cortex, and after a short period (from 4 to 30 ms) a second TMS pulse is applied to the other motor cortex. This TMS paradigm provides a unique opportunity to increase our understanding of the role of disconnection syndromes in cognition and neurological and psychiatric diseases. This has most commonly been described in stroke patients with an isolated unilateral lesion. Current thinking is that there is a net increase in excitability as observed in the unaffected hemisphere, a decrease in the affected perilesional cortex, partially explained by increased transcallosal inhibition to the affected hemisphere, and decrease to the unaffected side (Fregni et al., 2005). Recently, it has been proposed that the restoration of interhemispheric balance is a key factor in the recovery of motor control in patients with hemiparesis.

Local cortical excitability can be established also using a paired-pulse paradigm with a single coil. For example, a subthreshold conditioning stimulus 2 to 7 ms before a suprathreshold test stimulus reduces the amplitude of the test stimulus when given alone (termed "short interval intracortical inhibition"; SICI). With a longer inter-pulse interval ~7–10 ms, the test stimulus is facilitated (termed "intracortical facilitation"; ICF). This paired-pulse technique can probe local cortical network changes associated with pathology and interventions (e.g., drugs, brain stimulation), and in this way provides some mechanistic insight into net cortical excitability changes, such as with the MEP. The pathophysiology of various neurological and psychiatric diseases has also been investigated with paired-pulse TMS. For example, abnormalities in the paired-pulse curve (response at incremental inter-stimulus intervals) have been reported in Parkinson's disease, schizophrenia, depression, and obsessive-compulsive disorder (Greenberg et al., 2000; Pascual-Leone et al., 2002; Ridding et al., 1995). The results of paired-pulse curve can help to elucidate the pathophysiology of these neurological and psychiatric disorders, even if the findings are rather nonspecific.

When electromyographic activity is halted for some milliseconds after the elicitation of an MEP appears in the electromyography, this is called the silent period (SP). This occurs when the subject maintains muscle contractions and a single suprathreshold TMS pulse is elicited. Essentially, it is the time between the end of an MEP and the beginning of the following electromyographic activity (a resting period), and it is interceded by GABA receptors. Most of the SP is considered to be due to inhibitory mechanisms at the motor cortex, while spinal inhibitory mechanism is believed to contribute to the first 50 to 60 ms of this suppression. Patients who suffer from movement disorders undergo abnormally long or short silent periods. This parameter is beneficial in assessing pathophysiology and therapeutics of motor-based syndromes, as well as in cognitive disorders like autism, in which GABAergic activity (measured by the investigation of cortical inhibition) is involved.

Motor cortex mapping can be studied by investigating the MEP responses in the motor cortex area of a target muscle. Map area and volume, center of gravity, and optimal site are the parameters that will help to elucidate how the cortex is reorganized after injury and how the restoration of the corticospinal pathway leads to regaining motor function after neurological damage, such as stroke or spinal cord injury. An enlargement of the motor area representation and an increase of the MEP have shown a positive correlation with motor recovery (Rossini 2000; Thickbroom & Mastaglia, 2002).

Understanding Brain Function by Disrupting Activity: The Virtual Lesion

By moving away from primary cortical areas, such as the prefrontal cortex, or posterior parietal cortex, the same stimulus may elicit no observable or perceived response, but likely results in similar cortical activation. The brain activation therefore may or may not lead to activation of functional networks, but either way is not typically thought of as disruption to meaningful spontaneous activity. Such brain stimulation can, however, strongly disrupt functional pathways during voluntary brain activity. One of the most striking, simple, but well-studied examples of activity disruption is when a single suprathreshold pulse of magnetic or electric stimulation is applied over the target primary motor representation of a contracting muscle. The augmented evoked response (relative to at rest) is followed by a distinct period of quiescent muscle activity despite the same voluntary command of sustained muscle contraction. This disruption is not described under normal physiologic circumstances; it is unique to the synchronous pulse of electromagnetism. The phenomenon is thought to involve both cortical and spinal components, has an undefined onset but defined end (resumption of muscle contraction some 150 ms later), and is argued to represent GABA-B receptor–related inhibition. While this phenomenon is only detected using sensitive surface electromyography (very short time course), other examples are more obvious and functionally disruptive. A spectacular example of this is the disruption of voluntary speech when rTMS is applied to left-hemisphere eloquent language areas. Indeed, this has been approved by the US FDA as a technique to assist with pre-surgical tumor re-section planning, where surgery could potentially result in damage to speech and language areas, leading to aphasia postsurgery. While this will likely continue to be a useful clinical tool, allowing precision and functional relevance in an individually specific way, basic functions ascribed to cortical regions have long been known from classical lesion (postmortem) studies, and previous electrophysiological mapping studies. The ability to transiently/reversibly induce a lesion, using painless EM stimulation in the healthy brain, provides an exciting and exquisite ability to probe functional networks in real time in the awake human, and has begun to substantially improve our understanding of brain function.

The concept of a "virtual lesion" has become increasingly important in cognitive neuroscience, and numerous studies have been conducted using this model. This transient alteration of cortical target function, typically induced by single-pulse TMS, short trains of TMS, or tDCS, can be examined during a cognitive task (online mode), or by these neuromodulation protocols (rTMS/tDCS) prior to the task (offline mode). Though the results and validity of this method should be cautiously interpreted since the precise physiology of both the techniques and the behavior is incompletely understood, some useful, intriguing, and important findings have been demonstrated. A given cognitive task might be differentially affected (deterioration, improvement, or no change) by targeted brain stimulation, depending on whether or not neurons involved in the task become inhibited, excited, or remain unaffected by the electromagnetic stimulus. Nevertheless, the virtual lesion model has been demonstrated to effectively disrupt cognitive function, as well as enhance function, depending again on characteristics of the task and stimulation.

There are multiple examples of functional disruption by the virtual lesion. Low-frequency rTMS (excitability reduction effect) to the medial cerebellum can effectively disrupt the production of timed voluntary movements, illustrating a virtual-lesion cause-effect phenomenon not present with other suitable controls. This provides support to local functionally important areas, outside the cerebral cortex, that can be influenced by this technique. Transcallosal interactions for the control of voluntary hand function can be demonstrated using virtual lesions, for example a reduction in grip precision function resulting from a virtual lesion to the primary motor cortex ipsilateral to the active hand (which normally exerts exquisite inhibitory control on the homologous, active primary motor cortex contralateral to the hand). In the visual system, cathodal tDCS (excitability reducing) of the cortical motor threshold area can simultaneously enhance and suppress aspects of visual motion discrimination (improved discrimination at high contrast, impaired at low contrast), providing evidence for anatomical specificity of normal brain function, and indicating that EM stimulation can be used to influence function. This last point raises two important issues: first, that stimulation resulting in an improvement in one function might concurrently (or with a different time course) also change other functions; and second, that the outcome measures selected may or may not capture the full extent of stimulation effects. Evidence is steadily accumulating as to the different types and time course of stimulation effects, according to characteristics of the stimulation and the individual receiving the stimulation.

The concept of virtual lesions for understanding brain function is not limited to lower hierarchical sensory and motor brain function, but has been successfully used in executive function as well. For example, the role of specific parietal areas in arithmetic operations was recently demonstrated using the low-frequency rTMS virtual lesion model (Andres, Pelgrims, Michaux, Olivier, & Pesenti, 2011). When compared to a control site, stimulation over anatomically precise parietal cortex can disrupt math operations (longer response latencies) even if involving memory retrieval, such as with multiplication problems. This provides further support that EM stimulation can affect cortical operations in an anatomically specific way, and can be used to understand the role of brain regions in normal executive function.

The virtual lesion may not always have negative consequences. For example, in the healthy adult brain, enhanced visual spatial attention occurs (ipsilaterally) to rTMS-induced virtual lesions of human parietal cortex. Also, in the visual system, anatomically specific cortical stimulation (low-frequency rTMS) of the motion-perception areas MT/V5 can disrupt "spatial suppression", an effect usually associated with reduced motion perception and increased visual stimulus size, leading to enhanced motion perception in healthy subjects.

Knowing that the non-invasive EM stimulation techniques can influence local and network brain excitability and can secondarily influence function, it is plausible then that if a durable and lasting effect could be realized, function could be altered in a more sustained way, thus having potential clinical benefit. Pathological increases in excitability could be toned down and pathological reductions increased. Since experimental and clinical applications of rTMS for disruption use short stimulus trains, with few repeats, it is not thought to have a lingering effect on excitability change, much beyond the observed function deficit itself. Using established neuromodulation protocols involving longer total exposure to the EM stimuli (number of pulses—rTMS, static field duration—tDCS), it is possible to have enduring and functionally meaningful changes in excitability, as is the focus of the following section.

Enhancing Brain Function With Electromagnetic Stimulation

Neuromodulation employs advanced medical device technologies to enhance or suppress activity of the nervous system for the treatment of disease. These technologies include implantable as well as non-implantable devices that deliver electrical, chemical, or other agents to reversibly modify brain and nerve cell activity. Earlier in time, in 1940, a brief pulse of electrical current was being used to disrupt or "restart" the brain by inducing a seizure in patients with psychiatric disorders. The aim of ECT, which is one of the longest, better-established methods of brain stimulation, is to obtain the remission of the symptoms in patients with severe depression or schizophrenia when other treatments were unsuccessful. In ECT, electric currents pass through the brain and trigger a brief bilateral seizure, causing a reversal of symptoms of some mental illnesses. The mechanism of action is not totally clear, but it is known to affect multiple central nervous system components, such as hormones, neuropeptides, neurotrophic factors, and neurotransmitters. It also increases GABA transmission and receptor antagonism, which raises seizure threshold during ECT. Much of the stigma attached to ECT is based on early treatments in which high doses of electricity were administered without anesthesia, leading to memory loss, fractured bones, and other serious side effects. This technique is much safer today and is given to people while they are under general anesthesia. Although ECT still causes some side effects, it now uses electrical currents given in a controlled setting to achieve the most benefit with the fewest possible risks. Since then, many other neuromodulation techniques have been developed to change the neural circuits and to enhance brain function. Some of those procedures require surgery, with the implantation of the device in the brain or spinal cord, and some others are non-invasive, and each will be discussed in this section.

Invasive Neuromodulatory Interventions

As we know, neuromodulation is a very diverse term that includes non-invasive and invasive procedures that induce a reversible alteration of the nervous system. In addition to those techniques that require surgical interventions, we can include treatments that involve the stimulation of various nerves in the central nervous system, peripheral nervous system, autonomic nervous system, or deep cell nuclei of the brain that lead to the modulation of its activity. By definition, neuromodulation is a therapeutic alteration of activity either through stimulation or medication, both of which are introduced by implanted devices. These implanted devices are usually neural stimulators and drug delivery devices such as pumps. The disorders that can benefit from neuromodulatory interventions are very diverse and encompass acute and chronic pain syndromes, movement disorders, dystonia and spasticity, as well as epilepsy. An emerging subset of neuromodulation includes neuroprosthetics for either nerve regeneration or rehabilitation potential.

Deep brain stimulation (DBS), for example, consists of the implantation of electrodes in certain areas of the brain to produce electrical impulses that regulate abnormal impulses or affect certain cells/chemicals. A neurostimulator placed under the skin, usually near the collarbone, is connected to the electrodes from the stimulator. This technique delivers electrical current to the deep structures of the brain to treat a number of movement disorders, including Parkinson's disease, tremor, and dystonia. The current targets include the subthalamic nucleus, globus pallidus, and thalamus. Many reports in the literature can be found describing DBS for the treatment of depression, obsessive-compulsive disorder, anorexia, obesity, multiple sclerosis, and pain syndromes (Neumann et al., 2014; Quinn et al., 2014; Schlaepfer et al., 2014). Most recently, DBS has been at the forefront for the treatment of epilepsy.

Another very well recognized neuromodulatory intervention to treat epilepsy is the stimulation of the vagus nerve. Vagal nerve stimulation (VNS) is a technique in which a stimulator is implanted under the skin near the collarbone with a wire (lead) connecting the stimulator to the vagus nerve in the neck. Weak electrical signals travel along the nerve to the brain at regular intervals, preventing electrical bursts that cause seizures. The stimulator can be turned on and off by a handheld magnet, and it can prevent a seizure from happening if turned on at the correct time.

Other forms of neuromodulation can also target the spinal cord, such as spinal cord stimulation (SCS) in chronic pain patients. The spinal cord stimulator is a device that is used to apply pulsed electrical signals to the spinal cord. This therapeutic dose of electrical current to the spinal cord is used for the management of neuropathic pain. The most common indications include post-laminectomy syndrome, complex regional pain syndrome (CRPS), ischemic limb pain, and angina. There are scattered reports regarding the treatment of intractable pain due to other causes, including visceral/abdominal pain, cervical neuritis pain, spinal cord injury pain, post-herpetic neuralgia, and neurogenic thoracic outlet syndrome (Fagerlund et al., 2013; Goncalves et al., 2013; Naylor et al., 2013). Existing literature suggests that, in selected patients, SCS can produce at least 50% pain relief in 50%–60% of the implanted patients. Interestingly, with the proper follow-up care, these results can be maintained over several years. It is also used in motor disorders, where the lumbar spinal cord is a preferred target for the control of spinal spasticity or the augmentation of standing and stepping capabilities.

Surgically implanted devices are also effective for modulating the delivery of drugs to a desired target. This enables a lower dosage of the drug needed, as well as a decrease in side effects observed in systemic absorption. Furthermore, intrathecal implants are used in the treatment of pain syndromes such as those associated with nerve injury or cancer pain, as well as for the treatment of spasticity seen with stroke and spinal cord injury patients. In addition, intraventricular implants are used to deliver medication directly into the CSF or CNS for the treatment of epilepsy and pain.

Non-invasive Neuromodulation Therapies

In the past 10 years, many clinical neuroscience studies have focused on how dynamic interactions between different cortical regions underlie complex brain functions such as motor coordination, language, and cognition. Some of those studies using neuroimaging and neurophysiologic approaches have suggested that there exists a dysregulation in the dynamic brain networks in many neuropsychiatric disorders. The combination of NIBS and neuroimaging techniques has led us toward a greater understanding of those dynamic brain networks in health and disease. Brain stimulation techniques, such as TMS and tDCS, use electromagnetic principles to alter brain activity non-invasively, and to induce focal but also network effects outside the stimulation site. The combination of NIBS techniques with brain imaging techniques such as functional MRI (fMRI), positron emission tomography (PET), and EEG permit a causal assessment of that interaction between different network components, as well as their specific functional roles. The same techniques have been also used to explore hypotheses regarding changes in functional connectivity that occur during task performance in various diseases such as stroke, depression, and schizophrenia. In addition, in diseases characterized by pathologic alterations in either the excitability within a single region or in the activity of the different networks, these techniques provide a potential mechanism to alter cortical network function that correlates with clinical benefits.

Treatment of Motor Disorders and Combined Therapies

The neuromodulatory effects of non-invasive brain stimulation techniques are well established, and clinical improvements documented. However, the effects are typically short-lived (this depends on dose/exposure—and is in the order of 20 min to several weeks) and do not completely resolve symptoms. Thus, it was proposed that combining

NIBS with other therapies, such as drugs or behavioral therapy, might lead to a more prominent or enduring reduction in symptoms. The rationale and experimental findings for this concept in the motor systems are outlined below.

As discussed earlier, paired-pulse experiments are used for investigations into the nature of the cortical circuitry activated by TMS, and a variety of different methods exist to examine cortico-cortical connections, or connections to the motor cortex from other parts of the nervous system. With paired stimuli delivered over the motor cortex target muscle area, stimulus intensity and interval parameters can be manipulated to preferentially activate inhibitory or facilitatory cortical circuits. The rate/frequency of the pulses will determine if the effects are excitatory (for example, high frequency repetitive TMS, 10 Hz, or intermittent theta burst stimulation [TBS]) or inhibitory (low frequency rTMS, 1 Hz, or continuous TBS).

Also, epidural stimulation of the motor cortex induces an improvement in motor function in acute stroke. The aim is to promote the return of normal cortical excitability following the disruption caused by neurological damage. Long-term changes in cortico-motor excitability can be induced using repetitive TMS that are largely dependent on the frequency, duration, and intensity of stimulation.

Furthermore, other forms of non-invasive brain stimulation, such as tDCS, in combination with motor skill training have been shown to independently alter cortical excitability and enhance motor function in humans (Goodwill et al., 2013; Williams et al., 2013). In stroke motor recovery, the timing of tDCS application has shown important significance for function. If applied before robotic training, it can be beneficial for voluntary behavior and can change the nature of the training effect, and may lead to enhanced motor skill acquisition.

TDCS modulates the excitability of a targeted brain region non-invasively by altering neuronal membrane potentials and can be used to increase or decrease the excitability of neurons in a brain area, in order to alter function (a) for enhancement, or (b) to interfere, thus determining if that region plays an integral role in a specific motor/cognitive function. Unlike TMS, tDCS does not cause neurons to fire, but alters the *likelihood* that neurons will fire by hyperpolarizing or depolarizing brain tissue. Prolonged effects of tDCS have been attributed to LTP and LTD. It is known that in humans, 13 min of anodal tDCS over the primary motor cortex (M1) result in an increase in excitability up to 150%, which lasts up to 90 minutes.

Numerous research studies using tDCS have revealed that anodal stimulation can induce transient improvements in performance not only on motor task, but also in cognitive and linguistic tasks (which are described separately). In addition, by changing the polarity of the stimulation (cathodal stimulation) the excitability of the motor cortex can be decreased, meaning that the targeted neurons will be less likely to fire.

In neurological disorders such as stroke, where the pathophysiology is thought to be an imbalance in the interhemispheric excitability due to the lesion, rTMS and tDCS have been used to restore the lost balance, and thereby regain the lost function.

The affected hemisphere remains hypo-excitable, while the unaffected hemisphere is hyper-excitable. The tendency in clinical research studies has been to use NIBS techniques to down-regulate the healthy hemisphere (with cathodal tDCS or low frequency TMS) or up-regulate the affected stroke side (with anodal stimulation or high frequency TMS, for example). However, this change in brain excitability by itself does not lead to very sustained clinical effects; when behavioral training accompanies neuromodulatory techniques, the functional changes are proposed to be greater and more sustained.

In stroke recovery, upper limb robotic devices combined with NIBS tools have also shown great promise. Robotic-assisted devices are able to deliver a high amount of repeated movements that facilitate memory consolidation. They can also sense the amount of force a patient produces in a functional motor task and are able to adjust the amount of assistance accordingly, such that an independently non-attainable functional goal is achieved; as time goes on, the patient gains more control and independence and the robot reduces the assistance proportionally. Not only can robotic devices deliver intensive therapy, they also have precise instrumentation that measure kinematic and kinetic variables that allow for assessment of patient impairment and functional performance.

Despite the existing abundant literature. there is still a debate regarding which is the best NIBS tool or combination of tools to treat any given cognitive or motor dysfunction.

Treatment of Non-Motor Disorders

Non-invasive brain stimulation techniques have shown substantial promise for enhancing cognitive functions by the short- and long-term manipulation of neuroplasticity. While the observation of such improvements has been focused initially at the behavioral level with enhancements largely centered on the performance of basic tasks (as hand function or gait), it has been shown that the disruption and enhancement of other non-motor areas of the brain activity can also follow clinical improvements in very diverse neuropsychiatric diseases, as well as with demanding cognitive performance, such as complex mathematical calculations.

It has been shown, for example, that techniques like transcranial random noise stimulation (TRNS) applied on the bilateral dorsolateral prefrontal cortex (DLPFC) during 5 consecutive days, combined with cognitive training, enhances the speed of both calculation- and memory-recall-based arithmetic learning, confirming that TRNS can induce sustained enhancement of cognitive and brain functions.

There are other disorders, such as tinnitus, in which the pathophysiological basis is still not sufficiently clear, but is thought to occur due to a deafferentation-induced compensatory hyperactivity of auditory cortices within certain frequency representations, leading to maladaptive plasticity. In this case, the left temporoparietal area seems to be specifically involved, and disruption of its activity has been shown to reduce tinnitus. Therefore, neuromodulation via cathodal tDCS (inhibitory) or low-frequency rTMS (inhibitory) might be indicated to alter this pathological pattern of cortical activity.

tDCS is currently used as an exploratory treatment in numerous neurologic and neuropsychiatric disorders. With this technique, the area of stimulation will determine a change in different brain networks that can lead to an enhancement of different brain functions. For example, anodal tDCS to DLPFC elicits an improvement in working memory, while the stimulation of the M1 area improves motor learning (Brunoni & Vanderhasselt, 2014; Lally et al., 2013). If delivered to a primary motor area or to visual area V5, it can induce improvements in visuo-motor coordination. In addition, anodal stimulation of fronto-polar regions improves probabilistic classification learning, and over the left prefrontal cortical, tDCS leads to increased verbal fluency.

In non-motor disorders, a combination of brain stimulation tools with cognitive task is used to pursue a specific result. For example, a single TMS pulse can have a facilitatory effect when it is applied shortly before a cognitive task: a shorter latency for naming an object occurs when a single TMS pulse is given over Wernicke's language area 500–1,000 ms before the subject is shown the object (Töpper et al., 1998).

As we have suggested in other parts of this chapter, a combination of electromagnetic tools can help us elucidate the pathophysiology of several and diverse cognitive disorders, and ultimately can be used to treat them. Presently, one of the common applications of rTMS is for the treatment of depression, targeting the under-activation of the mood-regulating circuitry when stimulating the DLPFC. Also, studies using repeated sessions of high frequency rTMS over the DLPFC have suggested that it may be most effective in reducing the level of smoking and alcohol consumption. Also, other forms of neuromodulation in the spinal cord are available, such as percutaneous neuromodulation therapy (PNT), which has shown great capacity to relieve lower back pain, by applying electrical stimulation to deep tissues in the back (Rozen & Grass, 2005).

In summary, a substantial literature exists supporting the beneficial effects of non-invasive neuromodulatory tools as co-adjuvants of conventional therapy for diseases characterized by pathological alterations in either the excitability of one region of the brain, or in distributed networks. This is due directly to the potential of such techniques to alter cortical network function and structure in a beneficial manner. Despite the abundant promising clinical results obtained with these techniques, the different combinations of therapies that can be used, the best dose, exact intensity, frequency of stimulation, brain location, and many other parameters require further investigation.

Electromagnetic Stimulation in Cognitive Plasticity: Targets and Timing

Early attempts to improve motor dysfunction using NIBS were based on the premise that corticospinal excitability was altered in some proportion to the dysfunction, and that NIBS could positively alter the excitability and therefore positively influence function. This has been shown to be true on a number of occasions, using both magnetic and electrical stimulation (Bolognini et al., 2011; Edwards & Fregni, 2008; Lindenberg et al., 2010), although the relationship of corticospinal excitability and function is incompletely understood. How brain excitability is altered in disorders of higher cognitive function and the role of NIBS as a treatment tool are also unclear; however, a wealth of studies exist demonstrating enhanced cognitive processing and abilities in health and disease, particularly in psychiatric applications. Data supporting clinical improvement in medication refractory depression from rTMS to DLPFC have gained the most ground, with FDA approval in the United States, yet evidence exists for other applications including rTMS in obesity (Bou Khalil & El Hachem, 2013), craving in substance dependence (Jansen et al., 2013), attention in traumatic brain injury (Bonni et al., 2013), chronic pain (Rokyta & Fricova, 2012), and cognitive function in Alzheimer's disease (Nardone et al., 2014). A similar theme exists for clinical improvement using tDCS in psychiatry (for a review, see Mondino et al., 2014). In addition, promoting healthy brain function has been demonstrated, such as working memory improvement (Brunoni & Vanderhasselt, 2014) and even inducing "savant"-like capabilities in healthy subjects, as in bilateral tDCS application to DLPFC (Chi et al., 2010). Bilateral DLPFC TRNS improves learning and subsequent performance on complex arithmetic tasks (Snowball et al., 2013). In this example, 5 consecutive days of TRNS-accompanied cognitive training enhanced the speed of both calculation- and memory-recall-based arithmetic learning. These behavioral improvements were associated with defined hemodynamic responses consistent with more efficient neurovascular coupling within the left DLPFC. Testing 6 months after training revealed long-lasting behavioral and physiological modifications in the stimulated group relative to sham controls for trained and non-trained calculation material. These results demonstrate that, depending on the learning regime, TRNS can induce long-term enhancement of cognitive and brain functions. A separate study of tDCS targeting the left dorsolateral prefrontal cortex improved the ability to adapt gait and postural control to a concurrent cognitive task and reduced the cost normally associated with such dual tasking (Zhou et al., 2014).

Both the anatomical target and the timing of application might influence the effective augmentation of cognitive plasticity. It is generally accepted that there is anatomical target specificity for most stimulation effects. It is interesting, however, that in some sites, multiple benefits have been reported. For example, cerebellar tDCS can enhance accuracy (relative to anodal or sham stimulation) during a demanding subtraction version of a mental arithmetic task (complex task but not simple; Pope & Miall, 2012), can enhance the response to negative facial emotions (Ferrucci et al., 2012), and can enhance locomotor adaptation (Jayaram et al., 2012).

There is also accumulating evidence that brain-state matters, and "when" stimulation is applied will dramatically affect the neurophysiological and functional outcome. For example, with transcranial alternating current stimulation (tACS) in the human motor system, augmentation of corticospinal excitability is maximal if the frequency of stimulation reinforces present brain frequency, and is therefore different if applied at rest or during a cognitive task. tACS coincident with the idling beta rhythm of the quiescent motor cortex increases corticospinal output, although during motor imagery, the increase of corticospinal excitability is maximal with theta-tACS, likely reflecting a reinforcement of working memory processes required to mentally process and execute the cognitive task (Feurra et al., 2013). For paired associative stimulation (PAS), volitional activity can interact with the normal excitability increase observed at rest, causing a reversal of the effect (Elahi et al., 2014).

Similarly, paired TMS between cortical regions can also lead to changes in excitability changes outlasting the stimulation period—yet the direction of the change (increase or decrease) not only depends on the order of stimulus presentation, but whether the subject was at rest or engaged in a visuomotor task (Buch et al., 2011).

Brain stimulation can clearly have positive effects on cognitive processes. Such effects have some anatomical specificity and are largely influenced by brain state. These findings may guide future studies to optimize brain stimulation effects in cognition enhancement.

The Rise of Neuromodulation: Controversies, Ethics and Directions

While neuromodulation has been tried independently (e.g., in Eastern Europe), without the results being broadly communicated, rapid expansion of TMS came after its approval for the treatment of psychiatric disease. TDCS appeared to expand after one of the first modern publications using this method emerged in 2000, the *Journal of Physiology*. Regarding TMS, the application of rTMS for other treatment indications (e.g. stroke motor recovery) is now being sought; largely unreported but likely extensive off-label treatments are being tried across the United States in private clinics. For tDCS, since the publication of enhanced math ability around 2010 and improved gaming ability in military pursuits—and the associated media exposure (Falcone et al., 2012)—commercial opportunities, as well as home development of technologies and uncontrolled use, have commenced. This explosion in interest, while not completely unsubstantiated, is not well controlled or monitored. Consumers are proceeding blindly in technology, devices, and method. Indeed, it has been suggested that if some is good, more may be better. Evidence exists supporting that beyond a critical point, application of tDCS can have reverse effects than anticipated—speculated to be due to brain homeostatic mechanisms. The uncontrolled use, including potentially prolonged or addictive use, is unknown territory for risk/benefit. Cautionary notes have been written in leading journals (Bikson et al., 2013); however, since the home use of these devices is not regulated, the best we can do is try to inform people of the risks.

There has been an exponential rise in the number of publications on brain stimulation over the past two decades. Like many drugs discovered over the past century, the long-term effects, including genetic modifications, are poorly understood and undefined.

Similarly, the interventions' psychological impact (e.g. dependence, placebo, addiction) and interaction with other treatments/comorbidities, and so on, are not known (prolonged use, use in children?). The overwhelming majority of results suggest a positive effect for a wide range of brain functions and conditions. There are few null effects reported and relatively few adverse effects. That brain stimulation can work for so many brain functions, despite not a full understanding of the mechanisms or optimal use, could be suggestive of a publication bias (and popular media has distributed a glib and discrete message that this is easy and effective). Nevertheless, randomized double blind controlled trials continue to show positive effects, and these need to be taken seriously. Around the time of this publication, there were over 100 clinical trials registered at clinicaltrials.gov from across the globe, indicating a strong level of investigation, and a promising future for unraveling what therapies work and in which patients. Much work is currently being investigated to refine and understand both the method and the physiology, so that optimal stimulation paradigms can be applied in individuals.

The use of tDCS for the enhancement of brain function raises questions of ethics. Enhanced function in math ability can also be achieved by practice, quickness of thought, and memory—all achievable by dedicated effort and hard work. Similarly, motor skills and sports performance can be achieved by practice and effort. Will some people, seeking an advantage, use brain stimulation, with improved outcome for a given time input? Logically, those at disadvantage—such as with congenital or acquired neurological damage with overt or even subtle symptoms—should be given the opportunity for enhancement, if the adverse effect risk is low. But where on the normal distribution of cognitive or motor ability (e.g., two standard deviations below the mean) or professional duties (e.g., truck drivers, pilots, army, and stock market) should the line be drawn?

The answers to such questions are starting to be debated, and further work needs to be done here by those with expertise in medical science, ethics, and policy, before formal medico-legal decisions are made. In addition to those who take it upon themselves to alter their own brain function using such technologies, the onus also falls back on those applying the technique to others. This includes companies and individuals selling and promoting the devices, scientists testing the devices or protocols, and clinicians trying the devices for new indications or in new ways. Brain stimulation has an enigmatic and contemporary appeal, and thus lends itself well to powerful placebo effects and the potential for clinicians to abuse this for susceptible and desperate patients. Acknowledging that the mechanism is incompletely understood, but with a low risk profile and patient reports of benefit, it may be a reasonable treatment option (certainly the case for rTMS as used in depression), and is possibly akin to a drug given off-label as a viable treatment option. The gold standard clinical assessment of these techniques is likely to be the final phase of a clinical trial, including multicenter, randomized, and controlled clinical trial. However, this may not be the only method of understanding treatment effects, since many trials may not make it through the early stages for a host of factors extending beyond poor hypotheses and study design, to include financial and administrative factors. For these reasons, uncontrolled clinical applications on a large scale can inform much about effectiveness, tolerability, and feasibility, provided the clinicians effectively communicate their findings. For rTMS, established safety standards have been published for clinical and experimental work. Pertaining to the rTMS treatment for depression in the United States, the approval is circumscribed in equipment, method, and patient clinical profile. For less well-tested neuromodulation methods (e.g., tDCS), safety and efficacy guidelines are under development, while newer and emerging treatments (e.g., ultrasound) are still very experimental, and there are simply insufficient data to make judgments on clinical utility.[1] Knowing that a spectrum of evidence exists depending on the electromagnetic neuromodulation method and clinical indication, those responsible for applying stimulation need to explain to patients accurately the published risk/benefit, and where this is not known, the best available data should be described in lay terms such that patients can make informed decisions about the risk/benefit and potential alternatives.

While no globally accepted legal position exists on who can apply the stimulation (training of the clinician/scientist) and where the stimulation should occur (e.g., hospital or university, or home), several training courses have been established at recognized universities with a strong track record of pioneering this research field (e.g., Harvard Medical School and Oxford University). There are also company-sponsored device- and application-specific courses, and independent programs are being built into university courses. This commitment to the education and training of practitioners and scientists in the use of this technology is an important step forward as the number of uses and the diversity and number of device types grow. The parallel rapid expansion of technology with more precision of where/how we are stimulating (new imaging techniques/better existing techniques—and better understanding of brain response) means that there will be an ongoing need for education, as currently occurs in the medical field.

There are a number of challenges moving forward with the widespread implementation of EM stimulation across the world in health and disease, young and old. Yet, with the promising findings thus far, while acknowledging that techniques are still not optimal, the excellent safety profile arguably positions EM neuromodulation as one of the most compelling advances in human brain treatment, and a field worthy of excitement and pursuit of understanding.

Summary

In this chapter we have described the progressive understanding that the brain is not only a dynamic structure, but that it changes according to experience, and thus has the potential

---

1. With the recent public announcement of positive tDCS effects, combined with the mass deployment/availability of devices online, and limited accountability of companies, many people will be trying these devices in an uncontrolled environment—"open-source" testing with no way of capturing adverse events, or even positive effects. Perhaps the online environment (e.g., gaming) can be leveraged in the future to establish who is using these and to capture data on effectiveness and safety.

for substantial plasticity in health and disease. This plasticity is fundamentally adaptive and is important for human daily operations and existence (learning and memory), but it is also important in response to congenital or acquired pathophysiology and recovery from neurological insult, underlying much of the disability in society. Adaptive plasticity enables better interaction with the environment and society. We also discussed that maladaptive plasticity can be acquired, but potentially also reversed. Given that the brain is an electrical organ, and can respond overtly and discretely to electromagnetic fields, this opens up the possibility for the electromagnetic devices to probe brain circuitry, for both understanding and promoting adaptive plasticity. Great strides have been made in this field with both invasive and non-invasive EM stimulation. The field of NIBS has expanded rapidly in the last two decades, and a wealth of information is available regarding safety and efficacy in the treatment of various neurological disorders. As the technology develops in parallel with improved understanding of disease-specific pathophysiology and symptomatic correlates, we can anticipate that this field will continue rapidly expanding in the twenty-first century. With a precedent set using rTMS in the treatment of depression, it is anticipated that studies supporting other indications will follow. With the relatively low-risk profile of non-invasive stimulation and the accumulating evidence for efficacy in a variety of diseases of the nervous system, EM stimulation in the assessment and treatment of neurological disorders seems to be one of the most exciting and promising contemporary treatments in the field today.

References

Andres, M., Pelgrims, B., Michaux, N., Olivier, E., & Pesenti, M. (2011). Role of distinct parietal areas in arithmetic: An fMRI-guided TMS study. *NeuroImage, 54*(4), 3048–3056. doi: 10.1016/j.neuroimage.2010.11.009

Bashir, S., Edwards, D., & Pascual-Leone, A. (2011). Neuronavigation increases the physiologic and behavioral effects of low-frequency rTMS of primary motor cortex in healthy subjects. *Brain Topogr, 24*(1), 54–64. doi: 10.1007/s10548-010-0165-7

Batsikadze, G., Moliadze, V., Paulus, W., Kuo, M. F., & Nitsche, M. A. (2013). Partially non-linear stimulation intensity-dependent effects of direct current stimulation on motor cortex excitability in humans. *J Physiol, 591*(Pt 7), 1987–2000. doi: 10.1113/jphysiol.2012.249730

Bikson, M., Bestmann, S., & Edwards, D. (2013). Neuroscience: Transcranial devices are not playthings. *Nature, 501*(7466), 167. doi: 10.1038/501167b

Bolognini, N., Vallar, G., Casati, C., Latif, L. A., El-Nazer, R., Williams, J., & Fregni, F. (2011). Neurophysiological and behavioral effects of tDCS combined with constraint-induced movement therapy in poststroke patients. *Neurorehabil Neural Repair, 25*(9), 819–829. doi: 10.1177/1545968311411056

Boniface, S. J., Mills, K. R., & Schubert, M. (1991). Responses of single spinal motoneurons to magnetic brain stimulation in healthy subjects and patients with multiple sclerosis. *Brain, 114 (Pt 1B)*, 643–662.

Bonni, S., Mastropasqua, C., Bozzali, M., Caltagirone, C., & Koch, G. (2013). Theta burst stimulation improves visuo-spatial attention in a patient with traumatic brain injury. *Neurol Sci, 34*(11), 2053–2056. doi: 10.1007/s10072-013-1412-y

Bou Khalil, R., & El Hachem, C. (2013). Potential role of repetitive transcranial magnetic stimulation in obesity. *Eat Weight Disord.* doi: 10.1007/s40519-013-0088-x

Brunoni, A. R., & Vanderhasselt, M. A. (2014). Working memory improvement with non-invasive brain stimulation of the dorsolateral prefrontal cortex: A systematic review and meta-analysis. *Brain Cogn, 86C*, 1–9. doi: 10.1016/j.bandc.2014.01.008

Buch, E. R., Johnen, V. M., Nelissen, N., O'Shea, J., & Rushworth, M. F. (2011). Noninvasive associative plasticity induction in a corticocortical pathway of the human brain. *J Neurosci, 31*(48), 17669–17679. doi: 10.1523/JNEUROSCI.1513-11.2011

Caramia, M. D., Palmieri, M. G., Desiato, M. T., Iani, C., Scalise, A., Telera, S., & Bernardi, G. (2000). Pharmacologic reversal of cortical hyperexcitability in patients with ALS. *Neurology, 54*(1), 58–64.

Cheeran, B., Talelli, P., Mori, F., Koch, G., Suppa, A., Edwards, M., Rothwell, J. C. (2008). A common polymorphism in the brain-derived neurotrophic factor gene (BDNF) modulates human cortical plasticity and the response to rTMS. *J Physiol, 586*(Pt 23), 5717–5725. doi: 10.1113/jphysiol.2008.159905

Chi, R. P., Fregni, F., & Snyder, A. W. (2010). Visual memory improved by non-invasive brain stimulation. *Brain Res, 1353*, 168–175. doi: 10.1016/j.brainres.2010.07.062

Desiato, M. T., Palmieri, M. G., Giacomini, P., Scalise, A., Arciprete, F., & Caramia, M. D. (1999). The effect of riluzole in amyotrophic lateral sclerosis: A study with cortical stimulation. *J Neurol Sci, 169*(1–2), 98–107.

Doeltgen, S. H., & Ridding, M. C. (2011). Modulation of cortical motor networks following primed theta burst transcranial magnetic stimulation. *Exp Brain Res, 215*(3–4), 199–206. doi: 10.1007/s00221-011-2886-6

Edwards, D., Cortes, M., Datta, A., Minhas, P., Wassermann, E. M., & Bikson, M. (2013). Physiological and modeling evidence for focal transcranial electrical brain stimulation in humans: A basis for high-definition tDCS. *NeuroImage, 74*, 266–275. doi: 10.1016/j.neuroimage.2013.01.042

Edwards, D., & Fregni, F. (2008). Modulating the healthy and affected motor cortex with repetitive transcranial magnetic stimulation in stroke: Development of new strategies for neurorehabilitation. *NeuroRehabilitation, 23*(1), 3–14.

Edwards, D. J., Cortes, M., Thickbroom, G. W., Rykman, A., Pascual-Leone, A., & Volpe, B. T. (2013). Preserved corticospinal conduction without voluntary movement after spinal cord injury. *Spinal Cord, 51*(10), 765–767. doi: 10.1038/sc.2013.74

Edwards, D. J., Krebs, H. I., Rykman, A., Zipse, J., Thickbroom, G. W., Mastaglia, F. L., Volpe, B. T. (2009). Raised corticomotor excitability of M1 forearm area following anodal tDCS is sustained during robotic wrist therapy in chronic stroke. *Restor Neurol Neurosci, 27*(3), 199–207. doi: 10.3233/RNN-2009-0470

Elahi, B., Hutchison, W. D., Daskalakis, Z. J., Gunraj, C., & Chen, R. (2014). Dose-response curve of associative plasticity in human motor cortex and interactions with motor practice. *J Neurophysiol, 111*(3), 594–601. doi: 10.1152/jn.00920.2012

Elder, J., Cortes, M., Rykman, A., Hill, J., Karuppagounder, S., Edwards, D., & Ratan, R. R. (2013). The epigenetics of stroke recovery and rehabilitation: From polycomb to histone deacetylases. *Neurotherapeutics, 10*(4), 808–816. doi: 10.1007/s13311-013-0224-3

Escudero, J. V., Sancho, J., Bautista, D., Escudero, M., & Lopez-Trigo, J. (1998). Prognostic value of motor evoked potential obtained by transcranial magnetic brain stimulation in motor function recovery in patients with acute ischemic stroke. *Stroke, 29*(9), 1854–1859.

Fagerlund, A. J., Bystad, M. K., & Aslaksen, P. M. (2013). [Transcranial direct current stimulation for chronic pain]. *Tidsskr Nor Laegeforen, 133*(21), 2266–2269. doi: 10.4045/tidsskr.13.0003

Falcone, B., Coffman, B. A., Clark, V. P., & Parasuraman, R. (2012). Transcranial direct current stimulation augments perceptual sensitivity and 24-hour retention in a complex threat detection task. *PLoS One, 7*(4), e34993. doi: 10.1371/journal.pone.0034993

Ferrucci, R., Giannicola, G., Rosa, M., Fumagalli, M., Boggio, P. S., Hallett, M., Priori, A. (2012). Cerebellum and processing of negative facial emotions: Cerebellar transcranial DC stimulation specifically enhances the emotional recognition of facial anger and sadness. *Cogn Emot, 26*(5), 786–799. doi: 10.1080/02699931.2011.619520

Feurra, M., Pasqualetti, P., Bianco, G., Santarnecchi, E., Rossi, A., & Rossi, S. (2013). State-dependent effects of transcranial oscillatory currents on the motor system: What you think matters. *J Neurosci, 33*(44), 17483–17489. doi: 10.1523/JNEUROSCI.1414-13.2013

Fregni, F., Boggio, P. S., Mansur, C. G., Wagner, T., Ferreira, M. J., Lima, M. C., Pascual-Leone, A. (2005). Transcranial direct current stimulation of the unaffected hemisphere in stroke patients. *Neuroreport, 16*(14), 1551–1555.

Giacobbe, V., Krebs, H. I., Volpe, B. T., Pascual-Leone, A., Rykman, A., Zeiarati, G., Edwards, D. J. (2013). Transcranial direct current stimulation (tDCS) and robotic practice in chronic stroke: The dimension of timing. *NeuroRehabilitation, 33*(1), 49–56. doi: 10.3233/NRE-130927

Goncalves, G. S., Borges, I. C., Goes, B. T., de Mendonca, M. E., Goncalves, R. G., Garcia, L. B., Baptista, A. F. (2013). Effects of tDCS induced motor cortex modulation on pain in HTLV-1: A blind randomized clinical trial. *Clin J Pain*. doi: 10.1097/AJP.0000000000000037

Goodwill, A. M., Reynolds, J., Daly, R. M., & Kidgell, D. J. (2013). Formation of cortical plasticity in older adults following tDCS and motor training. *Front Aging Neurosci, 5*, 87. doi: 10.3389/fnagi.2013.00087

Gratton, C., Lee, T. G., Nomura, E. M., & D'Esposito, M. (2013). The effect of theta-burst TMS on cognitive control networks measured with resting state fMRI. *Front Syst Neurosci, 7*, 124. doi: 10.3389/fnsys.2013.00124

Greenberg, B. D., Ziemann, U., Cora-Locatelli, G., Harmon, A., Murphy, D. L., Keel, J. C., & Wassermann, E. M. (2000). Altered cortical excitability in obsessive-compulsive disorder. *Neurology, 54*(1), 142–147.

Hanajima, R., & Ugawa, Y. (1998). Impaired motor cortex inhibition in patients with ALS: evidence from paired transcranial magnetic stimulation. *Neurology, 51*(6), 1771–1772.

Haug, B. A., & Kukowski, B. (1994). Latency and duration of the muscle silent period following transcranial magnetic stimulation in multiple sclerosis, cerebral ischemia, and other upper motoneuron lesions. *Neurology, 44*(5), 936–940.

Hebb, D. (2002) *The organization of behavior, a neuropsychological theory*. New York: Psychology Press.

Hess, C. W., Mills, K. R., Murray, N. M., & Schriefer, T. N. (1987). Magnetic brain stimulation: Central motor conduction studies in multiple sclerosis. *Ann Neurol, 22*(6), 744–752. doi: 10.1002/ana.410220611

Iyer, M. B., Schleper, N., & Wassermann, E. M. (2003). Priming stimulation enhances the depressant effect of low-frequency repetitive transcranial magnetic stimulation. *J Neurosci, 23*(34), 10867–10872.

Jansen, J. M., Daams, J. G., Koeter, M. W., Veltman, D. J., van den Brink, W., & Goudriaan, A. E. (2013). Effects of non-invasive neurostimulation on craving: A meta-analysis. *Neurosci Biobehav Rev, 37*(10 Pt 2), 2472–2480. doi: 10.1016/j.neubiorev.2013.07.009

Jayaram, G., Tang, B., Pallegadda, R., Vasudevan, E. V., Celnik, P., & Bastian, A. (2012). Modulating locomotor adaptation with cerebellar stimulation. *J Neurophysiol, 107*(11), 2950–2957. doi: 10.1152/jn.00645.2011

Jayasekeran, V., Pendleton, N., Holland, G., Payton, A., Jefferson, S., Michou, E., Hamdy, S. (2011). Val66Met in brain-derived neurotrophic factor affects stimulus-induced plasticity in the human pharyngeal motor cortex. *Gastroenterology, 141*(3), 827–836 e821–823. doi: 10.1053/j.gastro.2011.05.047

Jones, E. G. (2000). NEUROwords. 8. Plasticity and neuroplasticity. *J Hist Neurosci, 9*(1), 37–39. doi: 10.1076/0964-704X(200004)9:1;1-2;FT037

Kobayashi, M., & Pascual-Leone, A. (2003). Transcranial magnetic stimulation in neurology. *Lancet Neurol, 2*(3), 145–156.

Kuo, H. I., Bikson, M., Datta, A., Minhas, P., Paulus, W., Kuo, M. F., & Nitsche, M. A. (2013). Comparing cortical plasticity induced by conventional and high-definition 4 x 1 ring tDCS: A neurophysiological study. *Brain Stimul, 6*(4), 644–648. doi: 10.1016/j.brs.2012.09.010

Lally, N., Nord, C. L., Walsh, V., & Roiser, J. P. (2013). Does excitatory fronto-extracephalic tDCS lead to improved working memory performance? *F1000Res, 2*, 219. doi: 10.12688/f1000research.2-219.v1

Lee, M., Kim, S. E., Kim, W. S., Lee, J., Yoo, H. K., Park, K. D., Lee, H. W. (2013). Interaction of motor training and intermittent theta burst stimulation in modulating motor cortical plasticity: Influence of BDNF Val66Met polymorphism. *PLoS One, 8*(2), e57690. doi: 10.1371/journal.pone.0057690

Lindenberg, R., Renga, V., Zhu, L. L., Nair, D., & Schlaug, G. (2010). Bihemispheric brain stimulation facilitates motor recovery in chronic stroke patients. *Neurology, 75*(24), 2176–2184. doi: 10.1212/WNL.0b013e318202013a

Ma, J., Zhang, Z., Su, Y., Kang, L., Geng, D., Wang, Y., Cui, H. (2013). Magnetic stimulation modulates structural synaptic plasticity and regulates BDNF-TrkB signal pathway in cultured hippocampal neurons. *Neurochem Int, 62*(1), 84–91. doi: 10.1016/j.neuint.2012.11.010

Mantovani, A., Rossi, S., Bassi, B. D., Simpson, H. B., Fallon, B. A., & Lisanby, S. H. (2013). Modulation of motor cortex excitability in obsessive-compulsive disorder: An exploratory study on the relations of neurophysiology measures with clinical outcome. *Psychiatry Res, 210*(3), 1026–1032. doi: 10.1016/j.psychres.2013.08.054

Mills, K. R., & Nithi, K. A. (1997). Corticomotor threshold is reduced in early sporadic amyotrophic lateral sclerosis. *Muscle Nerve, 20*(9), 1137–1141.

Mondino, M., Bennabi, D., Poulet, E., Galvao, F., Brunelin, J., & Haffen, E. (2014). Can transcranial direct current stimulation (tDCS) alleviate symptoms and improve cognition in psychiatric disorders? *World J Biol Psychiatry*. doi: 10.3109/15622975.2013.876514

Mulleners, W. M., Chronicle, E. P., Vredeveld, J. W., & Koehler, P. J. (2002). Visual cortex excitability in migraine before and after valproate prophylaxis: a pilot study using TMS. *Eur J Neurol*, *9*(1), 35–40.

Nardone, R., Tezzon, F., Holler, Y., Golaszewski, S., Trinka, E., & Brigo, F. (2014). Transcranial magnetic stimulation (TMS)/repetitive TMS in mild cognitive impairment and Alzheimer's disease. *Acta Neurol Scand*. doi: 10.1111/ane.12223

Naylor, J. C., Borckardt, J. J., Marx, C. E., Hamer, R. M., Fredrich, S., Reeves, S. T., & George, M. S. (2013). Cathodal and anodal left prefrontal tDCS and the perception of control over pain. *Clin J Pain*. doi: 10.1097/AJP.0000000000000025

Neumann, W. J., Huebl, J., Brucke, C., Gabriels, L., Bajbouj, M., Merkl, A., Kuhn, A. A. (2014). Different patterns of local field potentials from limbic DBS targets in patients with major depressive and obsessive compulsive disorder. *Mol Psychiatry*. doi: 10.1038/mp.2014.2

Parent, A. (2004). Giovanni Aldini: From animal electricity to human brain stimulation. *Can J Neurol Sci*, *31*(4), 576–584.

Park, C. H., Chang, W. H., Park, J. Y., Shin, Y. I., Kim, S. T., & Kim, Y. H. (2013). Transcranial direct current stimulation increases resting state interhemispheric connectivity. *Neurosci Lett*, *539*, 7–10. doi: 10.1016/j.neulet.2013.01.047

Pascual-Leone, A., Manoach, D. S., Birnbaum, R., & Goff, D. C. (2002). Motor cortical excitability in schizophrenia. *Biol Psychiatry*, *52*(1), 24–31.

Penfield, W. (1952). Epileptic automatism and the centrencephalic integrating system. *Res Publ Assoc Res Nerv Ment Dis*, *30*, 513–528.

Piccolino, M. (1998). Animal electricity and the birth of electrophysiology: The legacy of Luigi Galvani. *Brain Res Bull*, *46*(5), 381–407.

Pope, P. A., & Miall, R. C. (2012). Task-specific facilitation of cognition by cathodal transcranial direct current stimulation of the cerebellum. *Brain Stimul*, *5*(2), 84–94. doi: 10.1016/j.brs.2012.03.006

Quinn, D. K., Deligtisch, A., Rees, C., Brodsky, A., Evans, D., Khafaja, M., & Abbott, C. C. (2014). Differential diagnosis of psychiatric symptoms after deep brain stimulation for movement disorders. *Neuromodulation*. doi: 10.1111/ner.12153

Rakic, P. (2007). The radial edifice of cortical architecture: From neuronal silhouettes to genetic engineering. *Brain Res Rev*, *55*(2), 204–219. doi: 10.1016/j.brainresrev.2007.02.010

Ridding, M. C., Inzelberg, R., & Rothwell, J. C. (1995). Changes in excitability of motor cortical circuitry in patients with Parkinson's disease. *Ann Neurol*, *37*(2), 181–188. doi: 10.1002/ana.410370208

Rokyta, R., & Fricova, J. (2012). Neurostimulation methods in the treatment of chronic pain. *Physiol Res*, *61*(Suppl 2), S23–31.

Rossini, P. M. (2000). Is transcranial magnetic stimulation of the motor cortex a prognostic tool for motor recovery after stroke? *Stroke*, *31*(6), 1463–1464.

Rozen, D., Grass, G.W. (2005). Intradiscal electrothermal coagulation and percutaneous neuromodulation therapy in the treatment of discogenic low back pain. *Pain Pract*, *5*, 228–243.

Schlaepfer, T. E., Bewernick, B. H., Kayser, S., Hurlemann, R., & Coenen, V. A. (2014). Deep brain stimulation of the human reward system for major depression-ra-tionale, outcomes and outlook. *Neuropsychopharmacol*. doi: 10.1038/npp.2014.28

Snowball, A., Tachtsidis, I., Popescu, T., Thompson, J., Delazer, M., Zamarian, L., Cohen Kadosh, R. (2013). Long-term enhancement of brain function and cognition using cognitive training and brain stimulation. *Curr Biol*, *23*(11), 987–992. doi: 10.1016/j.cub.2013.04.045

Thickbroom, G. W., & Mastaglia, F. L. (2002). Mapping Studies. In *Handbook of Transcranial Magnetic Stimulation*, Chapter 12, pages 127–140, Arnold, London, England.

Töpper, R., Mottaghy, F.M., Brügmann, M., Noth, J., Huber, W. (1998). Facilitation of picture naming by focal transcranial magnetic stimulation of Wernicke's area. *Exp Brain Res*, *121*, 371–378.

Walsh, V., Pascual-Leone, A. (2005) *Transcranial magnetic stimulation: A neurochronometrics of mind*. Boston, MA: Bradford Books.

Williams, P. S., Hoffman, R. L., & Clark, B. C. (2013). Preliminary evidence that anodal transcranial direct current stimulation enhances time to task failure of a sustained submaximal contraction. *PLoS One, 8*(12), e81418. doi: 10.1371/journal.pone.0081418

Yang, S., Xu, G., Wang, L., Chen, Y., Wu, H., Li, Y., & Yang, Q. (2006). 3D realistic head model simulation based on transcranial magnetic stimulation. *Conf Proc IEEE Eng Med Biol Soc, Suppl,* 6469–6472. doi: 10.1109/IEMBS.2006.260877

Zhou, J., Hao, Y., Wang, Y., Jor'dan, A., Pascual-Leone, A., Zhang, J., Manor, B. (2014). Transcranial direct current stimulation reduces the cost of performing a cognitive task on gait and postural control. *Eur J Neurosci.* doi: 10.1111/ejn.12492

Index

Page numbers for primary discussions are in **boldface**. Page numbers for boxes are followed by b, figures by f, and tables by t, and footnotes by n and the note number.